Debriefing has emerged as one of the most controversial interventions in clinical psychology and psychiatry. At the scientific level, advocates and antagonists dispute its role in prevention and treatment, while in the field a new industry of professional counsellors applies debriefing, sometimes indiscriminately, to witnesses and victims of traumatic events. This book constitutes an unprecedented presentation and analysis of evidence for the efficacy, and otherwise, of psychological debriefing, in theory and application, and appraises current research findings on the proper use of such interventions.

With authoritative editorial guidance, the reader is taken through the controversies surrounding debriefing of various kinds, in various settings, and at various levels of organizational supervision and control. Contributors include many of the leading international authorities in post-traumatic studies, who draw on their first-hand experiences as investigators, and also witnesses, of traumatic events and their effects on those exposed to them. From major disasters affecting large numbers or even whole communities, to individual experiences of road traffic accidents, assault, or childbirth, the range of topics and points of view presented will make this an essential reference and guide for all practitioners – whatever their point of view.

Professor Beverley Raphael is attached to the Department of Psychological Medicine, University of Sydney, and is Emeritus Professor of Psychiatry for the University of Queensland. She is known worldwide for her work in bereavement and trauma studies, and her previous books, *The Anatomy of Bereavement* and *When Disaster Strikes*, were landmarks in the field.

John P. Wilson is Professor of Psychology at Cleveland State University and Director of the Center for Stress and Trauma in Cleveland. He is a consultant to the United Nations Humanitarian Task Force, and edited, with Beverley Raphael, *The International Handbook of Traumatic Stress Syndrome*.

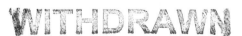

Psychological
debriefing

Theory, practice and evidence

Edited by

Beverley Raphael
University of Sydney and University of Queensland

and

John P. Wilson
Cleveland State University

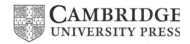

PUBLISHED BY THE PRESS SYNDICATE OF THE UNIVERSITY OF CAMBRIDGE

The Pitt Building, Trumpington Street, Cambridge, United Kingdom

CAMBRIDGE UNIVERSITY PRESS

The Edinburgh Building, Cambridge CB2 2RU, UK

40 West 20th Street, New York, NY 10011-4211, USA

10 Stamford Road, Oakleigh, VIC 3166, Australia

Ruiz de Alarcón 13, 28014 Madrid, Spain

Dock House, The Waterfront, Cape Town 8001, South Africa

http://www.cup.org

First published 2000

Printed in the United Kingdom at the University Press, Cambridge

Typeset in Utopia 8/12 pt [VN]

A catalogue record for this book is available from the British Library

Every effort has been made in preparing this book to provide accurate
and up-to-date information which is in accord with accepted standards
and practice at the time of publication. Nevertheless, the authors,
editors and publisher can make no warranties that the information
contained herein is totally free from error, not least because clinical
standards are constantly changing through research and regulation. The
authors, editors and publisher therefore disclaim all liability for direct or
consequential damages resulting from the use of material contained in
this book. Readers are strongly advised to pay careful attention to
information provided by the manufacturer of any drugs or equipment
that they plan to use.

ISBN 0 521 64700 2 paperback

Contents

Contributors

David Alexander
Centre for Trauma Research
Grampian Primary Care NHS Trust
Royal Cornhill Hospital
Bennachie
Aberdeen AB25 2ZH
Scotland

Ron Archer
c/o North Queensland Rural Health Training Unit
212 McLeod Street
Cairns
Queensland 4870
Australia

Keith Armstrong
Department of Veterans Affairs
Medical Center
4150 Clement Street
San Francisco, CA 94121
USA

Philip Boyce
Department of Psychological Medicine
Clinical Sciences Building
Nepean Hospital
PO Box 63
Penrith
New South Wales 2750
Australia

Vaughan J. Carr
Hunter Area Health Service
PO Box 833
Newcastle
New South Wales 2300
Australia

Claude Chemtob
Pacific Islands Division
Center for Posttraumatic Stress Disorder
Department of Veterans Affairs
1132 Bishop Street
Suite 300
Honolulu, HI 96813
USA

John Condon
Department of Psychiatry
Repatriation Hospital
Daw Park
South Australia 5041
Australia

Martin P. Deahl
City and Hackney Community Services NHS Trust
East Wing
Homerton Hospital
Homerton Row
London E9 6SR
England

Christine Dunning
University of Wisconsin-Milwaukeee
161 West Wisconsin Avenue
Suite 6000
Milwaukee, WI 53205
USA

George S. Everly Jr
International Critical Incident Stress Foundation
University of Maryland
10176 Baltimore National Pike
Unit 210
Ellicott City, MD 21042
USA

Raymond B. Flannery Jr
Department of Mental Health
Central Office
25 Staniford Street
Boston MA 02114
USA

Carol S. Fullerton
Department of Psychiatry
Uniformed Services University of the Health Sciences
F. Edward Hébert School of Medicine
4301 Jones Bridge Road
Bethesda, MD 20814
USA

Michael Hobbs
Oxfordshire Mental Healthcare NHS Trust
The Warneford Hospital
Warneford Lane
Headington
Oxford OX3 7JX
England

Brian Kelly
2nd Floor
Psychiatric Unit
Princess Alexandra Hospital
Ipswich road
Woolloongabba
Queensland 4102
Australia

Kerrie Kelly
PO Box 908
Kuranda
Queensland 4872
Australia

Justin A. Kenardy
School of Psychology
University of Queensland
Brisbane
Queensland 4072
Australia

Tom Lundin
Department of Neuroscience
Centre for Traumatic Stress Studies
Uppsala University Hospital
Sparrisgatan 2
S-754 46 Uppsala
Sweden

Richard Mayou
Department of Psychiatry
University of Cambridge
Cambridge CB3 9AN
England

Alexander McFarlane
Department of Psychiatry
Queen Elizabeth Hospital
28 Woodville Road
Woodville South
South Australia 5011
Australia

Jeffrey T. Mitchell
International Critical Incident Stress Foundation
University of Maryland
10176 Baltimore National Pike
Unit 210
Ellicott City, MD 21042
USA

Philip Morris
Queensland Health
Gold Coast District Health Services
Integrated Mental Health Service Executive Office
2nd floor
60 High Street
Southport
PO Box 554
Southport
Queensland 4215
Australia

Yuval Neria
Tel Aviv University
The Bob Shapell School of Social Work
Ramat-Aviv
Tel Aviv 69978
Israel

Coralie Ober
c/o Alcohol, Tobacco and Other Drug Services
Queensland Health
PO Box 48
Brisbane

Queensland 4001
Australia

Lorraine Peeters
PO Box 557
Malanda
Queensland 4885
Australia

Beverley Raphael
Centre for Mental Health
New South Wales Health Department
Locked Mail Bag 961
North Sydney
New South Wales 2059
Australia

Robyn Robinson
Trauma Support Consultants Pty Ltd
586 Drummond Street
North Carlton
Victoria 3054
Australia

Arieh Y. Shalev
Department of Psychiatry
Hadassah University Hospital
PO Box 12000
Jerusalem 91120
Israel

Melissa R. Sigman
Department of Psychology
Cleveland State University
Cleveland, OH 44115
USA

Derrick Silove
Psychiatry Research and Teaching Unit
Level 4
Health Services Building
The Liverpool Hospital
Liverpool
New South Wales 2170
Australia

Zahava Solomon
Tel Aviv University
The Bob Shapell School of Social Work
Ramat-Aviv
Tel Aviv 69978
Israel

Paul Stallard
Avon and Wiltshire Mental Health Care NHS Trust
Child and Family Therapy Service
Royal United Hospital (North)
Combe Park
Bath BA1 3NG
England

Cynthia Stuhlmiller
Academic Department of Psychiatry
St George Hospital Campus
7 Chapel Street
Kogarah
New South Wales 2217
Australia

Jane Turner
Department of Psychiatry
Mental Health Centre
K floor
Royal Brisbane Hospital
Herston
Queensland 4029
Australia

Robert J. Ursano
Department of Psychiatry
Uniformed Services University of the Health Sciences
F. Edward Hébert School of Medicine
4301 Jones Bridge Road
Bethesda, MD 20814
USA

Kelley Vance
Department of Psychiatry
Uniformed Services University of the Health Sciences
F. Edward Hébert School of Medicine
4301 Jones Bridge Road
Bethesda, MD 20814
USA

Lemming Wang
Department of Psychiatry
Uniformed Services University of the Health Sciences
F. Edward Hébert School of Medicine
4301 Jones Bridge Road
Bethesda, MD 20814
USA

Rod Watts
Auckland Rehabilitation Service
54 Carrington Road
PO Box 44037
Pt Chevalier
Auckland 1002
New Zealand

Lars Weisæth
Division of Disaster Psychiatry
Insitute of Psychiatry
University of Oslo
Building 20
Sognsvannseien 21
0320 Oslo
Norway

John P. Wilson
Department of Psychology
Cleveland State University
Cleveland, OH 44115
USA

Eliezer Witztum
Beer-Sheva Mental Health Center and Division of Psychiatry
Ben Gurion University of the Negev
Beer Sheva
Israel

Ruth Wraith
Women and Children's Health Care Network
Flemington Road
Parkville
Victoria 3052
Australia

Introduction and overview: Key issues in the conceptualization of debriefing

Beverley Raphael and John P. Wilson

Introduction: Models of debriefing

There is significant conceptual and definitional confusion in the use of the term debriefing. The word 'debriefing' is in very common usage, its popular meaning being that of 'telling about what has happened'. There is also a sense of reviewing or going over an experience or set of actions, to achieve some sort of order or meaning concerning them. Being debriefed implies being enabled or assisted to achieve such a review.

Debriefing as a technical term, implying a specific and active intervention process, has developed with more formal meanings. Foremost there has been the concept of 'operational debriefing'. This is a structured process following an exercise or event that reviews the actions taken, the contribution of various workers or participants, and the degree of success or otherwise of the operation. The purpose of this review is to learn from the experience, and so further develop skills to deal with similar or related events in the future. Operational debriefing is usually a formal process occurring some time after the action or event and may deal with equipment, activities, fulfilment of functions and roles, and so forth. It is at times also carried out more informally, as part of an operational team's activities, led by a designated person. It has often been recognized that such discussion has clarified the experience for those involved. It has also been suggested that it may have promoted a sense of mastery of the situation and team morale through the review of achievements. Some team leaders also suggested that it could be helpful to their personnel as they could, through this process,

obtain a better perspective, or even 'get things off their chests'. Thus there was, even before other debriefing concepts were developed, a sense that there may have been personal benefits for those involved in the process. These advantages were also seen as including the strengthening of the team, who had 'all gone through this together', shared the experience, and could come to sense a common meaning in it, or to understand their roles and actions in the event.

Another paradigm that has been recently re-examined and found to be useful is that of 'historical group debriefing', developed by the US military historian S. L. A. Marshall to obtain a history of combat episodes in World War II and described by Shalev (Chapter 1) as a model for debriefing soldiers. This model promotes a group environment for describing the experience and bringing together the different perceptions in ways that may lessen distress and provide some shared sense of meaning. It was first developed in a purely historical concept but was observed to benefit those involved. It had no formal structure and made no interpretations.

In the 1960s Caplan (1964) proposed a model of crisis intervention to deal with stressful life experience when normal coping mechanisms were overwhelmed, and linked this to the possibility of preventing untoward psychological outcomes of such stressors. This was a brief intervention framework and, while not the same as debriefing, probably set a context wherein other brief models of intervention to prevent adverse stress outcomes were likely to develop.

The concept of debriefing itself developed into what was known as psychological debriefing in the 1970s. A number of different models of this procedure evolved with respect to emergency, military or incident response workers and their needs. Several of the contributors to this book describe their views on how and why this new domain of psychological debriefing in its various manifestations evolved and link this to different theoretical views and possible rationales for debriefing.

The most widely used model of debriefing is that developed by Jeffrey Mitchell and known as Critical Incident Stress Debriefing (CISD). This form of psychological debriefing has a specific structure and format, and has been developed for the management of critical incident stress experienced by emergency service workers. It has more recently been expanded to encompass a programme of interventions known as Critical Incident Stress Management (CISM).

Dunning (1988) (see Stuhlmiller and Dunning, Chapter 22) has reviewed the various models of psychosocial debriefing and described a number of varieties, including those that were more specifically educational. She classed these as didactic and psychological and the latter were subdivided into CISD and a continuum of care approach with coping-skill building and cognitive restructuring. These other frameworks do not appear, however, to have had widespread usage; perhaps they have not been seen as widely applicable because they have had a lower profile than CISD.

Among the meanings of debriefing are those corresponding to its relationship to briefing of personnel to deal with an incident or event. This relates to the preparation, training and briefing of workers such as police, military, rescue and disaster personnel to deal with emergencies or other extraordinary situations. There is much to suggest that the adequacy and effectiveness of such training and preparation may mitigate the stressor aspects of the experience, and even diminish the risk of subsequent morbidity, in terms of stress-related health phenomena such as sleep disturbance, and social malfunctioning.

Briefing and debriefing may be linked processes, incorporated into the operations of an emergency or military workforce, or those of other groups exposed to psychological stressors. In this way they are 'integrated' into the workplace system. In other instances they may be described as a health or even mental health programme, and seen as helping with the management of workplace or critical-incident type stress. Here they may be integral parts of an occupational health and safety programme, or even a stress management programme. Debriefing may therefore be seen as multifaceted and viewed as applicable to a range of work environments' critical incidents.

Debriefing has extended far beyond its original contexts and is now widely applied to almost any life experience, even those that may be relatively positive. This may seem to apply a pathologizing framework to the inevitable and stressful experiences of life, perhaps contributing to the view that we are a stressed and traumatized society. On the other hand, debriefing is frequently driven by altruistic and human responses in the wish to help others who have suffered, to undo what has happened to them, to comfort and 'make things right'. Debriefing, with trauma counselling, may be seen as the centrepiece of the new 'trauma' industry, as a source of revenue and effective activities. Or it may be seen as the 'magic bullet' of preventive intervention, to prevent the suffering and chronic morbidity that may follow traumatic life experiences. What the majority of the contributors to this volume make clear, however, is that there is much belief and goodwill and valuable theoretical development, but a dearth of systematic hypotheses building on established science and tested in empirical studies with appropriate methodologies. However, as is the case in the development of scientific data, we must await the outcome of proper research to know what types of debriefing are appropriate under different circumstances. Clearly, there is a phenomenon of debriefing at work and classification of the mechanisms will unfold in due time.

It could be suggested that the understanding of stress generally, and traumatic stress in particular, has shown significant growth in the last two decades, especially with the rapid expansion of high-quality scientific studies. This research has validated earlier clinical frameworks. Debriefing is provided with a belief in its value, in ways that could be said to be similar to earlier understanding of traumatic stress syndromes. The scientific underpinning of any acute intervention such as debriefing needs also to evolve to validate its relevance to acute post-trauma response and to ultimate recovery.

To date this has not occurred. However, it is the purpose of the contributions in this book to lay foundations and suggest directions for future critical scientific research.

Each of the authors in this volume has made a significant contribution to the evolution of the field of debriefing. They bring diverse theoretical, research and practical experience to the great debriefing debate.

Core debriefing issues

Core debriefing issues include the frameworks in which debriefing may be conceptualized: for example, its narrative modality, as crisis intervention, as psycho-education, as stress management, as prevention, as therapy and as an integrated intervention. Also relevant are the events, stressors or experiences to which debriefing interventions may be applied – appropriately or inappropriately – for example critical incidents, traumatic stressors, bereavement, separation or dislocation, chronic stressors, disasters. The relation of debriefing to theoretical understanding of these stressor experiences is relevant in terms of the nature of the reactive processes in each instance, the rationale and timing of debriefing interventions, and elucidating for whom they may be effective.

Narrative or talking through the experience

Weisæth (Chapter 3) suggests that much talking through of experiences happens naturally, as in veterans' clubs, or as part of the natural behaviour of groups after experiencing a major incident. Ursano et al. (Chapter 2) show how natural talking, which occurred more frequently in those with high exposure and high post-traumatic stress disorder (PTSD) symptoms (Ursano et al., 1996), did not lead to any reduction of these symptoms when assessed seven months later. The narrative tradition is a strong one as McFarlane (Chapter 24) suggests, but here, as in psychotherapy research more generally, there is inadequate information about the degree to which 'telling the story' solves the problem, despite a profound belief that it will. It is of interest that indigenous peoples value a narrative model to resolve loss, but resolution of loss involves very different phenomenological processes, as is discussed below.

Numerous authors quote Pennebaker & Susman's (1988) work in support of their debriefing hypotheses, but this was carried out in less aroused subjects. There is a certain naturalness in talking about what has happened – but not for everyone. As some contributors point out, it may not be the best coping mechanism for all people, nor at all times. It is particularly important to consider the value of talking about distress and emotional reactions (which may include helplessness) when the individual must continue to function and deal with ongoing critical incidents or continuing horror, violence and so forth. A number of workers agree that this may not be appropriate. Interventions should therefore be tailored to individual and situational requirements. As Wilson and Sigman (Chapter 4) suggest, a person-situation model is necessary to define appropriate responses and evaluate their effectiveness.

Shalev (Chapter 1) points out that arousal and distress are potentially critical pathogenic elements in moving from a normal reaction to a stressor to PTSD. His studies show that decreasing arousal and high levels of distress may therefore be key preventive mechanisms. Yet there is considerable anecdotal evidence that arousal may actually be heightened for some persons after debriefing, and it may therefore be that the re-exposure in the talking through of the incident during debriefing may have adverse effects for some. There appear to be no clear mechanisms available to recognize, and deal with, those for whom this may be the case. McFarlane (Chapter 24) suggests that a pharmacological intervention may be appropriate in some instances. A further issue is how much talking through resolves what has happened and assists with mastery of the experience, as compared to reinforcing helplessness. This question is not answered by any of the work presented – yet it is critical. Terr (1991) has recognized that the repetitive play of traumatized children does not assist resolution, but rather represents ongoing traumatization, with repeated and unsuccessful attempts at mastery and integration. It seems that some of those who experience a severe incident, trauma or disaster, become so powerfully fixated in their victim status that they become 'tellers' of their story – but no resolution occurs. Rather they remain locked into the incident, even though they may not appear outwardly stressed or symptomatic. This mode of coping may have been reinforced for them by powerful feelings of importance related to the event, which makes them feel significant in ways that they have not felt before. Nevertheless, it is not resolved if they are still locked in time to this event and to these narratives of what happened. There are self-disclosures that facilitate healing and those that serve only to maintain defences against helplessness and injury.

A general belief that it would be better to talk about it is held by the public and by mental health professionals who believe that it will help people to recover. As the evaluation studies of Robinson (Chapter 6) and others demonstrate, those in emergency services provided with debriefing generally identify it as helpful to them in providing an opportunity to talk about what has happened. Those who have not had a chance to talk about their experience formally may feel they have been deprived of something that would have been helpful. However, as Watts (Chapter 9) and others show, the perceived helpfulness of debriefing does not correlate with outcome and indeed Ørner's more recent studies suggest that it is most helpful to, and most used by, those who might be considered to need it least (Avery & Ørner, 1998).

It can safely be said that the debriefing movement has contributed to 'making it alright' for men, in particular, to talk about their traumatic wartime or other experiences, and that this in itself may have contributed positively towards lessening the negative sanctions in all-male environments against emotional expression and recognition of personal distress. It has been shown frequently that the coping styles of men and women differ and that women talk more readily with others about their problems and share their feelings, while men use more active coping styles – action oriented and at times acting out. In the limited data available, there has been inadequate analysis on utility of debriefing models by gender, although Ursano et al. (Chapter 2) note that women may more readily use such a medium.

Some suggest that the pendulum may now have swung too far away from denial of the effects of psychologically traumatic experiences, with even minor experiences being identified as stressors that must be dealt with by debriefing or trauma counselling, and an excessive adoption of victim status in a stressed society. There is much to suggest that talking in groups is potentially negative when disparate individuals are drawn together. Some whose exposure has been minor may be traumatized by the vivid accounts of those more intensely involved. This emphasizes the importance of some type of screening or selection relevant to any process where group debriefing is offered.

'Natural' talking with family, primary confidant and friends takes place over time and has been studied by Ursano et al. (Chapter 2). This is generally perceived as an important part of the gradual integration and shaping of the memories of the experience. Some experiences are perceived as being too terrible to talk about, particularly with family members. Armstrong (Chapter 21) uses family settings as part of the model of multiple stressor debriefing. Further work is needed to determine when talking through is perceived as helpful and with whom, what is perceived to be helpful and unhelpful in response, and how patterns of talking through correlate with outcome, both in natural social interactions and in professional settings.

Earlier work on conjugal bereavement explored this narrative model, and it was found that the perceived unhelpfulness of social network support for talking about the bereavement, in situations seen theoretically to be important in the resolution of the loss, correlated with negative mental health outcomes. Where individuals were at risk in this way, professional interactions meeting these needs could to some degree prevent negative outcomes (Raphael, 1977). This suggests that an individual's readiness for talking through may need to be adapted both cognitively and emotionally to the subject's need and pace, and it may be that different stressors and their different reactive processes will similarly need to be taken into account.

Studies indicating that debriefing is helpful (e.g. Robinson, Chapter 6) suggest that telling of one's experience is valued, and that group sharing of personal narratives about a traumatic experience may at times contribute to a group knowledge and understanding of what has happened. This seems most likely to lead to learning, and to be helpful when it is for groups who are briefed, trained and work together. In a debriefing framework it is reported by many, including Mitchell and those using his model, to lessen job turnover and sick leave, and to improve other indicators of workplace stress. However, neither in the military, nor elsewhere, is there any available systematic data from controlled trials to show that it prevents PTSD; Mitchell and Everly (Chapter 5) also point out quite clearly that it is not intended as an intervention for the prevention or treatment of PTSD.

Crisis intervention or critical incident stress debriefing

Recently, debriefing has taken on a crisis intervention mantle as part of its contextualization of potential benefit. Debriefing has a more formal structure of intervention as proposed by Mitchell and those using his framework. While this model has been adapted to be less formal than was initially proposed, it still sits within an institutional framework. Equating debriefing with crisis intervention, as initially described, is not entirely inappropriate. Crisis intervention in Caplan's (1964) model was formulated in social and psychological terms and looked at natural gatekeepers, the use of social networks, and focussed, short-term intervention. Thus there could be said to be some similarities. However, debriefing as originally proposed was more to do with a one-off intervention, and could be said to differ in that it was formalized, structured and did not rely on social network interventions, except in terms of peer support. Moreover the definition of a crisis was somewhat different – a crisis arose when one's normal coping mechanisms could not deal with particular life problems. Debriefing is typically provided in the immediate aftermath of an event, when the individual cannot be said to have had an opportunity to demonstrate or fail to demonstrate coping and adaptation, except perhaps in those circumstances where high levels of ongoing distress or dysfunction make it clear that adaptation is not yet occurring.

The crisis intervention model also suggested that most people would resolve crises with minimal assistance, but that there were those who could be identified as at high risk, for instance through personal resources being totally overwhelmed or social networks failing. Interventions should focus on these groups. However, it is usual for debriefing to be provided for all who have experienced a particular event or stressor. It may even be, in many circumstances, that those likely to be in greatest need do not avail themselves of debriefing, perhaps through the denial, resistance and avoidance that are part of acute stress reactions.

Models of debriefing might fit within a crisis intervention framework. However, crisis intervention that has been shown to be effective has not been applied to situations where debriefing is routinely applied, nor in formats that fit with debriefing. A number of studies of the crisis intervention model per se in randomized controlled trials have been carried out. These studies include: bereavement crisis intervention for high-risk bereaved widows (Raphael, 1977), crisis intervention for those at risk following motor vehicle accidents (Bordow & Porritt, 1979), and crisis intervention in association with illness and injury (Viney et al., 1985). Debriefing has been shown in contributions to this book (e.g. Watts, Chapter 9; Hobbs and Mayou, Chapter 10) and elsewhere (e.g. Bisson et al., 1997; Wessely et al., 1998) to be ineffective in each of these contexts, and potentially to be associated with increased morbidity, even though perceived as helpful. It should be noted in the bereavement research quoted above that perceived helpfulness did not correlate with outcome – perceived unhelpfulness did, negatively. This has not been investigated in the debriefing literature. Furthermore, the crisis interventions usually take place in the weeks after the event, and most usually in the form of a number of sessions for individuals – not groups, although the latter are also used. The sessions are informed by understanding of individual dynamics and vulnerability.

Thus it may be concluded that, although debriefing could be seen within a framework such as crisis intervention, particularly in its critical incident stress management format, there are many dichotomies. What both procedures have in common is that both conceptually deal with disruptions to coping in normal persons who have experienced some degree of disequilibrium caused by a stressful life event. But the mantle of crisis intervention does not help the cause of debriefing, or its ubiquity. The formats are different, the focus and timing frequently differ and where randomized controlled trials of crisis intervention exist, debriefing has been shown to be ineffective and possibly harmful to some.

Debriefing as education or psycho-education

Dunning (1988) has highlighted the different models of debriefing and the strong educational basis of some as compared with others. This review throws into light both the potential effects of debriefing in educating workers in reactions to severe experiences and ways of coping. Such an educational framework can scarcely be criticized per se. Recognition of the importance of education prior to incidents is clearly demonstrated by a number of contributions. Earlier writing by Ursano et al. (1996) highlighted these values. Weisæth (Chapter 3), in particular, places emphasis on the 'learning' that may occur with proper leadership in groups and for individuals who successfully master a highly stressful traumatic experience. Further, elite military units undergo rigorous training for expectable challenges in warfare. Such training can build repertoires for mastery and efficacy through rehearsal and conditioning.

A number of important issues can be highlighted when one examines education and learning in relation to traumatic circumstances. The traditional CISD model teaches those involved the psychological symptoms they may expect to have and what is a 'normal reaction to an abnormal experience'. The learning in such presentations is passive and not active. Educational theory, particularly that of adult learning, emphasizes the value of active learning and problem solving. This would appear to be more inherently part of models such as those proposed by Weisæth (Chapter 3), Shalev (Chapter 1), Alexander (Chapter 8), Lundin (Chapter 13) and Armstrong (Chapter 21), where learning from debriefing may be better 'owned' by those participating.

Learning in debriefing is thus probably a critical issue, as in any intervention – but what is learned from whom? As noted above, those involved may learn symptoms, or pathological syndromes, and identify

with these – in much the same way medical students do with the illnesses they study. They may 'learn' that everyone needs assistance – not, as is known from catastrophes in many different circumstances, that human resilience is a powerful force, even against the greatest odds, and that the personal battle to deal with stressor experiences may make some even stronger (Tedeschi & Calhoun, 1996). They may learn that all stress should be medicalized, even though it is a 'normal response to abnormal circumstance'. This of course is not necessarily due to debriefing, but debriefing may be one instrument of a social movement driving perceptions of a stressed or traumatized victim society.

Learning, on the other hand, in those formats more oriented to adult learning may build on the strengths, and recognition, of each individual's pathway to mastery, as well as those of others. This also raises the question of what should be the focus of any teaching and learning in order to promote coping.

Clearly these matters are at present hypothetical and research is needed to clarify positive and negative learning in relation to debriefing-type interventions. Where this learning sits with respect to the overall learning of the individual is also important. If previous learning about how to deal instrumentally and personally with stressful life circumstances appears established, what does the learning of debriefing do to contribute further to this? Is it necessary, and how is it applied to the individual good? It is known that past experience with similar events/traumata is helpful in many instances (when these have been successfully dealt with), and that this personally acquired learning may 'inoculate' to some degree to protect against the next stressor.

Debriefing as stress management

Shalev (1994) has described debriefing as fitting more within the stress management framework. This is possibly a useful way of viewing these interventions, particularly as they now encompass a whole spectrum of workplace-related responses to stressful incidents. This is particularly relevant when one considers the findings reported by Mitchell and his colleagues (Chapter 5).

The interventions are for stresses encountered in emergency work; they are also aimed at less overwhelming stressors – 'critical incident stress' as opposed to 'traumatic stress'. They seek to help workers to function and to return them effectively to their workplace, avoiding adverse health and social effects. Their chapter claims success in this, which concurs with other findings that debriefing is not 'suitable' for overwhelming circumstances, where it does not appear to have helped. The concept of stress inoculation is also taken up in some stress management frameworks where it is part of preparatory training to deal with stressful circumstances to act out such events in role play.

Indeed Mitchell and colleagues (Chapter 5) do identify their programme, apparently appropriately, as CISM. It is only open to question what is a 'critical incident', and when does this on the one hand become a 'traumatic incident' or on the other merge with ordinary 'life events'. This definitional aspect varies frequently in different presentations on this issue. The clearest workplace stress management paradigm in this context is perhaps that of Flannery et al. (1991) in the Assaulted Staff Action Program, which encompasses building the stress management capacity of the system in a model of positive expectancy using the CISD paradigm.

Research in a stress management focus could be useful in testing the effectiveness of interventional systems such as CISM in organizations, as it is an institutional response that could allow pre- and post-test and longitudinal monitoring of cohorts. This would greatly increase understanding of the value of the paradigm. It should of course examine positive adaptive processes and outcomes as well as negative: stress as challenge and learning, and stress as vulnerability and inducing of pathology.

Debriefing after which events?

Horowitz's (1976) original model of stress response syndromes included bereavement as a traumatic stressor. Dislocation, distress, illness episodes and diagnoses, military service, peace-keeping activities and so forth have all been a focus of debriefing. Even child-

birth has been a focus for debriefing as identified by Boyce and Condon (Chapter 19). Wilson and Sigman (Chapter 4) describe a matrix model that highlights the multiplicity of stressors and thus decisions about interventions, and suggest that a typology of debriefing needs to be developed based on a rationale of empirical factors associated with risk, threat and injury to self and others.

This highlights the confusion between a model of debriefing developed for dealing with emergency workplace stressors of a critical kind and the spread of debriefing interventions alleged to have utility in almost every circumstance. This is exemplified as well in discussions such as those of Wraith (Chapter 14) where she emphasizes a distinction for children between events that the child might experience which are not traumatically damaging (e.g. to development) as compared with those that are. Yet there are no operational frameworks that assist well with this process. Wilson (1989) highlighted the multiplicity of stressors and their differential effects and Wilson and Sigman's (Chapter 4) chapter acknowledges these and the decisions they may involve for interventions, although still contextualizing such interventions as debriefings.

Loss stressors and life threat

The need to consider what is relevant for intervention is highlighted particularly by a consideration of the stressors of bereavement and life threat. Elsewhere it is argued that the former lead to loss reactions and the latter to traumatic stress reactions (Raphael, 1986, 1997). The phenomenology of normal reactions to the loss of a loved one is now well studied, particularly in its evolution over time, from the period following the 'event'. Factors that influence the course of, and vulnerability to, pathology as opposed to adaptation are relatively well explored. Sudden, unanticipated and untimely bereavements are known to be associated with higher risk for adverse outcomes. Perceived unhelpfulness of the social support network is also a factor. Very high initial distress may be predictive of poorer outcomes. The phenomena are different from those of traumatic stress reactions (Raphael & Martinek, 1997). There is substantial evidence that crisis intervention and grief counselling in various formats are effective (Parkes, 1980). The only study that shows a negative effect of intervention for outcome is that of Pollack et al. (1975), which provided an intervention at the earliest possible time (in the immediate 24–48 hours following the loss). These reports highlight the specific needs associated with an appropriate response to loss as a stressor, even though it is also recognized that the risk factor paradigms may be similar in some ways to those of trauma.

It is, of course, possible that bereavements may in and of themselves be highly traumatic. Experience with disaster circumstances and other instances where bereavements also encompass life-threatening aspects such as gruesome, mutilating horrendous deaths, life threat to the bereaved person, feelings of profound helplessness in the face of violent death, and so forth have provided some insights into the interventions needed. These recognize that the trauma stressor components may need to be dealt with separately and in terms of their specific phenomenology; frequently the traumatic stressor effect should be tackled first and then the bereavement. But there is no evidence to suggest that a debriefing format is helpful or even adequate in these circumstances. It may in fact actively interfere with a necessary phase of denial and numbing as the individual's ego cushions against the excessive stress experienced.

Thus it may be concluded that different levels, patterns and timing of interventions are relevant in relation to these two stressors (trauma and loss), even when they co-occur, and that the debriefing model is not appropriate in the light of current understanding.

Separation/dislocation stressors

The intense distress of separation from a primary attachment figure may occur as a result of an incident, particularly one affecting families, i.e. separation of those who are normally in close and emotional interaction. The distress may be part of a reaction to the loss of this person by death or other means. But those closely attached may also be separated by natural or human-engendered forces in community disasters, war or violence. More prolonged dislocation from home and

community may follow – for instance, in the case of refugees. Dislocation stress involves also the loss of normal sources of support, coping and understanding. Debriefing per se may be inappropriate to deal with acute separation distress where information, support, protection and attempts at reunion, bringing together or finding the outcome for the separated are critical. Debriefing in this context is unlikely to diminish the distress and may even add to it (Raphael, 1986).

The chronic stressors of dislocation, for example the loss of community or home from a disaster, or loss of country and culture as a refugee, may be the background upon which other stressful occurrences take place. Whether or not a debriefing model is then appropriate is contentious because, as noted below, it may seem a superficial, and even glib response, which does not recognize either the context of trauma sustained, or the interaction of acute incidents with this.

Chronic stressors and traumatization

Those supporting debriefing have never suggested that it is an appropriate response to chronic stressor situations or to chronic traumatization. Nevertheless, critical incidents and even traumatic incidents to which debriefing may be applied may not infrequently occur on such a background for affected individuals or groups. This is well highlighted in the discussion of the possibility of debriefing for indigenous populations in the chapter by Ober et al. (Chapter 17). Chronic transgenerational and ongoing traumatization have effects that must be recognized and cannot be dealt with superficially or briefly. Two things are relevant. First, political or broader community support, action and restitution may be central to outcomes with such chronicity. Secondly, an acute incident, or an acute intervention may open up this past and contribute to ongoing psychological traumatization. This may lead to negative outcomes, failure of current hard won adaptation, the need for more skilled and in-depth interventions, or new opportunities for dealing with these experiences. Debriefing is rarely cognisant of such issues, and much of it is taken up and practised with little recognition of these possibilities and their significance.

Disasters

Disasters may encompass a multitude of stressors both for those directly affected and for those who would assist them. Yet here the debriefing model may be too basic to deal with all such experiences at both community and individual level. As shown by Kenardy and Carr's (Chapter 12) contribution and to a degree by those of Watts (Chapter 9) and Lundin (Chapter 13), debriefing is not appropriate for survivors, although some other group support and information may be. The chaos of disaster may require an acute mental health intervention, but this is more likely to be in the context of support, safety, triage and provision for subsequent follow-up.

Wholesale provision of debriefing for populations after disaster cannot be justified, although other interventions may be (Singh & Raphael, 1981). Debriefing for emergency personnel who are briefed for disaster response may be an appropriate usage, but this also needs to be reviewed in terms of some of the contexts outlined above.

Thus it may be concluded that the broad term 'debriefing' (or the new all encompassing 'debriefings') does not provide any adequate framework for the complexity and differences in the nature of interventions that may be appropriate in relation to different stressor experiences and the adaptive and maladaptive reactions to those. A matrix understanding as suggested by Wilson and Sigman (Chapter 4) may be helpful, as may a multiple stressor model. Empirical research to back such approaches is sorely needed. However, different types of intervention, group and individualized, focussed to deal with vulnerabilities in those at high risk, and frameworks that recognize and facilitate growth, resilience and mastery are all required, as is research into their effectiveness. In addition, a sophisticated understanding of background stressors, strengths and dynamics can allow a more appropriate response to individual need.

Mass trauma, violence and conflict

Bringing together the multiple stressors that may occur in the setting of human rights violation, mass trauma, torture, refugee status and in already devastated and deprived settings is difficult. Nevertheless, these are relevant as the greatest burden of psychological traumatization and life stress occurs in such settings. Workers providing for basic needs may not see the relevance of mental health, or the relevant language may not recognize psychological trauma, or it may be seen as a traumatized transposition. Silove (Chapter 25) has drawn together a framework for responses in such settings which encompasses the domains of, security/safety, attachment, justice, identity/role, and existential meaning. This makes it clear that traditional debriefing models are inappropriate as an acute response in such settings, and that a more holistic response will be required. Clearly, there is a need for further systematic research to support the relevance and utility of this framework. The usefulness of such integrative concepts is recognized when the human needs involved in situations of trauma are dealt with more holistically.

Debriefing for whom?

This question is highlighted by a number of contributors to this book. For instance, Solomon et al. (Chapter 11) question the possibility of negative effects for those who are depressive and likely to be subject to negative ruminations. Other personality facets and coping styles may be influential in adaptation, and debriefing may interact positively or negatively with these – for instance, emphasizing emotional reactions for those for whom this is, either at this time or generally, not helpful. Chemtob (Chapter 16) is helpful in defining 'survival mode' psychological distortions used by individuals as a necessary adaptation. He emphasises the importance of understanding individual specific ways of responding to life events, such as survival strategies. Another question not adequately addressed anywhere is the significance of debriefing-type interventions for those who are psychologically vulnerable or indeed physically ill (see Turner and Kelly, Chapter 18).

Cultural rituals may supplant the need for formal debriefing because these are culturally specific prescriptions that involve similar processes. Weisæth describes this with Fijian peace keepers and Silver &

Wilson (1988) have described this elsewhere with native Americans (see also Chapter 4).

Social structures and class may be influential, as many studies have shown that the well educated and affluent are less vulnerable to negative outcomes, possibly in many different ways. Is debriefing necessary for them and if so what model? Debriefing assumes that all are equal in a group, but ultimately it is often not a group of equals and the interventions may be inappropriate or unnecessary for some and inadequate for others.

Children are a group requiring particular attention, in that the widespread use of debriefing now extends to them, both in school settings and in their families. Wraith (Chapter 14) sensitively analyses some of these issues from the point of view of her experience. She suggests that an individualized approach is essential, taking into account the child's development, family and other contexts. She describes a two-stage model, which is for stressed but untraumatized children, who require an individual approach. Instead she suggests a form of immediate intervention which she sees as 'psychological first aid', followed by 'clinical debriefing'. It is also seen as vital that interventions do not override the natural healing and recovery. As children frequently have little previous learning in how to cope with these stressors such learning may be important for development, as long as it does not damage it. Similar issues may apply with respect to development for adolescents, as Stallard (Chapter 15) suggests, as there are still likely to be cognitive and emotional challenges to be mastered in reaction to severe stress.

Of particular importance in the question of 'For whom?', is that of the roles fulfilled in an incident that is seen to require debriefing. These may be emergency service roles ranging from police, fire and rescue workers, ambulance, emergency medical teams, to those who provide back-up to the front-line workers, those involved in practical tasks of recovery, the body handlers, patients, health care staff, counsellors and so forth. The evidence for the uptake of debriefing is most cogent with the emergency services and military, where its use is now widespread. There is the need for evidence of its value in other settings and a number of trials suggest that it may have little benefit, or even be

potentially negative, for those directly involved as victims of accidents (e.g. motor vehicle), burns, general populations affected by disasters such as earthquakes, and so forth. Health care staff may not take up debriefing opportunities in the emergency settings, although they may in mental health settings. Nurses may use debriefing formally but rely on informal networks for their major support. Some studies show no benefit for body handlers (e.g. Deahl, Chapter 7), others suggest benefit in an integrated model (e.g. Alexander, Chapter 8), with more active learning. The general body of information provided by the contributors to this volume and elsewhere would seem to be that if there is benefit for debriefing, it is most likely to be for those who have been trained and briefed for emergency service, military or other paramilitary-type groups that have existing social structures with role differentiation.

Thus at present there is little evidence and few controlled trials to support the traditional format of debriefing, or CISD, even in a CISM framework, as being helpful for all critical life experiences and for everyone involved. The format may be applicable in institutional settings such as the emergency services and the military as a paradigm to change traditional models of coping, when and where this is seen as relevant to mental health outcomes. Even here, however, there must be awareness of individual need, coping styles, and potential negatives. It is therefore critical that research in this field is published in peer-reviewed journals. The emergency services and the military provide ideal settings for research that can examine, in depth, background factors, individual coping styles, and event characteristics and post-event variables, including the range of interventions, to determine possible relationships of any effects to positive and negative outcomes over time. This could validate the scientific reality of the person–environment interactional model and the effectiveness or otherwise of debriefing interventions.

Timing of debriefing interventions

The original model of debriefing emphasized the earliest possible intervention, i.e. in the first 24–48 hours, then at 72 hours and eventually even in the first week post event. As suggested above, this timing may or may not be appropriate. Shalev (Chapter 1) suggests that if debriefing is offered early, the stress and trauma may still be operating and those affected may still have to deal further with, say, the battle or disaster. Prolongation of distress may occur without lessening of arousal, and if debriefing in any way contributes to this, it may enhance or even create a 'catastrophic memory'. Of considerable interest too are personal accounts suggesting that debriefing might have been helpful at a later time, that it was not at the right time for that person. Such testimonials point to differences in readiness for psychological interventions in the acute period.

Two contributions in this volume present the use of a debriefing model at a later stage. Chemtob (Chapter 16) describes work with hurricane victims six months or more after the disaster and reports positive outcomes with helpers, teachers and children as well as school environments. Stallard (Chapter 15) reports debriefing adolescents three months after a school minibus accident, with some positive outcome in decrease of intrusion phenomenology. It is interesting that both these studies involve children and young people who may be secure enough to deal with their stressful experience only when reintegrated into normal family and school environments. This could also fit with McFarlane's (1987) finding that their reactions may be delayed beyond the immediate post-disaster period, and may be influenced by the behaviour of those around them, particularly that of parents. Whether this later intervention is usefully seen as a form of debriefing might be challenged but both Stallard and Chemtob have identified this as the model used, and suggested that it is a valid conceptual basis.

In respect of acute traumatic stress effects, a recent review by Solomon (1999) has highlighted the effectiveness, for those acutely stressed, of interventions that commence two weeks or more after the incident. This is measured against the failure to show benefits, in terms of prevention of PTSD and other post-trauma morbidity, of earlier interventions such as debriefing. She suggests that this allows time to identify those who really need such interventions; it may also be that they are more ready for it at this later stage. This is similar to findings for post-bereavement interventions and may

be the basis of more effective models to deal with these more severe stressor situations, as compared with critical incident stress.

What can be stated is that there is little research and even less identification of considerations of timing in terms of any scientific knowledge of response to stress generally and critical incident stress in particular. With respect to response to traumatic stressors there is considerable concern about what is known of the neuroendocrinology and psychophysiology of this response. It is suggested by Shalev (Chapter 1), however, who has studied this stress response that historical group debriefing, which is more fact finding and linked to operational debriefing, has produced decreased levels of anxiety and distress. Ursano (personal communication) suggests that debriefing may provide a humanistic outreach 'splint' and protect those affected in an acute period of distress. Interventions may increase or decrease arousal, distress and other responses in required directions, but, in general, research has not even systematically considered, let alone adequately tested, debriefing, or indeed other interventions, for impact on anxiety, arousal and distress, nor has the relevance of the timing of debriefing interventions been systematically examined.

Debriefing as psychotherapy

Mitchell and Everly (Chapter 5), Robinson (Chapter 6) and Dyregrov (1997) are emphatic that their debriefing model is not psychotherapy. Yet it shares some characteristics with psychotherapeutic techniques such as group psychotherapy, behavioural and cognitive-behavioural therapies, and even psychodynamic models, for example the use of group process, exploration of experience, examining cognitive distortions, provision of information, emotional expression or even catharsis, reconfronting stressful experiences, education and support.

Debriefing is usually provided as a one-off intervention, but there may be repeats. It may be part of a range of psychosocial interventions as noted above, for instance in the CISM model. But it is not provided as an intervention for those with identified problems, i.e. as treatment for a disorder, and thus has quite different aims as well as operations. It might hope to lessen psychosocial morbidity, but as this is usually not definably present when debriefing is provided it cannot be seen as a treatment intervention. It may, however, be seen on the spectrum of interventions (Mrazek & Haggerty, 1994) as a selective or indicated preventive intervention of the psychosocial kind.

Debriefing as prevention

Debriefing interventions have been suggested to have positive and potentially preventive benefits. In addition, there is a pervasive belief that providing debriefing after traumatic incidents will prevent the development of PTSD. As yet, there is no evidence to support this hypothesis. Debriefing is also believed to prevent more broadly based psychosocial morbidity. Mitchell's review (Chapter 5) and that of Robinson (Chapter 6), suggest intervention results in decreased sick days, less job turnover, and other effects of workplace stress, which fits with a stress-management paradigm. More evidence is needed from randomized controlled trials to demonstrate such effects, and those committed to debriefing agree with the need for further research. Both situational difficulties and reluctance to have a nonintervention control group because of the social demand for debriefing, and belief in its effectiveness, create problems in achieving methodological rigour. Whether debriefing interventions may prevent other morbidity, such as substance abuse or other anxiety or depressive disorders, has not been explored. As part of a spectrum of preventive approaches it may be that it can contribute some preventive effects – but further research would be required to answer this.

Shalev (Chapter 1) identifies key issues in preventing post-trauma morbidity as the reduction of distress or arousal. His historical group debriefing has been shown to achieve this for at least some participants. Whether this correlates with the prevention of PTSD is not yet reported. Weisæth's (Chapter 3) studies suggest that group stress debriefing may lead to enhanced feelings of self-competence, which he sees as central because the threat to self-esteem may, he believes, be the most severe threat for soldiers. Again, however, preventive effects are not yet established. Alexander's work (Chapter 8) suggests that there may have been preventive benefits but the methodology does not allow validation. Watts' (Chapter 9) studies show that, even though perceived as helpful, debriefing did not prevent negative psychological outcomes. The same is true of Hobbs and Mayou's (Chapter 10), Kenardy and Carr's (Chapter 12) and Lundin's (Chapter 13) work. Flannery's study (Chapter 20) is one of the few to replicate possible preventive benefits but there is a need for further controlled trials. Like Alexander's work (Chapter 8), there is a structural system effect and ownership. Boyce and Condon (Chapter 19) also suggest preventive effects in obstetric settings but acknowledge that these interventions should really be a routine part of good clinical care.

It is also inferred that debriefing may allow screening for those at higher risk of PTSD and serve a prevention function in this way as suggested, for instance, by Mitchell and Everly (Chapter 5) and Chemtob (Chapter 16). While this is theoretically possible, few situations of debriefing appear to have been subjected to any formal and systematic screening to identify those who might be vulnerable on the basis of established knowledge. There is clearly a need to define not only what is meant by debriefing, but what is its purpose and the criteria by which it can be defined.

Because preventive interventions are often most likely to demonstrate these effects with high-risk populations, reducing the risk to that of lower-risk groups when they are effective, debriefing could ideally be trialled with those at heightened risk. Because the causative matrix is so complex, as highlighted by Wilson and Sigman (Chapter 4) and specifically by Turner and Kelly (Chapter 18) for a health workforce, it seems likely that complex methodologies and use of core methods and measures would be necessary. This is supported by McFarlane's proposal (Chapter 24) for an international network of research collaboration to answer these questions.

Debriefing as an integrated intervention

Many of the contributions above discuss the importance of integrating debriefing processes and interventions into other organizational systems or structures.

Shalev (Chapter 1) discusses integrating it with something more like history-taking or operational debriefing in military settings. Weisæth (Chapter 3) speaks of integrating it with the team leaders' functions in full-time and reserve emergency response teams. Ursano et al. (Chapter 2) consider how much normal talking may reflect a debriefing aspect integrated into everyday life. Alexander (Chapter 8) reports on debriefing integrated in a mental health, occupational health and safety response system. Lundin's work (Chapter 13) also points to an integration of debriefing with peer response. In health care settings, both Turner and Kelly (Chapter 18) and Boyce and Condon (Chapter 19) suggest that debriefing intentions may be better achieved through integration into good clinical care. Flannery's (Chapter 20) debriefing model is also an occupational health and safety integration. Armstrong's (Chapter 21) debriefing is integrated with the longer-term, and multiplicity of, response for families post disaster. Mitchell and Everly (Chapter 5) suggest separate systems, integrated as part of the emergency service response system and part of an occupational health and safety framework.

This integration is an interesting evolution, suggesting a normalizing and holistic framework. Integration with cultural response systems is also a possible requirement, e.g. with indigenous populations where a holistic approach is also likely to be required. This integration paradigm fits with findings on post-disaster intervention (Singh & Raphael, 1981) where this psychological intervention was viewed as more appropriate when provided alongside other practical support, a finding repeatedly noted in anecdotal reports. Furthermore, attempts to provide a separate crisis intervention for those presenting to an emergency department were unsuccessful because those surveyed considered that they should be able to have their psychological support for these issues oriented alongside other care, and indeed during the screening process (Singh et al., 1987).

It may be concluded, therefore, that what has evolved as a separate (and frequently expensive) intervention system may more appropriately be integrated with other responses. That as an acute preventive, therapeutic or other intervention there is no evidence as to its benefit with broader populations outside emergency-type services. Nevertheless, modifications for a broader approach and application as an integrated model for emergency and military services may be its most appropriate role. The tasks of future research into debriefing are increasingly evident, but require commitment for the scientific advance of this field. Just as the field of trauma research has evolved in recent decades, there is a need for critical and soundly based research into debriefing, research that explores the reasons it is valuable, the beliefs that drive it, the forms it should take, and the processes that are relevant for which group and in which settings, as suggested by Wilson and Sigman (Chapter 4). However, extensive further research will be required to ensure first that no harm ensues, and, secondly, that resources are used for benefit in these and other settings.

REFERENCES

Avery, A. & Ørner, R. (1998). First report of psychological debriefing abandoned – the end of an era? *Traumatic Stress Points*, International Society for Traumatic Stress Studies, **12**, Summer.

Bisson, J. I., Jenkins, J. A. & Bannister, C. (1997). Randomised controlled trial of psychological debriefing for victims of acute burn trauma. *British Journal of Psychiatry*, **171**, 78–81.

Bordow, S. & Porritt, D. (1979). An experimental evaluation of crisis intervention. *Social Science and Medicine*, **13**, 251–6.

Caplan, G. (1964). *Principle's of Preventive Psychiatry*. New York: Basic Books.

Dunning, C. (1988). Intervention strategies for emergency workers. In M. Lystad (Ed.) *Mental Health Response to Mass Emergencies* (pp. 284–320). New York: Brunner/Mazel.

Dyregov, A. (1997). The process in psychological debriefings. *Journal of Traumatic Stress*, **10**, 589–605.

Flannery, R. B., Fulton, P., Tausch, J. & DeLoffi, A. Y. (1991). A program to help staff cope with psychological sequelae of assaults by patients. *Hospital and Community Psychiatry*, **42**, 935–8.

Horowitz, M. A. (1976). *Stress Response Syndromes*. New York: Jason Aronson, Inc.

McFarlane, A. C. (1987). Posttraumatic phenomena in a longitudinal study of children following a natural disaster. *Journal of the American Academy of Child and Adolescent Psychiatry*, **16**, 764–9.

Mrazek, P. J. & Haggerty, R. J. (1994). *Reducing Risks for Mental Disorders: Frontiers for Preventive Intervention Research*.

Washington, DC: National Academy Press.

Parkes, C. (1980). Bereavement counselling: does it work? *British Medical Journal*, **281**, 3–10.

Pennebaker, J. W. & Susman, J. R. (1988). Disclosure of traumas and psychosomatic processes. *Social Medicine*, **26**, 327–32.

Pollack, P. R., Egan, D., Vandebergh, R. & Williams, W. V. (1975). Prevention in mental health: a controlled study. *American Journal of Psychiatry*, **132**, 146–9.

Raphael, B. (1977). Preventive intervention with the recently bereaved. *Archives of General Psychiatry*, **34**, 1450–4.

Raphael, B. (1983). *The Anatomy of Bereavement*. New York: Basic Books.

Raphael, B. (1986). *When Disaster Strikes: How Individuals and Communities Cope with Catastrophe*. New York: Basic Books.

Raphael, B. (1997). The interaction of trauma and grief. In D. Black, M. Newman, J. Harris-Hendricks & G. Mezey (Eds.) *Psychological Trauma: A Developmental Approach* (pp. 31–43). London: Gaskell/Royal College of Psychiatrists.

Raphael, B. & Martinek, N. (1997). Assessing traumatic bereavements and PTSD. In J. P. Wilson & T. M. Keane (Eds.) *Assessing Psychological Trauma and PTSD* (pp. 373–95). New York: Guildford Press.

Shalev, A. (1994). Debriefing following traumatic exposure. In R, Ursano, B. McCaughey & C. Fullerton (Eds.) *Individual and Community Responses to Trauma and Disaster: The Structure of Human Chaos* (pp. 201–19). Cambridge: Cambridge University Press.

Silver, S. M. & Wilson, J. P. (1988). Native American healing and purification rituals for war stress. In J. P. Wilson, Z. Harel & B. Kahana (Eds.) *Human Adaptation to Extreme Stress: From Holocaust to Vietnam* (pp. 337–55). New York: Plenum Press.

Singh, B. & Raphael, B. (1981). Post-disaster morbidity of the bereaved: A possible role for preventive psychiatry? *Journal of Nervous and Mental Disease*, **169**, 203–12.

Singh, B., Lewin, T., Raphael, B., Johnson, P. & Walton, J. (1987). Minor psychiatric morbidity in a casualty population: identification, attempted intervention and six month follow up. *Australian and New Zealand Journal of Psychiatry*, **21**, 231–40.

Solomon, S. (1999). Inventions for acute trauma response. *Current Opinion in Psychiatry*, **12**, 175–80.

Tedeschi, R.G. & Calhoun, G. (1996). The posttraumatic growth inventory: measuring the positive legacy of trauma. *Journal of Traumatic Stress*, **9**, 455–71.

Terr, L. C. (1991). Childhood traumas: an outline and overview. *American Journal of Psychiatry*, **148**, 1–20.

Ursano, R. J., Greiger, T. A. & McCarroll, J. E. (1996). Prevention of post-traumatic stress: consultation, training and early treatment. In B. A. van der Kolk, A. C. McFarlane & L. Weisæth (Eds.) *Traumatic Stress: The Effects of Overwhelming Experience on Mind, Body and Society* (pp. 441–63). New York: Guilford Press.

Viney, L., Clarke, A., Bunn, T. & Benjamin, Y. (1985). An evaluation of three crisis intervention programs for general hospital patients. *British Journal of Medical Psychology*, **58**, 75–86.

Wessely, S., Bisson, J. & Rose, S. (1998). A systematic review of brief psychological interventions ('debriefing') for the treatment of immediate trauma related symptoms and the prevention of posttraumatic stress disorder (Cochrane Review). *The Cochrane Library*, **3**. Oxford: Update Software.

Wilson, J. P. (1989). *Trauma, Transformation and Healing*. New York: Brunner/Mazel.

PART I

Key conceptual framework of debriefing

Stress management and debriefing: historical concepts and present patterns

Arieh Y. Shalev

'They had been brought to the last extremity of hope [yet they showed] a passionate conviction that it would be all right, though they had faith in nothing, but in themselves and in each other'. (Manning, 1990/1930, Introduction, p. xii)

EDITORIAL COMMENTS

Shalev challenges simplistic notions of debriefing as it is frequently applied and outlines its development in the historical contexts of understanding psychological trauma and post-trauma morbidity. He emphasizes the need to be responsive to the diversity of human responses in such situations, the significance of distress and arousal, and the psychological and neurochemical responses in the early post-trauma period. His conceptualization notes the need to consider the traumatogenic effects of extreme stress such as its undesirability, uncontrollability, unpredictability and inescapability. He suggests that prolonged distress during a critical post-trauma period may enhance or even create a 'catastrophic memory' through neuroendocrine mechanisms. The essence of preventing post-trauma morbidity is therefore to reduce distress and arousal.

Traditional approaches, which open up the expression of emotion, make interpretations of response, or describe symptomatic presentations, may be inappropriate. Furthermore, debriefing may be offered where the trauma or stress is continuing, or when other stressors such as loss and dislocation have also occurred. Because any intervention at this early stage may impact on a relatively small segment of the causative matrix,

long-term evaluation may be inappropriate as a method of judging debriefing effectiveness. Beneficial effects may occur, as his research suggests, by following the original model of debriefing ('historical group debriefing'), which is more a fact-finding model of debriefing, similar to operational or instrumental debriefing. This explores the narratives of individuals in the group, accepting their memory of their experience, and makes no interpretation. In his studies such interventions have been shown to reduce the high levels of anxiety of some group members and to provide a more homogeneous and less distressed outcome for group members overall. There was an increase in self-efficacy. He also suggests that this type of experience may lessen the loneliness and detachment that may create problems for those traumatized.

The overall message of this chapter is that 'debriefing' should sit in the spectrum of response to those who have suffered severe psychologically traumatic experiences. But it should not be viewed simplistically because of what it may achieve – taking into account the spectrum of distress, reducing this may be the most important humane and preventive measure.

Shalev is clear on the importance of supporting and not negating the human response to others' suffering at this time. Debriefing is one format that can provide a structure for this. It should be used only to achieve appropriate effects such as the human and caring reduction of distress. This is the key element and this type of intervention is only relevant if it achieves this and is validated by appropriate evaluation. As he states 'both the accuracy of the initial hope and the strength of the negative evidence must be questioned'.

Why early interventions?

The main reason for conducting early treatment interventions after traumatic events is a moral one. Army commanders may also wish to conduct such interventions to reduce loss of personnel. State economists may expect them to reduce the burden of financial compensation given to victims. The medical profession would be pleased to see them reducing the prevalence of long-term morbidity. Yet these are auxiliary goals. The main point is that many survivors and witnesses of extreme events suffer: afflicted, anxious, depressed and dismayed, their pain may also become permanent. Morally, such human conditions should not be left unattended.

The same moral reason requires that early interventions effectively reduce human suffering. It does not dictate, however, which type of treatment should be administered, nor its timing or duration. The latter two are practical or pragmatic considerations. Pragmatism, however, is often obscured by theory, especially when theory becomes dogma. In the area of traumatic stress, a salient example of salutary theory turned into dogma is the early, front-line, treatment of combat stress casualties, the rigid implementation of which during the Vietnam war has been severely criticized (e.g. Camp, 1993) and has not resulted in known beneficial effect on the prevalence of chronic stress disorders (Bourne, 1978; Kulka et al., 1990). A treatment modality can aso become the subject of blind belief, in which case its implementation is uncritically preferred over that of other alternatives. This is both pragmatically and morally wrong. Has this become the case with debriefing?

The practical reasons for choosing debriefing, amongst other interventions, are all too obvious. Debriefing is relatively inexpensive and easy to deliver. It is said not to 'medicalize' emotional problems, and is readily acceptable to most relevant institutions. Other practical reasons, however, are debatable: debriefing does not create a stable commitment between the health care giver and his or her client(s). The practice is easily reducible into semi-structured 'do-it-yourself' instruction protocols, and, given the lack of convened standards, the implementation of any such protocol is

relatively immune to quality control. Finally, the expected long-term mythical efficacy of this intervention can be used to defer judgement about its effect until it is too late, and, meanwhile, refrain from additional diagnostic and treatment efforts.

Needless to say, the term debriefing refers to a heterogeneous array of interventions, which may include various degrees of abreaction, cognitive reconstruction, suggestion, self-diagnosis and education. Hence, a conceptual basis for debriefing as such is very elusive, as each component of this ensemble may have a rationale for itself (e.g. Shalev, 1994). Indeed, the healing theories behind abreaction (Freud, 1957/1917) or disclosure (e.g. Pennebaker & Susman, 1988) differ from those of graded exposure or teaching coping skills. Hence, the core of the argument for or against debriefing can not be theoretical and must remain empirical.

If one argues empirically, efficacy is, obviously, the central issue. Beyond efficacy, however, acceptability and the availability of adequate alternatives should also be considered. Debriefing has been accepted as a standard to meet obligations by many of the institutions that expose their members to stressful events, and this should not be overlooked. So far no viable alternatives has been shown to fare better (for a review, see Shalev, 1997b). In that regard, this chapter responds to the half-expressed plea, by a traumatized help-professional who, having been exposed to a massacre in Central Africa, could only say when she came back, overwhelmed, 'We even didn't get debriefing.', i.e. there was no help. If debriefing has become a synonym for help, then the cynical reply 'Debriefing wouldn't have helped you anyway.' is as unprofessional as the uncritical implementation of this technique as a cure for all. Hence, justice must be done not only to the construct of debriefing but also to those who are asking us professionals to provide a solution to their all too obvious distress.

For and against debriefing

The practice of debriefing has received substantial attention during the last two decades. Consequently this area has now been researched and documented in an intense, if somewhat scattered, way. Far from yielding a consensus, however, the cumulative results convey discontent and criticism. These are related mainly to the simultaneous presence of two diverging assertions: one clearly favouring debriefing and the other completely denying its beneficial effect and therefore its reason for existence.

One of the bitter disappointments came from a series of studies that failed to show a reduction in long-term psychopathology among survivors 'treated' in this way (e.g. Bisson & Deahl, 1994; Deahl et al., 1994; Raphael et al., 1995; Kenardy et al., 1996). Indeed, earlier views, according to which one or a few debriefing sessions could have long-term effects, may have been premature. However, there seems to be a general sense, often amongst survivors (see e.g. Robinson et al., 1997) that debriefing is worth while and beneficial. Hence, both the accuracy of the initial hope and the strength of the negative evidence must be questioned.

Possibly the best criticism of the initial expectations from debriefing relies on a series of recent studies that have shown that chronic disorders result from the combined effect of many contributing factors, and that whatever happens immediately following exposure (including the treatment provided) may have only a limited effect on the final outcome of traumatization.

As to the above-mentioned negative evidence, it comes mostly from retrospective studies without random assignment to treatment groups, studies that employed cursory measurement of trauma exposure (if at all), and were characterized by extremely long time-lags between treatment and measurement of outcome, by poor control for the resulting confounds (time effect, intercurrent life events), and by the absence of very essential continuity of care. The hypothesis to be prove by such a design (i.e. that the effect of one or a few hours of debriefing will be stronger than anything else before, during or after the traumatic event) has a very low probability, and obviously was not confirmed. Similar arguments may apply to the studies reporting positive outcomes. By analogy, if one were to evaluate the effect of the most potent antidepressant by measuring depressive symptoms one year after cessation of treatment, in a heterogeneous group of initially depressed and nondepressed individuals who received only one pill, very little in the recorded result would be pertinent to the question of efficacy. Rather than telling us about the quality of the agent itself, such results reflect the inadequate dose, the heterogeneity of the initial sample, the time-lag between treatment and evaluation and many other variables. Specifically, a sensitizing effect of debriefing (i.e. group members becoming more aware of their experiences and their emotional responses), when not followed by further elaboration, or if followed by other stressful experiences, may turn from being potentially beneficial to becoming harmful. Importantly, such hypothetical interactions cannot be identified by measuring a global outcome remotely.

Hence better understanding of the complexity of traumatic events, modest expectations from isolated interventions, and better integration of debriefing into the overall care for trauma victims would yield better arguments either for or against practising these interventions. Given the current pressure for evidence-based practice, the long-term survival of debriefing really depends on defining its relevant dimensions and finding a valid yardstick by which to measure them.

This chapter attempts to contribute to the survival of debriefing by arguing that these interventions should not be viewed as treatment for trauma but rather as stress management techniques. It also argues:

1. that in the absence of immediate and measurable relief in distress there is no ground for assuming a long-term effect of debriefing;
2. that the presence of short-term effect does not necessarily assure a long-term effect;
3. that debriefing affects individuals by modulating their concrete and symbolic relationship with the larger group;
4. that loneliness and isolation are particularly frequent among traumatized survivors, and are very harmful;
5. that the traumatogenic elements of stress, i.e. its being undesirable, intense, unpredictable, uncontrollable and inescapable, continue to operate during the period in which debriefing is applied; and
6. that, notwithstanding its exact protocol, debriefing should specifically address these elements.

Table 1.1. Historical appraisal of post-traumatic stress disorder (PTSD)

- The original formulation of PTSD borrowed its cardinal symptoms from earlier descriptions of acute grief
- The dynamic of loss overshadowed that of fear, exhaustion, surrender or annihilation
- Psychological processes, previously identified with recovery from loss, were assumed to be essential for healing traumatic stress disorders
- The failure to engage in such processes was to be responsible for PTSD
- Conscious levels of mental processing received more weight than other functions such as acquired fear conditioning, implicit learning
- The early responses to traumatic stress were considered as normal responses to 'outstanding' or 'abnormal' stressors
- The contribution of a priori and a posteriori factors was shunned
- The essence of prevention was in properly 'metabolizing' and 'integrating' the meaning of traumatic experience

Early psychological interventions and their historical context

Historically, the psychodynamic dimensions of the immediate aftermath of stressful exposure have been perceived as central for the development of subsequent disorders (Table 1.1). The original formulation of post-traumatic stress disorder (PTSD), for example, borrowed its main symptom clusters, 'intrusion' and 'avoidance', from earlier descriptions of loss and subsequent mourning (Freud, 1957/1917; Lindemann, 1944). Psychological processes, previously described in 'traumatic loss', were assumed to be essential for recovery from 'traumatic stress'. The failure to engage in such processes was similarly perceived as leading to protracted psychopathology, PTSD being explicitly interpreted as a form of 'impacted grief' (Horowitz, 1974). Stress, in fact, was confounded with loss, with many of its inherent elements (e.g. alarm, surrender (or freezing), exhaustion, exposure to grotesque scenes, chaotic responses) being ignored. Conscious integration was also perceived as the main road to recovery, while other levels of mental processing (e.g. fear conditioning, implicit memory) were largely ignored. Such appraisal has led to the assumption that early and appropriate elaboration of the traumatic event, by the survivor, prevents its long-term effect.

The birth of PTSD was also tainted in the 1960s by the specifics of the Vietnam War, amongst which the failure to address the psychological needs of combatants was particularly salient. The description of the Vietnam veterans' unaccommodating and hostile homecoming

(e.g. Lifton, 1973) and their sudden relocation from 'fox holes to continental US' are amongst the founding metaphors of the field of traumatic stress. Indeed, the treatment package delivered by military psychiatrists in Vietnam had very little room for psychological elaboration and abreaction (e.g. Bourne, 1973), as most medical efforts were either preventive (e.g. shorter duration of service) or doctrinal (e.g. ban on backward evacuation of combat stress casualties). The lack of early psychological care was therefore perceived as a direct cause for the high prevalence of mental disorders amongst veterans.

Additionally, the contribution of prior risk factors (biological, prior life events, prior psychopathology) to post-traumatic disorders was underappreciated. Indeed, such explanation was shunned, because the fact of prior vulnerability reduced the explanatory power of combat exposure itself and was seen as playing into the hands of those who tended to argue that only those previously sick (alias 'degenerates' Witztum et al., 1996) do not endure the challenge of combat.

The recognition of posterior risk factors (e.g. relocation, loss, re-exposure; Hobfoll, 1989; Solomon et al., 1993) was equally underappreciated. Importantly, it was also believed that the initial response to a traumatizing event was essentially normal; that a traumatic stressor was one that would induce distress in almost everyone (American Psychiatric Association, 1980); and that given proper treatment, normal recovery should naturally follow (for a critical review, see Yehuda & McFarlane, 1995). The burden of the causation and the essence of healing were, therefore, linked

Table 1.2. Biological theories of early causation

- Memory for events is consolidated during the period that immediately follows trauma
- Elevated level of the stress hormone adrenaline contributes to memory consolidation
- Adrenergic activation is associated with better recall of aversive information
- Levels of the stress hormone cortisol, during adversity, modulates the effect of noradrenaline on memory
- Information recorded shortly after an event may distort and affect its long-term recall
- Prolonged distress during a critical period enhances or even creates a catastrophic memory.
- The essence of prevention is in reducing distress and arousal

with working through the effect of the trauma (Table 1.2).

Debriefing was developed in such a historical context. Yet, other treatment interventions based on similar assumptions were developed as well. A salient example is the belief that chronic PTSD could be successfully treated by going back to the original incident and properly 'metabolizing' it. Such belief assumed, via misreading of Freud's assertion about the atemporality of unconscious (childhood) traumata and their later healing via psychoanalysis of adults, that psychologically traumatic events create atemporal recollections, frozen in the survivor's mind, and reversible at any stage. The practice of explorative therapies for PTSD prevailed, therefore, for more than 20 years, and has only recently been criticized as nonefficacious as a result of data collected in inpatient programmes of the Veterans Administration in the USA (Johnson et al., 1996; see comment by Shalev, 1997a).

Similar in its spirit was an attempt to help to reduce post-traumatic symptoms in Israeli combat veterans with PTSD by carefully re-exposing them, in mutually supportive peer groups, to the military environment, three years after the Lebanon war (1982). This enthusiastic and well-meant experiment only aggravated the condition of those involved, as shown by comparing them with a group of veterans with PTSD who did not participate in the programme (see e.g. Solomon et al., 1992).

Debriefing, therefore, is one of many treatment interventions related to the earlier understanding of stress disorders. Recent knowledge (e.g. Yehuda & McFarlane, 1995; Shalev, 1996) has challenged these assumptions, and thereby the ability of mental process-ing alone to bring about recovery. Yet, the

importance of the early response has not been denied. To the contrary, neurobiological theories (Post, 1992) and recent psychophysiological findings (Shalev et al., 2000) support the idea that the immediate aftermath of exposure is of critical significance. Memories of events may be consolidated during that time (Pitman, 1989). Elevated level of the stress hormone adrenaline contributes to consolidation of aversive learning (McGaugh et al., 1984; Cahil et al., 1994). Abnormally low levels of the stress hormone cortisol may further enhance the effect of noradrenaline on memory consolidation (Bohus, 1984; Yehuda et al., 1993). Information provided during the period that follows exposure may irreversibly affect the content of long-term memory (Loftus, 1979). These considerations converge into assuming that distress during the immediate aftermath of traumatization is indeed, pathogenic.

The accent, however, is on reducing psychic distress and physiological arousal, as means of preventing further pathology. Experiments have shown, in fact, that elementary fear responses can be acquired and maintained, in midbrain structures of the central nervous systeem, on the basis of poorly elaborated and certainly non-verbal signals (see e.g. Armony & LeDoux, 1997). If such is the case with trauma-related learning, then interventions would be beneficial to the degree that they reduce perceived adversity and the associated arousal. Importantly, a reduction of distress is a target for treatment, and not a specific technique, such that any intervention that would reduce arousal may be appropriate.

Complexity of traumatic events and individual responses

Distress during extreme events has been so well documented in literature and poetry (e.g. Manning, 1990/1930: Sasoon, 1963/1930) that a professional re-take can only reduce the direct truthfulness of such testimony:

Discussing exposure to death it is suggested

that it is infinitely more horrible and revolting to see a man shattered and eviscerated than to see him shot . . . 'and one sees such things; and one suffers vicariously, with the inalienable sympathy of man for man'. . . . 'One forgets, but he will remember again later, if only in his sleep' . . . the unburied dead festering, fly blown corruption, the pasture of rats . . . (Manning, 1990/1930, p. 11)

Yet the clarity of narratives seems to be lost when one comes to empirically define and measure human trauma. Inconsistencies between definitions of a 'trau-matic event' in successive versions of the American Psychiatric Association's *Diagnostic and Statistical Manuals* can illustrate this point: Traumatic stressors were originally defined as extreme and outstanding (American Psychiatric Association, 1980). Such apprai-sal has been eroded since (e.g. Breslau & Davis, 1987; Breslau et al., 1991), and the current appraisal of trau-matic events (American Psychiatric Association, 1994) is overinclusive to the point of seemingly embracing anything from childbirth (e.g. Wijma et al., 1997) to having endured the Nazi Holocaust. The current prop-osition includes, in addition, a mandatory dimension of response to the stressor, such that an event is now formally traumatic only for those individuals in whom it immediately provokes fear or horror.

Clinical reality, however, shows that some individ-uals who later become very sick, do not present with strong emotional responses during the few days that follow exposure (e.g. Shalev et al., 1993). Even those who 'break down' (e.g. soldiers in combat) show 'poly-morphous and labile' symptoms, including agitation, depression, numbing, or irritability (e.g. Solomon, 1993): 'a passing parade of every type of psychological and psychosomatic symptom' (Grinker & Spiegel, 1945).

How can one make sense of this array? Possibly by realizing that despite yielding more reliable observa-tions, the reality of events and the observable behav-iour that follows may be less important than the under-lying psychological dimensions. Defined that way, an event carries higher risk for traumatic responses when, for the individual involved, it is (a) unexpected (b) unacceptable, (c) intense, (d) uncontrollable and (e) inescapable (Foa et al., 1992; Bolstad & Zinbarg, 1997). Experimental literature shows, in fact, that the degree of control and the possibility of escape during stress modulate the expression of stress hormones in the brain (e.g. Voigt et al., 1990). In other words, while data pertaining to entire groups show statistical corre-lation between the intensity of the early response and subsequent PTSD, at an individual level the data have rather low specificity: most survivors who express early symptoms are likely to recover normally (see e.g. McFarlane, 1988; Shalev et al., 1997). Indeed, more recent studies (e.g. Ehlers & Steil, 1995) suggest that the way in which such symptoms are appraised by the individual determines their long-term outcome. An-other predictive factor that may not translate to overt behaviour is the amount of concrete and symbolic losses related to the traumatic experience (Hobfol, 1989).

It ensues that, within individuals exposed to poten-tially traumatic events, some may have extremely bad experiences and others may not. For example, a female survivor of a terrorist incident, in which a bus over-turned down a steep valley on its way to Jerusalem (Shalev et al., 1993), expressed an increased sense of self-confidence, stating that under the worst of circum-stances she acted with unexpected self-composure and effectiveness. She was the daughter of a Holocaust sur-vivor. In contrast, a younger male survivor of the same incident experienced piercing guilt for not having stopped the action, expressed as intrusive nightmares and daydreams. He had broken his hip during the inci-dent and therefore could not rescue himself nor other-wise modulate the effect of the stressor.

While clearly reflecting differences in sense of con-trol and self-efficacy, the overt behaviour of these two survivors may also be misleading. We could assume, for example, that the ecstatic lady described above was merely counter-reacting to a previously acquired sense of great vulnerability, and that the valiant young man was, in fact, starting to process new knowledge about his physical and psychological boundaries. Should a debriefing officer intervene and (a) throw the lady back to her catastrophic self-image (e.g. by having her share the dreadfulness of other people's experiences) and (b) cut short the youngster's appropriate processing of the event (by challenging a budding insight)? For those who conduct debriefing the presence of such complexity is a major problem.

Symptoms may, in addition, have different functions at different stages. In an earlier study (Shalev et al., 1996) we described a significant link between experiencing dissociation, during the traumatic event and subsequent PTSD. Dissociative experience predicted PTSD above and beyond the severity of events and the early responses. Data have been collected on an individual basis, one week following trauma.

We revisited the construct of peritraumatic dissociation, using the same rating scale (Marmar et al., 1994), in a debriefing study (Shalev et al., 2000), where data were collected two days after combat exposure, in groups of infantry soldiers of the Israel Defence Forces (IDF; see below). Not surprisingly, higher levels of dissociation were observed in soldiers with more intense combat exposure. Yet, dissociative symptoms significantly correlated with better evaluation of the group's and of individuals performance during combat. Hence, two days after exposure, i.e. exactly when most debriefing interventions are to take place, dissociation seemed to be associated with better appraisal. A recent study of rape victims similarly found that dissociation was associated with reduced physiological responses to reminders of the trauma (Griffin et al., 1997). Should debriefing challenge dissociative and distancing defences?

Heroic appraisal of acts and events may similarly be protective to some individuals, providing a sense of purpose and a symbolic way to transcend the direct experience of horror and disgust. One day after being severely injured, a recent immigrant to Israel, who had survived a terrorist act, said 'Now I have become part of this country's history.' Certainly, such 'defences' may later collapse, yet while they last they may be protecting the individual from extreme, uncontrollable emotions.

Such is also the case of early numbing, which the individual may productively maintain until better opportunities for feeling occur. It has been a common experience, amongst front-line soldiers, during the 1973 Yom-Kippur War, to be at home for 24 hours leave, yet experience numbing and distancing from previously loved activities. 'I sit in a lawn chair, by the University swimming pool, as I always loved to do', commented a student on leave, 'yet nothing is the same. I wonder what am I doing here, what are other people doing? I am there, but not truly so.' Psychiatrists who were attached to combat units used to warn soldiers who were going home that they may not be able to 'ease their defences' (i.e. could expect problems in experiencing emotions, particularly intimacy), yet that such symptoms were not unusual and did not reflect a mental problem (S. Tyano, personal communication). In challenging the heroic meaning of facts and events, and in deliberately seeking emotions, can debriefing inappropriately disturb the protective shield of those who are still numb or dissociated?

Importantly, traumatic events do not end upon termination of the impact phase (Raphael, 1986). Most such events continue, in fact, beyond the actual presence of a threat. Intractable pain may follow physical injury (Schreiber & Galai Gat, 1993). Losses may become fully apparent upon recovery. Humiliating impregnation may follow ethnically motivated rape (see e.g. Kozaric-Kovacic et al., 1995). Unexpected hostile homecoming may shatter painfully achieved self-control and resilience (Lifton, 1973). Debriefing would often occur during a period of ongoing traumatization, where further adversity is expected or actually occurring. 'Therapeutic flexibility' has been wisely recommended for interventions conducted at the early stages of the response to trauma (Rosser & Dewar, 1991).

Coping, crisis and loneliness

After trauma, some individuals may find themselves in a situation of crisis; that is, in a state where their coping resources are overtaxed and dysfunctional. Effective coping has been defined as (a) reducing distress, (b) enabling continuation of task-oriented activity, (c) preventing negative self-perception, and (d) enabling maintainance of rewarding interpersonal contacts (Pearlin & Schooler, 1978). Defective coping, therefore, would lead to disabling distress, negative self-perception and inability to enjoy rewarding interpersonal contacts. The importance of the last of these cannot be overestimated: in many traumatized patients the first overwhelming experience is one of total loneliness and isolation (see e.g. Dasberg, 1976). Again the older literature portrays the essence of belonging, as during the murderous Battle of the Somme, 1916 (Manning 1990/1930, Introduction, p. xii):

They had been brought to the last extremity of hope [and yet showed] a passionate conviction that it would be all right, though they had faith in nothing, but in themselves and in each other.

or

These apparently rude and brutal natures comforted, encouraged and reconciled each other to fate, with a tenderness and tact which was more moving than anything in life.

Feeling detached and isolated within such groups deprives an individual of the essential support of his or her peers. Not being 'emotionally tuned' in a group, may be one expression of such isolation. In a recent study of debriefing (Shalev et al., 1998), we assessed levels of anxiety and self-efficacy in 39 infantry soldiers, shortly after combat, and found them unequally distributed, with few individuals expressing outstanding levels of distress and detachment from all the others. Figure 1.1 presents the frequency distribution of state-anxiety scores before and after debriefing. As can be seen, the group is much more homogeneous following debriefing, as those who had had the highest scores previously became closer to most others.

Prematurely 'closing' the story

Isolation may also lead to premature closure of one's own incomplete and idiosyncratic narrative of a traumatic event, in which case those with more catastrophic views lose the opportunity to correct such views by listening to others. The following account is drawn from a session of debriefing, conducted a few days after combat exposure.

Company A. walked straight into an enemy ambush, at night, on a rocky hill where nothing was expected to happen. It all began at once: small weapons fire at very close range. The commanding officer and the radio operator were hit immediately. Another officer must have run forward and was also killed. In the darkness no one knew exactly what was going on. Fire seemed to come from all directions. Hand grenades were thrown, and soldiers who heard them coming warned their buddies. A sergeant took command. He thought that he had identified a source of fire and instructed the machine gunner to climb on a heavy boulder and fire back. The man was hit as soon as he reached a firing position. His body rolled down, his weapon remaining on the boulder. Other men started returning fire and throwing hand grenades. One managed to operate the radio. Then everything was silent again. The enemy seemed to have vanished.

While the fire was still going on, the medic ran forward to treat the wounded. In the dark he found the second officer, lying on the ground, and manually checked his body for wounds. His hands found two large bleeding holes in the officer's back. The officer was dead. The medic then left him and turned to treat the commanding officer, who was lying next to him. Unable to do more without light, he put a bandage over the commander's open abdominal wound and kept conversing and reassuring him. They must have communicated that way for several minutes – the medic will never be able to give an accurate estimate of time elapsed. When, at last, he could safely use a torch he then tried to insert an i.v. line but it was already too late: all veins had collapsed. A field surgeon, who arrived with a rescue team, attempted to surgically find a deeper vein, but the man died in their hands.

The company promptly left the area. According to military routine, they counted the remaining ammunition and underwent a series of fact-finding debriefings. The main witnesses, however, were in the hospital, hence many questions remained

State Anxiety Scores Before Debriefing

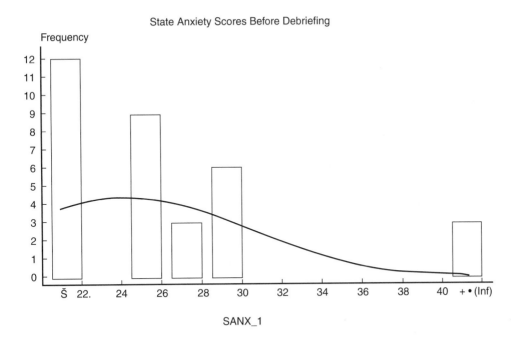

SANX_1

State Anxiety Scores After Debriefing

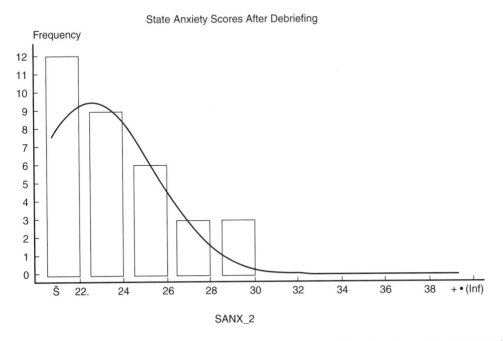

SANX_2

Figure 1.1. Frequency distribution of state anxiety scores before and after debriefing. (From Shalev et al., 1998, Copyright *Military Medicine*, International Journal of AMSUS.)

unanswered. No one could tell how the shooting started or where it had come from. Information about the commanding officer's injury came in later: an autopsy revealed a liver injury, which caused slow but fatal bleeding. These facts, however, did not reach the medic until quite late, leaving him with a piercing sense of incompetence and guilt. Another company searched the battlefield the next morning. They found the body of an enemy. Their grasp of the topography of the hill, however, was very different from the impression of the company's soldiers during the fight. The two versions never matched completely. Consequently, most men were left with uncertainty about actions and errors, which they could neither confirm nor dispel.

Visits to families of the killed-in-action are customary, and most survivors went to see the bereaved parents, where each of them was asked, repeatedly, to describe the action. By the third day after the incident, therefore, many had a 'definitive' version of the event, shaped by telling of the story again and again. Group debriefing revealed, however, that the individual versions differed. One soldier, for example, believed that both officers were killed by one bullet coming from an 0.5 in. machine gun. Others, however, considered this to be totally impossible. The medic remembered that the company commander died within 20 minutes of his injury, whereas the field surgeon's estimate was 45 minutes.

Comparison between versions became a very stressful experience. Five days after the incident the wounded radio operator was released from the hospital. He seemed to clearly remember that they had heard a word spoken in Arabic, that the commander subsequently shouted 'enemy ahead – open fire' and fired his M-16. This thoroughly contradicted what everyone had believed to be true until then – namely that the first shot to be fired was from the enemy. As the radio operator was relating his story a member of the group angrily left the room, saying that he couldn't listen to nonsense any longer. His own version seems to have been made and reshuffling the cards was too

upsetting. Interviewed at this point, some soldiers indicated that they were having nightmares and were suffering from increased alarm reaction. Others were reconstructing, again and again, their own recollections, trying to make sense of memory gaps and to reconcile paradoxical information.

This vignette illustrates how partial and incomplete pictures of an event settle and become the 'true' memory for each individual. It also shows how both strength (participating in families' grief) and weaknesses (loneliness) coexist at this stage. Such may be the case of many survivors: a mixture of effective and ineffective coping; a volatile combination of attempts to self-regulate and establish autonomy along with the desire to belong and to be taken care of. Importantly, joining the group does not provide a warranty for positive long-term outcome, as groups may be re-exposed, or may further 'catastrophize' the event. Indeed, once a group has defined itself as traumatized then belonging to it may lead (or may depend) on individually adopting the identity of a victim. Cohesion, therefore, is nondirectional, and may either reduce or enhance the expression of psychopathology.

A parsimonious approach to debriefing: cognitive reconstruction of events

In the above it has been argued the inherent complexity of traumatic events and their aftermath creates major constraints to productively practising debriefing. The appropriateness of theory-driven group interventions, at a stage at which individual responses are so diverse, has also been questioned. Specifically, some of the psychological ingredients of such interventions, such as disclosing emotions, 'psychologizing' the meaning of events and addressing some frequent responses as being 'symptoms', may not be productive. Indeed, the extent to which the latter are necessary is unclear: more parsimonious techniques may, in fact, be as effective.

Hence, when in 1991, our group initiated a study of debriefing in combat soldiers on the Lebanon border of Israel, we sought an alternative that would leave enough degrees of freedom to participants, not impose an alien (i.e. psychological) discourse on situations that are otherwise perceived as martial and operational, and yet have the group review the event and build a common narrative. We borrowed the model from S. L. A. Marshall's historical group debriefing (Marshall, 1944, 1947; Spiller 1980, 1988; Shalev, 1994). Marshall's technique consists of a systematic review of the event, by all the participants, without advice, interpretation or deliberate intervention. The effect of detailed cognitive reconstruction could, therefore, be studied, as such.

Historical group debriefing (HGD) would combine aspects of institutional fact-finding debriefing with psychological understanding of human performance under stress. Institutional, fact-finding debriefing is regularly practised, by numerous institutions, for purposes of gathering information and learning. Apparently instrumental, such team meetings may have a tremendous psychological impact, as they convey a formal meaning to events and deeds, and turn often mild preliminary appraisal into a stable meaning proposition (e.g. success, breakthrough, failure, cowardice). Fact-finding debriefing, in the IDF, is practised by military professionals – often by the group's natural leaders. Importantly, the focus is mostly operational, such that only facts that are relevant to learning expedient lessons are explored.

HGD was developed, during World War II, by the chief historian for the US army, Brigadier General Samuel Lyman Atwood Marshall. Its primary goal was to gather historical data, yet the technique was said also to have had profound psychological effects on participants (Marshall, 1947). As is often the case, the practice of HGD had a theory behind it. Surprisingly, Marshall's theory of ground combat was psychological as much as tactical. It assigned equal value to mental and physical elements, and articulated individual responses with elements of group psychology.

Marshall theorized that the battlefield presents the soldier with scant and ambiguous information. Enemy positions and allied forces are under cover. Sources of threat (e.g. artillery, weapon positions, mines) are camouflaged or hidden. The soldier's capacity to 'overcome his fears' depends, therefore, on his ability to 'feel the presence of others' and maintain a sense of belonging to a group. Individuals in combat, accordingly, can

function effectively only as members of a group. Conversely, the group can function only as long as its individual members maintain a sense of belonging. The forces underlying such mutual dependence were assumed to be both emotional and cognitive, paralysing fear being the direct consequence of 'fragmentation of the information' within the group.

Marshall seems to have grasped another attribute of distressed cognition, namely the individual's inability to identify and make sense of the overall pattern of a stressful event. He assumed, therefore, that no participant had the 'full story'. Consequently, he sought to obtain the 'historical truth' of combat by gathering a group narrative. Moreover, he seems to have trusted the testimony of commanding officers no more than that of privates, both being individual witnesses. He therefore did away with group hierarchy, at least for the duration of an interview: 'The word of a superior as to what a man (or a group) did should not be allowed to prevail against the direct testimony of the man himself' (Marshall, 1944, p. 204).

Marshall's debriefing sessions lasted several hours. They took place soon after combat. All members of the fighting group were invited to participate and 'describe the combat with all the possible details' in a 'strict chronological path'. All available testimonies were collected for each stage. Soldiers' thoughts and feelings were of particular interest as 'the moral side of war' was considered to be as important as its 'purely physical side' (Marshall, 1944, p. 210). Finally, the interviewer was to pay 'warm interest and respectful attention' to the unfolding narrative as 'He cannot obtain the interest of the company and its complete participation unless he conducts himself as a student rather than as a teacher.' The expression of emotions, such as that towards deceased buddies, received 'respectful attention' but no advice or interpretation was offered.

Conducting debriefing in this way, Marshall found that the sessions often became, for the participants, a 'morale building experience' and a 'spiritual purge' (Marshall, 1944, p. 215). Indeed, the technical elements of HGD are designed to allow each participant to disclose his or her own version and compare it with those of others. There are no conclusions, no lessons, and none of the versions is considered as 'true' or 'final'.

Indeed, the coexistence of many views is being validated.

The intervention conducted by us on the Lebanon front implemented Marshall's technical principles of exhaustive chronological review, temporary suspension of military ranks, tolerance of ambiguous information, and equal interest in cognition, emotion and action. No other intervention was included: the sessions started by describing the immediate preparation to combat and ended when the event was fully described. All the participants signed an informed consent, and were free to abstain or to leave the sessions at any moment. Their identities remained confidential. All those whom we asked to participate agreed to do so, but two left the sessions before the end. Thirty-nine individuals completed the study. All had participated in short engagements, in which their group took casualties (from one injured in action to several killed in action). The average age of the group was 19.4 years (range 18.5 to 24 years). The average length of the session was 2.5 hours. Ratings of symptoms of anxiety (Speilberger et al., 1970), intrusive thoughts and avoidance (Horowitz et al., 1979), peritraumatic dissociation (Marmar et al., 1994), combat exposure (Lund et al., 1987), self-efficacy (Bandura, 1982) and combat evaluation were collected before and immediately after the session.

The intensity of symptoms of intrusion and avoidance before debriefing resembles those previously observed in civilian trauma survivors (Shalev et al., 1996) and reflects an intense preoccupation with the event. Changes in the distribution of anxiety scores were presented above (Figure 1.1). Avoidance scores correlated positively with anxiety, and, as stated above, dissociation scores correlated positively with combat evaluation. Importantly, the sessions were followed by statistically significant reduction in anxiety and increase in self-efficacy (Shalev et al., 1998). These results confirmed, therefore, the assumption that the simple fact of reviewing the event by the group (a) can significantly reduce distress and (b) increases the homogeneity of the group.

Summary and conclusion

The main arguments against considering the long-term effect of debriefing as a valid measure of the efficacy of this technique relates to the complex aetiology of stress disorders and the relatively small proportion of the total causation that any brief psychological intervention is likely to affect. It is historically true that the role of psychological factors, operating during the immediate aftermath of traumatization has been perceived as cardinal in the development of subsequent stress disorders. Yet more recent information suggests that reducing arousal, shortly after exposure, may be as important as clarifying and working through the meaning of exposure. Accordingly, the traumatizing elements of the immediate post-event period, such as controllability, self-regulation, intensity of emotions, as well as loneliness and detachment from others, are to be the first concern of those practising debriefing, indeed of any person involved in early treatment of potentially traumatized individuals. Preliminary data are reported, suggesting that distress is unequally distributed amongst survivors. These data imply that those with higher levels of distress are more likely to feel, and be perceived as, different from the others. Finally, a study of debriefing in military units has been presented in support of the argument that simple reconstruction of a group narrative is sufficient to effectively reduce anxiety in recently exposed combat soldiers.

All the above may point to new directions in administering debriefing and measuring its effect. These may include an evaluation of short-term effect of debriefing and isolation of specific components of the technique and detailed study of each. Most importantly, it has been argued that the short-term success of any technique is not sufficient to assure its long-term effect. Debriefing, therefore, should be one of many measures made available to survivors whose health one wishes to protect.

Acknowledgements

This work was supported by a US Public Health Service Research grant MH-50379. My thanks are due to members of the Centre for Traumatic Stress, Tuvia Peri,

Dalia Brandes and Rivka Tuval for thoughtful comments, and to Ms Debra Erez for editorial assistance.

REFERENCES

American Psychiatric Association (1980). *Diagnostic and Statistical Manual of Mental Disorders*, 3rd edn. Washington, DC: American Psychiatric Press.

American Psychiatric Association (1994). *Diagnostic and Statistical Manual of Mental Disorders*, 4th edn. Washington, DC: American Psychiatric Press.

Armony, J. L. & LeDoux, J. E. (1997). How the brain processes emotional information. *Annals of the New York Academy of Sciences*, **821**, 259–70.

Bandura, A. (1982). Self-efficacy mechanisms in human agencies. *American Psychologist*, **37**, 122–47.

Bisson, J. I. & Deahl, M. P. (1994). Psychological debriefing and prevention of post-traumatic stress – more research is needed. *British Journal of Psychiatry*, **165**, 717–20.

Bohus B. (1984). Humoral modulation of learning and memory processes: physiological significance of brain and peripheral mechanisms. In A. Delacour (Ed.) *The Memory System of the Brain, Advances in Neuroscience* (pp. 337–64). Singapore: World Scientific.

Bolstad, B. R. & Zinbarg, R. E. (1997). Sexual victimisation, generalised perception of control, and post-traumatic stress disorder symptom severity. *Journal of Anxiety Disorders*, **11**, 523–40.

Bourne, P. G. (1973). Foreword. In C. R. Figley (Ed.) *Stress Disorders among Vietnam Veterans* (pp. vii–ix). New York: Brunner/Mazel.

Bourne, P. G. (1978). Military psychiatry and the Vietnam war in perspective. In P. G. Bourne (Ed.) *The Psychology and Physiology of Stress* (pp. 219–36). New York: Academic Press.

Breslau, N. & Davis, G. C. (1987). Posttraumatic stress disorder. The stressor criterion. *Journal of Nervous and Mental Diseases*, **175**, 255–64.

Breslau, N., Davis, G. C., Andreski, P. & Peterson, E. (1991). Traumatic events and posttraumatic stress disorder in an urban population of young adults. *Archives of General Psychiatry*, **48**, 216–22.

Cahill, L., Prins, B., Weber, M. & McGaugh, J. L. (1994). Beta-adrenergic activation and memory for emotional events. *Nature*, **371**, 702–4.

Camp, N. M. (1993). The Vietnam War and the ethics of combat psychiatry. *American Journal of Psychiatry*, **150**, 1000–10.

Dasberg, H. (1976). Belonging and loneliness in relation to mental breakdown in battle. *Israeli Annals of Psychiatry and Related Disciplines*, **14**, 307–21.

Deahl, M. P., Gillham, A. B., Thomas, J., Searle, M. M. & Srinivasan, M. (1994). Psychological sequelae following the Gulf War: factors associated with subsequent morbidity and the effectiveness of psychological debriefing. *British Journal of Psychiatry*, **165**, 60–5.

Ehlers, A. & Steil, R. (1995). Maintenance of intrusive memories in posttraumatic stress disorder: a cognitive approach. *Behavioural and Cognitive Psychotherapy*, **23**, 217–49.

Foa, E. B., Zinbarg, R. & Rothbaum, B. O. (1992). Uncontrollability and unpredictability in post-traumatic stress disorder: an animal model. *Psychology Bulletin*, **112**, 218–38.

Freud, S. (1957/1917). Mourning and melancholia. *The Complete Psychological Works of Sigmund Freud*, standard edn, vol. XIV. London: Hogarth Press.

Griffin, M. G., Resick, P. A. & Mechanic, M. B. (1997). Objective assessment of peri-traumatic dissociation: psychophysiological indicators. *American Journal of Psychiatry*, **154**, 1081–8.

Grinker, R. R. & Spiegel, J. P. (1945). The neurotic reactions to severe combat stress. In *Men under Stress*, (pp. 82–4). Philadelphia: Blackiston.

Hobfoll, S. E. (1989). Conservation of resources. A new attempt at conceptualizing stress. *American Psychologist*, **44**, 513–24.

Horowitz, M. J. (1974). Stress response syndromes: character style and dynamic psychotherapy. *Archives of General Psychiatry*, **31**, 768–81.

Horowitz, M. J., Wilner, N. & Alvarez, W. (1979). Impact of event scale: a measure of subjective stress. *Psychosomatic Medicine*, **41**, 209–18.

Johnson, D. R., Rosenheck, R., Fontana, A., Lubin, H., Charney, D. & Southwick, S. (1996). Outcome of intensive inpatient treatment for combat related posttraumatic stress disorder. *American Journal of Psychiatry*, **153**, 771–5.

Kenardy, J. A., Webster, R. A., Lewin, T. J., Carr, V. J., Hazell, P. L. & Carter, G. L. (1996). Stress debriefing and patterns of recovery following a natural disaster. *Journal of Traumatic Stress*, **9**, 37–49.

Kozaric-Kovacic, D., Folnegovic-Smalc, V., Skrinjaric, J., Szajnberg, N. M. & Marusic, A. (1995). Rape, torture, and traumatization of Bosnian and Croatian women: psychological sequelae. *American Journal of Orthopsychiatry*, **65**, 428–33.

Kulka, R. A., Schlenger, W. E., Fairbank, J. A., Hough, R. L., Jordan, B. K., Marmar, C. R. & Weiss, D. S. (1990). *Trauma and the Vietnam War Generation: Report of Findings from the National Vietnam Veterans Readjustment Study*. New York: Brunner/Mazel.

Lifton, R. J. (1973). Home From the War. New York: Basic Books.

Lindemann, E. (1944). Symptomatology and management of acute grief. *American Journal of* Psychiatry, **101**, 141–8.

Loftus, E. F. (1979). *Eyewitness Testimony*. Cambridge, MA: Harvard University Press.

Lund, M., Foy, D., Sipprelle, C. & Strachan, A. (1987). The combat exposure scale: a systematic assessment of trauma in the Vietnam war. *Journal of Clinical Psychology*, **40**, 1323–8.

Manning, F. (1990). *The Middle Part of Fortune*. London: Penguin Books. (Orginally published 1930.)

Marmar, C. R., Weiss, D. S., Schlenger, W. E., Fairbank, J. A., Jordan, K., Kulka, R. A. & Hough, R. L. (1994). Peri-traumatic dissociation and post-traumatic stress in male vietnam theatre veterans. *American Journal of Psychiatry*, **151**, 902–7.

Marshall, S. L. A. (1944). *Island Victory*. New York: Penguin Books.

Marshall, S. L. A. (1947). *Men under Fire: The Problem of Battle Command in Future War*. New York: William Morrow.

McFarlane, A. (1988) The longitudinal course of posttraumatic morbidity: the range of outcomes and their predictors. *Journal of Nervous and Mental Diseases*, **176**, 30–9.

McGaugh, J. L., Liang, K. C., Bennet, C. & Sternberg, D. B. (1984). Adrenergic influence on memory storage: interaction of peripheral and central systems. In G. Lynch, J. L. McGaugh, & N. M. Weinberger (Eds.) *Neurobiology of Learning and Memory* (pp. 313–32). New York: Guilford Press.

Pearlin, L. I. & Schooler, C. (1978). The structure of coping. *Journal of Health and Social Behavior*, **22**, 337–56.

Pennebaker, J. W. & Susman J. R. (1988). Disclosure of trauma and psychosomatic processes. *Social Science and Medicine*, **26**, 327–32.

Pitman, R. K. (1989). Post-traumatic stress disorder, hormones, and memory. *Biological Psychiatry*, **26**, 221–3.

Post, R. M. (1992). Transudation of psychosocial stress into the neurobiology of recurrent affective disorder. *American Journal of Psychiatry*, **149**, 999–1010.

Raphael, B. (1986). *When Disaster Strikes: How Individuals and Communities Cope with Catastrophe*. New York: Basic Books.

Raphael, B., Meldrum, L. & McFarlane, A. C. (1995). Does debriefing after psychological trauma work? *British Medical Journal*, **310**, 1479–80.

Robinson, H. M., Sigman, M. R. & Wilson, J. P. (1997). Duty-related stressors and PTSD symptoms in suburban police officers. *Psychological Report*, **81**, 835–45.

Rosser, R. & Dewar, S. (1991). Therapeutic flexibility in the post disaster response [editorial]. *Journal of the Royal Society of Medicine*, **84**, 2–3.

Sassoon, S. (1963). *Memoire of an Infantry Officer*. London:

Faber and Faber. (Originally published 1930.)

Schreiber, S. & Galai Gat, T. (1993). Uncontrolled pain following physical injury as the core-trauma in post-traumatic stress disorder. *Pain*, **54**, 107–10.

Shalev, A. Y. (1994). Debriefing Following Exposure to Trauma. In R. J. Ursano, B. G. McLaughey & C. S. Fullerton (Eds.) *Individual and Community Responses to Trauma and Disaster* (pp. 201–19). Cambridge: Cambridge University Press.

Shalev, A. Y. (1996). Stress versus traumatic stress: from acute homeostatic reaction to chronic psychopathology. In B. A. van der Kolk, A. C. McFarlane & L. Weisæth (Eds). *Traumatic Stress. The Effects of Overwhelming Life Experiences on Mind Body and Society* (pp. 77–101). New York: Guilford Press.

Shalev, A. (1997a). Treatment of prolonged posttraumatic stress disorder – learning from experience. *Journal of Traumatic Stress*, **10**, 415–23.

Shalev, A. Y. (1997b). Treatment failure in acute PTSD: lessons learned about the complex neurobiology of the disorder. *Annals of the New York Academy of Sciences*, **821**, 372–87.

Shalev, A. Y, Schreiber, S. & Galai, T. (1993). Early psychiatric responses to traumatic injury. *Journal of Traumatic Stress*, **6**, 441–50.

Shalev, A. Y., Peri, T., Canetti, L. & Schreiber, S. (1996). Predictors of PTSD in injured trauma survivors: a prospective study. *American Journal of Psychiatry*, **153**, 219–25.

Shalev, A. Y., Freedman, S., Brandes, D., Peri, T. & Sahar, T. (1997). Predicting PTSD in civilian trauma survivors: prospective evaluation of self-report and clinician administered instruments. *British Journal of Psychiatry*, **170**, 558–64.

Shalev, A. Y., Peri, T. & Rogel-Fuchs, Y. (1998). Historical group debriefing after combat exposure. *Military Medicine*, **163**, 494–8.

Shalev, A. Y., Pitman, R. K., Orr, S. P., Peri, T. & Brandes, D. (2000). Prospective study of responses to loud tones in trauma survivors with PTSD. *American Journal of Psychiatry*, **157**, 255–61.

Solomon, Z. (1993). *Combat Stress Reaction*. New York: Plenum Press.

Solomon, Z., Shalev, A., Spiro, S., Dolev, A., Bleich, A., Waysman, M. & Cooper S. (1992). The effectiveness of the Koach Project: negative psychometric outcome. *Journal of Traumatic Stress*, **5**, 247–64.

Solomon, Z., Laor, N., Weiler, D., Muller, U. F., Hadar, O., Waysman, M. et al. (1993). The psychological impact of the Gulf War: a study of acute stress in Israeli evacuees [letter]. *Archives of General Psychiatry*, **50**, 320–1.

Speilberger, C. D., Gorsuch, R. L. & Lushen, R. E. (1970). *Manual for State Trait Inventory*. Palo Alto, CA: Consulting Psychological Press.

Spiller, R. J. (1980). *S. L. A Marshall at Fort Leavenworth 1952–1962*. Fort Leavenworth, KS: The Combined Arms Center.

Spiller, R. J. (1988). S. L. A. Marshall and the ratio of fire. *Royal United Service Institute for Defence Studies Journal*, **133**, 63–71.

Voigt, K., Ziegler, M., Grunert-Fuchs, M., Bickel, U. & Fehm-Wolfsdorf, G. (1990). Hormonal responses to exhausting physical exercise: the role of predictability and controllability of the situation. *Psycho-neuroendocrinology*, **15**, 173–84.

Wijma, K., Soderquist, J. & Wijma, B. (1997). Post-traumatic stress disorder after childbirth: a cross-sectional study. *Journal of Anxiety Disorders*, **11**, 587–97.

Witztum, E., Levy, A. & Solomon, Z. (1996). Lessons denied: a history of therapeutic response to combat stress reaction during Israel's War of Independence (1948), the Sinai Campaign (1956) and the Six Day War (1967). *Israeli Journal of Psychiatry and Related Sciences*, **33**, 79–88.

Yehuda, R. & McFarlane, A. C. (1995). Conflict between current knowledge about posttraumatic stress disorder and its original conceptual basis. *American Journal of Psychiatry*, **152**, 1705–13.

Yehuda, R., Southwick, S. M., Krystal, J. H., Bremner, D., Charney, D. S. & Mason, J. W. (1993). Enhanced suppression of cortisol following dexamethasone administration in posttraumatic stress disorder. *American Journal of Psychiatry*, **150**, 83–6.

2

Debriefing: its role in the spectrum of prevention and acute management of psychological trauma

Robert J. Ursano, Carol S. Fullerton, Kelley Vance and Lemming Wang

EDITORIAL COMMENTS

This chapter explores two important parameters relevant to debriefing: who attends debriefing when this is a voluntary procedure (as it usually is); and does 'natural debriefing' through 'talking' have a beneficial effect? The former concept is important, for if debriefing is to be useful it should reach those in greatest need. The groups' research found that those with greatest exposure, with past disaster experience, and with good social support were more likely to seek debriefing after disaster exposure, and women more so. Those who do not attend may be at risk through lack of support networks and because they have had potentially no 'mitigating' effect of prior experience.

In a separate study the authors examined 'natural talking' after a disaster and attempted to evaluate whether or not this made a difference. They found that high levels of talking response with social networks were associated with high exposure and high education and high post-traumatic stress disorder (PTSD) symptoms. However, at the follow-up assessment seven months after the disaster, there was no indication that this talking had led to a decrease in symptomatology and levels of PTSD and depressive symptoms, which were found to be related to high levels of exposure as assessed earlier.

Ursano and his group conclude that these findings indicate 'several cautions for the real-world application of formal debriefing'. These include the need to identify potential high-risk groups and that further studies are needed to explore the 'talk' aspect of debriefing in both formal and natural circumstances.

There appears to be little evidence that talk reduces the symptoms that may follow trauma, although it may affect other outcomes such as distress, disability, time lost from work, health care utilization and family and work performance. Thus they challenge the concept of 'talking' as a cure or prevention.

These studies have identified conceptual issues in the debriefing debate: issues that need to be subject to further critical analysis and research appraisal.

This chapter really emphasizes the core conceptual issues that must still be clarified in terms of 'debriefing interventions' and how here as elsewhere, intervention frameworks are often far behind and may bear little relationship to the developing research in the aetiology, phenomenology and course of post-traumatic morbidity.

Introduction

Disasters and traumatic events occur most often in the complex context of multiple stressors including life threat, loss, bereavement, injury and exposure to death and the dead. Together these produce the experience of terror (Holloway & Fullerton, 1994). Each type of stressor effects the individual's picture of his or her present life, future and even past, which is reconstructed from a new vantage point. In addition, the complex trauma of a disaster, a war or a rape – also effects the recovery environment – the world of family and friends, instrumental and emotional supports, as well as material resources. If there is no food to eat after the mud slide, no way to travel to work to earn money after the earthquake, or no fuel with which to stay warm in the winter of a war in one's country, then the interventions necessary to decrease emotional arousal, sadness, fear and physiological dysregulation are far more than interpersonal support of any kind. Similarly, the risk of coccidiomycosis after an earthquake in the western USA (Ursano, 1997), the injuries that accompany an aeroplane crash, immune system alterations due to changes in sleep or eating habits or changes in risk-taking behaviours resulting in accidents after exposure to of war (Bullman & Kang, 1994; Kang & Bullman, 1996) can be the outcomes of most concern to both the psychological and physical health of trauma victims.

Debriefing: a piece of the trauma pie

Because of the complex interaction of individual and environment the treatment of disaster victims is multifaceted and must include community interventions, resource management, medical care, community restoration as well as individual-, group- and family-focussed interventions. Psychiatric interventions following trauma or disaster are based on the principles of preventive medicine and include organizational and community consultation and outreach programmes with the goals of identifying high-risk groups, promoting recovery and minimizing performance breakdown and group disruption (Ursano et al., 1996). In this network of assistance, debriefing has often been used by clinicians as an early intervention with groups exposed to traumatic events. The principles of debriefing are equally applicable to individuals and to families.

Debriefing is a systematic process of education, emotional expression, cognitive reorganization through the provision of information, fostering meaningful integration and group support through identifying shared common experience. Debriefing often makes use of naturally occurring groups. Historically, debriefing occurred on the battlefield, immediately after an event. S. L. A. Marshall, a name synonymous with the early roots of debriefing (for a review, see Shalev, 1994; see also Chapter 1, this volume), structured debriefing sessions to gain accurate historical facts about the experiences of soldiers in combat units.

This method was thought to have a beneficial effect on the participants and, in particular, to facilitate rapid return to duty. Debriefing makes use of the group's natural resources as suggested by the wartime notion of buddy support, i.e. support from peers is important to individual recovery following trauma.

The structure and type of modern debriefing is multidetermined by, for example, goals, group leadership and training, the type and severity of trauma, leadership and organizational support, the structure of the group, who attends and degree of participation in the group. In general, debriefing is based on the hypothesis that the cognitive structure of the event is modified through retelling and by experiencing an emotional release that prevents or reduces the risk of more serious stress reactions. Sharing and education of those experiencing a common trauma (Raphael, 1986), informing participants of the reactions of others (Dunning, 1990), and promoting ventilation of feelings through expression of emotions and the response of others (Dunning, 1990) are all proposed goals of debriefing. In addition, enhancing group cohesion and the general mobilization of social support have been described as important outcomes (Shalev, 1994).

The science of debriefing: if it works, prove it

The rapid growth of debriefing appears to attest to its popularity. However, systematic evaluation of the acute and long-term effectiveness of debriefing is lacking (Raphael et al., 1995). Of those limited studies that have attempted to evaluate the effectiveness of debriefing, methodological and conceptual differences have made it difficult to generalize from one population to another; for example, variations in the format of debriefings, differences in organizational culture, varying symptomatology of the subjects, psychiatric comorbidity, and multiple types of stress exposure have made evaluation of the effectiveness of these interventions challenging. One of the most detailed follow-up studies is that of Kenardy et al. (1996). This study reported that those who were not debriefed showed a more rapid reduction of their General Health Questionnaire scores over time. Examination of the characteristics of the subjects in this study suggest that personality, sensitivity and neuroticism may increase reactivity following the trauma with debriefing (Kenardy et al., 1996). In contrast, Chemtob et al. (1997) showed positive effects of debriefings given six months after Hurricane Iniki.

Dyregrov & Mitchell (1992) studied 101 individuals from five different groups (emergency room personnel, firemen, police, university personnel, and trauma workshop participants), to assess their use of 11 coping mechanisms. They found that the strategy judged most important was maintaining contact with other helpers. On the basis of these findings the authors suggested that broad-based programmes with an emphasis on peer support should supplement other techniques (Dyregrov & Mitchell, 1992; Holaday et al., 1995). Social support is often gained through feedback from one's peers. Recent social theory suggests that anxiety may motivate people to affiliate in order to gain more information about the appropriateness of their thoughts and feelings aroused by a stressful situation. Schachter (1959) observed that his subjects preferred to share the company of persons facing the same stressful situation. This support process is thought to develop when peers have the opportunity to share their stressful experiences and highlights the stress-moderating impact of empathy, normalization, and validation (Schachter, 1959; Gottlieb, 1996). Other studies have shown that primary care health care givers tend to ignore both their own symptoms and their social supports (Shalev et al., 1993) and that greater structured support among mental health care professionals leads to better outcomes (Fullerton et al., 1992; Fullerton & Ursano, 1994).

The protective effects of peer support include the sense of control and personal efficacy that are gained from the reciprocal helping process. Pennebaker & O'Heeron (1984) and Silver & Wortman (1980) have observed the positive impact of emotional ventilation on mood states. Janoff-Bulman and colleagues found that support groups assist individuals to re-establish meaning when life crises have shattered their assumptions about the world (Silver & Wortman, 1980; Pennebaker & O'Heeron, 1984; Janoff-Bulman, 1992; Gottlieb, 1996). Coates & Winston's (1983) studies showed that emotional ventilation mitigated feelings of deviance and depression, producing a normalizing effect that would not be likely to have occurred through interactions with individuals who had not been subjected to the same stressful encounter (see also Gottlieb, 1996). In the broadest sense, the debriefing models that have evolved as interventions following a disaster can be thought of as formalized group support. The social and interpersonal nature of the group are intuitively the ideal environments for the repair of safety and trust as well as self-esteem and intimacy. (Allen & Bloom, 1994).

Formal debriefing versus natural debriefing

If formal debriefing has an effect, is it also reasonable to believe that 'natural debriefing' – the normally occurring interpersonal processes of talking to friends and significant others about the trauma, and hearing of the universality of the stress response from coworkers – should also facilitate recovery following trauma (see Figure 2.1). Fullerton & Ursano (1997) have shown that caregiving by spouses of disaster workers is common (and stressful). Community leaders in the provision of rest, respite, 'grief leadership' and the management of the meaning of traumatic events may also foster a safe and secure recovery environment. But who talks to whom and whether it is helpful is not known. In a study of dental workers at the disaster in Waco, Texas, McCarroll et al. (1996) showed that those with previous disaster experience were more likely to talk to their colleagues (as against spouses) about their experiences, while those without previous experience were more likely to talk to spouses or significant others (than to their colleagues). It seems reasonable therefore that, if debriefing as a formal intervention is to work, we should be able to show that talking to intimates about a disaster or traumatic event leads to reduced levels of post-traumatic symptoms.

In this chapter two questions are addressed: (1) 'Who attends formal debriefings?' and (2) 'What is the effect of the natural debriefing process (e.g. talking to friends, significant others and coworkers)?' Preliminary findings from two disaster studies are presented and the implications for training and further research on the natural debriefing process following trauma and disaster are discussed.

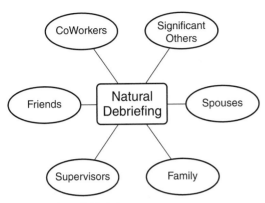

Figure 2.1. Natural debriefing.

Debriefing following disaster: who attends?

An important factor in planning disaster interventions is who attends debriefing – this is nearly always volunteer. Unfortunately, few empirical data are available in this area. Yet, for planning disaster interventions for large-scale populations as well as small, it is critical.

The Ramstein Air Force Base annual air show, Flugtag, was held on 28 August 1988. Approximately 300 000 attended, including Air Force members and families and civilians from the community. The atmosphere when the show began was festive, an annual event bringing Air Force families together. The much anticipated Flugtag ended in an atmosphere of horror, shock and chaos as three jets in the show collided in mid-air, burst into flames and fell on the watching families below. The first memory for many was of a huge fireball falling to earth. Burning debris from the crash was dispersed over a wide area, killing 70 members of the crowd and injuring more than 500 others. The extent of death and injury created pandemonium at the scene. Victims were lying on the ground everywhere. As the result of heroic efforts, all injured were evacuated within 90 minutes to area hospitals. Of the more than 500 injured, many sustained severe burns, facing a prolonged recovery period. In some instances, family members were unable to locate victims for several days because severity of the burns delayed body identification. After the disaster, several types of debriefing were offered on a voluntary basis including short debrief-

ings, Marshall-type debriefings and large-group debriefings/educational meetings.

A first cohort of medical care workers from two military bases, Ramstein AFB and Landstuhl Army Regional Medical Center ($n = 254$), were surveyed approximately 2 months after the Ramstein AFB disaster (October–November 1988, and again at approximately 6 months (March–April 1989), 12 months (September 1989), and 18 months (April 1990). Recruiting methods differed somewhat at the two locations. Workers at the health clinic dispensary at Ramstein AFB were contacted by post. At Landstuhl Army Hospital, a more comprehensive medical facility, health workers were contacted on a day when all were required to come for their influenza inoculations. Because of its importance as a military evacuation hospital, personnel at Landstuhl were more likely to have had previous experience with victims from other disasters than those at Ramstein. Follow-up surveys at 6, 12 and 18 months were distributed and returned by post. All subjects participating in the study were provided with a description of the study and responsibilities involved in participation, after which written informed consent was obtained. In this chapter, the focus is on findings from Time 1 (two months post disaster).

In order to understand better who chooses to attend debriefings, we examined the cohort of 254 medical care personnel who responded to the disaster and agreed to participate in our study. Thirty-five per cent of the subjects were at the air show at the time of the disaster. Nearly 40% of the subjects attended some type of debriefing, including four who were seen in brief mental health visits for debriefings; 60% had no debriefing. Nearly 74% had family or friends who were attending the air show at the time of the disaster. The majority of participants were male (64%), enlisted (68%), married (62%), Caucasian (76%), and had at least some college education (85%). Mean age was 32 years. Nearly 77% of this military medical group had some prior disaster experience.

Exposures to the Ramstein disaster were varied and multiple. Of the 254 participants, 53% reported directly treating disaster victims, 34% worked in the emergency room, 36% worked with child victims, 53% worked with burn victims, 27% had a disaster victim patient die, 37%

Table 2.1. Formal debriefing: who attends? Predictors from Ramstein air disaster

High disaster exposure	People with high levels of disaster exposure are 3.1 times more likely to attend a debriefing then those with low levels of exposure
Female gender	Females are 2.7 times more likely to attend a debriefing than males
Previous disaster experience	Those with previous disaster experience are 2.7 times more likely to attend a debriefing then those without prior disaster experience

talked to families of disaster victims and 12% had family or friends who were victims. For each individual their types of exposure were summed, creating an exposure scale that ranged from 0 to 6, with 29% scoring zero. Exposure scale scores were highly correlated with the number of victims treated. We created a high/low exposure scale with 60% showing 'low exposure' and 40% scoring 'high exposure' (i.e. three or more victims treated).

Those who attended a debriefing were significantly more likely to be female (54% female versus 31% male). However, there was no difference in age, education, race, marital status or rank between those who attended a debriefing and those who did not. Those who attended a debriefing also reported higher perceived social support from friends. Those with prior disaster experience were much more likely to attend a debriefing compared with those who did not have previous experience. Those who attended a debriefing were significantly more likely to be in the high exposure group, to have greater exposure scores and to have treated more victims.

In order to examine these variables in a multivariate manner, we used logistic regression and entered gender, prior disaster experience and exposure (high/low) simultaneously. Being female, having prior disaster experience, and having high exposure remained significant predictors of choosing to attend a debriefing, even with each adjusted for the other (see Table 2.1). Because we were also concerned that perhaps these predictors were confounded by the level of social support one expects from friends, we examine the data including 'perceived social support friends'. The findings were essentially unchanged.

On the positive side, this indicates that those with high exposure, a group at higher risk of psychiatric

illness, will gravitate to attend debriefings regardless of previous disaster experience and gender. The less exposed may feel that they are less in need of debriefing than those with high exposure, as evidenced by our finding that those with low exposure were less likely to attend a debriefing. On the negative side, it is important to note that this means that those without previous disaster experience, who in other studies have been shown to have greater symptom levels (McCarroll et al., 1996), are not seeking help. Interestingly, the data also indicate that those who see friends as good support (high-perceived social support friends) also tend to attend debriefings. Therefore, as in many psychosocial studies, those 'who have, get', e.g. those who already view friends/coworkers as support will seek debriefing. Perhaps this increases the probability of successful outcome to debriefing; however, so far there is no evidence for this. Outreach programmes to encourage individuals to attend debriefing should target those who do not usually see friends as supportive, males, those without prior disaster experience and those with lower levels of exposure.

Natural debriefing: the talking cure?

If debriefing works, it is reasonable to hypothesize that those who naturally talk more to intimates will also recover more quickly and show fewer symptoms than those who do not. In order to test this hypothesis we asked (1) 'Do disaster workers talk to intimates about the disaster?'; (2) 'If they do, who is likely to be talking and who is not?'; and (3) 'Is talking to intimates associated with lower symptoms and better outcome?' We conducted a preliminary investigation of the effects of talking on recovery from trauma in disaster workers after a mass casualty aeroplane crash.

Table 2.2. Natural debriefing: who talks? (Sioux City air disaster)

Demographics[a]	
Older	Older subjects are more likely than younger subjects to talk about the disaster with either spouse/significant other, coworker and/or another person
Higher education	People with a higher education level were more likely than those with a lower level of education to talk about the disaster with either spouse/significant other, coworker and/or another person
Married	Those who are married are more likely than nonmarried people to talk about the disaster with either spouse/significant other, coworker and/or another person
Exposure[b]	People with higher levels of disaster exposure are more likely than those with lower levels of exposure to talk about the disaster with either spouse/significant other, coworker and/or another person

Time 1 = two months post disaster; $n = 207$.

[a] Gender and race were not significant predictors of Total Talk.

[b] Exposure = mean of physical danger, worked with survivors, worked with dead, worked with families (of survivors and/or dead), problems with disaster work, and difficult choices

United Airlines aeroplane crash: Sioux City, Iowa

It was late afternoon, 19 July 1989, when a United Airlines DC-10 carrying 296 passengers and crew crash-landed at Sioux City, Iowa, following a mid-air malfunction that caused complete failure of the plane's hydraulic system. Casualties included 112 people who died. Rescue personnel were alerted approximately half an hour before the attempted landing, which occurred on an unused runway at the Sioux Gateway Airport; they awaited the landing just off the runway. Upon touchdown, the plane broke apart and burst into flames. The wreckage was scattered on and off the runway and in adjoining corn and soybean fields. Some victims, still in their seats, were thrown from the aircraft; others died in the burning fuselage. Of the 184 survivors, more than 70 literally walked away from the crash.

Our research/consultation group initiated a longitudinal follow-up of the disaster workers and provided consultation to the community. One month after the disaster, we distributed 440 surveys to the Sioux City Air National Guard disaster workers; 212 surveys were completed and returned by the disaster workers, of which 207 were usable (48% return rate). The median return date for these surveys was two months post disaster. Of these, 161 completed Time 2 (seven months median return date) questionnaires (response rate 78%). Of time 1 responders, 88% were male, 98% were white, 70% were married and 75% had completed some college education. Their average age was 37 years and 82% were enlisted members of the Air National Guard (18% officers). The sample at Time 2 was highly similar to that at Time 1. There were no significant differences between those who completed Time 2 surveys and those who dropped out.

Frequency of talking about the disaster to disaster exposure

In order to address talking to intimates, we first examined who reported that they were talking to spouse/significant other, coworker, or an 'other' at Time 1 and again at Time 2. ('In the past week, have you talked about the disaster with ____?') We created a Talk Scale by summing responses to these three. This created a scale that ranged from 0 to 3. As might be expected, Talk scores supported the inference that talking about the disaster was the norm. At Time 1, the mean of the Talk Scale was 1.56. At Time 2 mean Talk score was somewhat lower. At Time 1, those who were older, more educated, married and officers reported higher scores on the Talk Scale. There were no differences on gender or race (see Table 2.2). There were no differences on age, gender, race, education, marital status or rank, associated with Time 2 Talk scores.

Table 2.3. Natural debriefing: predictors of outcome (Sioux City air disaster)

PTSD[a]	People with PTSD at Time 1 were more likely than those without PTSD to talk about the disaster with either spouse/significant other, coworker and/or another person
IES[b]	People with higher IES Total and Intrusive symptoms at Time 1 were more likely than those with lower IES Total and Intrusive symptoms to talk about the disaster with either spouse/significant other, coworker and/or another person

[a] DSM-IV PTSD Scale (Ursano et al., 1995).
[b] Impact of Event Scale, IES (Horowitz et al., 1979).

The relationship of talking about the disaster to disaster exposure

We examined the relationship of disaster stressors exposure to Talk Scale scores. At Time 1, subjects were asked if: (1) they had been in physical danger; (2) they had worked with or assisted disaster survivors; (3) they had worked with the dead from the disaster; (4) they had contact with survivors or victims families; (5) they had encountered problems in accomplishing their rescue work; and (6) they had experienced difficult choices in their rescue work. Responses for these items were summed to yield a score for each subject that ranged from 0 to 5. Exposure scale scores were positively associated with Talk Scale scores for both Time 1 and Time 2.

In order to address intercorrelations among demographic variables and with exposure, we performed multiple regression analyses with Talk score as the dependent variable. Because rank was correlated with both education and age we dropped rank from further analyses. We then examined marital status, exposure, age and education as simultaneous predictors of Talk. Both exposure and education were significant predictors after controlling for the other variables. When we examined the same variables as predictors for Time 2, the outcome was similar, although education was only suggestive. Because age was highly correlated with marital status these results should be interpreted conservatively.

The relationship of talking about the disaster to outcome

We examined the relationship of Talk scores to outcome. Outcome measures (Time 1) included post-trau-

matic stress disorder (PTSD), measured with the DSM-IV PTSD Scale (Ursano et al., 1995; Fullerton & Ursano, 1997) and the Impact of Event Scale (IES) (Total, Intrusion and Avoidance) (Horowitz et al., 1979). At Time 2, outcome measures included PTSD (Keane Minnesota PTSD scale with 14 as the cut off for PTSD) (Keane et al., 1984) and the Zung depression scale (Zung, 1965) both in its index form and in its case identifying scoring, no depression versus mild/moderate/severe depression. At Time 1, those with PTSD reported higher Time 1 Talk scores. The Time 1 Talk scores were also positively correlated with IES Total and IES Intrusion. Time 1 Talk scores were not significantly related to Time 2 PTSD or depression scores.

In order to control for potential confounds of exposure and demographics, we carried out further analyses which showed that marital status and exposure remained significant factors with Talk and exposure associated with greater risk for PTSD. For PTSD at Time 2, the same analysis showed that Talk score (at Time 1) was not a significant predictor, although exposure and marital status continued to be significant. Results of models for Time also showed greater talk to be significantly associated with greater intrusion and total intrusion/avoidance symptoms. These findings are summarized in Table 2.3.

Conclusions

So what have we learned? Who attends a debriefing is important, since attendance is nearly always voluntary. We found that those with high exposure and females were more likely to attend a debriefing. Those without experience were less likely to attend. These results are similar to those found in dental professionals studied after the Waco disaster in Texas (McCarroll et al., 1996): those with previous disaster experience were more likely to seek peer support. (In that study, those without previous disaster experience were more likely to seek support from their spouse or significant other.) How individuals feel in relation to other group members may be an important mediating variable in where support is sought – either from peers in formal or natural debriefing or from family. For those with no previous disaster experience, group cohesion and how new members are integrated into the group may have particularly important implications for whether a new group member turns for support to their peer or work group. These 'talk resources' – family and peers – can be complementary to each other, but it appears that they are often chosen as alternative options.

The process of deciding to attend a debriefing or of using 'natural debriefing', here defined as the natural process of seeking opportunities to talk about a disaster and its effects on oneself and others, may also have implications for sensitization versus inoculation to future disaster stress. There is conflicting evidence in the literature regarding the contribution of past experience to behavioural and psychological responses to disaster. One point of view maintains that past experience may inoculate the worker against some of the adverse effects of exposure to traumatic events (Weisæth, 1989; Raphael, 1986; Norris et al., 1994; Raphael et al., 1996), decrease anticipatory stress (McCarroll et al., 1993, 1995), or help to assimilate the event. In a study of 58 nonprofessional and 57 professional firefighters who jointly fought a large hotel fire that claimed 14 lives, firefighters with previous experience integrated the event better than the inexperienced firefighters and 58% reported that more extensive training and preparation would have helped their performance (Hytten & Hasle, 1989). The alternative position is that cumulative exposure may increase sensitization to traumatic stimuli and may be associated with a breakdown in coping (Mitchell & Bray 1989; Moran & Britton, 1994). Beaton & Murphy's (1995) research with firefighters and paramedics failed to show any effect of past experience on stress. This suggests that the relationship between past experience and stress effects is complicated, perhaps curvilinear, with cumulative experience

being protective up to a certain level of exposure after which it may contribute to sensitization and adverse effects. The type of support obtained after a disaster may also be an important mediating variable and needs further study.

In the study reported here, we operationalized natural debriefing as reporting talking to coworkers or intimate family members about the disaster. Our talk measure was actually a measure of the 'talk network' – rather than frequency of talking – but it would be surprising if these were not highly correlated. Our results indicate that first and most importantly, but not unexpectedly, talking about a disaster to friends and intimates, even two months after the event, is common. Talking decreased at the seven-month follow-up. Those who were older, more educated and married were more likely to be talking about the disaster two months after the event, but by seven months no demographic variables predicted greater talk. Those who were more highly exposed to the disaster also reported greater talk scores at both two and seven months. Those with less exposure – who are also less likely to attend a debriefing – may need encouragement to talk about their disaster experience with intimates as well as to attend debriefings. Our results also indicate that, if talking matters to recovery, those with less education may be less likely to use this form of self-help. This finding is similar to much work in psychotherapy, where those who are more comfortable with talking about problems – in contrast to 'fixing' or being directed – are more likely to use this kind of treatment.

Curiously, higher Talk scores were related to increased PTSD, intrusive and avoidance symptoms at two months (as was being single and greater exposure to the disaster). This finding is somewhat unexpected and cannot provide support to debriefing as an intervention that effects psychiatric symptom levels. Factors other than talk may be important to the success or otherwise of debriefing after trauma and disaster. For example, the listener's response is central to the concept of emotional expression. Listening in a nonjudgemental manner may be a critical component of successful debriefing. Formal debriefing is certainly a much more complex process than only 'talking' and may offer additional advantages over 'talk'.

However, at the same time, talking is an ongoing, readily available process that is often an outcome of a debriefing. If for this reason alone, caution should be used in prematurely advocating debriefing as a post-disaster intervention. Debriefing may also have effects unrelated to psychiatric illness and symptoms – effects on performance recovery or decreased disability or increased 'happiness' that are not often measured in psychological outcome studies. Debriefing, like sleep medication or pain medication, may have little or no impact on standard health measures but still be an important intervention to limit pain, discomfort and disability.

Natural debriefing has potentially both psychological and practical advantages over formal debriefing – including saving on personnel resources (Drabek & Kay, 1976; Erikson, 1976) and being readily and continuously available. Mutuality or helping each other is a potential resource that is often the target of disaster interventions. Disaster mental health workers have generally believed that it is important to stimulate a disaster-exposed group's own resources for comforting and providing emotional and practical support to each other – resources both at work and at home. Often even the victim's and families' need for information is neglected (Winje & Ulvik, 1995). The presentation and delivery of information about what has happened, with whom, how, where, and when are important elements in initiating cognitive processing of the traumatic event. Correct, simple and repeated information can be very important.

It is important to note that all respondents in our study were military personnel previously screened for good health and having at least a high school education. Although this factor may limit the generalizability of our findings to some populations, findings here may be most applicable to police, firefighters, emergency medical personnel, and employees in certain industries. Similarly, because these populations are healthy and well educated, the findings may represent better possible outcomes for the variables studied here (attending a debriefing, talk relation to outcome) than might be seen in other less-screened populations.

This study indicates several cautions for the real world application of formal debriefing. For example,

further study is needed of who attends formal debriefings. This will help to identify potential high-risk groups. Similarly, whether talk is associated with fewer or greater psychological symptoms is extremely important to understanding the outcome, mechanisms, and risks of debriefing. Future studies of natural debriefing should: (1) control for trait factors of talk that are present prior to disaster exposure, for example the effect of talking may be different in those who usually use talking as a stress reduction strategy; and (2) control for initial level of symptoms when examining the effects of natural debriefing. In studies of debriefing, a wider range of outcome measures may be indicated to include psychological 'pain' (e.g. well-being), disability, days lost from work, health care utilization and family and work performance. Data are much needed on the natural debriefing that occurs before and after any formal debriefing; this is necessary to understand better the mechanisms underlying debriefing and its outcomes.

REFERENCES

Allen, S. N. & Bloom, S. L. (1994). Group and family treatment of post-traumatic stress disorder. *Psychiatric Clinics of North America*, **17**, 425–37.

Beaton, R. & Murphy, S. (1995). Working with people in crisis: research implications. In C. Figley (Ed.) *Compassion Fatigue: Coping with Secondary Traumatic Stress Disorder in Those Who Treat the Traumatized*, Vol. 1 (pp. 51–81). New York: Brunner/Mazel.

Bullman, T. A. & Kang, H. K. (1994). Posttraumatic stress disorder and the risk of traumatic deaths among Vietnam veterans. *Journal of Nervous and Mental Disease*, **182**, 604–10.

Chemtob, C. M., Tomas, S., Law, W. & Cremniter, D. (1997). Post-disaster psychosocial intervention: a field study of the impact of debriefing on psychological distress. *American Journal of Psychiatry*, **154**, 415–17.

Coates, D. & Winston, T. (1983). Counteracting the deviance of depression: peer support groups for victims. *Journal of Social Issues*, **39**(169).

Drabek, T. E. & Key, W. H. (1976). The impact of disaster on primary group linkages. *Mass Emergencies*, **1**, 89–105.

Dunning, C. (1990). Mental health sequelae in disaster workers: prevention and intervention. *International Journal of Mental*

Health, **19**, 91–103.

Dyregrov, A. & Mitchell, J. T. (1992). Work with traumatised children – psychological effects and coping strategies. *Journal of Traumatic Stress*, **5**, 5–17.

Erikson, K. T. (1976). Loss of communality at Buffalo Creek. *American Journal of Psychiatry*, **133**, 302–5.

Fullerton, C. S. & Ursano, R. J. (1994). Healthcare delivery in the high stress environment of chemical and biological warfare. *Military Medicine*, **155**, 54–9.

Fullerton, C. S. & Ursano, R. J. (1997). Posttraumatic responses in spouse/significant others of disaster workers. In C. S. Fullerton & R. J. Ursano (Eds.) *Posttraumatic Stress Disorder: Acute and Long-term Responses to Trauma and Disaster* (pp. 59–76). Washington, DC: American Psychiatric Press, Inc.

Fullerton, C. S., Wright, K. M., Ursano, R. J. & McCarroll, J. E. (1992). Psychological responses of rescue workers: fire fighters and trauma. *American Journal of Orthopsychiatry*, **62**, 371–8.

Gottlieb, B. H. (1996). Theories and practices of mobilising support in stressful circumstances. In C. L. Cooper (Ed.) *Stress, Medicine, and Health*, vol. 1 (pp. 339–74). Boca Raton, FL CRC Press.

Holaday, M., Warren-Miller, G., Smith, A. & Yost, T. E. (1995). A preliminary investigation of on-the-scene coping mechanisms used by disaster workers. *Journal of Mental Health Counselling*, **9**, 347–59.

Holloway, H. C. & Fullerton, C. S. (1994). The psychology of terror and its aftermath. In R. J. Ursano, B. G. McCaughey & C. S. Fullerton (Eds.) *Individual and Community Responses to Trauma and Disaster: The Structure of Human Chaos* (pp. 31–46). Cambridge: Cambridge University Press.

Horowitz, M., Wilner, N. & Alvarez, W. (1979). Impact of Event Scale: a measure of subjective stress. *Psychosomatic Medicine*, **41**, 209–18.

Hytten, K. & Hasle, A. (1989). Firefighters: a study of stress and coping. *Acta Psychiatrica Scandinavica* (Suppl.) **355**(80), 50–5.

Janoff-Bulman, R. (1992). *Shattered Assumptions*. New York: Free Press.

Kang, H. K. & Bullman, T. A. (1996). Mortality among U.S. Veterans of the Persian Gulf War. *New England Journal of Medicine*, **335**, 1498–504.

Keane, T. M., Malloy, P. F. & Fairbank, J. A. (1984). Empirical development of an MMPI sub-scale for the assessment of combat-related posttraumatic stress disorders. *Journal of Consulting and Clinical Psychology*, **52**, 888–91.

Kenardy, J. A., Webster, R. A., Lewin, T. J., Carr, V. J., Hazell, P. L. & Carter, G. L. (1996). Stress debriefing and patterns of recovery following a natural disaster. *Journal of Traumatic Stress*, **9**, 37–49.

McCarroll, J. E., Ursano, R. J., Ventis, W. L., Fullerton, C. S., Oates, G. I., Friedman, H., Shean, G. L. & Wright, K. M. (1993). Anticipation of handling the dead: effects of gender and experience. *British Journal of Clinical Psychology*, **32**, 466–8.

McCarroll, J. E., Ursano, R. J., Fullerton, C. S. & Lundy, A. C. (1995). Anticipatory stress of handling human remains from the Persian Gulf War: predictors of intrusion and avoidance. *Journal of Nervous and Mental Disease*, **183**, 700–5.

McCarroll, J. E., Fullerton, C. S., Ursano, R. J. & Hermsen, J. M. (1996). Posttraumatic stress symptoms following forensic dental identification: Mt. Carmel, Waco, Texas. *American Journal of Psychiatry*, **153**, 778–82.

Mitchell, J. T. & Bray, G. P. (1989). *Emergency Services Stress*. Englewood Cliffs, NJ: Prentice Hall.

Moran, C. & Britton, N. (1994). Emergency work experience and reactions to traumatic incidents. *Journal of Traumatic Stress*, **7**, 575–85.

Norris, F. H., Phifer, J. F. & Kaniasty, K. (1994). Individual and community reactions to the Kentucky floods: findings from a longitudinal study of older adults. In R. J. Ursano, B. G. McCaughey & C. S. Fullerton (Eds.) *Individual and Community Responses to Trauma and Disaster: The Structure of Human Chaos* (pp. 378–400). Cambridge: Cambridge University Press.

Pennebaker, J. W. & O'Heeron, R. C. (1984). Confiding in others and illness rate among spouses of suicide and accidental death victims. *Journal of Abnormal Psychology*, **93**, 473–6.

Raphael, B. (1986). *When Disaster Strikes: How Individuals and Communities Cope with Catastrophe*. London: Hutchinson.

Raphael, B., Meldrum, L. & McFarlane, A. C. (1995). Does debriefing after psychological trauma work? *British Medical Journal*, **310**, 1479–80.

Raphael, B., Wilson, J. Meldrum, L. & McFarlane, A. C. (1996). Acute preventive intervention. In B. A. Van der Kolk, A. C. McFarlane & L. Weisæth (Eds.), *Traumatic Stress: The Effects of Overwhelming Experience on Mind, Body, and Society* (pp. 463–80). New York: Guilford Press.

Schachter, S. (1959). *The Psychology of Affiliation*. Palo Alto, CA: Stanford University Press.

Shalev, A. (1994). Debriefing following traumatic exposure. In R.J. Ursano, B. G. McCaughey & C. S. Fullerton (Eds.) *Individual and Community Responses to Trauma and Disaster: The Structure of Human Chaos* (pp. 201–20). Cambridge: Cambridge University Press.

Shalev, A. Y., Schreiber, S. & Galai, T. (1993). Early psychological responses to traumatic injury. *Journal of Traumatic Stress*, **6**, 441–50.

Silver, R. L. & Wortman, C. B. (1980). Copying with undesirable life events. In J. Garber & M. E. Seligman (Eds.) *Human Helplessness: Theory and Applications* (pp. 279–92). New York: Academic Press.

Ursano, R. J. (1997). Disaster: stress, immunologic function, and health behaviour. *Psychosomatic Medicine*, **59**, 142–3.

Ursano, R. J., Fullerton, C.S., Kao, T. C. & Bhartiya, V. (1995). Longitudinal assessment of posttraumatic stress disorder and depression after exposure to traumatic death. *Journal of Nervous and Mental Disease*, **42**, 36–42.

Ursano, R. J., Grieger, T. A. & McCarroll, J. E. (1996). Prevention of post-traumatic stress: consultation, training and early treatment. In B. A. Van der Kolk, A. C. McFarlane, & L. Weisæth (Eds.) *Traumatic Stress: The Effects of Overwhelming Experience on Mind, Body, and Society* (pp. 441–63). New York: Guilford Press.

Weisæth, L. (1989). The stressors and the post-traumatic stress syndrome after an industrial disaster. *Acta Psychiatrica Scandinavica*, **80**, Suppl. 355, 25–37.

Winje, D. & Ulvik, A. (1995). Confrontations with reality: crisis intervention services for traumatized families after a school bus accident in Norway. *Journal of Traumatic Stress*, **8**, 429–44.

Zung, W. W. K. (1965). A self-rating depression scale. *Archives of General Psychiatry*, **12**, 63–70.

3

Briefing and debriefing: group psychological interventions in acute stressor situations

Lars Weisæth

EDITORIAL COMMENTS

This chapter by Lars Weisæth brings a very thoughtful appraisal of the significance of debriefing for different groups of personnel. The model presented is based on extensive traumatic stress research and experience and appraisal of the use of supportive and preventive interventions in disaster and trauma situations. It highlights the relation of debriefing to briefing and suggests that formal debriefing should be provided only for those who have been 'briefed' to deal with an incident, disaster or violently traumatic experience. This approach focusses on the potential value of what is called group stress debriefing (GSD) for professional rescue and emergency response teams, who are trained and mobilized. It may also have some value for those who are 'reservist' teams. He emphasizes, however, that its key principles may be incorporated into the leadership role of the team leader and he or she may be specifically trained to implement the model in the team's functional response and standdown. There may, in fact, be negative consequences, with intrusion of health personnel between the team leader and team members, and it is suggested that these health personnel (trained debriefers) should be used only in high-risk situations: for instance death of significant numbers of team members, witnessing of people dying and being unable to save lives, and feelings of failure in the rescue operations. Other groups, for instance natural groups, random groups or victim groups may need an individualized approach and other methods of prevention or trauma intervention to be provided – not a formal and structured group process.

Weisæth also describes the historical evolution of concepts relevant to debriefing – for instance the talking through of the traumatic experience, and suggests that veterans' clubs and other informal group processes have served such a function for a long period. The essential elements of 'debriefing' are seen as linked to theories of catharsis and emotional release, but he rightly questions whether or not this is the most effective coping in certain circumstances, and points to the need for further research about the timing and appropriateness of interventions. One potential advantage of the rapid and extensive uptake of debriefing, however, may be the encouragement of men in very masculinity-based organizations to discuss and share their feelings. Central to the potential effects of any debriefing are clarifying misperceptions about the event and its consequences, initiating communication amongst the participants, reinforcing and deepening the learning experience, strengthening group cohesion, recognizing and accepting emotion and stress reactions, facilitating grief work, and preparing the group for continued action.

He also suggests that debriefing may fulfil the wish for magic help in times of crises, dealt with in earlier times through ritual and religion, and cautions against intruding debriefing in group cultural rituals and processes that have been traditionally used to deal with traumatic experiences. The role of the commander is critical, as is comrade or 'buddy' support. However, failure to be able to fulfil the necessary role in the incident, through either unaccountable or accountable factors, is frequently what needs to be worked through and is a factor associated with later morbidity.

Research reported in this chapter describes findings from two disasters involving both full-time and reserve personnel and shows that, as with other studies, those receiving debriefing perceived it as helpful, and that the majority of people in both groups talked through the experiences with others, usually in groups. It was felt to have helped professionally and increased self-competence. Self-esteem Weisæth sees as a central issue and threat to self-esteem may be the most severe stress for a soldier. He also reports that the greatest fear experienced by the majority of soldiers is the fear that they will not be able to stand up to the combat experience, and this is more so for commanders. It is frequently reported as being even more fear-arousing than risk of death or mutilation.

Weisæth concludes that group stress debriefing can be effective in 'transforming subjective experience to learning experience' and that 'injury or threat to self-esteem' is a 'crucial dimension that needs to be addressed in the GSD' – this refers to the repair of both individual and team confidence – 'to get the group to accept reality and that, everything considered, the group had done as well as it could'.

Introduction

In our view, group stress debriefing (GSD) is an early intervention method for personnel groups exposed to a single task or repetitive tasks related to stressful events that carry a high potential for psychotraumatic effects. GSD is one element within a stress management programme. We prefer to reserve the term 'debriefing' for interventions with personnel who were briefed about their task, since the concept of *de*briefing indicates that briefing preceded the operation. A briefing commonly informs and instructs a team, crew or larger organization about goals and means in an operation to be put into action.

In addition to the short briefing given immediately before the operation, the personnel have, over a long time, been educated and trained in specific roles, codes of conduct, and standing operating procedures, to act according to definite plans.

The group stress debriefing examines what really happened and the actions carried out (to the extent that a technical debriefing has not already done so) and compares these with what had been expected and what had been planned, and the response to these experiences. Individual debriefing is similar in many respects and will be carried out if a single person has been exposed to severe operational stress. This concept of GSD is more comprehensive than processes where the goal is 'to reach a full understanding of what you have taken part in', which may be sufficient for persons who have simply shared an experience that could be traumatic.

The inflation of the term debriefing in today's usage to cover interventions after nearly all sorts of traumatic events, directed towards all sorts of people, including victims, often persons who were totally unprepared for what happened to them and given no task to perform, we consider to be confounding, deceptive and potentially harmful.

The way GSD is to be carried out depends on the pre-existing group structure, the group's level of professionalism and competence, its level of preparedness for the task-related event in question, and under what conditions the GSD is to be implemented.

On the basis of these characteristics, this chapter starts by describing five categories of such groups and some of the implications for GSD. Then there is a short historical excursion in the Western world in search of some of the traditional values of which it may be important to be aware when working with GSD. From there it concentrates on the rationale for using the group as an arena for preventive interventions, particularly for GSD in the strict sense of the term, which is likely to be relevant mainly for groups at levels 1 and 2 described below.

Group level 1: the professional team

The personnel at this level are highly selected, have a high level of pretraining, strong team spirit and full-time preparedness jobs. Their stress resilience is high and to them emergency work carries moderate to low risk of severe psychic traumatization.

High-risk situations for this group of personnel may, however, be seen after difficult operations that go wrong, with loss of control and particularly when the reason is individual or team failure, or there is direct exposure to danger with high mortality among team members. Severing the ties with his or her group after the exposure is associated with particularly high prognostic risk for a traumatized person in this kind of group.

Examples of such teams are military squads, rescue helicopter crews, firefighting units, rescue teams and emergency medical personnel. Such teams have certain comparative advantages for both handling and processing the effects of severe stress exposures, and accordingly GSD can be part of an ongoing internal group process. With a few exceptions, we see no need for clinician-guided GSD at this group level; in fact, outside preventive intervention may disturb the group's normal adaptive process. We see, however, an important role for health and mental health expertise as a part of the pretraining programme, including training for GSD for such groups, as advisers to commanders, and for early and adequate individual and even group intervention in high-risk cases.

Group level 2: the reserve team

The reserve team has personnel with a mobilization status in case of emergency, crisis or war. Although on a day-to-day basis they are employed in regular, ordinary work, personnel in this category are selected and pretrained for special emergency tasks and have undergone unit exercises. A proportion may have previously worked in full-time professional teams (group level 1).

Risk of psychic traumatization is higher than at group level 1, the most significant risk factors being deficiencies in selection of personnel, their pretraining, preparedness, planning and organization. Most effective prevention therefore would be improved selection and preincident training, training with equipment and preparedness. Examples of such teams are military reservists, industrial firefighting units, Red Cross Volunteer Rescue Corps and personnel within disaster medical preparedness organizations. In some countries preparedness for disasters and military defence depend on large numbers of such reservist personnel. This personnel category may therefore constitute a significant

proportion of the total population.

The goal for group 2 level should be to approach level 1 in competence, including familiarity with coping strategies for traumatic stress. The main role for health professionals is therefore to encourage that development. In reality, however, the level of competence in stress management for members of these groups is often so lacking that health personnel have a broader role, including that of leading GSD.

Group level 3: natural groups

The 'natural' groups consist of people who constitute a stable social network, but are not cohesive teams as are those of group levels 1 and 2; they are mobilized for emergency work without having much pretraining or any particular responsibility to be prepared. They may or may not be given a short briefing before they are put to work. Examples are employees of companies hit by major accidents, road workers digging victims out of an avalanche, and sailors picking up dead from the sea after a maritime disaster.

The risk of traumatization is higher than for group level 2. As the ability to use the group as a forum for GSD may be very limited among these personnel, their need to go through the process of comparing expectations with the real experience of the disaster or incident is less. At this level there is a need for the assistance of health personnel with experience in traumatic stress, less as leaders of GSD in the strict sense of the term but rather as facilitators of group discussions about the stressful event, and as providers of relevant information and guidance.

Group level 4: random groups

Random groups are made up of individuals who happen to be on the spot when an emergency situation arises, and spontaneously engage in rescue and helping efforts.

The risk level is yet higher than in the groups described above. Since the people in these random groups have had no formal responsibilities beforehand for emergency work and have lesser role demands to live up to, their needs differ from the personnel described in group levels 1 to 3 and it is highly questionable whether the talking-through process deserves to be termed debriefing.

However, some of the techniques of GSD may well be applied. Although their membership in the random group is of brief duration, it seems to be feasible for preventive work to utilize the group setting and probably also to reinforce the group aspect of the experience for the single individual. Professional health personnel could play a considerable role in potential prevention work for random groups.

Group level 5: victims groups

As the term describes, victim groups consist of persons who are victimized together. Quite often, the first rescue and other helping efforts for those worst hit originate in this group. Some persons within the group may have made considerable rescue efforts during the so-called isolation period, i.e. before help arrives from the outside. They are likely to be at lower risk than the rest of the group.

The risk of psychic traumatization in the group is substantial if the exposure has been severe. Again, the term debriefing is not appropriate for describing the kind of group intervention that may be carried out afterwards. Basically, individuals at this level ought to be met as the victims they are, and provided with interventions both at the group and individual levels.

The debriefing model described in the following is based on experience and traumatic stress research over many years, and less on systematic intervention research evidence.

So far research results on the effect of group stress debriefing are contradictory (Robinson & Mitchell, 1993; Bisson & Deahl, 1994; Deahl et al., 1994; Mitchell & Everly, 1995; Raphael et al., 1995). Consequently there is a strong demand for randomized controlled trials. In this respect group stress debriefing is no exception, whether as a positive or negative example. The practice of group stress debriefing shares with many other methods of preventive psychiatric interventions, a shortage of statistical data on its short- and long-term effects.

Some observers suspect that psychological debriefing is here to stay, whatever the outcome of trials. Palmer (1995) goes on to state that perhaps it always has been with us and quotes from Homer's *Odyssey* to prove his point: 'for when a man has endured deeply and strayed far from home he can cull solace from the rehearsal of old griefs. And so I will meet you questioning' (Homer, reprinted 1991). The many years which Odysseus spent on his journey back to his home and the many perils he encountered have been interpreted as a metaphor for a soldier's working through his traumatic war experiences. Homer's *Illiad*, the first book in Western literature and compulsory reading for educated young men during the centuries, has been regarded as a realistic description of how the experience of combat may affect a man's mental state.

Palmer's (1995) point that debriefing has always been with us is also illustrated by the fact that veterans have always had clubs and associations where they could share memories, talk endlessly about their experiences and constantly exchange supportive communications. Veterans who are deprived of such buddy groups sometimes express frustration and use neighbours and other friends as listeners. These examples from literature and the ways in which veterans organize their lives may be illustrations of the human need to recapitulate and share traumatic memories, presumably in order to avoid encapsulation of painful impressions.

The historical perspective is also useful for understanding the ambivalence towards disclosing emotional pain and sharing stressful experiences with others. It is well recognized that the history of traumatic stress is extraordinary (Herman, 1992; Raphael, 1996). It is probably unique both for a scientific field of enquiry and for a clinical practice; the important insights about the very existence of psychic trauma and the risk of psychic trauma to mental health have been denied and forgotten, actually again and again. That the suffering individuals need to avoid reminders of their traumatic exposure is only a part of the explanation. More important are needs in the society at large to retain a sense of safety and to avoid taking on responsibility for what has happened and the consequences. Another factor of importance and relevance for our topic is that emotional reactions to severe events may be equated with psychological vulnerability, particularly in groups dominated by certain male values, an issue to which we now turn.

Some historical glimpses

Since modern Western societies have important roots in the ancient Greek society, it might well be that some of its concepts and values still have an impact on us. Even a cursory investigation of history with regard to help-seeking behaviour and expression of emotions provides findings that appear strikingly familiar to us today. For example, in Aristotle's *Ethics*, the concepts of *megalopsykhia* and *autarkeia* were important. *Megalopsykhia* is a set of values, one of which implies that it is not very acceptable for the proud person to receive help. Ideally he should offer his services to others, while needing help would indicate dependence and even subordination. *Autarkeia* was the ideal of being self-sufficient. Friendship for men with *megalopsykhia* basically meant mutual admiration. Friends should be bothered as little as possible when one was troubled; friends should be seen when one enjoyed good fortune.

Some of the influential philosophical schools developed further these ideals about how to handle difficult life circumstances. The stoic's ideal was *apatheia*, the stoic calm and freedom from suffering. Many stoics have demonstrated that it is possible to free oneself from strong perceptual impressions and thereby achieve greater self-control in difficult situations.

At other times there were other attitudes to emotional expressiveness in the male role. 'No one rode with dry eyes', writes the author of *The Song of Roland*, the 'chançon de geste', the song about the battle at Roncevaux when Charles the Great, his nephew Roland and their companion Franks fought their tragic battle in Spain. 'A hundred thousand men broke out crying... The army wept'. The emperor's grief is severe, 'because such is the custom among Franks', and 'his tears flow when he sees the dead'.

Historical descriptions of heroes in war frequently stress how openly they expressed their sadness and grief. Recent studies by historians have confirmed that during certain historical periods crying in males was common; to cry was an expected response to tragic events. In fact, for male leaders crying was a public act; to express strong emotions was considered to be a sign of strength and masculinity. Thus grief leadership is nothing new. The last drastic change in the Western male role appears to have been an effect of Victorian influence during the nineteenth century. Within a few decades, from being considered an appropriate male grief reaction in public, crying became feminized and privatized, something reserved for the private domain only (Englund, 1991).

Fearlessness in the face of danger probably always has been an ideal for men. But even the Norse sagas, notorious for their innumerable accounts of heroic Viking warriors calmly facing death, offer one revealing observation that points to a more sophisticated understanding of fear: 'that er hraeddr madr sem ekki thorir at skjalva' [A man who does not dare to tremble is a really scared man].

Modern research findings (Duck, 1988) support the traditional impression that male friends do not express and share emotions to the same degree as girls and women do with their female friends. Since men are more open about their feelings when talking to a female friend, there is something about the interaction between males that works counter to sharing feelings in a more intimate relationship. In fact, these differences in social style between the sexes develop early in life: boys prefer to play in groups, girls in pairs or in groups of only three. Boys keep company by uniting about group activities, while girls select one or two 'bosom friends'. Girls use talking as a tool for cooperation; boys are more aggressive in their verbal interactions (Rutter & Rutter, 1993).

This is not the place to discuss the nature of these differences between the sexes and whether their origins are biological, psychological or social. But they seem to us to have some implications for how a group setting can be used to facilitate the working through of a possibly traumatic experience.

Beliefs and rituals

In mediaeval Europe, the Catholic Church offered very strong supportive measures that probably went a long way to help people cope with the ever-present threat to life by the three servants of death: war, starvation and plague. It is probably no coincidence that the sixteenth and seventeenth centuries, the period after the Reformation, became 'the centuries of fright'. Preserving the physical body had become the central goal in life while in previous times preservation of the soul had played the important role. Compared with what a priest can do for the soul, the medical doctor is a rather helpless person. The soul may have eternal life, the body is always in the long run fighting a losing battle. For a person who does not merely *have* a body, but *is* a body, in the end there is no rescue, no solution and no comfort. The modern fear of death is therefore a constant and untreatable condition.

Protestantism ripped away some earlier supportive structures in order to ease the individual's direct access to have a largely private affair with his God. The move from collective to individual reached its highest in individuals belonging to the Lutheran tradition.

In mediaeval times suffering was seen as God sent, and there was then always the hope that grief could turn to joy. If illness and suffering could not be eliminated through treatment or miraculous cure, it was always possible to give it meaning (von Achen, 1992). The method was 'imitatio Christi', which meant to imitate Christ, particularly the way in which he endured his suffering. If the ill person managed to live with illness, he or she could be awarded a relatively high social status, even when suffering from leprosy or other illnesses that at other times have been stigmatizing. Thus, two strategies were applied, mobilizing the resources of the sick person as well as the support from the social environment.

Learning about the rituals that played important roles historically makes one wonder to what extent the many new types of intervention introduced today to help people in times of crises also have ritual aspects. For the mediaeval person the saints were important as go-betweens. For each illness a particular saint had particular qualities to help that illness or to protect against it. For example, the holy Florian protected against fire. If one's house burnt down in spite of prayers to Florian, the holy Barbara would have a strong say in the salvation of those who had perished because of the fire. For those who survived with burn injuries, there was the holy Laurentius to thank: 'If I recover, I shall contribute to the Laurentius church that is being built' (von Achen, 1992). The wish for magic help is probably no less for modern humans in severe crisis, and the priestly role may be vacant in a less religious society like ours. The mental health professional working with the acutely traumatized was once advised to be 'honest about his failures and modest about his successes' (Main, 1946). It is still good advice.

Transcultural aspects

The shifting attitudes towards, and coping strategies dealing with, pain and suffering in Western culture throughout the ages have parallels in the different ways that cultures across the world help people to cope with severe life events. There have been timely warnings about the export of Western psychological practices, of which GSD is one, to various peoples affected by psychic traumas worldwide. It is pointed out that Western psychological ideas are part of Western culture, which is becoming increasingly globalized (Summerfield, 1995).

This is not the place to discuss this issue further, but we will mention one case where transcultural aspects played an important role when we evaluated the appropriateness of GSD.

In 1996, a team from our institution was asked by the United Nations (UN) to provide early screening and give advice about interventions for the Fiji Battalion in UNIFIL, the peacekeeping UN military operation in South Lebanon. The Fiji Battalion Headquarters at Qana had been shelled by artillery and more than 100 civilians who had sought refuge there had been killed by the shelling. Among their traditional ways of coping with severe stress, the Fiji culture has the ceremonial use of kawa drinking, a mild intoxicant, in intense group settings. Observing the obvious value that the interactions in the group had in coming to terms with what had passed made us drop ideas about GSD because we realized that they had their own format for group processing and that a traditional GSD might have disturbed their own way of working through. Individual screening and advice to commanders became our intervention methods.

The rationale for using a group setting

Group stress debriefing, group therapy and the therapeutic community, three important types of group interventions in psychiatry, had their development spurred by World War II (Marshall, 1944). This development, as it took place in British military psychiatry during the war, has been well described (Ahrenfeldt, 1958), as was how it influenced civilian psychiatry after the war (Main, 1989).

Using the group as a systematic forum for interventions, as a method of improving the quality of life and in the hope of prolonging life was first described by a New England internist, Joseph Hershey Pratt (1907). The first group analytical studies were published in the 1920s (Burrow, 1925). According to Herlofsen (1996), looking back on World War II, it was self-evident that higher-level systems, such as the group, small as well as large, would come to supplement the traditional individual approaches of clinical psychiatry. Hundreds of doctors and psychiatrists entering the army experienced the limitations of the medical model of individual illness and personal treatment. Many men soldiered on effectively, carried by well-run units with high group morales, while they had manifest signs of personal breakdown and refused to report sick. In the words of Main (1989, p. 127): 'In the Army the individual was cared for, trained, and valued highly, but only as a contributor to group purposes, and for the survival of his group as a whole he must be risked, perhaps even to lose his life.'

Danger tends to make people seek company and protection in groups. Few life experiences reinforce small-group cohesion as much as a shared feeling of danger. The strength of the group bonding may be hard to estimate fully unless one has been at the front and experienced war-like circumstances and witnessed this group phenomenon oneself. Belonging to a group creates boundaries to the outside world and makes the individual feel safe and strong.

Similarly, the small group is a place to re-establish order, trust and a feeling of safety. A group provides social support by offering a sense of belonging, inclusion, identity, acceptance, friendship, emotional contact, communication, information, practical help and social control (Manning & Ingraham, 1987, Tyler & Grifford, 1991; Herlofsen, 1994). As a containing and caring environment the group may be seen as a re-creation of the original maternal environment. But if emotions in the aftermath of a traumatic event run so high that the ability to work through is compromised, the group is not a perfect place to communicate and integrate experiences. Another limitation of a group is the sacrifice of individuality and autonomy that the members must make.

It has already been stated that the pre-existing character of the group is important for how GSD is carried out, and that the professional team and the reserve team, according to our model, share characteristics and goals, although there are also some differences. The use of GSD in these settings needs to take the above issues into account.

Professional and mobilized reserve teams

Professionals and mobilized reserves are prepared for emergency situations through their selection, education, training, exercises, daily routine work and more or less frequent experiences with similar stressful operations. These professionals are likely to carry out planned systematic team work. Some characteristics of these uniformed units are specialist skills, shared identity, mutual reliance and strong *esprit de corps*. The main factor in building and maintaining their self-esteem is based upon intraprofessional evaluation criteria, and thus they are themselves best qualified to evaluate the quality of their own performance. High motivation and dedication to their work, pride, independence and the need to be self-contained are primary characteristics, and a strict hierarchical structure is usually balanced by strong bonding.

It is necessary to qualify for membership in these kinds of group, and also to confirm to specified health requirements. Failing health may mean loss of abilities necessary for work and have serious consequences for further career and group membership.

The main research findings in traumatic stress studies of these groups are that these tight-knit groups have a high resilience to stress impacts, such as disaster rescue operations or exposure to war stress (Weisæth,

1989). They are not immune to stress effects, but membership of these groups provides a much higher stress tolerance than single individuals can build. This will be elaborated in the following. They tend to accept each others' stress reactions and, because every member is important for the group to function, they prefer to tolerate disturbing stress reactions rather than exchange the person for a newcomer. The group's stress resilience increases with the quality of its leadership, cohesion, motivation, discipline, equipment and medical support. Mental health professionals may have failed to meet this kind of resilience if they previously have been exposed only to patient populations during their training and practice. The highly selected population that most clinical training provides may create the wrong impression of human vulnerability and resilience, and, for example, contribute to the notion that stress exposures inevitably lead to stress reactions, or that a strong stress reaction necessarily needs to be treated.

Another characteristic of personnel at levels 1 and 2, particularly of team leaders, is that their training often includes extensive and intensive training in group psychology, social psychology and organizational sociology. Military and police academies, for example, have taught these subjects for a long time. The military tradition has been to include these subjects under the heading 'Military leadership', which demonstrates how obviously important they have been seen to be. Professionals at this level tend to be very eager to learn about task-related stress and rapidly define these aspects as a part of their needed expertise. Mental health professionals would be wise to appreciate these background qualifications when they collaborate with such organizations.

A consistent finding, however, in research on stress effects of comparable exposures by groups of levels 1 and 2, is that, although professionals are more resilient, significant levels of psychiatric morbidity can develop among professionals when they encounter tasks that turn out to be impossible, for example rescue operations in disasters with high mortality. Findings from two studies of rescuers will be used to illustrate this point.

In an offshore oil rig disaster in 1980 with a mortality of 58% among the victims we compared the stress reactions and coping problems during the rescue work among personnel from the National Norwegian Rescue Service (group level 1) with those of oil platform personnel participating as mobilized reserves (group level 2) (Ersland et al., 1989). Although one-third of the rescuers were exposed to severe risk to their own lives during the operation, other stressors, such as witnessing people dying and being unable to save lives, were the crucial stress experiences. As for disturbing stress reactions experienced during the rescue operation, significant differences were found between the professionals and the mobilized reserves on the following criteria: experiencing uncertainty, anxiety, restlessness and hyperactivity. There was a strong relationship between experiencing strong stress reactions during the rescue operation and the risk of suffering from mental health problems nine months post disaster when 17% of the professional rescuers and 25% of the nonprofessionals reported poor mental health.

Discriminative analysis indicated that the following six types of reactions were predictors of mental health problems among rescuers: uncertainty, restlessness, anxiety, irritation, discouragement and apathy. The rescuers who had participated frequently in rescue work displayed a lower prevalence of poor mental health compared with those who had seldom participated and also those who had not participated at all: only 4.3% of those who had often taken part compared with 26.2% those who had never participated previously.

The need to work through the emotional disaster experiences was reported more frequently by those in the poor mental health group (91%) compared with the others (54%). Little opportunity to do so was reported more frequently among those reporting poor mental health (29%) compared with the others (11%). Despite this, the rescuers in the poor mental health group had actually shared their own emotional reactions and feelings more frequently with others than those who reported unchanged mental health, although half of them had done so only a few times. A total of 88% of the rescuers reported a need to work through the emotional disaster experiences by sharing their feelings with others. The opportunity to work through the painful emotional feelings with others was reported as very good or reasonably good by 85% of the rescuers, 15% reporting little opportunity. Sixty-four per cent of the rescuers reported that they had shared their own reactions and feelings with other people after the disaster, and 26% had done so frequently. The effect of sharing painful emotional feelings with others was reported as 'good' by 21% of the rescuers, 'reasonably good' by 42%, as of 'little effect' by 17% and of 'no effect' by 20%.

In a study of reserve firefighters (group level 2) involved in a very demanding rescue operation of more than 100 hotel guests trapped in a high-rise building fire, the most significant stressors reported to have been experienced during the exposure were all related to fear of failure in the rescue operation (Hytten & Hasle, 1989).

In the aftermath, post-traumatic stress scores were significantly higher among men without practical experience in fire rescue work than among men with such experience.

The GSD was carried out in conjunction with the professional fire brigade. One beneficial effect of this procedure was that the tendency of the reservists to focus more on the deceased, those they had failed to rescue, than on the vast majority who had been rescued was counterbalanced. This demonstrates the ability of the professionals to evaluate their own performance in a balanced way, while the reserve teams lacked that competence.

Another modification of the way the GSD was carried out was that an anaesthesiologist was brought in to explain why those deceased by carbon monoxide poisoning may have minute pupils, which, in combination with a pink skin colour, made them look alive. It had been a disturbing experience for firefighters who had to make difficult decisions on priorities between living and deceased in their rescue work. This use of medical expertise was justified, since the professional fire brigade personnel, although familiar with the phenomenon, were at loss to explain the mechanisms that could account for it, and a need for that was expressed during the debriefing. Belenky et al. (1996) reported medical emergency situations from the Gulf War where medical expertise was clearly needed in the GSD for medics and soldiers.

All the firefighters in our study reported that they had talked a great deal about their experience with other people, either in a formal debriefing session or in a group with fellow workers. As reported from most debriefing studies where self-reporting methods have been used, the evaluations were positive. Out of 39 men who participated in debriefing sessions as many as 38 stated the debriefing had helped them to some degree ($n = 14$), or to a higher degree ($n = 24$). Two-thirds claimed that the rescue effort had been professionally useful and as many felt that their selfconfidence had increased. Enhanced group cohesion, more knowledge about people's responses and a different priority of values were also mentioned as positive effects of this fire rescue experience.

As described above, medical doctors in the military organization with its tight-knit groups and strong group cohesion and identity, group morale and leadership were the first health professionals not only to understand the protective power of being members of a well-disciplined group, but also the destructive psychological effect of becoming separated from the group. To carry out strong social obligations in the face of severe danger, which is what military combat is all about, creates the strongest bonding between men: one for all, and all for one. Nowhere will it be more obvious that one's life depends on one's buddy, and this dependency is mutual. The extent to which losing the respect of team mates constituted a severe threat to self-esteem became obvious when, during the World War I, the increased risks to the soldiers' mental health associated with evacuation procedures to the rear was documented. To remove a soldier from his group significantly reduced the chances that he would benefit from early treatment and return to duty, and it increased the risk to his long-term mental health. (Other soldiers who have coped with their battle anxieties supported by comradeship and affection may be left alone and vulnerable when their friends are killed in battle.) The three illness and prognostic risk factors stimulated by premature evacuation of a combat-stressed soldier from the front are: separation from the group, which may be felt as if he or she is letting down comrades, unit, the cause, and himself; removal from the group, which is the medium with those human resources to ensure recovery, namely the commander and comrades; and, finally, evacuation may satisfy a primary gain, that of increasing the chances of survival, which may be difficult to give up.

The threat combat poses to self-esteem is a most severe stress on the soldier. As many as 50% of soldiers have as their greatest fear the risk that they may not be able to stand up to the combat experience, and among commanders it is even more dominating, and surprisingly often reported as more fear arousing than the risk of death or mutilation (Shalit, 1988).

The main focus on the forward psychiatric treatment which was developed during the World War I was that the intervention should be carried out close to the front, as early as possible and with a strongly expressed expectation that the soldier's function would soon return to normal (proximity, immediacy, expectancy (PIE)). Another acronym conveying the same principles is BICEPS (brevity of treatment, immediacy, centrality, expectancy, proximity, simplicity). It is emphasized that a combat stress reaction should be seen as a temporary and reversible reaction that causes a temporary reduction of functional capacity in a previously normal person who is overwhelmed by severe stressors. For group levels 1 and 2 the GSD should be seen in the context of the knowledge and skills in self-help they have acquired in their training and in the comrade support that is another anchor in their coping strategies.

In our studies of responses during the exposure, one research finding was that most of the variance in a person's cognitive, emotional and behavioural responses during exposure to extreme stress was his or her level of competence, i.e. the sum of education, training, exercises and real-life experiences (Weisæth, 1989). The functional element in competence was the application of skills in the critical situation. In a study that compared professionals and nonprofessionals involved in body handling in a mass death situation, the professionals (pathologists and police investigators) appeared to handle their stress by problem-focussed coping (U. F. Malt & L. Weisæth, unpublished data), i.e. the professional person is likely to use job skills and task orientation to cope. Few reported that they had to use energy to maintain their emotional control, very much in contrast to the nonprofessionals. Such findings may be of interest in studying the need for emotional ventilation afterwards, but the implications are not yet clear to us. High risk for traumatization for well-trained rescue professionals may be limited to situations where they have a heavy responsibility but fail to succeed in their rescue work. Difficult operations go wrong because rescue workers are unable to apply their full capacity for various reasons. In our practice we have seen up to 50% psychiatric morbidity in group 2 persons after such events. Dysfunctional factors included absence of operation preparedness, lack of group organization and efficient leadership, and scarcity of equipment. To be helpless in combination with heavy responsibilities in their role as rescuers appears to give rise to a high-risk cluster.

Comrade support

In trauma studies of persons who have been exposed to severe stress as members of groups, it seems to be a regular finding that talking to comrades is rated very highly, often on top of any scale (before spouse, group leader and professional helper). The explanation given is usually that 'talking to them is talking to someone who knows what it was like' (Weisæth, 1984). Like other social systems comrade groups provide: social support; emotional support; evaluative support in which the person is given feedback from the environment on how his or her behaviour is perceived; information support, practical advice and guidance on how problems at work can be solved; and instrumental support, direct help in carrying out a task.

Buddy aid has high availability, it is free and there is a need for referral. In contrast to the professional secrecy, the buddy has a secrecy based on general morale. A friend-to-friend relationship is based upon independence and has a mutual character with a divided responsibility for what takes part in the encounter (Dittman, 1999).

Group stress debriefing: from subjective experience to learning experience

Group stress debriefing, in the formal and modern manner, may be traced historically to the after-action interviews carried out by Brigadier General S. L. A.

Marshall when he studied the performance of American soldiers during World War II. When Marshall tried to get a coherent and complete picture of what had taken place during a battle by interviewing single soldiers he discovered, as have many trauma therapists, that the picture was very fragmented. Thus, he had the idea of having the soldiers talk to him in a group setting. Clearly, Marshall's interest as a historian was to establish the facts about the stressful event; he was not really interested in the emotional aspects or whether the establishment of a correct picture of what had happened would be helpful for the soldier (Shalev & Ursano, 1990).

In the absence of solid evidence that the various prescribed forms of GSD have preventive effects, thinking and practice has been directed more towards factors that make groups function well, and that seem to facilitate a rapid return to full capacity after particularly stressful events (Shalev, 1994). Hopefully, this procedure neutralizes risk factors for adverse developments. According to this view, the purpose of GSD is:

- To clarify misconceptions about the event and its consequences.
- To initiate communication about the event among the participants.
- To reinforce and deepen the learning experience.
- To strengthen group cohesion.
- To recognize and accept emotions and stress reactions.
- To facilitate grief work.
- To prepare the group for continued action.

Institutions such as the military, police force, etc. appreciate most of these goals, not the least the idea that talking in a group may increase the learning effect of an operative experience. Learning at the experimental level is a particularly intense way of internalizing aspects of reality. The processing that preferably should take place may be described as the transformation of a subjective experience to a learning experience (German: *Erlebnis zu Erfahrung*).

Stress management – a leadership responsibility

It is an old army principle that an officer's first concern should be the welfare of his men. Persons unfamiliar with military life will often be surprised at the extensive and basic care for personnel that military leadership includes: blisters, cold, wet clothes, lack of sleep, fatigue, nervousness, food, hot drinks, and hygiene are all of concern to the officer. Early signs of illness and injury are important for the commander's evaluation of a person's operational capacity. It is of course the front-line conditions of war that are the background for these traditions which have created a male leadership role which emphasizes also the nurturing, caring, fatherly role. Thus stress management is an important and integrated part of a basic and total care system. In the military, stress management is a leadership responsibility: in fact it is a very great part of the leadership, both before, during and after operations. The role of the medical corps, i.e. of the military health personnel in preventive psychiatry is essentially to motivate the organization and to help to train the soldiers in matters relating to traumatic stress. The commander as leader is central and the main strategy is to work through the officer in order to reach the personnel. There is an old principle saying, 'Don't get between a leader and his men'. Outside interventions are also likely to threaten basic leadership principles that are summarized as 'the three classical C's': control, command and communication. Most officers are very eager to improve their skills and appreciate advice. Considering what has been described above it should come as no surprise that advocating GSD has been an easy task at group level 1; GSD has for some time been a topic taught at Norwegian military academies. At one academy we had the skill-training component, i.e. the practice in leading GSD as a natural follow-up to the cadet's encounter with dead bodies at an institute of pathology, which is also a part of their regular training. Another training situation was 'the hell week' at the army ranger course.

If a professional leader, soldier, police officer or firefighter, is entrusted to lead operations in which he or she is responsible for matters of life and death to personnel, why should he or she not be trusted to be able to lead a group stress debriefing afterwards dealing with what they have gone through? The philosophy of modern leadership, emphasizing both instrumental and emotional aspects of leadership, is consistent with, indeed very much along the lines of GSD principles.

Prevention methods, such as forward psychiatry principles, are often recognized or 'discovered' when adaptive coping strategies are studied, in other words in studies of health maintenance rather than in studies of pathological mechanisms. Then the interventions are applied by health personnel, as the medical corps practised forward psychiatry during World War I.

Ideally, there should be a transfer of competence in the skills and strategies of prevention from health personnel to responsible leaders and those primarily affected. This is what happened with forward psychiatry; its principles became part of military leadership and part of comrade support. In our experiences with military and civilian group, levels 1 and 2, we find that group stress debriefing as an intervention method can go the same way. Furthermore, there are good reasons to assume that GSD has been practised by good leaders at all times, but probably in a less prescriptive form than, for example, Critical Incident Stress Debriefing (CISD).

One of the questions that remains unanswered is the timing of GSD in operations of long duration with more or less continuous or ongoing stress and few and brief breaks. Should GSD be applied during a pause or should it wait until the entire operation is over? Many professionals, including medical doctors and military personnel, have tasks where it is essential to be able to time correctly when to be instrumental and when to be empathic, and more in contact with one's own feelings and emotional reactions in others. Research has yet to shed light on regulating factors and the risks involved in trying to manipulate them when it comes to these kinds of long-lasting stress exposure.

The role of mental health professionals

We see a role of mental health professionals primarily in education and training of group levels 1 and 2 about traumatic stress and GSD whenever possible. In the absence of solid evidence that clinician-guided GSD is more effective than the peer group process we cannot readily recommend interventions from the outside. Some of the advantageous factors in cohesive groups are easily disturbed by external intrusion, for example the finely tuned balance in the relationship between the skilled leader and his group members. The presence of clinicians in a group process may misleadingly give the impression that the interventions are therapeutic. Acceptability is a *sine qua non* for the person who is responsible for GSD. A social worker who offered GSD to helicopter crews after a maritime disaster was rejected with the statement: 'We don't want to be pitied.' Other unintended effects of using clinicians may be that preventive work is seen as too difficult for the nonprofessional helper, and some leaders may be relieved of responsibility by calling in external experts. Furthermore, in principle we think that clinicians should be held in reserve for situations where the illness risk is high and not in the range usually seen in group levels 1 and 2. Clinicians are a scarce resource. At the least, high-risk groups should have the highest priority.

Over the last two decades however, the practice of GSD has been spreading with amazing speed. The method is usually advocated as an effective intervention to prevent the development of the syndromes in the post-traumatic stress spectrum, such as post-traumatic stress disorder and burnout. Mitchell & Everly (1995) emphasize that CISD is not to be considered equal to therapy. It appears, however, that CISD may be applied not only as a primary preventive method but as a secondary preventive method as well, since post-traumatic stress reactions of significant intensity are dealt with in the group when this debriefing is being carried out.

The rapid spread of a preventive intervention method to different cultures, countries and groups has been said to attest to its value (Dyregrov, 1997). But the same could be said about diazepam (Valium) in the 1960s. In spite of our somewhat expectant and critical attitude, it is interesting and in many ways promising that GSD as a method has been so acceptable as a way of facilitating talking in groups dominated by traditional male values. In our experience, however, the highly structured, prescriptive forms of GSD, while on the one hand providing the sense of predictability and control that such groups tend to value, may on the other hand violate the freedom of the individual group member to deal with themes of his or her experience, and responses to them, at his or her own tempo.

In general, the axiom of early intervention has to be challenged as long as there are insufficient data to support it in a convincing way, and even more so when professional health workers carry out the interventions and not lay people. For example, the value of catharsis is often taken for granted. For males, probably more than for women, when it come to GSD practice one has to ask whether strong emotional reactions are compatible with the sense of mastery of the situation. There are particular ways of dealing with emotions in particular subcultures, which was perhaps what Graham Greene hinted at with his term 'the military abbreviation of a smile'. It is true, however, that at times the military system has shown that it could not take the condition of a suffering soldier seriously unless there was a physical symptom, and that emotional repression was identified as the essence of manliness. In training group levels 1 and 2 in GSD we generally tend to be less prescriptive and to put less emphasis on the so-called 'emotional phase'. Furthermore, since these groups have often gone through a technical debriefing already, it is less important to spend much time on establishing a picture of what actually happened. The 'fact phase' is sometimes difficult because there may be harmful effects of disclosing all horrible aspects that only some of the group experienced. For example, when debriefing military helicopter crews it is important to realize that the cockpit personnel is a subgroup that may have had frightening experiences or information during a critical situation that the rest of the crew may not need to share. In such cases separate debriefing sessions should be held.

The essence of debriefing

As exemplified also in this chapter, most studies point to very general factors as being important when participants evaluate their experience of GSD. Being together in the same group, talking to colleagues, experiencing the fact that others had similar stress reactions as oneself, etc. are frequently reported (Ørner, 1996). At this point it may also be relevant to refer to research on psychiatric ward experiences which shows that patients often report as helpful aspects of the treatment programme that the clinicians do not value highly, and

that treatment regimens often turn out to reflect what the preferences of the therapists would have been, if *they* had had need of help.

In our work with GSD for group levels 1 and 2 we have gradually come to consider injury or threat to self-esteem as a crucial dimension that needs to be addressed in the GSD. This psychological problem is a natural reaction to failure, for whatever reason, to carry out an assignment in a successful way. This is the situation in which we find GSD is most needed. As already emphasized, GSD is a part of what is meant by leadership and the responsibility of the leader to take care of personnel.

To repair individual and team confidence is therefore an important task. In order to do that, the true picture of all the circumstances needs to be known, the 'what went wrong' needs to be acknowledged. Next, the acceptance that it did not go well, 'that it could not be done', is the main theme. This phase implies a cognitive reinterpretation of what happened. Much time is usually spent on working through the discrepancy between the expectancies created by their past experiences and the briefing, and what actually took place. According to general stress theory, this discrepancy is of course a very essential part of the stressor–stress response relationship.

The goal is to get the group to accept reality and that, everything considered, the group had done as well as it could. The emotional reactions of guilt and shame, because they are socially induced, are best dealt with in the social group situation that a GSD provides.

Finally, because the team did not function as it should in the failed operation, there is a sense of discontinuity or disruption of the team. To re-establish the team and its cohesiveness and identity is therefore important, and GSD is often helpful in this matter.

REFERENCES

Ahrenfeldt, R. H. (1958). *Psychiatry in the British Army in the Second World War.* London: Routledge & Kegan Paul.

Belenky, G., Marcy, S. C. & Martin, J. A. (1996). After action critical incident stress debriefings and battle reconstructions following combat. In J. A. Martin, L. Sparacino & G. Belenky

(Eds.) *The Gulf War and Mental Health: A Comprehensive Guide* (pp. 105–14). New York: Praeger Press.

Bisson, J. J. & Deahl, M. P. (1994). Psychological debriefing and prevention of post-traumatic stress. *British Journal of Psychiatry*, **165**, 717–20.

Burrrow, T. (1925). The group method of analysis. *Psychoanalytical Review*, **14**, 268–80.

Deahl, M., Gillham, A. B., Thomas, J. et al (1994). Psychological sequelae following the Gulf War. Factors associated with subsequent morbidity and the effectiveness of psychological debriefing. *British Journal of Psychiatry*, **165**, 60–65.

Dittmann, S. (1999) *Comrade Support: A Guide.* Oslo: HQ Defence Command Joint Medical Services, Department of Psychiatry.

Duck, S. (Ed.) (1988). *Handbook of Personal Relationships: Theory, Research and Interventions.* Chichester/New York: John Wiley.

Dyregrov, A. (1997). The process in psychological debriefings. *Journal of Traumatic Stress*, **10**, 589–605.

Englund, P. (1991). Om gråtens historie [The landscape of the past.] (pp. 221–61) [On the history of crying]. In *Förflutenhetens Landskap.* Stockholm: Atlantis.

Ersland, S., Weisæth, L. & Sund, A. (1989). The stress upon rescuers involved in an oil rig disaster. "Alexander L. Kielland" 1980. *Acta Psychiatrica Scandinavica*, **80**, Suppl. 355, 38–49.

Herlofsen, P. H. (1994). Group reactions to trauma: an avalanche accident. In R. J. Ursano, B. G. McCaughey & C. S. Fullerton (Eds.) *Individual and Community Responses to Trauma and Disaster: The Structure of Human Chaos* (pp. 248–66). Cambridge: Cambridge University Press.

Herlofsen, P. H. (1996). Group treatment in the aftermath of trauma. In E. L. Giller & L. Weisæth (Eds.) *Clinical Psychiatry: Post-Traumatic Stress Disorder* (pp. 315–28). London: Bailliere Tyndall.

Herman, J. C. (1992). *Trauma and Recovery.* New York, Basic Books.

Homer (reprinted 1991). *The Odyssey,* Book XV. Oxford: Oxford University Press.

Hytten, K. & Hasle, A. (1989). Fire fighters: a study of stress and coping. *Acta Psychiatrica Scandinavica* **80** (Suppl. 355), 50–5.

Main, T. F. (1946). Discussion: forward psychiatry in the Army. *Proceedings of the Royal Society of Medicine*, **39**, 140–2.

Main, T. (1989). The concept of the therapeutic community. In J. Johns (Ed.) *The Ailment and Other Psychoanalytic Essays by Tom Main* (pp. 123–41). London: Free Association Books.

Manning, F. J. & Ingraham, L. H. (1987). *An Investigation into the Calue of Unit Cohesion in Peacetime.* In G. Belenky (Ed.)

Contemporary Studies in Combat Psychiatry (pp. 47–67). New York: Greenwood Press.

Marshall, S. L. A. (1944). *Island Victory*, Harmondsworth, Middx: Penguin Books.

Mitchell, J. T. & Everly, G. S. (1995). *Critical Incident Stress Debriefing (CISD).* Ellicott City, MD: Chevron Publishing.

Ørner, R. (1996). Intervention strategies for emergency response groups: a new conceptual framework. In S. E. Hobfoll & M. W. de Vries (Eds.) *Extreme Stress and Communities: Impact and Intervention* (pp. 499–521). Dordrecht: Klüwer Academic Publishers.

Palmer, I. (1995). Response to treatment varies. [Letter.] *British Medical Journal*, **311**, 510.

Pratt, J. H. (1907). The class method of treating consumption in the homes of the poor. *Journal of the American Medical Association*, **49**, 755–9.

Raphael, B. (1996). Social re-integration and political action. In E. L. Gillet & L. Weisæth, (Eds.) *Clinical Psychiatry: Post-traumatic Stress Disorder* (pp. 329–51). Bailliere Tyndall, London.

Raphael, B., Meldrum, L. & McFarlane, A. C. (1995). Does debriefing after psychological trauma work? *British Medical Journal*, **310**, 1479–80.

Robinson, R. C. & Mitchell, J. T. (1993). Evaluation of psychological debriefings. *Journal of Traumatic Stress*, **6**, 367–82.

Rutter, M. & Rutter, M. (1993). *Developing Minds. Challenge and Continuity Across the Life Span.* Harmondsworth, Middx: Penguin Books.

Shalev, A. Y. (1994). Debriefing following traumatic exposure. In R. J. Ursano, B. G. McCaughey & C. S. Fullerton (Eds.) *Individual and Community Responses to Trauma and Disaster: The Structure of Human Chaos* (pp. 201–19). Cambridge: Cambridge University Press.

Shalev, A. Y. & Ursano, R. J. (1990). Group debriefing following exposure to traumatic stress. In J. E. Lundberg, U. Otto & B. Rybeck (Eds.) *Proceeding Wartime Medical Services.* (pp. 192–201). Stockholm: Forsvarets forskningsanstalt, FOA.

Shalit, B. (1988). *Konfliktens och stridens psykologi.* [The Psychology of Conflict and Combat.] Stockholm: Liber.

Summerfield, D. (1995). Debriefing after psychological trauma. Inappropriate exporting of Western culture may cause additional harm. *British Medical Journal*, **311**, 509.

Tyler, M. P. & Grifford, G. K. (1991). Fatal training accidents: the military unit as a recovery context. *Journal of Traumatic Stress*, **4**, 233–49.

von Achen, H. (1992). Det farlige liv. Middelalderens håndtering av lidelse, sykdom og død. [The dangerous life. Coping with suffering, illness and death in the medieval age]. In I.

Øye (Ed.) *Liv og helse i middelalderen* [Life and Health in the Medieval Age] (pp. 22–48). Bergen: Bryggen Museum.

Weisæth, L. (1984). *Stress Reactions to an Industrial Disaster*. Oslo: University of Oslo, Medical Faculty.

Weisæth, L. (1989). A study of behavioral response in an industrial disaster. *Acta Psychiatrica Scandinavica*, **80**, suppl. **355**, 13–24.

4

Theoretical perspectives of traumatic stress and debriefings

John P. Wilson and Melissa R. Sigman

EDITORIAL COMMENTS

In this chapter, Wilson and Sigman emphasize the complexity and diversity of responses to extreme events, and the need to take those factors into account. Debriefing they suggest is one of a spectrum of post-trauma interventions that may be encompassed in frameworks such as Critical Incident Stress Management, crisis intervention and many others. However, the focus in this chapter is on a thorough examination of the theoretical underpinning of all such interventions and indeed the critical and unanswered questions that this whole field generates. The authors describe a range of components from education to counselling in the response set of debriefings and see these as being on a spectrum that includes, or is linked to concepts such as crisis intervention. They also emphasize the need to define the conceptual pillars of debriefing, building on the experience of applying such techniques as well as any empirical findings. The more complex the situation the greater is the need for a 'complex decision-making protocol to design helpful interventions and identify the appropriate timing of these'. In the balance of the equation questions arise as to pathologizing the experience as opposed to facilitating true coping and resilience, and also the expectancies potentially raised by debriefing processes. They propose a person–environment interactional process in response to, and resolution of, trauma and that debriefing should be conceptualized within this framework.

Cognitive appraisal and coping style are influential. The authors list potentially traumatic events and the stressor components that may be embedded in these, and emphasize that some events contain multiple types of stressors that compound individuals' responses. A critical event matrix may enable the delineation of high-risk situations, high-risk reactions and high-risk persons. Furthermore, it could provide a framework for targeting specific components with modules of interventions, thus providing a focussed and potentially individualized response. Evaluation needs to take into account the components and their targeting and aims, for instance for death encounter, and loss, in traumatic bereavements. Timing, support, expression and education are such components in Mitchell's model, and goals might range from functioning to learning to prevention. This chapter is of great value in identifying the complexity of the individuals' experience in circumstances that lead to stressor and traumatic effects; it also emphasizes that there are multiple and variable stressor experiences, individuals and environments which will all influence response and outcome. The authors conceptualization of a matrix for decision-making for clinical or other interventions, for management and for research, can be helpful in taking this field forward. This is particularly relevant when many approaches have been inappropriately simplistic.

Finally, Wilson and Sigman conclude that events that are the subject of debriefings are often chaotic and ambiguous, making it even more difficult to organize an effective set of interventions. This is all the more reason for both qualitative and quantitative evaluations to be developed, and utilized in interagency and international contexts to allow appropriate development of conceptualization and research in this field of acute interventions. As Wilson and Sigman conclude, 'it is important to maintain an attitude of scientific enquiry ... one that is in keeping with the common sense and wisdom of clinical tradition'.

Introduction

Traumatic stressors and their consequences to human life are profound in terms of the depth of impact for psychic integration, ego-states and spiritual well-being. The acute and long-term effects of trauma for psychosocial functioning and life course development are diverse but include both pathological and non-pathological outcomes. Clearly, there is a spectrum of stress response syndromes (Wilson & Raphael, 1993) as well as of potential interventions that may facilitate the recovery and healing from the adverse effects of trauma and disaster (Raphael, 1986). The purpose of this chapter is to examine theoretically the concept of psychological debriefings as forms of intervention following exposure to traumatic stressors.

A theoretical framework for understanding the concept of psychological debriefings requires a complex model of the factors that affect the application of the social–psychological processes that define different types of debriefing. By definition, a debriefing refers to a form of follow-up to an event that has occurred. Afterwards, information is obtained by a person or group about the event itself. One of the semantic difficulties in using the term 'debriefing' and studying the efficacy of different applications of debriefing processes to traumatic events is that the words themselves have many possible connotations.

To begin, we must recognize that the term briefing is defined 'as a process to supply with all the pertinent instructions or information (e.g. to brief pilots before a flight)'. Thus a debriefing is a process of learning about that event for which a person or group was briefed. Clearly, there are many situations involving trauma and disaster for which individuals have not been briefed or prepared psychologically for the events which they subsequently encountered. Hence the term debriefing takes on a different meaning and qualitative nature in such situations. For example, in assisting persons who were the victims of a tornado that did not

allow for advanced warning and preparation, the disaster workers may provide aid, assistance, counselling and other forms of intervention, such as Critical Incident Stress Debriefing (CISD). Indeed, as noted by Mitchell and Everly (see Chapter 5) the term 'crisis intervention' often refers to a multicomponent process at different levels of individual, group or organizational functioning. In recognition of this fact, there has been an attempt to characterize the nature of the multicomponent elements that exist in different situations involving traumatic stress, disasters or other forms of stressful life-events. Moreover, the multicomponent elements of crisis intervention have implications for timing the on-set and off-set of the interventions, the length of the procedure or process, the degree of standardization or structure of the process, the criteria for deciding who should or should not participate in the intervention process, and the issues of follow-up and monitoring the effectiveness of the interventions employed. Everly & Mitchell (1997) made a useful attempt to review and reconceptualize the diversity of techniques and approaches under the rubric of Critical Incident Stress Management (CISM), a generic term that includes such processes and techniques as CISD, peer counselling, defusing, demobilization, community outreach or disaster intervention programmes, education about stress, trauma and disasters. Thus it may be seen that from the earliest thinking about crisis interventions and psychological debriefings (e.g. Lindemann, 1944; Caplan, 1964) to the present day controversies concerning the application of debriefings (Raphael et al., 1995), there has been an evolving knowledge base that has accumulated through practical need (e.g. disaster intervention), clinical insights (e.g. crisis intervention, counselling centres), programmatic efforts (e.g. CISM teams for trained duty responders such as emergency management teams, police, and firefighters), and empirical studies of debriefing procedures during or after a disaster.

As with any scientific body of knowledge, there are areas in which empirical and clinical data are conflicting, contradictory or simply missing from the extant literature. Clearly, this is the case when it comes to understanding and critically evaluating the efficacy of psychological debriefings. On the one hand, there are studies such as that of Everly & Boyle (1997) in which a meta-analysis of five published studies from 1991 to 1997 revealed a beneficial effect of CISDs. These five studies involved different types of traumatic events (e.g. ferry sinking, mass shooting, hurricane, urban riots, etc.). The studies measured stress, post-traumatic stress disorder (PTSD), depression, a broad range of psychiatric symptoms and anxiety reactions. The statistical analysis generated significant effects for the debriefing procedure. On the other hand, Raphael et al. (1995) have raised important questions about whether such interventions are appropriate because they are short term in nature and do not tell us whether the procedures facilitate or impede the naturally occurring processes of healing and recovery.

In order to build a generic and comprehensive model of psychological debriefings, many factors must be incorporated into the structure. This chapter attempts to identify the core elements and mechanisms that serve as the strata resting underneath the phenomena of post-traumatic psychological debriefings. This is not an easy task because the phenomena of disasters, critical events and traumatic stressors are multidimensional in nature. Consideration of critical interventions thus becomes as complex and complicated as the events themselves. Clearly, it cannot be assumed uncritically that one type of debriefing or psychological intervention will be appropriate to all situations, nor that such situations may or may not warrant a form of individual or group process to provide aid and assistance. Therefore, in an attempt to specify the factors required for a theoretical model of debriefings, we do not subscribe to or endorse, any particular model that has been developed in recent decades. Rather, references are made to those models, developed from applied experiences by their adherents, that appear to be a part of the larger set of factors making up the conceptual pillars of the debriefing processes.

The next section of this chapter presents a critical event matrix analysis of psychological debriefings, i.e. a set of factors that can be placed into a conceptual matrix to identify the mechanisms, processes and factors germane to understanding the potential effects of debriefings and various types of intervention. However, before presenting these dimensions for discussion, it is useful to examine questions that confront clinicians, researchers and specialists who work in the field of traumatic stress and those interested in the phenomena of post-traumatic interventions.

Some critical questions concerning debriefings

In what situations are short-term or brief interventions appropriate or inappropriate?

When does an intervention such as a debriefing facilitate or impede in the normal stress response recovery process?

What are the range, form and processes of debriefings and interventions that are applicable to the diversity of stressful events?

What methods and techniques should be used to assess and monitor the outcome of debriefing processes?

What criteria define a successful debriefing?

What criteria determine whether the form of intervention should be used at the individual, group or cultural level?

How does the magnitude (e.g. small catastrophic) and complexity (e.g. single event – multistressor components) influence the nature and type of intervention procedures?

What are the criteria that define standards of care in debriefing?

What types of assessment procedure and psychometric measure should be used in outcome studies?

How does one identify persons, reactions and situations that constitute significant risk for adverse effects of exposure to traumatic events?

What does exposure to death and bereavement mean in terms of acute or long-term effects and what types of intervention help or hinder the processes of adaptation following traumatic bereavement?

What are the implicit assumptions about the need for debriefings and interventions?

Are persons assumed to develop stress-related pathologies or does human resilience suggest alternative formulations on the nature and type of intervention, if any at all is necessary?

Linking briefings and debriefings after trauma

Weisæth (1995), in an important contribution on the role of debriefings and the prevention of long-term adverse consequences of traumatic stress exposure, noted that the concept of debriefings must be connected to an antecedent set of events. However, it is often the case in disasters and other forms of trauma that there are no 'briefings' for what has transpired to adversely impact on the lives of the survivors or victims. This fact is most important since natural and technological disasters, genocidal warfare, terrorist activities and other traumatic events often contain multiple stressors that are frequently unpredictable, chaotic and random in nature. Further, the complexity and multiplicity of such experiences produce a broad range of emotional impacts on the psyches of the survivors. As observed by Smith & North (1993), such disasters often contain horrific sensory and perceptual experiences, which may later haunt the survivor with PTSD, anxiety or depressive states. When considering what should constitute a helpful debriefing intervention, the diversity of needs must therefore be considered in terms of psychological triage. Clearly, not all survivors will require the same type or degree of assistance. In that sense, complex, multistressor disasters or critical incidents require a complex decision-making protocol to design helpful interventions and to identify the appropriate timing of these.

To state the problem of linking briefings to post-event debriefings somewhat differently, the attempt to establish a one-to-one, before and after connection with implications for intervention, runs the risk of oversimplifying what may be enormously complex circumstances defining the nature of the traumatic event. In this regard, the issue of debriefing is conceptually less useful than such questions as:

1. What interventions are immediately useful to promote coping and the nonpathological stress response sequence?
2. What types of emotional difficulties can be anticipated post event and planned for accordingly?
3. What types of psychological assessments and empirical measures should be used to assess state or risk and protective factors, if any?
4. What are the phasic differences in symptom manifestation and coping patterns among the survivors and rescue responders.
5. Does 'too much' intervention effort, even if well intentioned, potentially compound a complicated event by adding secondary stressors?
6. Are there multiple critical periods in which particular interventions have their most specific effects?
7. How can survivors or rescuers mobilize peer-based support to promote resiliency and healing from within the group rather than by outside interventions?

Above and beyond these considerations are the well-known factors inherent in crisis interventions, which include timing of commencement of intervention, duration, frequency of contact, intensity of the process for individuals or groups, expectancies and voluntary versus nonvoluntary participation, and appropriateness or otherwise of the conceptual basis of intervention. Finally, the context or milieu of the debriefing relates significantly to the expectancies imparted in the process. Since traumatic events, disasters and critical incidents are part of the everyday reality of human experience, pathologizing the expected nature of the stress response sequence may not be as helpful as facilitating positive coping and resilience. By definition, a debriefing or crisis intervention is a short-term social–psychological process and not a form of long-term treatment. As will be discussed later, the recognition of this fact can then lead to 'targeted' interventions derived from a critical event matrix analysis for a traumatic situation. However, the issues of the appropriateness and effectiveness of these still remain.

The spectrum of interventions

The issue of the link between briefing and debriefings points to the need to delineate further the spectrum of interventions that are possible after a traumatic event. As noted by Mitchell and Everly (Chapter 5), psychological debriefings anchor one end of the spectrum of interventions that are possible. At the other end are other forms of intervention that include community-based services, governmental and nongovernmental assistance, grass-roots action-planning committees, consultative reviews, special programmes of children and families, school-based crisis management programmes, specialized post-traumatic counselling programmes, educational programmes, specialized bereavement counselling and traditional psychotherapy. As reviewed by Raphael (1986) and Horowitz (1986), the overall goal of intervention efforts is to facilitate a working through of the stressful event at both the individual and community level in order to promote integration, stabilization and healthy coping. Moreover, in the larger context of the spectrum of interventions, a theoretical model can also encompass the idea of systematic interagency planning and cooperation to coordinate targeted interventions. Wilson (1995) has written on the possible models of interagency networking in order to promote pro-active planning of different types of preventative and intervention strategies. Thus, considering the spectrum of interventions that can be employed after a traumatic event or disaster situation, the concept of debriefing takes on a more robust meaning as a component of these rather than simply a short-term intervention process (Ursano et al., 1996).

The issue of delineating the spectrum of interventions after a traumatic experience has other implications at the clinical, applied and research levels. First, what practice guidelines are necessary to provide a consistent standard of care within the field? Secondly, what is the most accountable dissemination vehicle for the practice guidelines? Thirdly, what types of research study are needed to monitor the quality and effectiveness of different interventions?

A theoretical framework for traumatic stress and psychological debriefings: a person–environment model of traumatic reactions

A theoretical framework for understanding the applications of psychological debriefings is, of necessity, multidimensional as well as interactional in nature. A person–environment interaction model (Aronoff & Wilson, 1985; Wilson, 1989) is a useful way to specify and explain how person variables (e.g. personality, age, intelligence, defensive styles, traits, etc.) influence the reactions and cognitive processing of traumatic events. Wilson (1989) has presented in detail an interactional paradigm of post-traumatic stress syndromes. Implicit in this model are multiple interaction effects between situational variables (e.g. stressor events, dimension of trauma, experienced nature of trauma, the structure of trauma in terms of complexity, post-traumatic events and sequelæ) and person variables, which determine the patterns of individual subjective responses and adaptation to traumatic experiences. A person–environment interactional model is quite useful when conceptualizing the application of debriefings to traumatic events. Traumatic events are not equivalent; they vary along many dimensions and contain different types of stressor (Green, 1993) that have differential impacts on people. Traumatic events are appraised and processed differently by people who vary in cognitive style and ego-defences. Clearly, there are different appraisals, perceptions and attribution made by people to the same traumatic event. Cognitive processes occur during and after the termination of a traumatic event and vary along such dimensions as perceptual denial or avoidance, perceptual and cognitive distortion, degrees of accurate appraisal, use of dissociative processes and the level of intrusive overload present in traumatic memory.

The interaction between person and situation variables implies that the post-event information processing (e.g. recall, memory, sensory-perceptual encoding of stressor phenomena, sense of chronology of experience, etc.) will be distributed statistically among those involved in the traumatic event. A clear implication of this model is that, whatever the form of debriefing or other intervention, there will be expectable degrees of diversity among the reactions reported by the participants. However, the more uniform, specific, discrete and limited are the stressors comprising the nature of the trauma, the greater is the expected degree of similarity in reported reactions to that experience.

A person–environment interactional model of traumatic events also specifies the typologies of traumatic events and stressor dimensions that are experienced directly or indirectly by a person (Wilson, 1995). Tables 4.1 and 4.2 illustrate these typologies.

Table 4.1. A typology of traumatic events

- Childhood abuse
- Domestic and family violence
- War trauma and civil violence
- Natural disasters
- Technological, industrial, toxic disasters
- Political oppression, torture, internment
- Duty-related trauma (police, fire, rescue workers)
- Mass genocide, holocaust
- Physical illness, terminal disease trauma
- Occupational, workplace trauma
- Traumatic loss, bereavement
- Anomalous trauma

Table 4.1 classifies 12 distinct types of potentially traumatic events and Table 4.2 classifies five distinct dimensions of stressors that may be typically embedded in a traumatic event. At the core of traumatic stressor dimensions are threats, injuries or exposures that pose a risk to self, others, physical integrity, the biosphere and the built environment. Further, it is possible that some types of traumatic event contain multiple types of stressor that may intensify, compound and make more severe an individual's reactions and problems of adaptation following the event. In constructing a theoretical framework for debriefing models of intervention, therefore, it must be recognized that there is broad range of complexity to traumatic events and their impact on individual well-being. Similarly, there are differences in individual subjective responses to the threshold levels of stressors. Some people are more vulnerable than others to distressing psychological impacts at lower threshold levels. Conversely, there are resilient people who can tolerate relatively high levels of stressor impact without adverse impacts on functioning (Wilson, 1995).

Moreover, a person–environment model specifies that there will be a critical event matrix that comprises high-risk situations, high-risk reactions and high-risk persons (Weisæth, 1995). Thus, using typological classification of traumatic events and the trauma-specific stressors embedded within them, an interactional theoretical framework allows for the construction of a critical event matrix which, of course, subsumes a capacity to scale threshold levels with categories for determining high-risk situations, persons and reaction patterns to trauma.

As applied to psychological debriefings, the complexity of traumatic situations along the dimensions discussed above could lead to research studies that not only generate information about the critical event matrix and its properties but also produce information about (1) what types of debriefings are useful, (2) for what types of persons, (3) under what situations, and (4) at what point in time after the event. Stated differently, all crisis interventions are targeted processes designed to assist those who have experienced a crisis, traumatic event or a disaster. From the perspective of a critical event matrix for risk assessment, targeted interventions such as debriefings should be adaptive and flexible enough to meet the particular needs of those involved in the stressful life experience. Similar to the concept of trauma-specific behavioural manifestations in PTSDs, psychological debriefings ideally would be target-specific interventions that comprise modules that could be tailored and adapted to the unique demands characterising a given event requiring a debriefing mechanism.

Table 4.2. Traumatic stressor dimension: direct or indirect experience and impact to the self

- Threat or injury to self, personality, identity and physical integrity
- Threat or injury to others that is witnessed directly or indirectly
- Threat or injury to physical integrity, bodily function or health
- Threat or injury to the earth, biosphere, the built or modified environment, which is experienced directly, witnessed as a bystander, or afterwards at or near the location
- Threat, traumatic bereavement/loss or injury to personal relationships, attachments and social networks of personal significance

Similarities and differences in traumatic events and stressor impacts

It is a truism to say that traumatic events are differentiated from each other on the basis of the stressor dimensions that define them. As noted above, stressor impacts may occur at individual, group or community levels. Stressor events can be categorized in many different ways: type of event; duration; frequency; severity; level of injury or damage produced to persons and the environment; potential for re-occurrence; social-psychological, societal and cultural changes produced by the event; short versus long-term consequences to health, well-being and stability of the social fabric, and so on. Green (1993), in a similar analysis, proposed eight generic dimensions of trauma: (1) threat to life or limb, (2) severe physical harm or injury, (3) recept of intentional injury/harm, (4) exposure to the grotesque, (5) violent/sudden loss of a loved one, (6) witnessing or learning of violence to a loved one, (7) learning of exposure to a noxious agent, and (8) causing death or severe harm to another. When applied to the analysis of stress debriefings, it becomes apparent that these dimensions may be crossed in a matrix to compare a set of issues of consideration in planning for a particular debriefing situation. For example, ongoing genocide in places such as Bosnia or Cambodia during the Pol Pot regime contained stressor experiences that were prolonged, severe, frequent with a high potential for reoccurrence, and produced social, political and cultural changes. Further, all eight of Green's (1993) generic stressor dimensions were in evidence to varying degrees. When one is reviewing a form of debriefing, therefore, there are clearly multiple considerations in terms of who is being targeted for a psychological debriefing from the perspective of the critical event matrix analysis. A related issue as regards who receives a debriefing is the question of the timing of the intervention. As is well known in the development of PTSDs (Wilson & Raphael, 1993), there may be immediate (acute), delayed or long-term effects to traumatic exposure. Thus, in terms of models of debriefings, assessment needs to be made of the proper timing of the intervention to achieve maximally effective results. In related ways, research should sample the severity of reactions and benefits or adverse effects of debriefing interviews to determine the pathways, patterning and resolution of stress-related symptoms at a given time post event.

The confrontation with death

While it is the case that traumatic events differ from each other in terms of stressor dimensions, special attention should be placed on critical incidents that involve a death encounter (Raphael, 1986). A recent study (Robinson et al., 1997) found that, among trained professional responders, exposure to situations involving a death encounter rated as the most stressful and disturbing type of event to which they had responded in the line of duty. Further, in terms of predicting PTSD symptoms, this factor had the highest value in a statistical regression analysis. Similarly, in his seminal writings on Hiroshima. Lifton, (1993) coined the term 'death immersion' to characterize the survivors' depiction of the ultimate horrors witnessed after the atomic bomb that exploded and destroyed the city of Hiroshima. Clearly, the confrontation with death and dying not only conveys images and experiences that form the basis of traumatic memories, but it also attacks human vulnerability that is normally protected by healthy ego-defences.

A model of debriefings needs to specify the risk factors associated with death encounters, for such experiences have complexity to them as well. Images, such as the dead in Cambodia, Rwanda, Bosnia and Hiroshima speak to the widespread impact of genocide and/or ethnic cleansing. Natural and technological disasters, such as the explosion of TWA flight 800 killing all on board, leave traumatic imprints to survivor families and rescue workers who handle the body parts, debris and personal belongings of the victims. Further, death encounters may lead to traumatic bereavement (Raphael &d Martinek, 1997), which may require special forms of intervention either in the wake of the trauma or at a later time. For example, a recent study found that trauma associated with the unexpected death of a loved one had long-term consequences for the experience of mourning. It was also found that in some cases of traumatic bereavement there were long-term effects to identity as well as symptoms of PTSD and a complicated bereavement cycle. Considering these results, it may be that any 'debriefing' initially should address issues of post-traumatic reactions associated with trauma related to the loss, and that later interventions should be focussed to help to process the experience of mourning. The complexity of traumatic bereavement points to the interrelationship between trauma and bereavement and the importance of carefully timed interventions to assist the survivor most effectively.

Criteria for defining a successful debriefing

A theoretical model of debriefing also needs to specify as clearly as possible the criteria for defining a successful procedure. An implicit assumption made by those who extol the virtues of debriefings is that they help victims or rescuers to ventilate emotions and begin a process of sharing information about the stressful event, which may have short- and long-term salutary effects for mental health and well-being. While verbal reports about the efficacy of a debriefing may be of value, they cannot always be accepted at face value, since some participants in the debriefing may not disclose personal concerns, stress reactions or symptoms in the wake of a traumatic event for several reasons including social pressure to say desirable things about the debriefing or owing to avoidance, numbing and emotional constriction in the early period after the event. Criteria defining a successful debriefing must therefore determine a set of common measures (criteria) that could be applied across different stressful events to ascertain which mechanisms worked best for the participants.

Everly & Mitchell (1997), after a review of the literature, proposed a five-stage model that is useful in terms of identifying the parameters that should be considered: (1) stabilization of the situation, (2) acknowledgement of the crisis or stressful event and its impact on self and others, (3) facilitating understanding, and (4) homeostatic functioning. Further, in their model of CISM they identified four factors as fundamental to crisis response: early intervention, psychosocial sup-

port, opportunity for expression, and education (Everly & Mitchell, 1997, p. 71).

These four factors are useful to a theoretical model of debriefings, since they are dimensions for which outcome criteria could be developed. For example, early intervention post event implies a time-from-event dimension. So, what criteria define success at early, middle and later time? Similarly, psychosocial support may have multiple connotations. Should support be at the individual or group level and for how long? And by what types of technique of intervention (e.g. peer counselling, one-to-one counselling, eye movement desensitization and reprocessing catharsis, etc.)? Moreover, it is both logical and sensible that opportunities for expression and educational learning about such phenomena as PTSD and normal reactions to abnormal events is potentially palliative. But what criteria define opportunities for expression? Is it one session, ten sessions or the ability to access mental health resources at a self-determined place? Finally, while education about reactions to traumatic events appears helpful, which criteria define what is educational and what is not in the context of debriefing situations? What 'education' may in fact 'educate' people provided with it to develop symptoms of PTSD, as opposed to a process of recovery? Is there the possibility of creating standardized training modules that could be employed in a common way that would allow more precise evaluations to be made?

The issue of establishing criteria for defining a successful or unsuccessful debriefing is more than theoretical. To advance the knowledge base on debriefings, it is important to attempt to delineate the relative criteria – create operational measures and/or definitions that then can be employed in research studies using different methodological approaches to address hypotheses in carefully constructed research studies (e.g. quasi-experimental, longitudinal and epidemiological). Finally, attempting to determine criteria for evaluating the efficacy of a debriefing is related to the goals that are established for a particular situation. Clearly, goals may vary depending on organizational priorities. Weisæth (1995, p. 315), in his review, listed ten goals that are common to debriefings: (1) make group ready for the next task; (2) strengthen and deepen learning from the event; (3) clarify misconceptions of the event and its consequences; (4) recognize, accept and discuss connected feelings and other stress reactions; (5) reduce symptomatology that can produce long-lasting stress disorder, burnout, illness and behaviour disturbance; (6) identify persons at risk; (7) encourage and inform participants about where to turn if they need help; (8) increase participants' ability to help each other; (9) facilitate mourning and grief work; and (10) improve communication among participants.

The criteria for determining the efficacy of debriefing may be directly tied to the goals, which are defined for the situation. Some goals may have a higher priority and sense of urgency than others. For example, preparing a military combat unit for its next tactical operation may be more important than facilitating mourning and grief of a fellow soldier. In contrast, a United Nations (UN) health professional in Bosnia or Rwanda who has witnessed mass killing, illness and destruction may be at risk for burnout or PTSD and may need to ventilate personal feelings about his or her immersion into scenes of death and destruction in order to prepare for the next task or assignment. As noted by Weisæth (1995), there is a small but informative set of studies of high-risk persons, high-risk groups, high-risk situations and high-risk reactions that have been identified for traumatic events. For example, a high-risk person maybe one who is younger or who has a history of premorbid psychopathology or previous exposure to trauma. A high-risk situation often has multiple stressors and exposure to death, injury or threat to physical integrity. Similarly, high-risk reactions were found by Holen (1993) in a study of a North Sea oil rig disaster in which reactions such as cognitive impairment at the time of the event were more strongly associated with the development of PTSD symptoms. A theoretical model of debriefing must incorporate dimensions of risk (situations, reaction, persons and groups) and attempt to specify how these factors are part of a critical event matrix of debriefings within a person–situation interactional model. A further question arises as to where debriefing sits in respect of other interventions in such trauma contexts.

The diversity of traumatic events

As noted earlier in this chapter, traumatic events contain specific types of stressor experience. In that regard, there is a type of nonequivalence between traumatic phenomena and how each person perceives and processes the event. A theoretical model of psychological debriefings connected to extreme stress experiences needs to recognize these differences and somehow incorporate them into a critical event matrix analysis of debriefings. For example, the Everly & Mitchell (1997) model of debriefings was originally developed for paramilitary or highly cohesive small-group emergency responders. Yet, other critical incident events range from natural and technological disasters to mass genocide (Raphael, 1986; Wilson & Raphael, 1993). Military trauma is also a focus of debriefing (Solomon & Shalev, 1995). Further, there are single event critical incidents (e.g. a hotel fire, personal assault; motor vehicle accidents, etc.) that differ qualitatively in nature from those in terms of the victims' response as well as the requirements of the responders to provide assistance. A complex theoretical model of debriefings must therefore specify the quantitative and qualitative differences between events requiring debriefings and how the nature of the traumatic event, in a sense, dictates the targeted interventions that may be required to aid those in need of assistance, either as a direct victim or as a responder.

Conclusion

It must be recognized and understood that traumatic events, disasters and critical incidents are very often chaotic situations of enormous confusion, ambiguity and difficulty in organizing an effective set of interventions. At the level of the responder or practitioner, there is nearly always a sense of urgency to be helpful, compassionate and competent in delivering assistance to those in need. An obvious implication of this reality is that any model (theoretical or procedural) must be flexible enough to identify, accommodate and execute interventions that attempt to deal with the idiosyncratic nature of each critical incident event. While it is important for theoretical models to guide research and inform policy decisions, it is equally important for such models to guide researchers and practitioners as to the complexities that are consequential to the ultimate well-being of the clients being served. An obvious implication of this position, given current controversies in the field about the status of debriefings (Raphael et al., 1995) is that it is important to maintain an attitude of scientific enquiry towards debriefings, in keeping with the common sense and wisdom of clinical tradition. In this regard, the dearth of comprehensive, coordinated efforts to move systematically in scientific and applied ways to address the critical questions of the field is no longer a choice. Coordinated, programmatic efforts, within a sound and critical grounding embedded within a theoretical framework, are necessities for advancement of theory, research and application. If nothing else, lessons from the past 50 years have taught us that trauma and debriefings will always be interlinked. We have a natural propensity to process that which disturbs the soul, injures the self and damages our communities and social networks. The evolution and use of good psychological debriefings may be the twenty-first century equivalent to vaccinations. However, to know how useful and effective these 'psychological vaccinations' could be is unknown at present, nor has there been any adequate scientific consideration of their potential for adverse effects. Nevertheless, it is imperative to move beyond polemical debates and establish constructive interagency and international dialogue to advance the core questions confronting the field of traumatic stress. Understanding the mechanisms, processes, applications and utility of conducting interventions, and these include debriefings, after traumatic events will broaden the spectrum of knowledge and make informed choice possible for the greatest good for those who suffer from traumatic exposure.

REFERENCES

Aronoff, T. & Wilson, J. P. (1985). *Personality in the Social Process*. Hillsdale, NJ: Earlbaum.

Caplan, G. (1964). *Principles of Preventive Psychiatry*. New York: Basic Books.

Everly, G. S. & Boyle, S. (1997). A meta-analysis of the critical incident stress debriefing (CISD). Paper presented to the 4th World Congress on Stress, Trauma and Coping in the Emergency Services Professions, Baltimore, MD.

Everly, G. S. & Mitchell, J. T. (1997). *Critical Incident Stress Management (CISM): A New Era and Standard of Care in Crisis Intervention*. Ellicott City, MD: Chevron Publishing.

Green, B. (1993). Identifying survivors at risk: trauma and stressors across events. In J. P. Wilson & B. Raphael (Eds.) *International Handbook of Traumatic Stress Syndromes* (pp. 135–44). New York: Plenum Press.

Holen, A. (1993). The North Sea oil rig disaster. In J. P. Wilson & B. Raphael (Eds.) *International Handbook of Traumatic Stress Syndromes* (pp. 471–8). New York: Plenum Press.

Horowitz, M. J. (1986). *Stress-Response Syndromes*, 2nd edn. New York: Jason Aronson.

Lifton, R. J. (1993). From Hiroshima to the Nazi doctors: the evolution of psycho-formative approaches to understanding traumatic stress syndromes. In J. P. Wilson & B. Raphael (Eds.) *International Handbook of Traumatic Stress Syndromes* (pp. 11–24). New York: Plenum Press.

Lindemann, E. (1944). Symptomatology and management of acute grief. *American Journal of Psychiatry*, **101**, 141–8.

Raphael, B. (1986). *When Disaster Strikes: How Individuals and Communities Cope with Catastrophe*. New York: Basic Books.

Raphael, B. & Martinek, N. (1997). Assessing traumatic bereavements and PTSD. In J. P. Wilson & T. M. Keane (Eds.) *Assessing Psychological Trauma and PTSD* (pp. 373–95). New York: Guilford Press.

Raphael, B., Meldrum, L. & McFarlane, A. C. (1995). Does debriefing after psychological trauma work? *British Medical Journal*, **310**, 1479–80.

Robinson, R., Sigman, M. & Wilson, J. (1997). Duty-related stressors and PTSD symptoms in suburban police officers. *Psychological Report*, **81**, 835–45.

Smith, E. M. & North, C. S. (1993). Post-traumatic stress disorder in natural disaster and technological accident. In J. P. Wilson & B. Raphael (Eds.) *International Handbook of Traumatic Stress Management* (pp. 395–46). New York: Plenum Press.

Solomon, Z. & Shalev, A. (1995). Helping victims of military trauma. In J. Freedy & S. Hobfoll (Eds.). *Traumatic Stress* (pp. 241–61). New York: Plenum Press.

Ursano, R. J., Greiger, T. P. & McCarroll, J. E. (1996). Prevention of post-traumatic stress: consultation, training and early treatment. In B. A. van der Kolk, A. C. McFarlane & L. Weisaeth (Eds.) *Traumatic Stress: Effects of Overwhelming Experience on Mind, Body and Society* (pp. 441–63). New York: Guilford Press.

Weisæth, L. (1995). Disaster: risk and preventive intervention.

In B. Raphael & G. Burrows (Eds.) *Handbook of Studies on Preventive Psychiatry* (pp. 301–2). Amsterdam: Elsevier Science B. V.

Wilson, J. P. (1989). *Trauma, Transformation and Healing.* New York: Brunner/Mazel.

Wilson, J. P. (1995). Traumatic events and post-traumatic stress disorder and prevention. In B. Raphael & G. Burrows (Eds.) *Handbook of Studies on Preventive Psychiatry.* Elsevier Science B.V.

Wilson, J. P. & Raphael, B. (Eds.) (1993). *International Handbook of Traumatic Stress Syndromes.* New York: Plenum Press.

PART II

Debriefing: models, research and practice

5

Critical Incident Stress Management and Critical Incident Stress Debriefings: evolutions, effects and outcomes

Jeffrey T. Mitchell and George S. Everly Jr

EDITORIAL COMMENTS

Mitchell and Everly present a comprehensive review and update of their seminal and broadly applied model of Critical Incident Stress Debriefing, which they describe as a 'crisis intervention component of Critical Incident Stress Management: a comprehensive, integrated and multi-component crisis intervention system'. In defining debriefing in this context the authors emphasize its linkage as one of crisis intervention to other conceptualizations of this kind, and as but one component of a spectrum of potential trauma-related interventions. The components of critical incident stress management include preincident education/mental preparedness training, individual crisis intervention, support/on-scene support, demobilization after disaster or large-scale events, defusing, critical incident stress debriefing, significant other support services for families and children, and follow-up services and professional referrals as necessary.

Mitchell and Everly emphasize the model as a response system for the prevention and management of stress experienced by emergency response personnel and one implemented through and with the support of their organizations. In this context the model is reported to be effective in reducing stress, returning workers rapidly to functioning after exposure to critical incidents, and at times as reducing symptomatology afterwards.

One of the difficulties that arises, Mitchell and Everly acknowledge, is the confusion over terms and the failure of methodologies to evaluate their specific model of debriefing in the situation for which it was developed

(i.e. emergency services) and as part of a comprehensive stress management/crisis intervention framework. Nevertheless, they report on a number of studies specifically relevant to their model that support positive outcomes for it in a number of contexts.

Unfortunately, much of this material is not widely available and, as they acknowledge, as for negative outcome studies, there is a need for greater methodological rigour. The sum of these studies suggests a high level of perceived helpfulness and positive perception by personnel of the provision of such an overarching programme in terms of their organization's commitment, beneficial effects in terms of decreased sick days and staff turnover, positive experiences for staff, and decreased symptom reports for some who have received it.

As the authors suggest stronger, systematic analysis of these and other findings, with critical appraisal of their focus, populations and methodological limitations, could contribute further to this field. Although the authors systematically outline many components that are seen in the crisis intervention mode, the relative effectiveness or otherwise of their intervention system in addressing each of these is not yet defined. Nevertheless, their work in the field leads them to conclude that their model is valuable and effective in the emergency service settings for which it was developed.

Mitchell, as the person who, more than any other, has pioneered the debriefing movement, is now in an ideal position to contribute to a collaborative and critical scientific approach. This can bring together experience, practice, passion and science to respond effectively to the range of stressors that critical incidents bring, both to emergency services and to the broader community. Debriefing, bred out of the altruistic response to human suffering, is strong enough to sustain such appraisal and can only benefit from such advances. As Mitchell and Everly conclude 'no single study starts out as the last word in CISM'. This approach is complex, and should be utilized and evaluated, as it was intended, as a multicomponent intervention strategy, and be neither provided nor studied simplistically.

Introduction

For anyone who plays the game of golf, it would be unreasonable to attempt to play a round using only one golf club. The game requires the skilful use of numerous and functionally diverse golf clubs to meet effectively the challenge of the course.

Similarly, for those who practice the specialty of crisis intervention, it would be unreasonable to attempt to intervene amidst the complexities of a psychological crisis using only one form of crisis intervention technology, for example only debriefings. Rather, intervention in a psychological crisis requires the skilful use of numerous and functionally diverse crisis intervention technologies to meet effectively the challenge represented by the acute psychological crisis.

Mitchell and Everly have pioneered the use of a comprehensive, integrated and multicomponent crisis intervention system referred to as Critical Incident Stress Management (CISM). In this chapter, the comprehensive CISM system is described and reviewed.

Historical foundations of CISM

From a historical perspective, the provision of emergency psychological care has most often been referred to as crisis intervention. Indeed, crisis intervention is sometimes thought of as emotional first-aid (Neil et al., 1974).

In order to understand better the nature of crisis intervention, let us first offer a working definition of a psychological crisis. As the body struggles to maintain a physical homeostasis, or steady state, so the mind struggles to maintain a similar balance. A psychological crisis is a condition wherein the individual's psychological balance has been disrupted. There is, in effect, a psychological disequilibrium. More practically speaking, a crisis may be defined as a state of emotional turmoil wherein one's usual coping mechanisms have failed in the face of a perceived challenge or threat. Caplan (1969) denoted two types of crises: developmental and situational. Developmental crises are those associated with growing up and living through life's span (birth, childhood, adolescence, young adulthood, middle age, and old age and death). Situational crises are those which occur along the course of life (illness, accidents, disasters, threat, loss, grief, etc.).

Once we have developed an understanding of the nature of crisis, the goals of crisis intervention become more apparent. The goals of crisis intervention should include assisting the person in a crisis to return to a more steady state of psychological functioning (i.e. psychological homeostasis). Practically speaking, the primary goal of crisis intervention is to assist the person in returning to an adaptive level of independent functioning that approximates to the precrisis level of adaptation. At the very least, the goal of crisis intervention is a stabilization of acute symptomatology. The focus of crisis intervention is always the present crisis condition as opposed to past crises and/or chronic contributing factors (Caplan, 1964; Neil et al., 1974; Parad, 1996).

Among the first to systematically enquire into crisis intervention was Edward Stierlin (1909), who investigated the psychological aftermath of a major European mining disaster in 1906. Later, T. W. Salmon (1919) made a significant contribution to the literature via his recollections and analyses of psychiatric emergencies during World War I. From his work and that of Kardiner & Spiegel (1947), the three principles of crisis intervention – proximity, immediacy and expectancy – were derived.

Many modern writers point to Eric Lindemann's (1944) account of the Coconut Grove nightclub fire in 1943, in which 492 people lost their lives, as the beginning of modern crisis intervention theory and practice. He was later joined by Caplan and established the first crisis intervention centre in the USA and together they more clearly defined the nature of crisis intervention theory and practice.

By the mid 1950s Schneidman & Faberow (1957) were pioneering suicide prevention programmes based on crisis intervention theory and practice. They created a prototype for suicide prevention centres throughout the USA by their work in the Los Angeles area.

In the 1960s and 1970s there was a proliferation of walk-in clinics and telephone hotlines. The aim in the delivery of some of the mental health services by community mental health centres had shifted to a prevention-oriented crisis intervention format. The use of paraprofessionals was becoming widespread. Non-directive, client-centred counselling and basic problem solving and conflict resolution techniques were the most common crisis intervention processes available. As time passed, group interventions and multicomponent crisis intervention programmes were established (Everly & Mitchell, 1997).

The notion that crisis intervention should be multicomponent, which is the primary thrust of this chapter, is not new. Bordow & Porritt (1979) demonstrated that multicomponent crisis intervention was more effective for traffic accident victims in reducing distress than was a single-session psychological intervention. Interestingly, their data further showed that even the single-session psychological intervention was more effective in reducing distress compared with no intervention at all.

Mitchell (1981, 1982, 1983, 1986, 1988, 1992; Mitchell & Resnick, 1981) suggested that a multicomponent crisis intervention programme should be used to mitigate psychological distress amongst emergency services personnel and assist them in returning to normal duties. Mitchell (1983) described a logical and systematic multicomponent approach to mitigating stress and also intervention with distressed emergency personnel.

This multicomponent crisis intervention system was, unfortunately, initially referred to generically as Critical Incident Stress Debriefing (CISD). The label collectively referred to interventions such as individual crisis support services, a three-step small-group discussion called a 'defusing', a six-step (now a seven-step process) group discussion called a 'formal critical incident stress debriefing' and follow-up interventions. Later, Mitchell (1986, 1988, 1992) expanded this multicomponent approach to crisis intervention to include or-

ganizational support programmes, additional precrisis educational preparation and a psychological decompression technique called demobilization for use in large-scale operations.

As one might imagine, considerable operational confusion resulted from the redundant nomenclature wherein the term 'critical incident stress debriefing' was used to describe (1) a collective genre of crisis intervention techniques as well as (2) a specific formalized step-by-step group discussion process (Mitchell, 1983). It is important to note that the CISD group process was not designed as a stand-alone or one-off procedure. Instead, CISD was designed to be used only within the context of a comprehensive and multicomponent crisis intervention system known as Critical Incident Stress Management (CISM). Neither was it suggested that CISD was psychotherapy or a substitute for psychotherapy. CISD, like the entire field of CISM, is crisis intervention, not psychotherapy.

Mitchell & Everly (1996, p. 62) warn that 'Teams which do not pay attention to a comprehensive approach to critical incident stress management and, instead, think that one process such as the debriefing … is enough to support the people they serve are making a significant error. No one service can be equally applicable to all people in all circumstances at all times. Quality teams provide a variety of services to suit the needs of the people they serve'.

Raphael (1986) clearly emphasised the multicomponent nature of crisis intervention for victims of disaster as well as the emergency personnel and disaster relief workers. Her book states that programmes need to be developed to prepare people to manage the psychological impact of disaster. Additional support services should also be provided during the disaster. An umbrella of care for the workers, victims and community should be in place. This umbrella covers such strategies as triage and psychological first aid, psychosocial support, debriefings and referrals for more intense psychological care.

In 1993, Mitchell & Everly wrote a seminal text on multicomponent crisis intervention entitled *Critical Incident Stress Debriefing: An Operations Manual*. Despite its main title, the text served as a detailed operational guide to a broad-based crisis intervention system consisting of over 15 crisis intervention technologies. The text described the components of CISM such as education, individual crisis intervention sessions with peer counsellors, significant other support, professional referral systems, on-scene support services, defusings, demobilizations, CISDs, community outreach programmes, follow-up services, and research and development. Unfortunately, the manner in which the system was integrated was not clearly delineated.

In 1997, Everly & Mitchell consolidated and functionally integrated the multicomponent system initially described by Mitchell (1983, 1988, 1992) into a comprehensive seven-component crisis intervention programme. The words 'Critical Incident Stress Management' form part of the title to formalize the use of the term and to encourage crisis interventionists to grasp the concept that CISD is not a stand-alone process but merely one component of a larger, broader field.

The components of comprehensive CISM

In the early development of crisis intervention theory and practice, an individual consultation was the most common intervention. One improvement in the field of crisis intervention is that group processes, family interventions and a wide range of other services have been introduced and found to be helpful. These evolutions led to the development of the CISM approach.

CISM is a comprehensive, systematic and multicomponent approach to the management of traumatic stress in personal and work settings. It is a variation of the field of crisis intervention and thus shares the same goals and many of the same traditional and historic crisis intervention practices. It contains interventions that are useful before, during and after the occurrence of traumatic events. The interventions fall into three main categories:

1. Interventions for the individual:
   (a) general stress management education,
   (b) mental preparedness training,
   (c) on-scene support,
   (d) individual crisis intervention support,
   (e) referrals for psychotherapy.

2. Interventions for groups:
   (a) preincident education,
   (b) defusings,
   (c) demobilizations during disaster operations,
   (d) CISD,
   (e) follow-up meetings.

3. Interventions for the environment:
   (a) support for families,
   (b) organizational support,
      • consultations to management,
      • developing organizational commitment to stress management (screening of personnel, proper training, stress management education, good management practices, etc.).
   (c) community support,
      • community outreach,
      • community education,
      • crisis counselling and referrals.

The core components of a CISM programme are summarized in Table 5.1. Although originally developed for emergency services personnel, CISM is inherently flexible and therefore can be modified so as to be applicable to any organisation or constituent group.

Preincident education and mental preparedness training

No other CISM component can match education and training for its importance. Stress education courses should be instituted early when workers join organizations. It is best to teach people about stress in their orientation programmes rather than waiting until they encounter serious stress. Then, periodically throughout the length of their careers, in-service education sessions should be provided to keep workers abreast of new knowledge in the field of stress.

Psychological preparedness training is consistent with Caplan's (1964) notion of a primary prevention technology. Preincident education or mental preparedness training is designed to set the appropriate expectation for the crisis/disaster experience while enhancing the behavioural response to the crisis. The goals of psychological preparedness have been summarized by Everly (1995b) and by Everly & Mitchell

Table 5.1. Comprehensive Critical Incident Stress Management

---

1. Preincident education/mental preparedness training
2. Individual crisis intervention support/on-scene support
3. Demobilizations after disaster or large-scale events
4. Defusing
5. Critical incident stress debriefing (CISD)
6. Significant other support services for families and children
7. Follow-up services and professional referrals when necessary

---

(1997). They are (1) set appropriate expectations for actual experiences, (2) increase cognitive resources relevant to a crisis, and (3) teach behavioural stress management and personal coping techniques. When these goals are achieved, they may prevent psychological dysfunction and disorder (Solomon & Benbenishty, 1986; Hytten & Hasle, 1989; Weisæth, 1989a,b).

Individual crisis intervention and on-scene support services

The most commonly used crisis support intervention is that for individual crisis. There are clearly many such protocols. Everly & Mitchell (1997), for example, developed a five-step model for such intervention. There are many times when group crisis interventions (defusing or CISD) are not appropriate. This is especially so when only one or two of the personnel within an organization are affected by a traumatic event; after the defusings and CISDs are completed and when on-scene support services are required. Individual crisis intervention focuses on individual needs and does not interfere with the overall operations or with the general staffing of the operation. Individual crisis intervention services can be provided by professionals or specially trained para-professionals, and they can be provided immediately. They are designed:

(a) to stabilize a crisis situation,
(b) to mitigate the impact of the crisis experience,
(c) to assist the individual in mobilizing his or her own resources,

(d) to assist the individual in normalizing the crisis experience,
(e) to restore distressed individuals to normal functions rapidly (Mitchell, 1976; Mitchell & Resnick, 1981; Slaikeu, 1984; Mitchell & Bray, 1990).

Demobilization after disaster

A demobilization is a group intervention technology for use in disasters. It is best conceived of as a transitional intervention that allows for psychological and psycho-physiological decompression following disengagement from a large-scale crisis operation. The demobilization consists of a 10-minute informational lecture followed by 20 minutes of rest and food. Its use is reserved for large-scale, prolonged incidents or disasters. It is, therefore, the most rare of all of the crisis intervention services provided by CISM teams (Mitchell & Everly, 1996).

Defusing

This crisis intervention procedure is a small-group discussion of a traumatic experience, which takes place within a few hours of the ending of the traumatic event. Ideally, it is provided within 8 to 12 hours of a traumatic incident when the group members are most open to intervention. If this window of opportunity is missed, one-to-one (individual) services are provided and the CISD is arranged. The defusing consists of three main segments. It has a brief introduction, which motivates the personnel and outlines the guidelines that make the process run safely and smoothly. For example, the personnel are assured that the defusing team will not take notes or make reports of the discussion to anyone. What is discussed during the defusing is held in confidence. The second phase of the defusing is the exploration phase, in which the incident is described by the participants in broad terms. The third and final phase of the defusing is the information phase, in which the defusing team informs the participants. Information on the types of symptom that might be encountered is presented to the group members. Sometimes a defusing may be all that is necessary for a particular group. More typically it helps the team members to determine whether a CISD is necessary and it helps to reduce psychological discord and tension so that the team can have the time to properly set up the CISD (Mitchell & Everly, 1996; Everly & Mitchell, 1997).

Critical Incident Stress Debriefing

CISD is a structured group meeting in which a distressing traumatic event is discussed. The CISD is designed to mitigate the stress of a tragic event. It is also designed to accelerate the normal recovery processes of healthy (nonclinical), homogeneous populations who are experiencing normal reactions to an acutely distressing event. Although its goals are to mitigate the impact of a traumatic event and accelerate recovery, CISD is not a stand-alone process. It should always be used within the context of a complete stress management programme, namely CISM.

CISD is useful as a tool to identify members of the group who may need additional assistance, such as a referral for psychotherapy. The term 'Critical Incident Stress Debriefing' is a proper noun. It refers to the specific model of psychological debriefing developed by S. L. A. Mitchell in the USA during the late 1970s and early 1980s. CISD group intervention follows a specific seven-phase model which has (1) an introduction phase, (2) a fact phase, (3) a thought phase, (4) a reaction phase, (5) a symptoms phase, (6) a teaching/information phase, and (7) a re-entry phase. CISDs are provided by specially trained teams made up of peer support personnel combined with mental health professionals. The CISD process is often applied to groups within 24 to 72 hours after the ending of the incident. It may be provided later if the circumstances warrant a delay in the provision of the service.

The process is consistent with Caplan's (1964) formulation of the notion of secondary prevention. CISD is designed to mitigate the adverse psychological impact of a traumatic event by reducing the intensity and chronicity of symptoms subsequent to the trauma. It is also designed to facilitate psychological closure to a traumatic event. It is not designed to eliminate all of the stress symptoms that are associated with the traumatic event. In a CISD, when individuals are identified as needing additional support or psychotherapy, they are referred for such services (Mitchell & Everly, 1996; Everly & Mitchell, 1997).

Significant other support services for families and children

Providing support services to the members of an organization is, of course, very important, but without also supporting the environment in which the personnel live, the organization's members cannot be fully supported. When their families are cared for by the organization, personnel are more content and morale stays high. Stress is easier to tolerate if there is a supportive climate around the people in an organization. That climate can best be created by a programme of significant other support.

Education, spouse group debriefings, family crisis counselling and group support meetings for families are the most common types of intervention for family members (Mitchell & Everly, 1996; Everly & Mitchell, 1997).

Follow-up services and professional referrals

One of the great values of an organized systematic intervention such as CISM is that it provides a unique opportunity to do field assessments and triaging. A standardized CISM programme as part of a standing crisis plan ensures that everyone in the crisis will receive the opportunity for support either from peer counsellors or from professional mental health providers. CISM programmes do not compete with traditional mental health services. If implemented correctly, CISM programmes will enhance and complement the delivery of traditional employee assistance and traditional mental health services. Referrals may be made to psychological or psychiatric services, medical services, religious services, family support services, financial aid services, career counselling and legal services (Everly & Mitchell, 1997).

CISM was intended to be a comprehensive crisis intervention programme. Operationally, the term 'comprehensive' denotes a programme that spans the three phases of the crisis spectrum: (1) the precrisis phase, (2) the acute crisis phase, and (3) the post-crisis

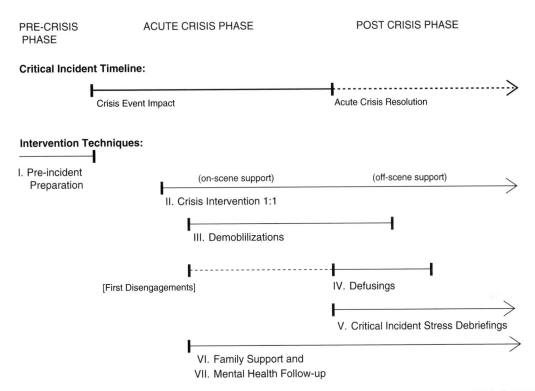

Figure 5.1. Critical Incident Stress Management intervention timeline. (Reproduced with permission from Everly & Mitchell, 1999.)

phase (Mitchell & Everly, 1996; Everly & Mitchell, 1997). The CISM programme proposed by Mitchell & Everly spans the crisis spectrum as illustrated in Figure 5.1. In sum, we agree with the recommendation of the British Psychological Society that crisis intervention should be an integrated and multicomponent approach (British Psychological Working Party, 1990).

Clearly crisis intervention techniques can be used in a variety of settings. The comprehensive crisis intervention system called CISM has many applications: it can be applied to entire organizations such as businesses or industries, emergency services organizations, schools and communities.

No matter where the programme is applied, the ultimate success of effective, comprehensive CISM in any organization relies heavily on the existence of an accepting and supportive administration that supplies an atmosphere of respect and dignity for its staff. Stress management starts with an appropriate screening programme that carefully selects the best candidates for positions within the organization. Overall stress management is encouraged in an organization by effective training programmes, which include general stress management education, mental preparedness training and pre-exposure stress management programmes. Good management practices maintain the health of the organization and contribute to the health and happiness of the personnel who serve that organization. Management's acceptance of a CISM team approach that includes the use of specially trained peer support personnel and mental health professionals is essential. The team must provide a wide range of individual, group and environmental services before, during and after critical incidents.

Without the positive atmosphere described above, any CISM programme will be impaired, suffer from demoralization and typically face failure in the applications of most of its crisis intervention and stress management procedures.

Putative mechanisms of action in CISM

The term 'mechanisms of action' refers to the mechanisms or processes through which any given intervention exerts its effect. In the study of psychopharmacology, for example, an understanding of the mechanisms of psychoactive drugs are considered to be essential to the viability and utilization of the drug. Drugs are sometimes prescribed for their side effects as well as their main effects. But, in general, the use of any drug is made more effective by understanding, not just whether it works, but why it works. The mechanisms of action for psychological and behavioural interventions are usually more subtle and less well understood than the mechanisms of action of drugs. Nevertheless, any intervention that exerts any effect at all must, by definition, have some mechanism of action that accounts for that effect. Psychological interventions most likely have many complex interacting mechanisms at the root of their effectiveness. While more complicated in terms of processes, understanding the mechanisms of action undergirding psychological and behavioural interventions is no less important.

The study of putative mechanisms of action is also important if we are to improve our interventions and continue to innovate. Such scrutiny teaches us why our interventions succeed and why they fail. It allows us to trouble-shoot complicated situations, as well.

The following paragraphs review and speculate upon the mechanisms of action which underlie the field of CISM.

Salmon (1919) as well as Kardiner & Spiegel (1947), writing about their experiences of emergency psychiatry in world wars, note that the emergency provision of care during a crisis is different from traditional clinical applications. From their analyses emerged the three principles of the crisis intervention process:

1. Proximity – close to or within the crisis venue.
2. Immediacy – rapid intervention.
3. Expectancy – setting appropriate expectations for treatment and returning to function.

Slaby and his coworkers (1975) identified the following key factors in successful crisis intervention:

1. Immediacy.
2. Innovation (i.e. creative and flexible intervention).
3. Pragmatism (i.e. practical, goal-directed, action-oriented intervention).

In a review of psychiatric therapies, Spiegel & Classen (1995) analysed the processes that underlie crisis intervention as follows:

1. Immediacy in timing of the interventions.
2. Social support, listening.
3. Ventilation of emotion (catharsis).
4. Commonality of experience as shared by those who participated in the same or similar crisis.
5. Cognitive processing of the crisis.
6. Anticipatory guidance (i.e. anticipating for the person in distress).
7. Educating, normalizing, teaching coping responses.

In 1970, Yalom studied and identified curative factors that facilitated improvement in his therapeutic groups. The factors perceived as most important by Yalom's respondents are as follows. They are listed in descending order of importance:

1. Interpersonal learning (i.e. learning to integrate information from others).
2. Catharsis (i.e. ventilation of emotions).
3. Cohesiveness (i.e. feeling as an integral part of a group).
4. Personal insights (i.e. learning about self from others' information).
5. Interpersonal teaching of others.
6. Existential awareness.
7. Universality (i.e. destruction of the myth of uniqueness).
8. Instillation of hope.

All of the factors listed in the sections above are potentially active not simply in therapy for groups and individuals, but in crisis intervention procedures as well.

More recently Wollman (1993) analysed the bases for the effectiveness of crisis intervention groups. His findings of helpful factors are as follows:

1. Group cohesion.
2. Universality.
3. Catharsis.

4. Imitative behaviour.
5. Instillation of hope.
6. Imparting of information (teaching).
7. Altruism.
8. Timeliness.
9. Existential factors.

A review of these factors reveals that, in Wollman's opinion, crisis intervention groups are effective for many of the same reasons that psychotherapy groups are effective, but with the added advantage of timelines (i.e. immediacy, in the language of crisis intervention).

Atle Dyregrov of Norway, has made extremely valuable contributions to the field of traumatic stress management. His excellent description of process issues in psychological debriefings presents a number of factors or mechanisms of action that influence the success or failure of the CISD group process (Dyregrov, 1997). He emphasizes the synergetic relationship between these facts. They are:

1. The degree of exposure to the traumatic event.
2. Leadership.
3. Structure and flow of the group meeting.
4. Participants (personalities, training, experience, prior traumas, support systems, etc.).
5. Nature of the group.
6. Organizational atmosphere (acceptance of support by the organization).
7. CISD environment (timing of CISD, physical surroundings, duration of the meeting, disturbances, etc.).

An alteration in any single factor can exert an influence on all of the other factors. Each factor or mechanism of action can enhance or inhibit positive CISD outcomes. Dyregrov's article sheds light on the complexity of the CISD process and the difficulties researchers will encounter should they employ simplistic research designs to explore CISD without regard to the complex interactions of numerous factors inherent in the CISD process.

In a specific examination of CISD group crisis intervention technology, Everly (1995a) identified 10 putative mechanisms of action (see also Mitchell & Everly, 1996). The following factors were on his list:

1. Early intervention.
2. Affective ventilation (catharsis).
3. Opportunity to put the crisis into words on a cognitive level.
4. Behavioural structure.
5. Psychological structure and progression.
6. Yalom's group processes (as noted earlier).
7. Support from one's peers.
8. Demonstration of caring.
9. Instillation of hope and a sense of control.
10. Opportunity for follow-up assessment and treatment, if appropriate.

As noted earlier behavioural and psychological interventions are not likely to derive their effectiveness from a single monolithic action (referred to as the main effect, in analysis of variance parlance). Rather, behavioural and psychological interventions are far more likely to derive their effectiveness from interacting factors or variables. Thus, they are interaction effects. As the effects of interacting variables are seldom additive, but are synergistically multiplicative, even rigorous components analyses are seldom capable of ascribing relative weights to interacting variables in a manner that is valid for all individuals. So, rather than estimate their relative values, we have simply chosen to offer the following factors as those that we believe are the four core process mechanisms of action upon which all of CISM, as a crisis response intervention system, rests. They are as follows:

1. Early intervention

CISM interventions are designed to be implemented during the acute crisis phase, in the form of in-the-field, on-scene support, as quickly after the crisis resolution as possible. There is simply nothing quicker by design. Early, if not immediate, intervention has long been recognized as an important aspect of crisis response.

Salmon (1919) and Kardiner & Spiegel (1947) noted the importance of rapid, emergency-oriented psychiatric intervention in World Wars I and II, respectively. More recently, Solomon & Shalev (1995) have suggested similar intervention strategies.

Lindy (1985) argued that after a traumatic event victims begin to insulate themselves from the world through the construction of a 'trauma membrane' or protective shell. The longer one waits to penetrate the shell, the more difficult it becomes, according to this formulation.

Earllier, Rapoport (1965) argued for the practical importance of early intervention, as did Spiegel & Classen (1995) in their review of emergency psychiatry.

Empirically, Bordow & Porritt (1979) were probably the first to test the importance of early crisis response. Their results support the conclusion that immediate intervention is more effective than delayed intervention.

Solomon & Benbenishty (1986) empirically analysed the three tenets of crisis response: proximity immediacy, and expectancy. Each of the three was found to exert a positive effect.

Lastly, Post (1992), in a most provocative paper, argued that earlier intervention may prevent a genetically based lowered threshold for neurological excitation from developing in response to trauma. Earlier intervention may thus prevent the development of a cellular 'memory' from being transmitted to excitatory neural tissues.

2. The provision of psychosocial support

All human beings require some form of support from others (i.e. psychosocial support). This may come in the form of esteem, friendship, respect, trust, aid in problem solving or merely listening. Crisis accentuates this need.

American psychologist Carl Rogers wrote cogently in his theory of self-psychology that all humans have an innate need for 'positive regard' (Rogers, 1951). They possess a need to be valued by others. Bowlby (1969) argued that there exists a biological drive for the bonding, or attachment, between humans, especially between mother and child. Similarly, Maslow (1970) has written most coherently that one of the basic human needs is that for social affiliation with others. According to Maslovian theory, many crises result from a loss of social support/affiliation.

Frank (1974), in his analysis of psychotherapy, argued that all psychotherapeutic improvement is based on the intervention's ability to reduce demoralization, especially through contradicting the notion of alienation. Individuals in crisis often feel alone, uniquely plagued, and abandoned.

By its very existence, any form of crisis response initiates the process of social support. Buckley et al. (1996) found an inverse relationship between social support and the prevalence of post-traumatic stress disorder in the wake of motor vehicle accidents. Bunn & Clarke (1979), in an early study of crisis intervention technologies, found that as crisis counselling services were provided, in the form of 20 minutes of supportive counselling, anxiety levels diminished. Dalgleish and others (1996) also confirmed the assumption that social support is inversely correlated with post-traumatic stress-related symptoms. Finally, Flannery (1990), in a comprehensive review of the role of social support in psychological trauma, found a general trend indicative of the value of social support in reducing the aversive impact of trauma.

3. The opportunity for expression

Bruno Bettleheim, an early psychotraumatologist, noted, 'What cannot be talked about can also not be put to rest' (Bettleheim, 1984, p. 166). Much earlier, according to van der Hart and his co-workers (1989), Pierre Janet (1889) had declared in the 1800s that successful recovery from trauma required the patient to verbally reconstruct and express the traumatic event.

The notion that recovery from trauma is predicated upon the verbal expression of not only emotion, but also cognitions, is virtually universal throughout crisis response literature. Spiegel & Classen (1995) in their review of crisis psychiatry, noted the importance of cognitively processing the crisis.

Pennebaker and others in an elegant series of empirical investigations demonstrated the true value of expression (Pennebaker, 1985, 1990; Pennebaker & Beall, 1986; Pennebaker & Susman, 1988). His investigations demonstrate the value of expression on not only psychological outcome measures but also physiological and behavioural measures.

4. Crisis education: expectancy and coping

The fourth and final mechanism of action we find operating in CISM is that of crisis education (i.e. setting appropriate expectations and teaching practical coping techniques).

People in crisis commonly experience a sense of being out of control. Recovery (i.e. the restoration of psychological homeostasis) is often dependent upon re-establishing a sense of control. The perception of control is enhanced through setting appropriate expectations and teaching effective instrumental coping behaviours (Everly, 1989; Bandura, 1997).

Investigations and formulations by Taylor (1983) and Bandura (1997) argued convincingly for the power of perceived control as a mitigation of crisis stress and psychological discord. In his review of control and stress, Everly (1989) concluded that understanding, as induced by information/education is a powerful stress reduction strategy. Further, Spiegel & Classen (1995) pointed out that cognitive processing of the crisis is also an important step towards resolution. The operational corollaries of these formulations, therefore, would be educational interventions so as:

1. To warn people in high-risk environments as to the nature of their risk exposure and how to cope with crisis situations if they do occur (Hytten & Hasle, 1989; Weisæth, 1989a; Jonsson, 1995) as is done in precrisis preparation protocols (Mitchell & Everly, 1996; Backman et al., 1997).
2. To teach crisis coping techniques during the crisis as a means of mitigating the crisis response, facilitating re-establishment of homeostasis, and increasing the sense of self-efficacy (Everly, 1989; Bandura, 1997).

We have now reviewed the concepts and mechanisms that are thought to serve as a foundation for CISM as a crisis response system. In the final analysis we have concluded that four fundamental elements, or processes, are present. They are summarized here because of their importance.

1. Early intervention.
2. The provision of psychosocial support.
3. The opportunity for expression.
4. Crisis education.

These factors are, we believe, the four cornerstones of CISM. Indeed, the search for mechanisms of action in psychological interventions is not an easy one. That which is most florid, is not always that which is most salient. Often the most potent mechanisms are latent, or obscured.

Research on CISM

Studies on debriefing

The results of studies on the effectiveness of a single intervention such as debriefing are mixed. Some studies have demonstrated negative results and some positive.

A number of studies indicate that debriefing services have no appreciable positive effect (Paton, 1995; Weisæth, 1989b: Griffiths and Watts, 1992; Searle & Bisson, 1992; Deahl et al., 1994). The negative outcome studies have methodological flaws that limit useful interpretation. The lack of standardized implementation of debriefing approaches considerably weakens the reported findings. There are also problems with studies that present data on different types of victim. Frequently the negative outcome studies fail to define the debriefing model used and also fail to clarify the type of training of those who provided the debriefings. Many of the negative outcome studies do not use standardized outcome measures or have substantially delayed post-test assessments. Subjects may have been exposed to additional traumatic events, which confounds the assessments of the original event.

There are three negative outcome studies that are frequently referred to and appear to summarize most of the negative findings in the field (McFarlane, 1988; Kenardy et al., 1996; Bisson et al., 1997). One should, however, be cautious in drawing conclusions about debriefings based on these studies. A thorough review of these papers reveals that the studies do not uniformly standardize the type or even the nature of the 'debriefing' process used. What is clear is that either the Mitchell model of CISD, as defined above, was not used, or it was substantially altered and therefore not evaluated, even though the contrary is often reported in the literature. When an independent variable is not adequately defined, the meanings of the study are obscured.

The McFarlane (1988) study found that there was a positive short-term effect for the 128 people who attended 'debriefings', but a greater likelihood of developing delayed post-traumatic stress disorder (PTSD). There were, however, confounding factors in the study. For example, 7% of the participants suffered bereavement and 23% endured property loss. That fact makes them primary victims, not the secondary victims for whom the debriefing process was developed. Another concern about the study is that there is a covariate. The negative, long-term effect (delayed PTSD) was found *only* when the subjects in the study had an elevated level of neuroticism.

Even greater caution should be employed when drawing conclusions from the Kenardy et al. (1996) study. The first evaluation was performed six months after the traumatic incident. There were no baseline data available. The study therefore ignores both historical and maturational effects. The authors themselves noted that the term 'debriefing' was not clearly defined and 'there was no control over the debriefing procedures'. (Kenardy et al., 1996, p. 47).

The Bisson et al. (1997) study found no appreciable positive effects of debriefing burn victims. The CISD process, however, was substantially altered from its intended purposes. For example, it was used on individuals not on groups as it was originally designed to be. In addition, the process was utilized out of the context of a comprehensive, systematic and multicomponent approach to traumatic stress management. In other words, it was employed as a one-off or stand-alone process, which is contrary to its original design. Furthermore, the Bisson study appears to presume that a psychological debriefing is equivalent to good psychiatric practice. CISD and other forms of psychological debriefings are crisis intervention strategies, not psychotherapy. In reference to this study, Dyregrov (1998, p. 4) says, 'If anything is measured in Bisson et al.'s study it must be the effect of a badly timed rapid conversation, and not a sound clinical intervention.'

Several Master's theses and doctoral dissertations indicate the positive results of CISD. The earliest study was performed by Lanning (1987). She identified six positive perceptions of debriefings for emergency personnel:

1. The debriefing prepared participants for stress symptoms they might encounter.
2. The debriefing enabled participants to accept symptoms and not feel that they were 'going crazy'.
3. Participants received support from other participants.
4. Some problems were resolved.
5. The participants felt safe in talking about their feelings and not having to hide them or be macho.
6. The mandatory debriefings did not make the participants feel singled out.

The lack of a randomized control group is certainly problematic in Lanning's study.

In 1988, Bohl explored the Mitchell model debriefing process. Her study involved a naturalistic randomized control group. That is, some personnel were given a debriefing and others, in an adjacent department, were not, even when they worked at the same incidents and experienced a similar exposure to the traumatic event. No evidence of systematic assignment error could be deduced. She found that a 90-minute CISD within 24 hours of the traumatic event was effective in lowering feelings of depression, anger, anxiety and stress-related symptoms. The positive benefits held at least up to the three-month post-event test (Bohl, 1988).

In a similar study, Bohl (1995) measured the effectiveness of CISD on 65 firefighters after a serious traumatic event. A group of 30 personnel received CISD 24 hours after the event and 35 did not. There does not appear to be selection or assignment bias in the study. An assessment performed three months later indicated that the debriefed group had lower levels of anger, anxiety and depression. In addition, there were fewer reported long-term symptoms of PTSD, such as nightmares, flashbacks or changes in sleep or eating habits. The study design was post-test only.

Rogers' (1993) doctoral dissertation evaluated the Mitchell model of debriefing. The analysis suggests that the CISD process was helpful in reducing psychosocial stress by generating a moderate increase in a feeling of being in control of one's reactions to the critical incident. Of the emergency personnel who received debriefings, 72% reported lowered symptoms after the debriefing and demonstrated better resolution of their traumatic stress reactions than those who were not debriefed. A problem with the study is that the participants had experienced different traumatic events, with variations on the intensity of the distress.

After the Los Angeles riots in 1992 researchers studied the impact of stress reactions on emergency medical services personnel and the effectiveness of CISD. Using the Frederick Reaction Index the researchers compared groups of emergency medical services personnel who had received debriefings with those who had not received the service after the same or very similar experiences in the riots. Those workers who were given an opportunity to participate in a CISD session scored significantly lower on the Frederick Reaction Index (an average of 10.7 compared with a mean of 14.3 for those not debriefed) (Wee, 1996; Wee et al., 1999).

Hannemann (1994), in her Master's thesis on CISD, evaluated the use of the Mitchell model debriefings with volunteer firefighters in Nova Scotia and concluded that there were eight dominant themes associated with CISD services:

1. The positive impact of the CISD process on the department.
2. The positive impact of the CISD process on the individual.
3. The value of ventilating.
4. The value of being able to express emotions.
5. The importance of getting the whole perspective.
6. The CISD helped firefighters to accept that they had done their best.
7. The CISD helped them to feel that they were not alone in their feeling.
8. The CISD produced a sense of bonding or brotherhood.

Hanneman's study was qualitative in nature. No control group existed and no comparative data analysis was performed.

In a study of 823 ambulance personnel in Australia, 64% were aware of the broad range of CISM services offered to them in the aftermath of tragedies. Of these, 97% felt that the services were important to them. Only 3% believed that the services were not important. When CISD services were evaluated by themselves, 82% of the personnel believed that the CISDs were helpful (Robinson, 1994). The absence of a control group limits the conclusions that can be drawn from this study.

After a mass shooting in Texas in 1991, Jenkins (1996) performed a controlled longitudinal assessment of the effectiveness of the CISD intervention. Recovery from the trauma appeared to be most strongly associated with participation in the CISD process. CISD was useful in reducing symptoms of depression and anxiety for those who participated in the CISD compared with those who did not.

Debriefings were used subsequent to Hurricane Iniki in Hawaii with several groups of disaster workers. A core CISM service (education) was added to the design of the study. Group education was provided in addition to the CISD. The research cohort was divided into two groups for pre-test and post-test comparisons. To provide a control group paradigm, a time-lagged design was employed wherein the pretreatment assessment of the second group was concurrent with the post-treatment assessment of the first group. Repeated analysis of variance (ANOVA) indicated the psychometrically assessed post-traumatic stress (Impact of Event Scale) was reduced in both groups as a result of the psychological debriefing intervention combined with additional traumatic stress education (Chemtob et al., 1997).

The debriefing intervention has been applied to adolescents in addition to adults. Stallard & Law (1993) compared adolescents who received debriefings to those who did not. They concluded, 'Psychological debriefings can be effective in reducing intrusive thoughts, possibly by validating the person's experience of the trauma, allowing a reinterpretation of their attribution and providing a forum in which emotions can be discharged' (Stallard & Law, 1993, p. 663). Debriefings may mitigate the intrusive thought pattern that is considered the most important aspect of the PTSD complex. In another study of traumatized children, debriefing significantly reduced the severity of post-traumatic stress reaction in those children who received debriefings. Children who were not debriefed did not fare as well (Pynoos et al., 1994).

In 1994, Scandinavia suffered its worst peace-time sea disaster in history with the sinking of the *Estonia*. Over 900 people perished. Nurmi (1997) contrasted three groups of emergency response personnel who received the CISD intervention with a group of emergency nurses who received support from supervisors, but no CISD. Data indicated that psychometrically assessed (Impact of Event Scale) symptoms of PTSD several days post incident were lower in each of the three groups that received the CISD than in the nursing group that did not receive the CISD. Nurmi noted that this was the largest application of 'Mitchell model' of CISD in Finnish history.

Similar positive results have been found in other professions. In a study of 219 nurses, 193 reported that the CISD process was helpful to them (Burns & Harm, 1993). Dyregrov (1989) found debriefings helpful with disaster workers and rescue workers (Dyregrov et al., 1992).

Everly & Boyle (1997) in an effort to assess the effectiveness of group crisis intervention subjected five investigations (Bohl, 1995; Jenkins, 1996; Chemtob et al., 1997; Nurmi, 1997; Wee et al., 1999) to meta-analysis. All five investigations used Mitchell's CISD model. In an aggregated sample six of 337, the mean Cohen's D was 0.86, indicative of a large positive effect attributable to the CISD intervention.

The debriefing literature indicates both positive and negative outcomes. How can that be? When different groups of researchers are coming up with vastly different results, several questions should be asked. Are they following the same procedures? In other words, are the debriefings the same? Have the service providers been adequately trained to perform services such as debriefings? Are they working with groups that have experienced roughly equal levels of trauma? In other words, are the same things really being measured? Have the researchers taken into account the complex interactions existing between a range of factors that influence the positive or negative outcomes of the CISD intervention? The answer is often, 'No'.

Answers to the above questions make a difference. Frequently, we conclude that the main factors in whether outcome data are positive or negative regarding debriefing are the training, skill and experience of the provider and not the process itself (Dyregrov, 1997). This is the same conclusion that many have reached regarding research in psychotherapy (Seligman, 1995).

Multicomponent crisis intervention studies

Multifactorial CISM-like crisis response programmes contain most, or all, of the CISM intervention concepts, but may not be thought of as CISM or referred to as CISM. As discussed above, the results of studies on a single crisis intervention process, namely the CISD, are mixed. On the other hand, studies that review a multicomponent approach to CISM produce more consistently positive results.

Blackwelder's (1995) evaluation of the 'Mitchell model' of CISD used in school districts discussed the effectiveness of CISM and the need for appropriate training of support staff. She concluded that there were improved effects when CISM-trained staff were used in support services, but when services were provided by untrained personnel, they were perceived to be ineffective.

Solomon & Benbenishty (1986), investigating the core crisis intervention principles of proximity, immediacy and expectancy, revealed that all three were positively correlated with soldiers returning to the fighting unit. Further analysis revealed that immediacy and expectancy were correlated inversely with the development of PTSD.

Brom et al. (1993) investigated primary victims of traffic accidents. A CISM-like programme combining practical help, information, support, reality testing, confrontation with the experience, and referral to psychotherapeutic treatment was evaluated. Scores on a checklist of trauma symptoms improved. The improvement suggests the effectiveness of the multifactorial CISM-like intervention.

Flannery and coworkers (1995) conducted a series of elegant studies testing the concept of multidimensional CISM as applied to workplace violence in three US state mental hospitals. Each hospital created a critical incident response team using solid CISM principles, including debriefings. The cumulative results of this well-controlled multisite study yielded strong evidence for the ability of CISM to reduce the harmful effects of workplace violence. Reduced sick leave, lowered accident claims and reduced staff turnover were reported as a result of the CISM programme.

Leeman-Conley (1990) conducted a revealing study applying CISM services to bank employees. She collected data on sick leave and compensation payments before and after a CISM programme was established. Her results indicated that the CISM programme yielded a 60% decline in sick leave and a 68% decline in compensation payments. What was intriguing about her data was the fact that the number of bank robberies actually increased after the CISM programme was established while the negative outcomes associated with robberies actually declined. Grainger (1995, p. 197), in another study of bank employees exposed to robberies, reported that 'Nineteen of the 22 victims attended critical incident stress debriefing and most found this valuable'. It should be noted that Grainger used components of CISM other than the debriefing.

Campbell (1992) wrote a doctoral dissertation on a CISM programme, which has been used effectively to support Federal Bureau of Investigation (FBI) agents after traumatic events. He found that, once a critical incident support programme was instituted in the FBI, agents reported improvements in several areas.

These responses not only reflected statistically significant pre–post change, and hence support for evaluation of the FBI's Post-Critical Incident Programme, but they resoundingly supported the value of the Post-Critical Incident Programme and the post shooting aspects of that programme. Not only has this programme provided these positive results, but there have been five specific areas that demonstrate the reduction of negative response. Each of these five areas was also statistically significant. These areas include no longer using agents as scapegoats, the reduction of the use of alcohol after shooting incidents, the positive adjustment to work, the reduction of insensitive responses by other members of the FBI, and no longer being isolated and alone ... (Campbell, 1992, p. 100)

...All of these responses supported the Post-Critical Incident Program and the efforts of the FBI to foster and enhance successful individual adjustment to trauma ... (Campbell, 1992, p. 100)

...The third general observation is that there is a need for a formalised response and debriefing process following critical incidents experienced by the FBI ... (Campbell, 1992, pp. 110).

In a study of a broad-spectrum CISM programme instituted for corrections officers in a New South Wales corrections facility, Ott & Henry (1997) found a substantial reduction in the cost of workers' compensation for stress-related conditions. The coordinated approach to stress management included a family support programme, a peer support crisis intervention programme, staff counselling with professional counsellors, a social club, a fitness programme, stress management and critical incident stress education programme, debriefings and rehabilitation services. The facility experienced a reduction in absences, enhanced communications between staff and contract professionals, and an accelerated return to work after traumatic events. The one-year (1994) costs for compensation before the programme was established was (Aus)$614 648. Once the stress programme was established the workers' compensation costs the next year dropped to (Aus)$51 178. Ott & Henry reported that the lowered costs have continued up to the time of their report (August 1997).

Manzi (1995) evaluated a residential CISM programme at the On Site Academy in Gardner, Massachusetts. The programme has been designed for people who have experienced psychologically disabling symptoms from some form of a traumatic event. The On Site Academy's constituency is the emergency services personnel of North America. The Academy employs a short-term residential variation of the CISM programme. A rationale for this is that these individuals, so adversely affected by trauma, still find themselves in the midst of a psychological crisis, regardless of how much time has actually passed since the actual traumatization. The core components of the programme are:

1. Training/education in stress and coping techniques.
2. CISD.
3. Paraprofessional peer support.
4. Individual counselling.
5. Eye movement desensitization and reprocessing (EMDR).
6. Other support services as required.

Manzi (1995) surveyed 108 graduates of the On Site Academy an average of 10 months after leaving the programme. Of 45 surveys returned, 100% reported that the On Site Academy had met their expectations and goals. In addition, 100% of the respondents reported that they would recommend the On Site Academy to others. Manzi's study revealed significant decreases in cognitive, physical, emotional and behavioural symptoms from pre-CISM to post-CISM.

Following a successful pilot project on nursing stress (Kirwan, 1994) in the Manitoba province of Canada, the Medical Services Branch of the Canadian government authorized the implementation of a national CISM programme for the Indian and Northern Health Services nurses. A full CISM programme was implemented. Subsequently these nurses were sampled to assess both the need and the effectiveness of the programme.

Survey and interview data were collected, analysed and reviewed by an independent evaluation organization (Western Management Consultants, 1996). Data were collected from nurses working in British Columbia, Alberta, Manitoba and Ontario. Of 582 nurses, 236 (41%) responded.

The study revealed that 65% of the nurses experienced at least one critical incident per year in the workplace. These critical incidents included, but were not limited to, death of a child, attempted or physical assault, breakins at nursing facilities, verbal threats, suicide or attempted suicide of patients.

The evaluation report (Western Management Consultants, 1996) stated that 99% of the field nurses indicated that the CISM programme reduced the number of days they were absent from work. Furthermore, the report concluded, 'Survey data suggest MSB [Medical Services Branch] CISM significantly reduced turnover among field nurses' (Western Management Consultants, 1996, p. 53).

Additional financial evaluations revealed a 7.09 financial benefit-to-cost ratio, which may be seen as an over 700% return on investment. The authors of the evaluation report concluded, 'It is evident that the quality of the existing programme is exceptional. The MSB programme is a state-of-the-art programme that should be emulated by other employers, and sets a standard by which alternatives should be judged' (Western Management Consultants, 1996, p. iv).

Since CISM services were originally introduced into the emergency services professions in the mid 1970s many thousands of people in many professional categories have experienced various aspects of the support services. The recipients of CISM services have been generally satisfied with the services and see these efforts as a practical means to mitigate stress in their work. The overall evaluation of CISM services by many thousands of emergency services personnel has been quite positive (Dyregrov, 1989; Dyregrov et al., 1992; Robinson & Mitchell, 1993; AAOS, 1996). Two studies in particular (Robinson & Mitchell, 1993; AAOS, 1996) indicate that over 90% of the hundreds of personnel in these studies who received CISD services evaluated the services as beneficial. The vast majority of the thousands of emergency personnel and others who have been helped by CISM services consider CISM helpful. According to Seligman (1995) such opinions are of value. The recipients of these programmes know what is working and they may tell us more than randomized efficacy studies.

Conclusions

Virtually every study, both negative and positive, is flawed by some methodological problems. Some contain more or less serious imperfections than others. Despite their flaws, each study offers another window, which sheds more light on the CISM field. Each study enhances our overall understanding of the intricate interrelationships of a multiplicity of factors that influence either the positive or negative outcomes of a wide range of CISM interventions. No single study stands out as the last word in the field of CISM. Many more studies will need to be conducted before we develop a more complete understanding of the factors that enhance the potential for positive CISM outcomes and diminish the potential for negative CISM outcomes.

This chapter should move the exploration of the entire field of CISM away from the previous misguided evaluations of single intervention strategies to a more appropriate investigation of multicomponent intervention strategies. The evidence presented in the sections above, particularly in the sections on Studies on debriefing and Multicomponent crisis intervention studies, offers several important lessons. First, a review of the studies on single-intervention strategies indicates mixed results. Some studies are negative and some are positive and they all have methodological flaws. Secondly, the application of simple research designs to interventions that are inherently complex and multi-component increases the potential for misinterpretations of the data. Thirdly, studies on multicomponent crisis intervention strategies are stronger and demonstrate consistently positive outcomes.

Finally, the studies reviewed in this chapter indicate that a comprehensive, systematic and multicomponent crisis intervention approach to traumatic stress, namely CISM, has an excellent potential for mitigating critical incident stress and restoring people to normal life functions. It is clear that no single stress intervention technique can be equally applicable or equally successful with all people, under all circumstances and at all times. Therefore, a broad spectrum of interrelated CISM interventions has been developed and it has already demonstrated consistently positive outcomes.

REFERENCES

AAOS (American Academy of Orthopaedic Surgeons, Department of Research and Scientific Affairs) (1996). Tales from the front: huge response to sound off on CISD. *EMT Today*, **1**(2), 3.

Backman, L., Arnetz, B., Levin, D. & Lublin, A. (1997). Psychophysical effects of mental imaging training for police trainees. *Stress Medicine*, **13**, 43–8.

Bandura, A. (1997). *Self-efficacy: The Exercise of Control*. New York: W. H. Freeman.

Bettleheim, B. (1984). Afterward. In C. Vegh (Ed.) *I Didn't Say Goodbye*. New York: E. P. Dutton.

Bisson, J., Jenkins, P. L., Bannister, C. & Alexander, J. (1997). Randomised controlled trial of psychological debriefing for victims of acute burn trauma. *British Journal of Psychiatry*, **171**, 78–81.

Blackwelder, N. L. (1995). *Critical Incident Stress Debriefing for school employees*. Ph.D. thesis. Ann Arbor, MI: UMI Dissertation Services.

Bohl, N. (1988). Effect of psychological intervention after critical incidents on anger, anxiety and depression. Ph.D. dissertation, California Graduate Institute.

Bohl, N. (1995). Measuring the effectiveness of CISD: a study. *Fire Engineering*, August, 125–6.

Bordow, S. & Porritt, D. (1979). An experimental evaluation of crisis intervention. *Social Science and Medicine*, **13**, 251–6.

Bowlby, J. (1969). *Attachment*. New York: Basic Books.

British Psychological Working Party (1990). *Psychological Aspects of Disaster*. Leicester: British Psychological Society.

Brom, D., Kleber, R. & Hofman, M. (1993). Victims of traffic accidents: incidence and prevention of post-traumatic stress disorder. *Journal of Clinical Psychology*, **49**, 131–9.

Buckley, T. C., Blanchard, E. & Hickling, E. (1996). A prospective examination of delayed onset PTSD secondary to motor vehicle accidents. *Journal of Abnormal Psychology*, **105**, 617–25.

Bunn, T. & Clarke, A. (1979). Crisis intervention. *British Journal of Medical Psychology*, **52**, 191–5.

Burns, C. & Harm, L. (1993). Emergency nurses' perceptions of critical incidents and stress debriefing. *Journal of Emergency Nursing*, **19**, 431–6.

Campbell, J. H. (1992). A comparative analysis of the effects of post-shooting trauma on special agents of the federal Bureau of Investigation. Ph.D. Dissertation, Michigan State University.

Caplan, G. (1964). *Principles of Preventive Psychiatry*. New York: Basic Books.

Caplan, G. (1969). Opportunities for school psychologists in the primary prevention of mental health disorders in children. In A. Bindman & A. Spiegel (Eds.) *Perspectives in Community Mental Health* (pp. 420–36). Chicago: Aldine.

Chemtob, C., Thomas, S., Law, W. & Cremmiter, D. (1997). Post-disaster psychological intervention: a field study of the impact of debriefing on psychological distress. *American Journal of Psychiatry*, **154**, 415–17.

Dalgleish, T., Joseph, S., Trasher, S., Tranah, T. & Yule, W. (1996). Crisis support following the *Herald of Free Enterprise* disaster. *Journal of Traumatic Stress*, **9**, 833–45.

Deahl, M. P., Gillham, A. B., Thomas, J., Searle, M.M. & Srinivasan (1994). Psychological sequelae following the Gulf War: factors associated with subsequent morbidity and the effectiveness of psychological debriefing. *British Journal of Psychiatry*, **165**, 60–5.

Dyregrov, A. (1989). Caring for helpers in disaster situations: psychological debriefings. *Disaster Management*, **2**, 25–30.

Dyregrov, A. (1997). The process in psychological debriefings. *Journal of Traumatic Stress*, **10**, 589–605.

Dyregrov, A. (1998). Psychological debriefing – an effective method. *Traumatology*, **4**.

Dyregrov, A., Thyhodt, R. & Mitchell, J. T. (1992). Rescue workers' emotional reactions following a disaster. In S. R.

Engelman (Ed.) *Confronting Life-threatening Illness*. New York: Irvington Publishers, Inc.

Everly, G. S. (1989). *A Clinical Guide to the Treatment of the Human Stress Response*. New York: Plenum Press.

Everly, G. S. (1995a). The role of the critical incident stress debriefing (CISD) process in disaster counselling. *Journal of Mental Health Counselling*, 17, 278–90.

Everly, G. S. (1995b). *A Psychological Trauma Prevention Program for the Kuwaiti Police*. Kuwait City: Social Development Office, Amiri Diwan.

Everly, G. S. & Boyle, S. (1997). A meta-analysis of the critical incident stress debriefing (CISD). Paper presented to the 4th World Congress on Stress, Trauma and Coping in the Emergency Services Professions, Baltimore, MD.

Everly, G. S. & Mitchell, J. T. (1997). *Critical Incident Stress Management (CISM): A New Era and Standard of Care in Crisis Intervention*. Ellicott City, MD: Chevron Publishing.

Everly, G. S. & Mitchell, J. T. (1999). *Critical Incident Stress Management (CISM): A New Era and Standard of Care in Crisis Intervention*, 2nd edn. Ellicott City, MD: Chevron Publishing.

Flannery, R. B. (1990). Social support and psychological trauma: a methodological review. *Journal of Traumatic Stress*, 3, 593–612.

Flannery, R. B., Hanson, M., Penk, W., Flannery, G. & Gallagher, C. (1995). The Assaulted Staff Action Program: An approach to coping with the aftermath of violence in the workplace. In L. Murphy, J. Hurrell, S. Sauter & G. Keita (Eds.) *Job Stress Interventions* (pp. 199–212). Washington, DC: APA Press.

Frank, J. D. (1974). *Persuasion and Healing*. Baltimore, MD: Johns Hopkins University Press.

Grainger, C. (1995). Occupational violence: armed hold up – a risk management approach. *International Journal of Stress Management*, 2, 197–205.

Griffiths, J. & Watts, R. (1992). *The Kempsey and Grafton Bus Crashes: The Aftermath*. East Lismore, New South Wales: Instructional Design Solutions.

Hanneman, M. F. (1994). *Evaluation of Critical Incident Stress Debriefing as perceived by volunteer firefighters in Nova Scotia*. Ph.D. dissertation. Ann Arbor, MI: UMI Dissertation Services.

Hytten, K. & Hasle, A. (1989). Firefighters: a study of stress and coping. *Acta Psychiatrica Scandinavica*, 80, Suppl. 355, 50–5.

Janet, P. (1889). *L'Automatisme Psychologique: Essai de Psychologie Experimentale sur les Formes Inférieur de l'Activité Humaine*. Paris: Felix Alcan.

Jenkins, S. R. (1996). Social support and debriefing efficacy among emergency medical workers after a mass shooting incident. *Journal of Social Behaviour and Personality*, 11, 477–92.

Jonsson, U. (1995). *Slutrapport Fran Globen-projektet*. Stockholm: Polishogskolan.

Kardiner, A. & Spiegel, H. (1947). *War, Stress and Neurotic Illness*. New York: Hoeber.

Kenardy, J. A., Webster, R. A., Lewin, T. J., Carr, V. J., Hazell, P. L. & Carter, G. L. (1996). Stress debriefing and patterns of recovery following a natural disaster. *Journal of Traumatic Stress*, 9, 37–49.

Kirwan, S. (1994). *Nursing Stress Pilot Project*. Winnipeg: Manitoba Provincial Medical Services.

Lanning, J. K. S. (1987). *Post-trauma recovery of public safety workers for the Delta 191 crash: debriefing, personal characteristics and social systems*. Ph.D. disseration. Ann Arbor, MI: UMI Dissertation Services.

Leeman-Conley, M. (1990). After a violent robbery . . . *Criminology Australia*, April–May, 4–6.

Lindemann, E. (1944). Symptomatology and management of acute grief. *American Journal of Psychiatry*, 101, 141–8.

Lindy, J. D. (1985). The trauma membrane and other clinical concepts derived from psychotherapeutic work with survivors of natural disaster. *Psychiatric Annals*, 15, 153–60.

Manzi, L. A. (1995). Evaluation of the on site academy's residential program. Unpublished research investigation submitted to Boston College.

Maslow, A. (1970). *Motivation and Personality*. New York: Harper & Row.

McFarlane, A. C. (1988). The longitudinal course of post-traumatic morbidity. *Journal of Nervous and Mental Disease*, 176, 30–9.

Mitchell, J. T. (1976). Rescue crisis intervention. *EMS News*, 4(3),4. Baltimore, MD: Maryland Institute for Emergency Medical Services Systems.

Mitchell, J. T. (1981). Acute stress reactions and burnout in pre-hospital emergency medical services personnel. Paper presented at the First National Conference on Burnout, November, Philadelphia, PA.

Mitchell, J. T. (1982). Recovery from rescue. *Response Magazine*, Fall, 7–10.

Mitchell, J. T. (1983). When disaster strikes . . . The critical incident stress debriefing process. *Journal of Emergency Medical Services*, 8(1), 36–9.

Mitchell, J. T. (1986). Teaming up against critical incident stress. *Chief Fire Executive*, 1, 24; 36; 84.

Mitchell, J. T. (1988). The history, status and future of critical incident stress debriefings. *Journal of Emergency Medical Services*, 13(11), 49–52.

Mitchell, J. T. (1992). *Comprehensive Traumatic Stress Management in the Emergency Department.* Monograph Series, *Leadership in Nursing.* The Emergency Nurses Association.

Mitchell, J. T. & Bray, G. P. (1990). *Emergency Services Stress: Guidelines for Preserving the Health and Careers of Emergency Services Personnel.* Englewood Cliffs, NJ: Prentice-Hall, Brady Publications.

Mitchell, J. T. & Everly, G. S. (1993). *Critical Incident Stress Debriefing (CISD): An Operations Manual for the Prevention of Traumatic Stress Among Emergency Services and Disaster Workers.* Ellicott City, MD: Chevron Publishing.

Mitchell, J. T. & Everly, G. S. (1996). *Critical Incident Stress Debriefing (CISD): An Operations Manual for the Prevention of Traumatic Stress Among Emergency Services and Disaster Workers,* 2nd edn revised. Ellicott City, MD: Chevron Publishing.

Mitchell, J. T. & Resnik, H. L. P. (1981). *Emergency Response to Crisis.* Bowie, MD: Robert J. Brady Company, Prentice Hall International.

Neil, T., Oney, J., Difonso, L., Thacker, B. & Reichart, W. (1974). *Emotional First Aid.* Louisville, KY: Kemper-Behavioural Sciences Associates.

Nurmi, L. (1997). The sinking of the 'Estonia'. Paper presented at the 4th World Congress on Stress, Trauma and Coping in the Emergency Services Professions, 2–6 April, 1997, Baltimore, MD.

Ott, K. & Henry, P. (1997). *Critical Incident Stress Management at Goulburn, Correctional Centre (A Report).* Goulburn, NSW: NSW Department of Corrective Services.

Parad, H. (1996). The use of time limited crisis intervention in community mental health programming. *Social Service Review,* **40**, 275–82.

Paton, D. (1995). Debriefing: social support and recovery from trauma. Psychologically speaking. Paper presented to the Australian Psychological Society (WA Branch), 1–3 June.

Pennebaker, J. W. (1985). Traumatic experience and psychosomatic disease. *Canadian Psychologist,* **26**, 82–95.

Pennebaker, J. W. (1990). *Opening Up: The Healing Power of Confiding in Others.* New York: Avon.

Pennebaker, J. W. & Beall, S. (1986). Confronting a traumatic event. *Journal of Abnormal Psychology,* **95**, 274–81.

Pennebaker, J. W. & Susman, J. (1988). Disclosure of traumas and psychosomatic processes. *Social Science and Medicine,* **26**, 327–32.

Post, R. (1992). Transduction of psychosocial stress onto the neuro-biology of recurrent effective disorder. *American Journal of Psychiatry,* **149**, 990–1010.

Pynoos, R. S., Goeenjian, A. & Steinberg, A. M. (1994). Strategies of disaster intervention for children and adolescents. Paper presented at the NATO Conference on Stress, Coping and Disaster in Bonos, France.

Raphael, B. (1986). *When Disaster Strikes: How Individuals and Communities Cope with Catastrophe.* New York: Basic Books.

Rapoport, L. (1965). The state of crisis: some theoretical considerations. In H. Parad (Ed.) *Crisis Intervention: Selected Readings* (pp. 22–31). New York: Family Service Association of America.

Robinson, R. C. (1994). *Follow-up Study of Health and Stress in Ambulance Services, Victoria, Australia,* Part I. Melbourne, Victoria: Victoria Ambulance Services.

Robinson, R. & Mitchell, J. T. (1993). Evaluation of psychological debriefings. *Journal of Traumatic Stress,* **6**, 367–82.

Rogers, C. (1951). *Client-centered Therapy.* Boston, MA: Houghton Mifflin.

Rogers, O. W. (1993). An examination of Critical Incident Stress Debriefing for emergency service providers: a quasi-experimental field study. Ph.D. dissertation. Ann Arbor, MI: UMI Dissertation Services.

Salmon, T. W. (1919). War neuroses and their lesson. *New York Medical Journal,* **109**, 993–4.

Searle, M. M. and Bisson, J. I. (1992). Psychological sequelae of friendly fire. Unpublished paper presented at the *Military Psychiatry Conference on Stress, Psychiatry and War,* Paris, France.

Seligman, M. E. P. (1995). The effectiveness of psychotherapy. *American Psychologist,* **29**, 965–74.

Shneidman, E. S. & Farberow, N. L. (1957). *Clues to Suicide.* New York: McGraw Hill.

Slaby, A., Lieb, J. & Tancredi, L. (1975). *Handbook of Psychiatric Emergencies.* Flushing, NY: Medical Examination Publishing.

Slaikeu, K. A. (1984). *Crisis Intervention: A Handbook for Practice and Research.* Boston, MA: Allyn and Bacon, Inc.

Solomon, Z. & Benbenishty, R. (1986). The role of proximity, immediacy, and expectancy in front-line treatment of combat stress reaction among Israelis in the Lebanon War. *American Journal of Psychiatry,* **143**, 613–17.

Solomon, Z. & Shalev, A. (1995). Helping victims of military trauma, In J. Freedy & S. Hobfoll (Eds.) *Traumatic Stress* (pp. 241–61). New York: Plenum Press.

Spiegel, D. & Classen, C. (1995). Acute stress disorder. In G. Gabbard (Ed.) *Treatments of Psychiatric Disorders* (pp. 1521–37). Washington, DC: American Psychiatric Press.

Stallard, P. & Law, F. (1993). Screening and psychological debriefing of adolescent survivors of life-threatening events. *British Journal of Psychiatry,* **163**, 660–5.

Stierlin, E. (1909). *Psycho-neuropathology as a Result of a Mining Disaster March 10, 1906.* Zurich: University of Zurich.

Taylor, S. (1983). Adjustment to threatening events. *American Psychologist*, **38**, 1161–73.

van der Hart, O., Brown, P. & van der Kolk, B. (1989). Pierre Janet's treatment of post-traumatic stress. *Journal of Traumatic Stress*, **2**, 379–96.

Wee, D. (1996). Research in critical incident stress management. Part 4. How effective is this? *Life Net*, **7**(2), 4–5.

Wee, D., Mills, D. M. & Koelher, G. (1999). The effects of Critical Incident Stress Debriefing on emergency medical services personnel following the Los Angeles civil disturbance. International *Journal of Emergency Mental Health*, **1**, 33–8.

Weisæth, L. (1989a). A study of behavioural responses to an industrial disaster. *Acta Psychiatrica Scandinavica*, **80**, Suppl. 355, 13–24.

Weisæth, L. (1989b). The stressors and post-traumatic stress syndrome after an industrial disaster. *Acta Psychiatrica Scandinavica*, **80**, Suppl. 355, 25–7.

Western Management Consultants (1996). *The Medical Services Branch CISM Evaluation Report.* Vancouver, BC: Western Management Consultants.

Wollman, D. (1993). Critical incident stress debriefing and crisis groups: a review of literature. *Group*, **17**, 70–83.

Yalom, I. (1970). *Theory and Practice of Group Psychotherapy.* New York: Basic Books.

6

Debriefing with emergency services: Critical Incident Stress Management

Robyn Robinson

EDITORIAL COMMENTS

This chapter presents a further view of the Mitchell's model of debriefing and Critical Incident Stress Management (CISM), setting it in a crisis intervention context. Robinson highlights the separation of this model from psychotherapy. She then goes on to differentiate it in professional and workplace terminology, as well as examining its historical context, current status and conceptual basis. The latter defines the social and health model in which it sits and its practical role in the emergency services. Here, its evolution is linked to changes in cultural attitudes towards the acceptance of the psychological trauma model, expansion of psychology and the development of the Mitchell model. She reviews evaluation studies in terms of acceptance of CISM in the emergency service workplace, the reported value of the service for recipients and empirical studies. The latter are reviewed with recognition of the methodological problems in those studies having negative, as well as those with positive, outcomes. The need for evolution of research design is emphasized in view of the complexity of trauma experience, response and other variables shaping outcomes. She also highlights her observation that many of the negative studies do not provide definitions of the model of debriefing used, and target groups other than emergency workers. She emphasizes the need for the evidence base to be broadened and the essential need for systematic and convergent evaluation using a variety of appropriate methodologies to investigate specific research and evaluation questions. She also summarizes from the point of view of experience as a practitioner, the poten-

tial effects and risks and the essential elements of a debriefing model. These might also be questioned and investigated in terms of the need to build a scientific base to justify their potential contribution.

Robinson clearly indicates that the programme she is describing is oriented at the stress people experience in their work, particularly emergency service workers. While both her chapter and that of Mitchell and Everly acknowledge that CISM may at times have evolved to broader use, its prime application is to emergency workers. Robinson also specifically emphasizes that, while CISM has been applied to other work situations, more is needed to identify and evaluate appropriate systems, and that its role is not for the broader community, or for primary victims or survivors, whose needs are likely to be both more intense and more individual.

She concludes by emphasizing the need for good-quality research, to understand better the strong perceptions of helpfulness and their significance, to define the model evaluated (e.g. Mitchell or other), and to address the complex tasks of furthering such science.

Overview

This chapter focuses on Critical Incident Stress Management (CISM) and Critical Incident Stress Debriefing (CISD) in emergency service agencies. In the first section, key terms are defined and then a brief background of emergency service CISM/CISD is described. The conceptual basis for CISM/CISD follows, with the context in which CISM and CISD are applied in emergency services. Evaluation studies of CISM/CISD are reviewed and comments are made about the difficulties that face research efforts in this area. There follows a summary of the effects and risks of CISM/CISD and, finally, a description of the essential elements of debriefing.

Definitions

This chapter begins with some definitions in order to avoid misinterpretation or ambiguity about key terms used in this field.

- *Critical Incident Stress Management (CISM)* is a comprehensive, multicomponent, well-integrated work-based programme that is designed to assist emergency service workers, or allied professionals, to deal effectively with the traumatic and highly stressful components of their work. CISM may also be described as 'trauma management programmes' and 'psychological support programmes'. The core elements are the comprehensiveness of the approach (preventative and remedial), that programmes are work based and that they focus mainly or exclusively on traumatic stress as opposed to general work stress or organizational stress.

  CISM programmes comprise many elements, including education (on trauma and its management), one-on-one counselling/support, group meetings, follow-up and partner support. They are fully described by Mitchell & Everly (1996) and Everly & Mitchell (1997). CISM programmes manage day-to-day traumatic events as well as large-scale incidents.
- *Critical Incident Stress Debriefing (CISD)* is but one component or intervention strategy of CISM. It is defined as 'a group meeting or discussion about a distressing critical incident. Based upon core principles of education and crisis intervention, the CISD is designed to mitigate the impact of a critical incident and to assist the personnel in recovering as quickly as possible from the stress associated with the event' (Mitchell & Everly, 1996, p. 8). The term is used here, as it was developed by Mitchell, to refer to a group and not an individual activity. CISD follows a seven-stage model and is conducted by a team of specially trained peers and mental health professionals.

- *A peer support person* is defined as 'an emergency service worker who has been specially selected and trained to provide a first line of assistance and basic crisis intervention to other emergency service personnel' (Robinson & Murdoch, 1998, p. 1). Traditionally, peer support has focussed on trauma, but more recently some peer programmes have been expanded to address job-related and personal problems of staff. Nevertheless, a focus on crisis is maintained.

Over recent decades, two professional 'branches' have developed that focus on trauma. The older of the two branches, pioneered by many well-known figures, has a generic orientation, and considers trauma as it may affect all people and all circumstances. The more recent branch, developed primarily by Dr Jeffrey Mitchell, focusses on workplace trauma and in the emergency services in particular. Each branch has its own professional body and a tendency towards its own language set (see Table 6.1). Thus different words tend to be used to describe similar notions and this has caused some confusion. In this chapter, the various words that appear to describe the same phenomenon will be treated as more or less equivalent: for example, traumatic stress and critical incident stress will be treated as having similar meanings.

Historical background

It has been recognized for many years that emergency service workers can face traumatic situations in the course of their job, especially in circumstances of disasters and major emergencies. In Australia, for example, the pioneering work of Raphael recognized the need for support to workers and helpers involved in a disaster, and described a psychological debriefing procedure in this context (Raphael, 1977, 1986, pp. 282–6). Specific applications to emergency service personnel are also made.

CISM programmes for emergency service workers (including, but not limited to, debriefing) were developed by Mitchell in the late 1970s to early 1980s in the USA. These were introduced into Australia, Canada and Norway in the mid-to-late 1980s and into many other

Table 6.1. Terms used to describe trauma and its management

	Professional branch	
	Traumatic stress	Workplace trauma
Stimulus	Traumatic event	Critical incident
Response	Traumatic stress	Critical incident stress
Management	Trauma management	Critical incident stress management
Professional society	International Society for Traumatic Stress Study	International Critical Incident Stress Foundation

countries soon after (Robinson, 1995). Since these pro-grammes were so successful, and the concepts so applicable to similar workplaces, other groups of professional workers adapted and adopted the emergency services model to their own circumstances. Consequently, today, there are many different programmes of psychological support in the workplace, which have been developed for a diverse group of populations including emergency service workers, defence force personnel, corrective services, hospital staff (both general and psychiatric), airline staff, employees from rehabilitation agencies, departments of education, health and welfare, industries with a high risk of industrial accidents (such as mining, deep-sea oil extraction and exploration), industries with risk of violence to staff (such as hold-ups in banks and gas stations), high-risk sports and others.

While there are common themes and similar principles running through the majority of modern programmes, there is also sufficient diversity in programme aims and processes to make it difficult to speak generically about these (see, e.g. Lewis (1994) for applications of the Mitchell model to nonemergency service populations). The Mitchell model and some other programmes (such as that of Armstrong et al. (1991)) have sufficient specificity to enable evaluation, but much of what is practised other than by the emergency services, in Australia at least, has not been fully described and documented, let alone assessed. It is important to understand that there is much diversity practised under commonly used terms such as debriefing, CISM and trauma management.

The above situation may well intensify, in the immediate future, due to a number of factors. First, the kinds of organization adopting trauma management

programmes appear to be increasing and programmes are being applied to a very diverse set of workplaces. For example, peer support personnel are being introduced into nonemergency service agencies. Secondly, trauma management programmes themselves are tending to develop in their size, scope and importance as a consequence both of their success within agencies and also the increasing body of knowledge about trauma, its impact and its treatment.

There are many issues raised by the expansion of CISM programmes into such a variety of organizations. However, those issues are beyond the scope of this chapter, which focusses on emergency services.

Current status

Deliberations about current CISM/CISD practices ought to distinguish the following kinds of programme and practice:

The Mitchell model as applied to emergency services

These are comprehensive programmes, with educational as well as post-incident support components, which are carried out by trained personnel according to specific protocols. They are early intervention programmes designed to assist personnel in dealing with critical incidents on a daily basis. While CISM is employed after disasters, the focus of programmes is on general trauma. The expected outcomes of CISM include reduction in acute stress response, facilitation of individuals 'coming to terms with' or 'processing' traumatic events, mobilization of own coping resources, mobilization of social support, facilitation of worker's return to work, enhanced workplace morale and positive impacts on the financial costs of unresolved stress as may be reflected in staff turnover, sick leave, workers' compensation and the like. The effects of these programmes are best assessed on a regular basis; the specific effects of particular interventions, such as CISD, are best assessed soon after the intervention, i.e. within weeks. Longer-term studies are also needed and here the effects of early intervention studied months or years afterwards needs to focus on the multiplicity of variables (of which early intervention will be but one) that can be expected to influence the individual at the time of assessment.

Alternative models as applied to emergency services

Alternative support programmes in emergency services need to be assessed on their merits, as occurs for the Mitchell model. While this statement may seem trite, in fact people may believe that they are assessing the Mitchell model but be studying a process that differs in fundamental ways and in reality reflects different practices.

The Mitchell model and modifications to it applied to nonemergency service workplaces

While there are studies and reports of the helpfulness of CISM programmes in institutions such as hospitals, banks, corrective services, etc., there may be other workplaces where CISM may not be as successful. For example, peer work may be seen as a logical extension for those who enter helping professions but may be less attractive for people whose vocation is less person centred.

Models and practices applied to members of the community

Much care is needed in applying the Mitchell CISM model to community groups. This is especially so where exposure to trauma has come about through the accident of people being thrown together at a particular time, or where there are communities of people with diverse needs and different levels of exposure to a traumatic event who may have little in common with others

so exposed. Time and experience will undoubtedly enable appropriate models of support to be developed, and these may well include elements of CISM.

Models and practices applied to primary victims/survivors

The CISM model may be quite unsuitable for primary victims/survivors. The needs of primary victims/survivors can be expected to be more intense and more individual. In addition, it is not possible to establish a planned and systematic response to trauma in the way that can be achieved with members of a workplace.

The conceptual basis of CISM/CISD

There are several bodies of literature relevant to the conceptual underpinning and understanding of CISM and CISD, namely those that focus on crisis intervention, on the nature of recovery from trauma and on process variables.

Crisis intervention

The major body of literature, and the one emphasized by Everly & Mitchell (1997) is that of crisis intervention. Crisis intervention was developed by Lindemann (1944), following support offered to victims of a fire in the Coconut Grove nightclub in Boston, Massachusetts. Caplan (1964) developed the focus of crisis intervention from one of loss and grief to that of broad-spectrum potentially stressful or traumatic events (Gilliland & James, 1997). Shortly after, various crisis intervention models were developed that widened the applications even further. While crisis intervention was initially developed for citizens after disasters (the Coconut Grove fire) it was subsequently developed for smaller-scale situations such as rape, violence, traumatic loss, and any situation that could overwhelm the coping strategies of individuals. In 1986, Parad predicted, 'There will be, I believe, continued experimentation with brief crisis therapy in non-social work settings such as child care centres..., employee assistance programmes in the workplace (think of the potential – there are over 100 million workers in the USA, many of them experiencing severe daily crises on and off the job), and schools' (Parad, 1986, p. 17).

The context in which crisis intervention was developed was of ordinary people faced with extraordinary events that overwhelmed their personal coping skills. As Hafen & Fransen (1985, pp. 18–19) argued, support intervention is 'unlike traditional methods of treatment for emotional problems ... it is earmarked by narrow goals of short duration. In a nutshell, crisis intervention is aimed at helping a person regain equilibrium – return to normal functioning – by providing emotional support during a time of emotional vulnerability'. Crisis intervention emphasizes prevention generally, which is evident in education about crisis management, as well as the attempts, by early intervention, to prevent the development of chronic unresolved problems.

The goals of crisis intervention have been variously described, but can be summarized in the following way:

to protect the individual from additional stress,
to minimize the impact of the crisis on the individual,
to mobilize the personal coping skills of the individual and the external support networks, and
to restore the individual to his or her precrisis level of functioning or higher.

CISM has all of the characteristics of a crisis intervention model. Education (prevention) is a key strategy and Mitchell wrote 'The CISD team is active in stress education and preventative programmes before a stressful event ever occurs' (Mitchell & Bray, 1990, p. 134). Intervention aims 'to reduce the impact of a critical incident and to accelerate the normal recovery of normal people who are suffering through normal but painful reactions to abnormal events' (Mitchell & Bray, 1990, p. 143). CISM also emphasizes getting people back to work.

Recovery from trauma

Knowledge about recovery from trauma is growing. One aspect of particular relevance is the value of talking about experiences. A developing body of knowledge

and argument suggests that humans need to express their thoughts and feelings in words (or writing) and that there is a time frame in which this should occur (see Pennebaker, 1990, 1993; van der Kolk et al., 1996). This may be part of making the experience 'real'.

Process variables

The skills and knowledge of the people who provide support are important variables in understanding outcomes. In the field of psychotherapy, it has been argued that the skills of the therapist are of great importance (Seligman, 1995). This should be no less true for crisis intervention. For example, Blackwelder (1995, p. xi) concluded that there are better effects when CISM trained staff are used in support services rather than untrained personnel. Dyregrov (1996) found that debriefings led by trained debriefers are more effective than those led by untrained people and, in a review of the processes of debriefing, stated that 'the background, training and personal qualities of the leaders are extremely important variables in making successful debriefings' (Dyregrov, 1997, p. 593).

Special attention may need to be given to the roles of peers in CISM programmes. Peers perform many tasks including education, one-on-one-support, small-group discussions or defusings, debriefings (together with mental health professionals), follow-up of staff and referral of staff to therapists, as appropriate. The value of lay persons in support roles has been ably demonstrated (Carkhuff, 1987) and, more recently, the value of peers has been described (see, e.g., Robinson, 1993, 1997; Tunnecliffe & Roy, 1993; Hanneman, 1994).

Peers assist the emergency service workers to talk about their experiences, to feel that they have been understood, and to assess their own coping skills. As Wilson (1989, p. 197) stated, it is often difficult for people who have experienced trauma to talk about what has happened, 'they fear that the mental health professional "will not understand" what they have gone through since "they were not there" and therefore cannot possibly understand "what it was like"'. In the emergency services, the people who are most likely to fully comprehend the plight of those who experience traumatic situations are fellow employees. In many instances, peers have been in similar situations. They can therefore readily relate to the situations of their colleagues and are generally perceived 'to understand'. The reason why understanding is important may be that it enables the individual to focus on relevant thoughts and feelings. If understanding is not present, the people so affected may be taken away from the task of dealing with their experiences and shifted towards trying to explain their feelings and behaviours to others. They may then also have to deal with additional feelings, such as anger, that were generated from unhelpful conversations.

There may also be logistical factors that enable peers to assist emergency service workers in their recovery. Peers are often flexible in the amount and timing of their contacts; they can be with workers for long periods of time in extreme circumstances and they can also maintain brief but continual contact as appropriate. It is possible for them to meet a worker on common ground or in mutually agreed informal settings. These arrangements may be conducive to frank discussions. Peers' ability to be on hand quickly may be particularly important in emergency services. Strong emotions can quickly become suppressed, bottled-up or dissociated over time and it may be very important for distressed individuals to talk to somebody quickly while emotions are keenly felt (Robinson & Murdoch, 1998).

There are two tasks ahead. First, the different bodies of knowledge need to be integrated, combining that which is known about the inner workings of the mind with that which is known about the ways in which the individual deals with his or her environment. Secondly, the general body of knowledge about trauma needs to be applied, differentially, to various groups or populations. For example, emergency service workers experience particular kinds of trauma, they have some expectation that their work will entail trauma, and they develop coping skills to deal with this. Thus, the impact and resolution of trauma on these personnel can be expected to have elements differing from those experienced by other people. It may be that the high coping skills of personnel (Robinson, 1984, 1986, 1993), combined with their need to control emotions so that they can perform their job, gives a narrow window of opportunity for personnel, post incident, to 'process' inci-

dents. This would make the quick support response advocated by crisis intervention theory particularly important. It would also explain, in part, the value of peers because they can provide rapid support.

CISM in emergency services

The introduction of trauma management programmes into emergency services has been very rapid and, in the main, highly accepted by workers. It is important to understand the reasons for this development. The following factors are suggested.

Cultural attitudes towards the acceptance of trauma

It has been suggested that people are ambivalent about acknowledging, validating and deliberating on those aspects of our existence that are emotionally difficult to comprehend and to contemplate – such as trauma. Herman (1992), for example, argued that in the field of trauma one finds, over time, waves of acknowledgement followed by waves of denial, and that these fluctuations apply equally to the professional and the general community. Our attention to trauma in the mid to late 1980s may in part reflect our being in a period where there has been a willingness to examine it.

Expansions in psychology

The general body of knowledge of psychology has greatly expanded over the past few decades. There is greater understanding of, and emphasis on, the mental and emotional aspects of human functioning as well as a greater knowledge of helping and counselling skills. The study of trauma has developed very rapidly. Psychological helping skills have, arguably, become more specialized, and with this specialization has come a greater diversity of people who are taking on the helping role. Parallel developments occurred earlier in the area of physical health where there was an expansion in the kinds of available assistance between a patient and a medical doctor (e.g. trained first aider, ambulance officer, nurse). So too, in the field of psychological health, there appears to be an introduction of different levels of assistance between a client and a mental

EMERGENCY SERVICE AGENCY

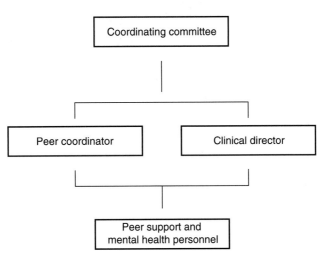

Figure 6.1. Organizational structure for CISM programmes.

health professional (mental health nurse, psychologist/ psychiatrist/social worker). Peers are one of several groups that appear to be filling this gap.

Mitchell's particular model

When Mitchell introduced CISM, he presented a model based solidly in crisis intervention theory. He described the intervention activities that are part of CISM, and also detailed the roles that people who would administer programmes must play and the organizational structure needed in order for programmes to function in the workplace. The comprehensive and yet easily understandable nature of this instruction, in my opinion, assisted people in implementing programmes. His work provided a mission to act to action-oriented people who were relieved that not only had the emotional pain associated with their job been recognized and validated but that an achievable solution had been presented in a way that maximized their control over themselves and the helping process.

The implementation of CISM programmes is fully described elsewhere (Mitchell & Everly, 1996), and a brief overview only is given at this point (see Figure

6.1). A management committee oversees the programme, which is administered by a peer coordinator in conjunction with a clinical director (mental health practitioner). A team of peer support personnel and mental health practitioners provide the CISM services.

Before any traumatic event occurs, it can be reasonably expected that there will have been:

field education on trauma, coping and the available CISM support services,
development of a trained team of peers and mental health professionals, and
development of protocols and policy to guide the ways in which critical incidents are managed.

Following an incident, there occurs a fairly exhaustive enquiry in order to determine the best possible course of action, CISD being but one option. In fact, in some emergency services, one-on-one support and defusings (shorter forms of debriefing offered within 24 hours) are now the preferred option.

Thus, in the emergency services, CISM is offered within a structure, which is described in protocols and policies and which should be known by all members of the agency (Robinson & Murdoch, 1996).

Evaluation studies of CISM/CISD

There are various kinds of evidence that demonstrate the value of CISM programmes.

Acceptance of CISM in the workplace and by the professional community

- New programmes continue to be started; established programmes continue to be maintained and expanded.

Anecdotal evidence suggests that many early programmes have continued into the current time. This has occurred despite scrutiny from within emergency services about the value of these programmes, and despite stringent national economies in many countries. There have been expansions of programmes across and within countries.

- Many programmes continue to base their policies and practices on the Mitchell model.

The Mitchell model, in its current form or with minor modifications, has continued as the model of choice for many current programmes (Tunnecliffe & Robinson, 1997). Some changes have been embraced, but these have generally been in line with the basic principles of Mitchell's model and the expanded role of peer support.

- Professional bodies have maintained a healthy and steadily increasing membership as well as healthy conference attendance.

The International Critical Incident Stress Foundation, and like-minded organizations such as the Canadian Critical Incident Stress Association and the Critical Incident Stress Management Foundation Australia, report growing membership and healthy conference attendance.

- Both peers and mental health practitioners continue to be trained in CISM and related interventions.

Training programmes for both peers and mental health practitioners are popular and this probably reflects the fact that participants find the training useful.

Reported value of services by recipients

- CISM programmes consistently yield very positive comments in surveys and studies.

Almost all surveys and studies that ask recipients about their opinions on CISM services and whether they find interventions to be helpful and beneficial reply in the affirmative. For example, a recent survey of ambulance officers in Victoria, Australia ($n = 755$, 60% response rate) rated the helpfulness of support services as follows: professional assistance 95%, peer support 95%, and debriefing/defusing 91%. This same study found that the perceived importance for services to continue were: for professional assistance 100%, peer support 98% and debriefings/defusings 97% (Robinson, 1997). Even studies cited as evidence for the lack of efficacy of debriefing report high perceived helpfulness of debriefing (Hytten & Hasle, 1989; Griffiths & Watts, 1992; Deahl et al., 1994; Kenardy et al., 1996).

Empirical studies

- A growing number of empirical studies show the benefits of CISM.

The number of positive outcome studies on CISD and CISM is growing. Reviews can be found by Mitchell & Everly (1996, 1997), Everly & Mitchell (1997) and Everly et al. (1999).

The next section classifies positive outcome studies according to the found benefits (see Table 6.2) and it can be seen that there is a broad spectrum of outcomes. Many studies have focussed on the reduction of the adverse effects of trauma, but some also demonstrate the value of CISM in enabling people to process trauma, to make sense of it, and to mobilize their personal and interpersonal coping strategies. The positive outcomes of CISD/CISM to organizations is also apparent from studies that show increased morale, improved work performances, and decreases in destructive behaviours of staff. As well, there are reported outcomes that demonstrate direct financial savings to organizations (reduced sick leave, reduced workers' compensation claims, less absenteeism and reduced staff turnover). The cost-effective studies are particularly

Table 6.2. Evaluation studies that find positive outcomes from CISM/CISD

Outcome	Studies
Reducing stress/trauma signs, less depression, less anxiety	Lanning & Fannin (1988), Ersland et al. (1989), Bohl (1991), Yule & Udwin (1991), Robinson (1993, 1997), Robinson & Mitchell (1993), Rogers (1993)[b], Stallard & Law (1993), Hanneman (1994)[a], Pynoos et al. (1994), Jenkins (1996), Wee (1996), Chemtob et al. (1997), Nurmi (1997)
Processing the event (expressing feelings, getting the facts etc.)	Dyregrov (1989), Burns & Harm (1993), Robinson (1993), Robinson & Mitchell (1993), Stallard & Law (1993), Hanneman (1994)[a], AAOS (1996), Richman & Blizzard (1996)
Mobilizing own resources and coping	Lanning & Fannin (1988), Rogers (1993)[a], Hanneman (1994)[a]
Mobilizing social support	Lanning & Fannin (1988), Campbell (1992)[a], Hanneman (1994)[a]
Work place improvement (higher morale and cohesiveness, less disruptive behaviour, enhanced work performance)	Campbell (1992)[a], Robinson (1993, 1997), Hanneman (1994)[a] Flannery & Penk (1996)
Cost-effectiveness of CISM programme (less sick leave workers compensation and staff turnover)	Leeman-Conley (1990), Flannery & Penk (1996), Ott & Henry (1997), Western Management Consultants (1997)
Positive CISM programme evaluation	Robinson (1993, 1997)

[a] Cited by Mitchell & Everly (1997).
[b] Cited by Everly & Mitchell (1997).

pleasing to see for, it is probably fair to state, many programmes (with their emphasis on confidentiality) have been slow to give funders the kinds of information that are needed in order for management to support programmes. For some managers in emergency services there has needed to be a 'leap of faith' (Ryan, 1996) to maintain and support programmes, for it has only been in recent times that empirical evidence has been gathered. Fortunately, there are now excellent examples of cost savings to organizations owing to the introduction of CISM programmes. For example, Western Management Consultants assessed the dollar value of a Mitchell CISM programme instigated for nurses in rural Canada. They were employed by the Canadian Health Authority to perform an independent evaluation and found that for every Canadian dollar spent on the CISM programme, (Can)$7.06 was saved as assessed through costs of sick leave, disability claims and staff turnover (Western Management Consultants, 1997). Ott & Henry (1997) reported a 92% reduction in stress-related compensation costs over a year, following the introduction of a staff care (CISM) programme at Goulburn Correctional Centre in New South Wales. Leeman-Conley (1990) reported a 60% reduction in sick days and 68% reduction in compensation payments and disability payments leave following the introduction of a staff support programme after hold-ups in the Commonwealth Bank of Australia.

Evaluation studies use a variety of designs. Self-reporting is commonly employed. Whereas earlier studies tended to used unstandardized instruments, more recent studies often employ known measures of trauma, anxiety and other variables. There are no 'pure experimental designs' with randomized groups, but comparison groups are reported by, for example, Bohl (1991), Wee (1996) and Chemtob et al. (1997). Here, in studies of debriefing, the groups of debriefed and non-debriefed people have formed through chance or through participants either deciding or declining to take part in debriefings. The effects of not wishing, or not being able, to participate in debriefings on outcomes can only be speculated upon and represent an unknown variable. Thus, in assessing the results of these studies, any methodological weaknesses also need to be taken into consideration.

Some comments need to be made with respect to the claims that debriefing is ineffectual and that debriefing may be harmful by leading to a delayed trauma response. The studies that claim that debriefing is ineffectual are based on findings of no difference on the General Health Questionnaire (GHQ) and/or Impact of Event (IES) scales between debriefed and nondebriefed subjects, namely: 195 'helpers' involved in the Newcastle, New South Wales, earthquake (Kenardy et al., 1996); 288 'helpers' involved in the aftermath of two bus crashes on the eastern coast of Australia (Griffiths & Watts, 1992); 58 firefighters who participated in a hotel fire rescue operation (Hytten & Hasle, 1989); 62 British soldiers with involvement in the Gulf War (Deahl et al., 1994); and primary burns victims (Bisson et al., 1997).

The studies from which it is claimed that 'debriefings make people worse' include a finding of higher IES score in debriefed versus nondebriefed 'helpers' in the Griffith & Watts (1992) study and a finding, in a study of 315 volunteer firefighters involved in the Australian Ash Wednesday bushfires in Victoria, of a correlation between being debriefed and the diagnosis of 'delayed onset' trauma response at 50 and 126 weeks post incident (McFarlane 1988).

A number of problems arise with these studies and with the conclusions that have been drawn from them (see also Robinson & Mitchell, 1995).

1. CISD is implemented and studied as an isolated procedure. CISD was conceptualized as one component of CISM and it is inappropriate to consider it other than in this context.
2. Comparisons are drawn between 'experimental' and 'control' groups without pretrauma baseline data (Griffiths & Watts, 1992; Deahl et al., 1994; Kennardy et al., 1996). This also occurs in studies that claim positive results for CISD/CISM; however, it is a more serious flaw in the negative outcome studies because it is likely that it is the more

highly traumatized people who undertake debriefings (or have debriefings organized for them) and thus have a higher trauma score prior to the debriefing than do nondebriefed people.

3. There is no description of the 'debriefing' intervention, the training or competence of the debriefers or their adherence to debriefing protocols. For example, Kenardy et al. (1996) stated that 'there was no standardization of debriefing services and procedures following the earthquake … we were not able to determine objectively the quality of the debriefing provided to each subject … we do not know to what extent the debriefing matched the model of Mitchell…'. Further they did not even know whether people in the 'debriefed group' had in fact received debriefing. Yet the authors go on to make conclusions about the process. The earlier Australian studies, cited above, are unlikely to have followed the Mitchell model because training in the model was not established at that time.
4. Debriefing is a relatively short intervention (two to three hours) usually held within a week of the traumatic incident. To assess its major impact, evaluation should be close to the debriefing (probably within weeks). Studies assess debriefings at nine months (Deahl et al., 1994), 12 months (McFarlane, 1988; Griffiths & Watts, 1992; Kenardy et al., 1996) and even longer time periods (McFarlane, 1988; Kenardy et al., 1996). The studies at 12 months are particularly unfortunate in their timing, given our knowledge of 'anniversary effects' and the inevitable confounding of this factor with study results. With long-term evaluation, the total support programme (or lack of it) ought to be assessed. It does not make sense to evaluate short-term crisis interventions years later, in isolation of other factors.
5. There are sometimes unrealistic expectations of debriefing. In the Deahl et al. (1994) study, there was assessment of soldiers who had experienced very gruesome events over a prolonged time. It is not surprising that a two-hour debriefing, if this was the sole support, which is assessed nine months later, revealed no impact on the GHQ and IES.
6. Some studies contrast groups receiving CISD with

groups that receive other kinds of support (e.g. Hytten & Hasle, 1989; Alexander, 1993). They are comparing different support systems and their conclusions do not invalidate CISM principles.

7. The criterion variables used to assess debriefing are often narrow. For example, the GHQ is essentially a measure of psychiatric impairment. A broader span of outcomes needs to be considered, as is evident from Table 6.2.

8. Some of the critical incidents studied are large-scale emergencies or disasters. While CISM applies to these, it is essentially more commonly used in day-to-day incidents with high impact.

9. Several of the authors whose articles have been quoted as being critical of debriefing in fact support the concept of debriefing in their articles. For example, Deahl et al. (1994) did not recommend discontinuing debriefings. Griffiths & Watts (1992, p. 75) cautioned against the conclusion that debriefings made people worse: 'those who were the most affected were more likely to attend debriefings and it is not indicative of the sessions making the personnel more affected in the long term'. McFarlane (1986, p. 563) wrote 'consideration should be given to the development of preventative strategies for such groups in future disasters, including a formal debriefing where information is given about the long term nature of post-traumatic stress disorder, and a follow-up of those defined to be at risk'. Nevertheless, both Watts (1994) and McFarlane (Raphael et al., 1995) express reservations about CISD at later times.

10. CISD was not designed for primary victims but for what may be referred to as secondary victims. Emergency service personnel are generally healthy people who mainly demonstrate strong coping skills. Their encounters with trauma are mostly in the course of their job and they have some expectations that this will occur from time to time. Primary victims are likely to show a different kind of trauma impact and one that is stronger and more prolonged than that experienced by emergency service workers. Thus the Bisson et al. (1997) article should be seen as a reference to primary victims, as is the McFarlane study where many of the volunteer fire-fighters were protecting their own homes, 23% suffered property damage and 7% experienced some bereavement (McFarlane, 1988). Some of the workers in the Griffith & Watts (1992) study were also primary victims.

As research and evaluation continues in the future, it may be useful to bear the following points in mind.

- The evolving nature of CISM/peer support programmes makes research difficult and complex, and patience is needed.

CISM programmes are evolving both within emergency services (e.g. increased roles of peer support, pro-active outreach to the field) and within other organizations. These extensions and expansions are a strength of CISM but make research difficult. For example, those focussing on CISD (and not on CISM) may be not only too narrow in their focus but also marginal. Many emergency services have for some time focussed on defusing and this is often used more frequently than debriefing. There is a problem that, in a rapidly evolving field which is very responsive to client feedback, formal research will lag behind practice.

- It is necessary to define what constitutes 'a model'.

With the exception of the Mitchell model and a few others (e.g. Armstrong et al., 1991), an emerging problem is that of defining models under review and also defining what constitutes a model. For example, Parkinson (1997) proposed that there is a separate CISM model developed by Dyregrov, but Dyregrov himself sees his practices as largely those of Mitchell (Everly et al., 1999). The defining of models is important because researchers need to know what it is that they are evaluating.

- Multiple methods of evaluation need to be employed.

Researchers in the field of evaluation, many decades ago, argued that any evaluation study should be concerned with the aims of that study in the first instance and that study design and methodology need to reflect study aims. Hence there has been caution against the advocacy of particular designs (or denigration of particular methods) in favour of a focus on what methods or designs can best answer the questions at hand. Evaluators have also long argued that the understanding of complex phenomena is often best achieved by collating information from a variety of sources and using a compilation of methodologies and designs. Thus the experimental paradigm, where it can be executed, will isolate variables under study (e.g. CISD) and examine their effects. This may be useful in some circumstances but it depends ultimately on the questions being asked.

• Definitions of evidence need to be broadened.

White has suggested that the recent debate on debriefing is an argument on what constitutes evidence (White, 1996) and this position has also been debated in evaluation circles for many years. Some of the controversy appears to centre on self-reporting, its credibility and the capacity to integrate recipient's verbalizations with psychological constructs. Information should be developed from a variety of sources, so it should not be suggested that self-reporting be the only kind of information to be sought. However, I would like to put the case for self-reporting and its importance. The feedback that emergency service workers provide about what is helpful and what needs to be changed within CISM programmes is part of a continuing and important feedback loop to programme administrators. As programmes develop, needs change. For example, as peer systems become trusted they tend to become better utilized. Emergency service workers are well able to appraise and articulate how and why interventions are helpful to themselves and, in their observations, to others. We trust emergency service personnel to make decisions that affect our well-being and even our lives, so that we can trust their capacity to articulate what they do and do not find helpful to them when they are in need of support themselves.

In summary, the development of empirical evidence is likely to take time because of the complexity of what is being studied and also because of the need for sensitivity in working with people who have been exposed to traumatic incidents. There are likely to be methodological and conceptual difficulties for researchers in this field. It is important to gather information from a broad variety of sources and examine this in its totality. Studies with obvious methodological or conceptual flaws should be excluded from the data bank. Conclusions need to be carefully drawn. For example, evaluations of bad debriefing practices should identify that what is being studied is bad practices. Where studies yield conflicting findings, attempts should be made to understand the reasons for the differences found. For example, sometimes conflicting findings may reflect differences in methodology or different assumptions about CISM and its aims.

The vast balance of evidence suggests that properly run CISM programmes, in emergency services and allied professions, are of very high value and are cost-effective to agencies. Nevertheless, more research is needed to explain why these interventions are as helpful as they are. Figley (1996), commenting on the general field of trauma, recently made the point that it is necessary to move past arguing and demonstrating that trauma traumatizes people towards developing a clearer view of what helps people and why. A similar argument can be advanced in the field of CISM. It is necessary to move beyond arguing that crisis intervention and CISM assist people and focus more on developing a better understanding of the central elements in helpful interventions and psychological constructs that explain them.

A summary of effects and risks of CISM/CISD

The major effects of well-run CISM programmes are summarized below, followed by a brief description of some of the pitfalls that may occur.

Effects

Reduction in signs of stress and trauma; reduction in anger, anxiety and depression.
Assistance in 'processing' the event (getting the facts together, ventilating emotions, verbalizing feelings and thoughts, etc.).
Mobilization of own coping strategies.
Mobilization of support networks.
Increase in morale and cohesiveness between people who work together; improved communication.

Improvement in work performance and reduction in destructive behaviours at work.

Perception that the 'workplace cares' by virtue of the provision of support services.

Perception of a safety net being there for all employees.

Reduction in sick leave, workers' compensation, staff turnover and legal suits.

Reduction in family disruption due to job stress.

Risks

Risks may be incurred if programmes are not properly established, run and monitored, if interventions are conducted by nontrained personnel or if there is a violation of the established protocols. Some of the potential problems from improperly run services are listed below.

CISM

Organizational problems in which the CISM programme is not accepted by the organization or unduly conflicts with existing support services.

Lack of management support such that any gains from CISM are cancelled out in time.

Lack of appropriate checks and balances to ensure that only the most appropriate people are selected as CISM team members, that there is appropriate initial and ongoing training, and that the the highest system of ethics and accountability is maintained.

Inappropriate use of CISM interventions, for example organizing debriefings for problems that debriefing was not designed to address (such as general organizational problems).

Using debriefing when another intervention (or no intervention) is more appropriate.

Ineffective communication infrastructure to properly maintain the CISM programme.

Inadequate financing and resourcing of programmes.

Using debriefing as *the* intervention instead of developing a comprehensive CISM programme.

Group activities: CISD and defusing

Where group activities are not conducted according to established protocols, the following may occur:

Retraumatization of group members from inappropriate listening to stories from others, or hearing of information too long after the incident.

Escalation of anger and conflict between members of a group where this is allowed to get out of control by people who misrun the group.

Inappropriate disclosure of material voiced in a group setting.

Ineffectual group sessions because the people running the group practice psychotherapeutic skills instead of crisis intervention practices

Lack of attention to teamwork skills such that team members compete with one another or do not work effectively as a team with one another.

Inappropriate groupings of people in a debriefing or defusing (e.g. combining people who mistrust one another; combining people with very disparate experiences of an event and/or exposure to varying degrees of intensity of the event).

Breaches of confidentiality.

The essential elements of debriefing

In keeping with the focus of this book, this section describes the essential elements of debriefing. Figure 6.2 depicts the individual in the context of his or her social environment, at a point in time when debriefing commonly occurs. The essential elements need to be seen within a time context and within a framework that considers the individual and his or her interaction with others, including a debriefing (if this occurs), the immediate social and work support network and the broader community.

• Timing.

The first two essential conditions are the presence of a critical incident and the timing of the support response. Crisis interventions need to occur soon after a critical incident. Along a time scale, crisis intervention may be the first helping response.

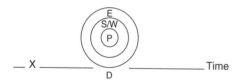

Figure 6.2. The individual and his or her environment post critical incident time. P, person; D, debriefing group; S/W immediate social and work environment; E, broader social context; X, critical incident.

The person

In the early stages after a trauma there are several tasks that face the individual.

- Understanding the facts of the situation, piecing together all bits of information, and forming a gestalt.

People often find it important to piece together the bits of information relating to a critical incident so that it is possible to get a sense of what happened over a period of time. This may be important in enabling people to complete an experience so that they can eventually begin to see it in its broader context (getting things into perspective) as something that has occurred in the past. One senses the struggle that people have when they are faced with a traumatic situation in which essential information is missing. For example, when people take their own lives it sometimes is not possible to ascertain whether this action was intended or not. Lack of that important piece of information can sometimes make it very difficult for those who remain to make sense of what happened and eventually 'let it go'.

- Connecting thoughts, feelings and pictures (especially if these have become or remain dissociated).

A common need, which many people seem to experience, is that of 'putting together' the memories of what was seen, thought, heard, felt and smelt. The integration of emotions is particularly important, though often a difficult task to achieve.

- Putting thoughts, feelings and pictures into language.

The verbalization of our inner psychological processes has been argued, by some, to be a central task in the recovery from trauma. Putting words to thoughts, feelings and visual experiences appears to enable the person to bring them under control and make them more manageable.

- Managing own stress responses and, in particular, establishing that one's response is 'normal'.

When people are confronted with unusual and difficult events, it appears to be very important for them to ascertain whether or not their reactions are similar to those of other people in kind, intensity and duration. To find out that one's own reactions are similar to those of others seems to be reassuring and to assist people in coping with their stress response. This can be particularly important for emergency service workers, where capacity to cope is of central importance.

The immediate social and work environment

Individuals do not operate in isolation but within a social context. The helpful roles that others in a debriefing group may play are many. Group members who are present at the debriefing, as well as the team members running it, can assist the individual in any or all of the four tasks listed above. They do so by providing information, listening, and offering their own experiences. The sense of developing an understanding of one's own response can be greatly assisted by others. However, the group can provide more than this including the following:

- Being understood and having people care about you in your time of need.

There appears to be a fundamental need that many, if not all, humans have, namely to share frightening and distressing experiences with others who have at least some understanding of what has been experienced and who feel some caring or concern that this has occurred. This has been well understood by religious helping groups as well as many renowned psychologists such as Carl Rogers. The basis for this human need can only be speculated upon, but may be an innate need and part of our social nature.

- Receiving information on trauma and coping.

Information on trauma and coping will assist an individual to understand his or her reactions and to mobilize coping strategies. Education is central to crisis intervention. It gives a cognitive hold on what people can do to manage themselves and their circumstances.

The broader social context

The broader social context also needs to be considered. The organization to which the individual belongs has an important part to play in the recovery process.

• Management support.

In those industries where workers often 'give much' of themselves, it may become particularly important for management not only to support but to be seen to support their staff in critical times. Too often, the negative results of perceived/actual lack of management support has been described, and this may be more distressing to a worker than the traumatic incident itself.

The debriefing (as part of CISM!)

Finally, the nature of the intervention itself is important.

• The CISD structure and process.

The CISD process is described elsewhere. When properly executed by people who have been appropriately trained in CISM, this allows for the processes described above to occur. However, CISD needs to be understood within the context of CISM, and CISM needs to be seen in the context within which the individual functions.

Conclusion

CISM is continuing to develop, and the helpfulness of peer support, in particular, is still finding its upper limit. The work of Mitchell and others has facilitated a major change in attitudes and practices that has mostly been widely welcomed, but perhaps not always fully understood by all. The debate around debriefing has highlighted the need for those involved in the field to be clear about their understanding and use of key terms and it has also highlighted the need for good research. Debriefing is but one component of comprehensive CISM programmes. It is important that research efforts clarify exactly what it is that is under review and that study conclusions relate to this. In particular, distinctions need to be made between the Mitchell model and others, and there needs to be clarification of programmes implemented in the workplace as opposed to programmes developed for primary victims and/or members of the public.

Emergency services continue to lead the field with respect to trauma management in the workplace. It is important that constructive forums for discussion and writing be developed and maintained so that new developments can be described and improved evaluation research implemented.

REFERENCES

AAOS (American Academy of Orthopedic Surgeons, Department of Research and Scientific Affairs) (1996). Tales from the front: huge response to sound off on CISD. *EMT Today*, 1(2), 3.

Alexander, D. (1993). The Piper Alpha oil rig disaster. In J. P. Wilson & B. Raphael (Eds.) *International Handbook on Traumatic Stress Syndromes* (pp. 461–70). New York: Plenum Press.

Armstrong, K., O'Callahan, W. & Marmar, C. (1991). Debriefing Red Cross disaster personnel: the multiple stressor debriefing model. *Journal of Traumatic Stress*, 4, 581–93.

Bisson, J., Jenkins, P., Alexander, J. & Bannister, C. (1997). Randomized controlled trial of psychological debriefing for victims of acute burn trauma. *British Journal of Psychiatry*, 171, 78–81.

Blackwelder, N. L. (1995). Critical incident stress debriefing for school employees. Ph.D. thesis. Ann Arbor, MI:UMI Dissertation Services.

Bohl, N. (1991). The effectiveness of brief psychological interventions in police officers after critical incidents. In J. Reese, J. Horn, J. & C. Dunning (Eds.) *Critical Incidents in Policing* (pp. 31–88). Revised. Washington, DC: US Government Printing Office.

Burns, C. & Harm. I. (1993). Emergency nurses' perceptions of critical incidents and stress debriefing. *Journal of Emergency Nursing*, 19, 431–6.

Campbell, J. H. (1992). A comparative analysis of the effects of post shooting trauma on special agents of the Federal Bureau of Investigation. Dissertation. Michigan State University.

Caplin, G. (1964). *Principles of Preventative Psychiatry.* New York: Basic Books.

Carkhuff, R. (1987). *The Art of Helping,* 6th edn. Amherst, MA: Human Resource Development Press.

Chemtob, C. M., Thomas, S., Law, W. & Cremniter, D. (1997). Post disaster psychosocial intervention: a field study of the impact of debriefing on psychological distress. *American Journal of Psychiatry,* **154,** 415–17.

Deahl, M. P., Gilham, A. B., Thomas, J., Searle, M. M. & Srinivasan, M. (1994). Psychological sequelae following the Gulf War: factors associated with subsequent morbidity and the effectiveness of psychological debriefing. *British Journal of Psychiatry,* **165,** 60–5.

Dyregrov, A. (1989). Caring for helpers in disaster situations: psychological debriefing. *Disaster Management,* **2,** 25–30.

Dyregrov, A. (1996). History and status of CISD. Paper presented at the 1st European Congress on Stress in Emergency Service Personnel and Peace Keeping Forces. 17–20 March, Sheffield, UK.

Dyregrov, A. (1997). The process of psychological debriefing. *Journal of Traumatic Stress,* **10,** 589–606.

Ersland, S., Weisæth, L. & Sund, A. (1989). The stress upon rescuers involvedin an oil rig disaster: 'Alexander L. Kielland,' 1980. *Acta Psychiatrica Scandinavica,* **80,** Suppl. 355, 38–49.

Everly, G. S. & Mitchell, J. T. (1997). *Critical incident stress management: A New Era and Standard of Care in Crisis Intervention.* Ellicott City, MD: Chevron Publishing.

Everly, G. S., Flannery, R. B. & Mitchell, J. T. (1999). Critical incident stress management (CISM): a review of the literature. *Aggression and Violent Behaviour,* in press.

Figley, C. (1996). Charles Figley: My traumatology. Workshop presentation, Melbourne, Australia.

Flannery, R. B., Jr & Penk, W. E. (1996). Program evaluation of an intervention approach for staff assaulted by patients: preliminary inquiry. *Journal of Traumatic Stress,* **9,** 317–24.

Gilliland, B. E. & James, R. K. (1997). *Crisis Intervention Strategies.* Pacific Grove, CA: Brooks/Cole Publishing Company.

Griffiths, J. A. & Watts, R. (1992). *The Kempsey and Grafton Bus Crashes: The Aftermath.* East Lismore, NSW: Industrial Design Solution, University of New England, NSW.

Hafen, B. Q. & Fransen, K. J. (1985). *Psychological Emergencies and Crisis Intervention.* Engelwood, CO: Morton Publishing Company.

Hanneman, M. F. (1994). Evaluation of critical incident stress debriefing as perceived by voluntary fire fighters in Nova Scotia. Ph.D. thesis Ann Arbor, MI: UMI Dissertation Services.

Herman, J. L. (1992). *Trauma and recovery.* New York: Basic Books.

Hytten, K. & Hasle, A. (1989). Firefighters: a study of stress and coping. *Acta Psychiatrica Scandinavica,* **80,** Suppl. 355, 50–5.

Jenkins, S. R. (1996). Social support and debriefing efficacy among emergency medical workers after a mass shooting incident. *Journal of Social Behaviour and Personality,* **11,** 477–92.

Kenardy, J. A., Webster, R. A., Lewin, T. J., Carr, V. J., Hazell, P. L. & Carter, G. L. (1996). Stress debriefing and patterns of recovery following a natural disaster. *Journal of Traumatic Stress,* **9,** 37–49.

Lanning, J. K & Fannin, R. A. (1988). It's not over yet. *Chief Fire Executive,* August/September/October, pp. 40–5, 58–63.

Leeman-Conley, M. (1990). After a violent robbery . . . *Criminology,* **4,** 4–6.

Lewis, G. W. (1994). *Critical Incident Stress and Trauma in the Workplace.* Muncie, IN: Accelerated Development, Inc.

Lindermann, E. (1944). Symptomotology and management of acute grief. *American Journal of Psychiatry,* **101,** 141–8.

McFarlane, A. C. (1986). Long-term psychiatric morbidity after a natural disaster. *Medical Journal of Australia,* **145,** 561–3.

McFarlane, A. C. (1988). The longitudinal course of posttraumatic morbidity, *Journal of Nervous and Mental Diseases,* **176,** 30–9.

Mitchell, J. T. & Bray, G. (1990). *Emergency Services Stress.* Englewood Cliffs, NJ: Prentice Hall.

Mitchell, J. T. & Everly, G. S. (1996). *Critical Incident Stress Debriefing: An Operations Manual for the Prevention of Traumatic Stress Among Emergency Services and Disaster Workers,* 2nd edn, revised. Ellicott City, MD: Chevron Publishing.

Mitchell, J. T. & Everly, G. S. (1997). The scientific evidence for critical incident stress management. *Journal of Emergency Medical Services,* **22,** 86–93.

Nurmi, L. (1997). Experienced stress and value of CISD among Finnish police officers (DVI) and emergency personnel in the Estonia ferry disaster. Paper presented at the 4th World Congress on Stress, Trauma and Coping in the Emergency Services Professions, Baltimore, MD.

Ott, K. & Henry, P. (1997). *Critical Incident Stress Management at Goulburn Correctional Centre.* Goulburn, NSW: Goulburn Correctional Centre.

Parad, H. (1986). Crisis intervention: past, present and future. Paper presented at the 1st National Conference on Crisis Intervention, November, Adelaide Victoria.

Parkinson, F. (1997). *Critical Incident Debriefing.* London: Souvenir Press (E & A) Ltd.

Pennebaker, J. W. (1990). *Opening Up: The Healing Power of Confiding in Others.* New York: William Morrow.

Pennebaker, J. W. (1993). Putting stress into words: health, linguistic and therapeutic implications. *Behaviour, Research and Therapy*, **31**, 539–48.

Pynoos, R. S., Goeenjian, A. & Steinberg, A. M. (1994). Strategies of disaster intervention for children and adolescents. Paper presented at the NATO Conference on Stress, Coping and Disaster, Bones, France.

Raphael, B. (1977). The Granville train disaster: psychological needs and their management. *Medical Journal of Australia*, 1303–5.

Raphael, B. (1986). *When Disaster Strikes: A Handbook for the Caring Professions.* Sydney: Hutchinson.

Raphael, B., Meldrum, L. & McFarlane, A. C. (1995). Does debriefing after psychological trauma work? *British Medical Journal*, **310**, 1479–80.

Richman, M. & Blizzard, C. (1996). *Tasmanian Emergency Services CISD Team Annual Report 1996–1997.* Tasmania: Tasmanian Emergency Services CISD Team.

Robinson, R. (1984). *Health and Stress in Ambulance Services*, Part I. Melbourne: Social Biology Resources Centre.

Robinson, R. (1986). *Health and Stress in Ambulance Services*, Part II. Melbourne: Social Biology Resources Centre.

Robinson, R. (1993). *Follow-up Study of Health and Stress in Ambulance Services Victoria, Australia 1993.* Melbourne: Victorian Ambulance Crisis Counselling Unit.

Robinson, R. (1995). Critical incident stress management in Australia. In G. S. Everly (Ed.) *Innovations in Disaster and Trauma Psychology*, vol. 1 (pp. 90–106). Ellicott City, MD: Chevron Publishing Corporation.

Robinson, R. (1997). *Evaluation of the Victorian Ambulance Crisis Counselling Unit, 1997.* Melbourne: Victorian Ambulance Crisis Counselling Unit.

Robinson, R. & Mitchell, J. T. (1993). Evaluation of psychological debriefing, *Journal of Traumatic Stress*, **6**, 367–82.

Robinson, R. & Mitchell, J. T. (1995). Getting some balance back into the debriefing debate. *Bulletin of the Australian Psychological Society*, **17**, 5–10.

Robinson, R. & Murdoch, P. (1996). *Position Statement and Standards of Practice for Psychological Debriefing and Defusing in Emergency Services.* Melbourne: Victorian Combined Emergency Services Critical Incident Advisory Committee.

Robinson, R. & Murdoch, P. (1998). *Guidelines for Establishing and Maintaining Peer Support Programs in Emergency Services.* Ellicott City, MD: Chevron Publishing.

Rogers, O. W. (1993). An examination of critical incident stress debriefing for emergency service providers: a quasi-experimental field study. Ph.D. thesis Ann Arbor, MI: UMI Dissertation services.

Ryan, D. (1996). The role of management in peer support programs. Paper presented at the 10th Anniversary Conference of the Victorian Ambulance Crisis Counselling Unit, Melbourne.

Seligman, M. E. P. (1995). The effectiveness of psychotherapy. *American Psychologist*, **29**, 965–74.

Stallard, P. & Law, F. (1993). Screening and psychological debriefing of adolescent survivors of life threatening events. *British Journal of Psychiatry*, **163**, 660–5.

Tunnecliffe, M. & Robinson, R. (1997). Peer support survey results. *Emergency Support Newsletter*, **3**, 2–3.

Tunnecliffe, M. & Roy, O. (1993). *Emergency Support: A Handbook for Peer Supporters.* Palmyra, Western Australia: Bayside Books.

van Der Kolk, B. A., McFarlane, A. C. & Weisæth, L. (1996). *Traumatic Stress: The Effects of Overwhelming Experience on Mind, Body and Society.* New York: Guilford Press.

Watts, R. (1994). The efficacy of critical incident stress debriefing for personnel. *Bulletin of the Australian Psychological Society*, **16**, 6–7.

Wee, D. (1996). Research in critical incident stress management. Part 4, How effective is this? *Life Net*, **7**(2), 4–5.

Western Management Consultants (1997). Evaluation of critical incident stress management services. Conference presentation at the 4th Congress on Stress, Trauma and Coping in the Emergency Services Professions, Baltimore, USA.

White, T. (1996). Critical incident stress debriefing: are we falling for our own propaganda? *Bulletin of the Australian Psychological Society*, **18**, 8.

Wilson, J. P. (1989). *Trauma: Transformation and Healing: An Integrative Approach to Theory, Research and Post-traumatic Therapy.* New York: Brunner/Mazel.

Yule, W. & Udwin (1991). Screening child survivors for post-traumatic stress disorders: experiences from the Jupiter sinking. *British Journal of Clinical Psychology*, **30**, 131–8.

7

Debriefing and body recovery: war grave soldiers

Martin P. Deahl

EDITORIAL COMMENTS

Combat and its effects are well established as stressors, but the particular aspects of the roles of certain groups of soldiers need further research. This chapter reviews what is known about the psychological impact of body recovery, and in particular the possible effects on soldiers whose role it is to recover the bodies of colleagues or those of the enemy. Deahl's research and understanding of this field is clearly heightened by his own experience of body recovery after the Kings Cross Underground fire in London. The special issues faced by soldiers who may recover bodies in situations of ongoing threat and factors that may mitigate the impact are the subject of this chapter.

A fortuitous naturalistic opportunity for research arose when two groups of soldiers could be compared: one had had debriefing; the other for operational reasons had not. The study found that debriefing did not mitigate the psychological distress experienced, which was very similar in the two groups. Factors that predicted ongoing distress included the degree of perceived threat experienced by the soldiers, and this was negatively correlated with previous 'real-life experience' of handling body remains. Past psychological problems also increased vulnerability, and only a small number had sought specialist help. Negative impact of this psychological morbidity on personal relationships was also found, indicating the significance of the morbidity described.

The author discusses possible explanations for the 'failure' of debriefing to produce beneficial effects, including the culture of tough mindedness in the mili-

tary, and the possibility that the soldiers may have achieved debriefing of their own through informally talking with colleagues, as they were encouraged to do.

The protective value of previous experience led the author to recommend a 'stress inoculation' training technique to prepare workers for body handling, and finding ways to reduce emotional identification with the victims.

The hopes that debriefing would prevent such problems are not validated by the findings of this study and the author acknowledges the need to evaluate better the appropriateness and effects of debriefing.

Like many of the contributors to this volume, Deahl supports the continuation of debriefing. This emphasizes the hopefulness of the wish to assist those who are psychologically traumatized. It should also demand the development of interventions that are not only humane but also effective.

Introduction

Of all the duties soldiers and emergency service workers are called upon to undertake in the service of their country following combat, disasters or accidents there is none potentially more distressing or unrewarding than body handling. Not only are workers exposed to sensory stimuli that shock and offend, but they also confront their own existential vulnerability and frailty. During combat there is the additional burden of realizing that death has been deliberately inflicted – often by one's own comrades. It is not a popular duty – one which carries considerable stigma and taboo that is often not subsequently disclosed or discussed with family, friends or colleagues, remaining an awkward semi-secret to be recounted only amongst the body handlers themselves.

My own personal experience of body handling was similar to that of many I have subsequently studied. As a bystander, and one of the first doctors present at the scene of the 1987 Kings Cross Underground fire in London it was assumed that I would know what to do! In the absence of a Coroner's Officer or access to the Public Mortuary, we commandeered a church hall opposite Kings Cross station, and I was asked to assist in the documentation, handling and identification of approximately 20 dead that had been brought from the scene of the disaster. Despite my medical degree, and like most of the other members of the emergency services that night, I had no training or preparation for this sort of work, which was completely beyond anything I could have imagined. I removed each body from its bag, placed it upon a table, carefully described any visible injuries and catalogued any personal effects, identifying the body wherever possible. During that night there was a great deal of extreme emotion ranging from ribald black humour to extreme irritability and angry outbursts. Nearby journalists bore the brunt of the anger, frustration and distress of the police and other emergency service workers. I recall subsequently finding some of the more macho police officers locked in toilet cubicles weeping inconsolably or found them wandering around in an apparent dissociative daze. I concealed my own feelings and emotions beneath a cloak of detached professional objectivity. Throughout, the Salvation Army made endless cups of tea by way of solace (Deahl & Domizio, 1987, p.19)! At that time I was a young trainee psychiatrist at the Maudsley Hospital and Institute of Psychiatry in London. When I returned to work the following morning and told my colleagues and seniors (some of the leading figures of British psychiatry) what I had done the night before, their response was to send for the chaplain to talk to me – they simply didn't know what to say or do! My own reactions and emotions that night as well as my observations of the emergency workers at the scene and the reactions of my colleagues stimulated my own interest in psychological trauma. I have since sublimated my own feelings into writing, lecturing and researching.

But what about the other people in the church hall with me that evening; how did they cope? My impression is that many resorted to heavy alcohol (mis)use to seek respite from the images and memories that haunted them. What does one say to mitigate the effects of such psychological trauma? Does psychological debriefing or any other form of intervention reduce the long-term consequences of psychological trauma? Can it do harm? Does it matter? In 1987 the answers to these questions were all unknown, although there were innumerable anecdotal reports suggesting that psychological debriefing was beneficial and intuitively this seemed right. It was not until 1991 during the Gulf War as a serving military psychiatrist that I had the opportunity, along with colleagues to test the efficacy of psychological debriefing.

Violent death is an inevitable consequence of natural and human-engendered disasters, aeroplane crashes, terrorist outrage and combat. Although these events are depressingly common in today's world, body handling is often a unique once-in-a-lifetime experience for those individuals called upon to deal with the aftermath of trauma. The lessons learnt in the light of their experience are all too often forgotten and future generations of workers and their managers make the same mistakes, often at considerable personal emotional expense.

Body handling as a stressor

Body handlers carry out diverse duties, which may involve prolonged as well as brief contact with the dead. This may include recovery, transport, identification, labelling and cleaning body parts as well as burial of the dead. They may be exposed to violent, abusive or grotesque death, which are all significantly associated with an increased risk of subsequent psychiatric disorder (Lifton, 1973; Laufer et al., 1984, 1985; Green et al., 1989).

Like many unpleasant situations in life, the expectation and anticipation of events can be as stressful as reality. Workers assigned to body-handling duties may have to wait hours or days contemplating their work before embarking on their task. Delays are frequent and may be due to a variety of factors such as securing and making safe the scene of a disaster, allowing foren-sic investigation, or securing the ground in a combat zone. The waiting period often results in significant stress and has been reported by some as being the most stressful part of an operation (Ersland et al., 1989). The longer the wait the more stressful the situation. Imagin-ation is often a poor reflection of reality and the actual duties may be considerably more or less disturbing than is anticipated. As a result of prolonged waiting in anticipation, workers may be in a state of considerable stress before even commencing their duties. High levels of arousal and stress prior to commencing duties may increase fatigability and contribute to general ill health, which in turn may contribute to psychological degradation, reduced working efficiency as well as in-creasing vulnerability to long-term psychological se-quelae. Previous experience of body handling, appears to mitigate against anticipatory stress as well as that of subsequent body handling which is considerably greater amongst younger and more inexperienced per-sonnel (Ersland et al., 1989; Jones, 1985; McCarroll et al., 1992; Deahl et al., 1994).

Research carried out on body handlers

The long-term individual psychological impact follow-ing exposure to violent death and body handling is poorly understood and little systematic research has been conducted in this area. Perhaps not surprisingly it is not a popular subject to contemplate or discuss amongst either the individuals involved or military and disaster planners. The unpredictability of disaster and combat create serious difficulties in conducting re-search in circumstances that are inevitably chaotic and where the operational imperative to prosecute a mili-tary operation or to save life is paramount. In addition the emergency services and rescue workers tend to work in cohesive tight-knit groups, generally suspi-cious of, and rejecting outsiders, especially mental health professionals. They often foster a macho image and are reluctant to admit distress or show signs of perceived psychological weakness – especially in front of their colleagues. Nevertheless, there is a body of research that suggests that rescuers and emergency service workers may themselves be traumatized by

confronting death in disaster or combat situations.

Taylor & Frazer (1982) studied the reactions of 100 personnel involved with the recovery and identification of the dead after the Mount Erebus aeroplane crash in Antarctica on the 28 November 1979. They demon-strated that one-third of the sample experienced transi-ent problems initially, and about 20% after three months. At 20 months there was still evidence of sub-jects being in distress, although their data did not allow formal psychiatric diagnosis. They suggested that the stress of body recovery and identification was a com-plex interaction between environmental and task stres-sors, job competency, perceptual and emotional defen-ces, management and follow-up support.

McCarroll et al. (1993) used a questionnaire to study the anticipated stress of body handling in male and female soldiers, both with and without prior experi-ence, and a group of college students with no prior experience of handling the dead. Inexperienced female soldiers and students demonstrated highest levels of anticipated stress. There were no gender differences amongst soldiers with previous body-handling experi-ence, whose mean scores were more than 10% lower compared to the inexperienced group. This finding was confirmed when the soldiers were then shown visual material of traumatic death. There was a highly signifi-cant correlation between anticipatory stress measured by questionnaire and stress scores on exposure to the visual material. Their findings suggest that 'stress in-oculation' by previous body-handling experience may be important in reducing anticipatory stress associated with disaster.

McCarroll et al. (1992) studied 562 US military per-sonnel assigned to mortuary duty during the Gulf War. Using the Brief Symptom Inventory (BSI) and Impact of Event Scale (IES) they found that, compared with the inexperienced and nonvolunteers, both previous body-handling experience and volunteer status were inde-pendently associated with significantly lower scores on depression, anxiety and somatization subscales as well as the global symptom score. Both volunteer status and previous body-handling experience were related to re-duced intrusion, avoidance and total IES scores.

In an attempt to characterize those aspects of body handling and traumatic death that workers find most stressful Ursano and colleagues have conducted extensive interviews with US body handlers involved in a variety of disasters. These studies include: the Dover Air Force Base Mortuary following the military air disaster of December 1985 in which 256 people were killed; the *USS Iowa* gun-turret explosion in 1989; Ramstein Air Base Flugtag disaster of 1988; United Airlines Flight 232 air crash in Sioux City, Iowa, in 1989; and Gulf War casualties in 1991 (Ursano & McCarroll, 1990; Ursano et al., 1990, 1992). Contact with children's bodies was intensely distressing to almost all involved irrespective of whether the workers had children themselves or not and irrespective of professional status including pathologists and medical examiners. Comments such as they 'hadn't lived' or they appeared 'innocent and had no control over what happened' were common. The discovery of children's toys at the disaster scene is a frequent source of distress, alerting rescue workers to the possibility of discovering children's bodies. Ursano reports a firefighter entering a smoke-filled room, feeling around and touching a dead infant, preferring to believe it was a dog.

Paradoxically natural-looking intact bodies with no visible cause of death were also reported as more distressing, as well as extremely grotesque remains such as decapitated or badly burned bodies or bodies that been submerged in water for a substantial time.

Accidental mutilation of the dead during handling is another powerful stressor. My most vivid personal recollection during the night of the Kings Cross fire was of removing the clothing of a young female, burned, but intact and without other obvious injury. As I removed what I thought were her tights I realised I was degloving the burnt skin from her legs. Another badly burned victim's arm broke off in my hand as I tried to remove the body from its bag. Many Gulf War body handlers were extremely upset by having to stand bodies upright in order to put them into bags and secure them with masking tape on the victims' head to keep them in the body bag.

Many individuals wear gloves – even if they are not having direct contact with the dead. These not only identify individuals as members of a group but appear to have both a real and symbolic protective role from the dead.

Unpleasant sensory stimulation (particularly smell) is universally distressing. Rescue workers often use scents and pleasant odours (which may include cigar smoke and burning coffee) to try to disguise the smell of decaying remains – usually without much success (Cervantes. 1988). Smells often persist in the imagination and many workers report being unable to wash the smell away for several days after their duties have been completed. Many workers are unable to eat meat after exposure to burned bodies. Although I did not suffer from PTSD following my experience at the Kings Cross tube fire, vivid (almost photographic) memories of that night were evoked when, 12 years later, I visited the scene of the 1999 Paddington railway disaster and encountered smells reminiscent of the Kings Cross scene.

Novelty, surprise and shock all contribute to the stress of body handling. The anticipation of opening a body bag (particularly when blood and body fluids are leaking from the bag) is troublesome and many experienced workers will make excuses to stand away or avert their gaze while the bag is being opened. Similarly, turning a body lying prone is also a cause of distress as the occiput is much stronger than the face and although intact often conceals a badly damaged face. Ursano reports that pathologists at Dover Air Force Base even X-rayed body bags to lessen the shock and surprise of the remains therein. Many experienced workers find the shock and surprise lessened by opening body bags in a hospital mortuary or other clinical setting where they have an increased sense of control. An experienced pathologist at the Kings Cross fire was acutely distressed in dealing with the dead at the scene, electing instead to go to the hospital to obtain gowns and gloves for the rest of us to wear.

Any factors resulting in increased identification with the dead generally result in greater distress. Soldiers in the Gulf War who were required to remove the personal effects of enemy dead, including personal correspondence and photographs of family and loved ones, found the experience intensely upsetting. Anything that identified the individual as human caused distress. Most soldiers found handling their own comrades, particularly those who had died as a result of 'friendly fire', more distressing than handling enemy dead. Dead women, particularly those who showed evidence of torture and sexual assault prior to death caused particular distress. It was not only the dead that caused distress, however, body handlers who witnessed unnecessary mutilation (namely, seeing allied soldiers playing football with the head of an enemy soldier) and witnessing looting by allied personnel (such as a senior officer taking wristwatches from the bodies of enemy dead) all caused additional distress. Following the latter incident, several Army War Graves Service (AWGS) personnel were reluctant to carry money or any other item of value in case they themselves were accused of looting. One soldier even tried to discard his wedding ring!

Not all studies have demonstrated increased psychiatric morbidity following body handling. Alexander (1993) using a case-control paradigm, failed to show any increase in psychopathology in a group of 35 policemen three years after the Piper Alpha oil rig disaster. He attributed the outcome to good organization and sensitive staff management policies. A similar finding was reported by Thompson & Solomon (1991), who reported low levels of distress in a group of police officers who volunteered for a victim recovery team. They attributed their findings to a variety of factors, including preparation, positive interpersonal relationships among team members, and debriefing.

Attempts to minimize morbidity following disaster and rescue work including body recovery and identification duties have resulted in calls for the provision of routine early psychological intervention in both victims and rescue workers alike. They have also led to the emergence of a disaster industry led by a variety of professional groups including psychologists, psychiatrists, social workers and lay counsellors, who have all sought to establish a role for themselves following traumatic incidents (British Psychological Society Working Party, 1990). In a survey of senior officers of UK emergency services, 72% reported some critical incident stress provision within their local service, although only 28% felt that sufficient attention was paid to this aspect of staff welfare (Ørner et al., 1993). Early interventions are intuitively appealing and a response to perceived need but whether or not they work is another matter. Numerous anecdotal reports suggest psycho-

logical debriefing in particular helps to reduce subsequent morbidity (e.g. Dyregrov, 1989; Armstrong et al., 1991). The uncritical acceptance of such claims has led to the widespread use of psychological debriefing after traumatic events, as well as leading to the relative neglect of other important issues such as training, preparation and other forms of intervention. Unfortunately there is little other than anecdotal evidence to demonstrate the effectiveness of debriefing and the vast majority of published studies suffer from serious methodological failings (Table 7.1).

Much published work has little relevance to body recovery and has concentrated on accident victims or members of the emergency services engaged in disparate (and often unspecified) activities at a disaster site and it is unclear to what extent the findings of research in one area of psychological trauma can be generalized to a highly specialized task such as body recovery. It is also unclear whether research findings in military personnel can be generalized to civilians. Prior to 1990 there had been no comparison or controlled studies of psychological debriefing in civilian or military body handlers. It was therefore serendipitous when, during the 1991 Gulf War, an officer serving with the British Army War Grave Registration Team spontaneously approached the psychiatric services soliciting help to minimize the distress and what he perceived would be the long-term psychological impact of their work.

Gulf War Graves Registration Team study

Despite the early allied victory, many soldiers in the Gulf War suffered potentially traumatic experiences: one such group was those soldiers employed in the AWGS. Working in small teams, their duties included the recovery, identification, and preparation for burial of both Allied and enemy war dead. The study was unusual in that for operational reasons one group of subjects received psychological debriefing and the other group did not, thereby creating a comparison group enabling the effectiveness of early intervention and psychological debriefing to be assessed.

We studied 74 British regular soldiers, serving with the AWGS (median age = 28 years, range 19–44), with a median length of service of nine years). Those soldiers

Table 7.1. Common methodological problems in psychological debriefing research

- Not prospective
- Small sample sizes
- Absence of control groups
- Varying degrees of exposure to trauma
- Absence of random allocation
- Other confounding variables ignored
- Low response rates
- Sampling bias
- Lack of uniformity of psychological debriefing
- Timing variance
- Questionnaire versus interview results

From Bisson & Deahl (1994).

who joined the AWGS in the UK received training that included preparation for the emotional and psychological consequences of their work. In the Gulf, AWGS required reinforcements; these were all volunteers recruited in the theatre of war, although some had little idea what they were volunteering for! The period of training was, by operational necessity, brief, but all the training for personnel recruited in the UK included exposure to dead bodies in a mortuary. Soldiers were given the opportunity to withdraw from the AWGS and one did.

A psychological 'debriefing' by welfare professionals (chaplains, psychologists, psychiatrists or social workers) was organized as soon as possible, either in the Gulf or on return to the UK; for one group this was not operationally possible. There were no significant differences between the groups in terms of age, rank, previous military experience (including previous body-handling duties) or marital status. The nature of the body-handling duties undertaken by the two groups was identical. The intervention included an educational component, in which the symptoms of post-traumatic stress were explained as a normal human reaction to abnormal stress, a small-group debriefing session with two welfare professionals, using the Dyregrov (1989) model, and finally advice on where to get help, if required. The emphasis was on the frequency and normality of any disturbing symptoms in an attempt to destigmatize and facilitate help-seeking.

Nine months after their return from the Gulf the subjects were sent three questionnaires by post. First, subjects completed a demographic questionnaire, which also sought details of past psychological problems, previous experience of body handling, and specific questions about their experiences and duties in the Gulf, details of health or emotional problems, relationship difficulties and help-seeking since the conflict. It also asked subjects to describe their subjective opinion of their Gulf experience and, if received, the psychological debriefing. Subjects also completed the General Health Questionnaire – 28-item version (GHQ-28) (Goldberg & Hillier, 1979). The GHQ is a reliable instrument designed to detect nonspecific psychiatric morbidity, which has been validated in a variety of settings, including work with disaster workers (McFarlane, 1988). Finally, subjects were asked to complete the IES (Horowitz et al., 1979). The IES is a 15-item self-report instrument designed to measure the two principal symptom groups found in post-traumatic stress disorder (PTSD), namely avoidance and intrusive repetitive images and thoughts. Chi-squared tests and confidence intervals (CI) were used to analyse categorical variables and analysis of variance (ANOVA) to establish the significance of differences between continuous variables.

Results

Sixty-two subjects completed the questionnaire ($n = 86$), and of the respondents 34% had a GHQ-28 indicating that they were likely 'cases' of psychiatric morbidity. Fifty per cent of respondents had an IES score of 12, or more, and 34% of the total scored over 20, indicating high levels of intrusive and avoidance symptoms in the PTSD constellation. There was a significant relationship between the GHQ 'caseness' and the traumatic stress symptoms. Forty-two respondents received a psychological debriefing either in the Gulf or on their return to the UK, and almost 50% reported that they found this helpful. In comparison with the 20 subjects who did not receive a debriefing, intrusive and avoidance symptoms were not significantly different. It was found that psychiatric caseness stress, and traumatic stress symptom levels were not significantly different for those who had had debriefing compared with those who had not.

There was no association between GHQ caseness (GHQ-28 score higher than 5) or IES (a score of > 12) and debriefing status. Fifty per cent of those debriefed were classified as cases on the IES, in comparison with 42.1% for those 20 subjects not debriefed. For GHQ-28, 37.5% of those debriefed were cases versus 33.33% for the nondebriefed.

There were also no significant differences in GHQ-28 or IES scores between those who received psychological debriefing in the Gulf immediately after the war or in the UK following post-operational leave.

There was a significant association between both overall GHQ-28 and IES scores and 'caseness' on either instrument and a subsequent change in close relationships, particularly separation from an established partner. Nine respondents reported separating from an established partner and another seven reported relationship difficulties.

Traumatic stress (IES) caseness was significantly less likely in those soldiers who had previous real-life experience of handling human body remains. Both scores were unrelated to numbers of bodies handled (median = 50), whether the bodies were of allied or of enemy soldiers, and whether the bodies were dismembered or intact. Both general and traumatic stress caseness was significantly more likely in individuals who perceived a significant threat to their own safety – that is, at some point during their experience in the Gulf they felt they were going to be killed. Soldiers who were cases on either measure were significantly more likely to have perceived their experience as unpleasant. Those with a past history of psychological problems were also more likely to show high scores. Despite their levels of symptoms, however, only 25% of those who were cases on general or specific symptomatology sought help for their problems after return from the Gulf.

These results show evidence of psychological morbidity in a group of fit young men nine months after their experiences during the Gulf War: this is comparable with the results of other studies in military and civilian populations. Of particular interest is the small number of individuals who actually sought help for the symptoms they reported. This probably reflects the prevailing culture in the armed forces and emergency services that emphasizes tough-mindedness and tends to militate against seeking help for psychological problems. It has been suggested that soldiers may accept their symptoms as an inevitable consequence of their experiences (O'Brien & Hughes, 1991) and either do not want professional help, perceive that professional help would not be useful, or may have high levels of perceived self-efficacy (Solomon, 1989). It is also well recognized that sufferers of PTSD avoid seeking help as part of the syndrome – to avoid reminders of the traumatic experience. The impact and clinical significance of the symptoms reported in this study are difficult to judge. It is not possible on the basis of these findings to distinguish distress from disorder and disability, but their association with the disruption of previously stable relationships suggests that they may be serious and that complacency over the suffering they cause would be inappropriate. In addition to relationship problems, PTSD is also known to be associated with, and may present as behavioural disturbance, work or disciplinary difficulties, and alcohol and other substance abuse. The symptoms of PTSD should always be actively sought in high-risk individuals, such as soldiers or emergency workers who may present with a variety of apparently unrelated problems and who are reluctant to volunteer the distressing intrusive and avoidance phenomena to which they are related, particularly if they have been involved in taboo activities such as body handling.

The failure of the psychological debriefing to significantly reduce morbidity is disappointing. This finding has since been confirmed in a number of replication studies following other types of psychological trauma (e.g. Bisson et al., 1997). Although the psychological debriefing was not rigorously standardized in terms of content and timing, it contained the same common elements and reflects the practical difficulties of gaining prompt access to individuals working under difficult circumstances. The need to regularly talk about their experiences had been emphasized to all the AWGS personnel during their training. It is possible that a formal intervention of this kind, by welfare professionals, offers little further protection from subsequent morbidity when informal debriefing within the teams is already established as normal working practice. Psychological debriefing may be more effective when carried out by individuals who have successfully survived body handling previously and been trained in the techniques of debriefing.

Although no beneficial effect was observed as a result of 'group cohesion' factors, in that soldiers who had previously worked together before the Gulf deployment had no less risk of morbidity, it is likely that the high morale and motivation of the force led to rapid integration and acceptance of new individuals within each team.

There was no apparent difference in post-traumatic morbidity between soldiers trained for body recovery in the UK and those trained in the Gulf; the longer UK training appeared to confer no advantage. This does not mean, however, that training is ineffective: the two groups worked closely together and their association with better trained and prepared comrades may have had indirect benefits on the less well-prepared group trained in the Gulf. Although soldiers with previous experience of body handling appeared to cope well, they represent a self-selected group; individuals who had found a similar previous experience distressing would be unlikely to volunteer for this type of duty.

Training techniques for body handlers should employ graded exposure, which may enhance the effectiveness of stress inoculation. It is also important that training should seek ways of reducing identification and emotional involvement with victims: e.g. not looking at faces, not remaining with individual bodies throughout the entire process of recovery, identification, placement in mortuary and hand over (Ursano & McCarroll, 1990).

It is of interest that morbidity was greater in those soldiers who felt their lives were at risk: this may reflect retrospective bias by a more distressed group but it serves as a reminder that military body handlers often work in hostile environments and subject to other potential stressors. The high questionnaire scores in those individuals who had previously sought help for emotional problems is interesting. This finding raises the potential importance of individual vulnerability and highlights the need for prospective studies to investigate whether there is a role for screeening individuals recruited into 'high risk' occupations.

A variety of premorbid variables such as a positive family or past personal psychiatric history, neuroticism and other personality factors, as well as social support have all been implicated as 'vulnerability factors' increasing the likelihood of PTSD developing following traumatic stress.

No study in this area of research is ideal and this has its share of methodological problems. Our results rely on self-report questionnaires, which, although valid and reliable, are less satisfactory than results obtained from a standardized, structured clinical interview. Reluctance to disclose symptoms may lead to an underestimate of true morbidity. Despite these reservations, the high response rate and the presence of a control group lend weight to the study and its findings.

Training and preparation of soldiers for war grave duties

There is ample evidence to suggest that training and preparation may significantly reduce the likelihood of long-term psychological sequelae after body-handling duties. However, training works only if it is realistic and our own study suggests that merely taking soldiers to a mortuary and exposing them to human remains may be insufficient. Perhaps the only truly realistic preparatory experience is previous body handling and in this regard perhaps soldiers should be sought who have had previous 'real' experience and who have not suffered subsequent psychological problems.

There is clear evidence that volunteers do better from the psychological point of view. Body handling is an extraordinary duty and is certainly not what soldiers expect to join the army for. Volunteers should be sought wherever possible – volunteers who have the opportunity of making an informed choice about whether to participate. It is important that the exact nature of the duties is explained as clearly and accurately as possible and not diminished in an attempt to persuade individuals to participate. Cohesive groups of individuals should be selected to undertake body-handling duties; groups who are already used to working together in a team rather than disparate individuals brought together for the occasion.

Prior to deployment body-handling teams should be clearly briefed regarding tasks and roles. Their activity should be broken down into a series of drills and routines with as much pre-exposure practice as possible. Wherever possible initial exposure should be as gradual as possible, particularly to the more severe stressors such as mutilated, grotesque and burned dead. Techniques should be taught in order to minimize identification with the dead, such as dehumanizing the victim, deliberately not looking at faces and ensuring that those individuals who recover the dead should not be responsible for identification or cataloguing personal effects. Individuals should have the minimum possible contact with any individual body and should not be allowed to accompany a particular body throughout the recovery, documentation and identification stages. General measures such as the use of role and ritual to provide a protective cloak of objectivity and emotional detachment cannot be overstated.

Of all the possible ameliorating factors informed, positive and assertive leadership is the single most important factor in minimizing the psychological impact of body handling. In addition to facilitating and maximizing group cohesion commanders and managers have responsibilities to ensure the physical well-being of their men which is a *sine qua non* psychological well-being. Physical fatigue should be minimized by ensuring shift patterns are adhered to and that their men take regular breaks during their duty; this is not always straightforward as body handlers and rescuers quite commonly work through their breaks and during rest periods out of a sense of 'wanting to get the job done' and 'duty' to the dead. During the course of their work, commanders and managers should facilitate regular 'inbriefings' allowing them to ventilate feelings and share experiences as well as allowing individuals who are clearly not coping to be identified. On these occasions regular praise and encouragement should be given, with emphasis on the importance of the work. The professional status of the group should be continually acknowledged and validated, allowing the body handlers the same protective objectivity and detachment enjoyed by others at the scene who automatically enjoy professional status, such as pathologists, forensic scientists and the coroner's officer. Commanders may employ 'grief leadership' techniques to legitimize distress and facilitate ventilation of feelings within the rest of the team, which should be acknowledged. It is all too easy to laugh or mock an individual for being weak and lacking moral fibre. The psyche varies in its ability to cope with trauma – if a soldier has difficulty coping with the task he should be allowed temporary respite and excused duties, the next day he may cope without difficulty and long-term psychiatric morbidity avoided. Strong leadership and use of a 'buddy' system in which inexperienced workers are paired with more experienced colleagues also protects against feelings of fear and the sense of personal isolation this engenders.

Following body-handling duties debriefing is important despite its apparent lack of long-term efficacy in preventing psychological reactions. Debriefing should include an educational component, putting the work in context and emphasizing its importance to the operation, the army, society and the families of the deceased. Psychiatrists and other mental health professionals should direct their effort towards educating commanders and managers rather than trying to deliver a service themselves. Debriefing should be one element of a comprehensive package of staff support that begins prior to the operation and concludes with long-term follow up to enable appropriate support and treatment arranged for those individuals who go on to develop psychiatric disorder as a result of their experience. Workers should be warned of the sorts of symptom they might expect and at what point and where they should seek help. There should also be an open discussion about the risks of alcohol misuse as well as the problem of broaching the subject with friends and families.

Body handling is an unpopular, unglamorous and distasteful activity. To undertake this requires courage and fortitude. Emphasis should be placed on the value of the work and the professionalism of the group. Body handling is not part of the job of a soldier, police officer or emergency worker. We nevertheless expect them to undertake this work on our behalf without complaint. We as professionals owe them a duty to educate and explore ways of minimizing the long-term impact of their distressing and unpleasant experience.

REFERENCES

Alexander, D. A. (1993). Stress among police body handlers: a long-term follow-up. *British Journal of Psychiatry*, **163**, 806–8.

Armstrong, K., O'Callahan, W. & Marmar, C. R. (1991). Debriefing Red Cross disaster personnel: the multiple stressor debriefing model. *Journal of Traumatic Stress*, **4**, 581–93.

Bisson, J. I. & Deahl, M. P. (1994). Psychological debriefing and prevention of post-traumatic stress. More research is needed. *British Journal of Psychiatry*, **165**, 717–20.

Bisson, J. I., Jenkins, P. L., Alexander, J. & Bannister, C. (1997). A randomised controlled trial of psychological debriefing for victims of acute burn trauma. *British Journal of Psychiatry*, **171**, 78–81.

British Psychological Society Working Party (1990). *Psychological Aspects of Disaster*. Leicester: The British Psychological Society.

Cervantes, R. (1988). Psychological stress of body handling, Part II and Part III: debriefing of Dover AFB personnel following the Gander tragedy and the body handling experience at Dover AFB. In R. J. Ursano & C. S. Fullerton (Eds.) *Exposure to Death, Disasters and Bodies*. Bethesda, MD. F. Edward Herbert School of Medicine, Uniformed Services University of the Health Services.

Deahl, M. P. & Domizio, P. (1987). Personal view. *British Medical Journal*, **295**, 1411.

Deahl, M. P., Gillham, A. B., Thomas, J., Searle, M. M. & Srinivasan, M. (1994). Psychological sequelae following the Gulf War: factors associated with subsequent morbidity and the effectiveness of psychological debriefing. *British Journal of Psychiatry*, **165**, 60–5.

Dyregrov, A. (1989). Caring for helpers in disaster situations: psychological debriefing. *Disaster Management*, **2**, 25–30.

Ersland, S., Weisæth, L. & Sund, A. (1989). The stress upon rescuers involved in an oil rig disaster. 'Alexander L. Kielland' 1980. *Acta Psychiatrica Scandinavica*, **80**, Suppl. 355, 38–49.

Goldberg, D. P. & Hillier, V. F. (1979). A scaled version of the GHQ. *Psychological Medicine*, **9**, 139–45.

Green, B. L., Lindy, J. D., Grace, M. C. & Gleser, G. C. (1989). Multiple diagnosis in post-traumatic stress disorder. The role of war stressors. *Journal of Nervous and Mental Disease*, **177**, 329–35.

Horowitz, M., Wilner, N. & Alvarez, W. (1979). Impact of Event Scale: a measure of subjective stress. *Psychosomatic Medicine*, **41**, 209–18.

Jones, D. J. (1985). Secondary disaster victims: the emotional effects of recovering and identifying human remains. *American Journal of Psychiatry*, **142**, 303–7.

Laufer, R. S., Gallops, M. S. & Frey-Walters, E. (1984). War stress and trauma. *Journal of Health and Social Behaviour*, **25**, 65–85.

Laufer, R. S., Brett, E. & Gallops, M. S. (1985). Dimensions of post-traumatic stress disorder among Vietnam veterans. *Journal of Nervous and Mental Disease*, **173**, 538–45.

Lifton, R. J. (1973). *Home from the War*. New York: Simon and Schuster, Inc.

McCarroll, J. E., Ursano, R. J., Fullerton, C. S. & Lundy, A. L. (1992). Dimensions of stress among mortuary workers. Paper presented at the 1st World Conference, The International Society for Traumatic Stress Studies, June, Amsterdam, the Netherlands.

McCarroll, J. E., Ursano, R. J., Ventis, W. L., Fullerton, C. S., Bates, G. L., Friedman, H., Shean, G. L. & Wright, K. M. (1993). Anticipation of handling the dead: effects of gender and experience. *British Journal of Clinical Psychology*, **32**, 466–8.

McFarlane, A. C. (1988). The longitudinal course of post-traumatic morbidity. The range of outcomes and their predictors. *Journal of Nervous and Mental Disease*, **176**, 30–9.

O'Brien, L. S. & Hughes, S. J. (1991). Symptoms of post-traumatic stress disorder in Falklands veterans five years after the conflict. *British Journal of Psychiatry*, **159**, 135–41.

Ørner, R. J., Paulson, R., Thompson, M., Pickles, M., Cook, C., Brown-Warr, R. & Stone, C. (1993). Critical incident stress management services in United Kingdom emergency services. Paper presented at the 2nd World Congress on Stress Trauma and Coping in Emergency Service Professionals, Baltimore, MD.

Solomon, Z. (1989). Untreated combat related PTSD – Why some Israeli veterans do not seek help. *Israeli Journal of Psychiatry and Related Sciences*, **26**, 111–23.

Taylor, A. J. W. & Frazer, A. G. (1982). The stress of post-disaster body handling and victim identification work. *Journal of Human Stress*, **8**, 4–12.

Thompson, J. & Solomon, M. (1991). Body recovery teams at disasters: trauma or challenge? *Anxiety Research*, **4**, 235–44.

Ursano, R. J. & McCarroll, J. E. (1990). The nature of a traumatic stressor: handling dead bodies. *Journal of Nervous and Mental Disease*, **178**, 396–8.

Ursano, R. J., Fullerton, C. S., Wright, K. M. & McCarroll, J. E. (Eds.) (1990). *Trauma, Disasters and Recovery*. Bethesda, MD: Uniformed Services University of the Health Sciences.

Ursano, R. J., Fullerton, C. S., Wright, K. M., McCarroll, J. E., Norwood, A. E. & Dinneen, M. P. (Eds.) (1992). *Disaster Workers: Trauma and Social Support*. Bethesda, MD: Uniformed Services University of the Health Sciences.

8

Debriefing and body recovery: police in a civilian disaster

David Alexander

Creation can come from the experience of destruction if lessons are learnt and practice changed. (Gibson (1996, p. 57))

EDITORIAL COMMENTS

This chapter provides a detailed discussion of Alexander's experience and research in the management of two groups of police officers involved in body handling and recovery after a major oil rig disaster. Of particular interest are the structures and processes that were set in place and appear to have contributed to positive outcomes. There is also the advantage for a programme of previous occupational health and safety research that allowed for a matched control group of officers to be identified. The structures included: careful preparation, including: support for the use of humour, and talking with colleagues; provision of defusing and debriefing by experienced and skilled senior police; back-up by the specialist mental health clinicians who were well known to the group, including the author, from previous work with them; pairing of younger and older workers; and a supportive general culture. These workers showed positive outcomes three months and three years later, believing that their work had enhanced their skills and self-confidence. They felt competent to do this type of work again. The workers reported the use of black humour and talking to colleagues as helpful strategies; good morale, interpersonal relationships and efficient organization were also seen to contribute positively. Keeping things to oneself was seen as neither helpful nor popular.

The findings are reviewed by Alexander, who is cautious in their interpretation, but highlights the multiple components that were potentially valuable. While further research may have helped to dissect out any potential contributions from the defusing or debriefing interventions the constraints of further research with such a population, in such circumstances, need to be fully acknowledged.

Some of the findings here reinforce hypotheses put forward by Weisæth's (Chapter 3): that is, the role of management and leadership in both strategies for mitigating stressor effects and in provision of debriefing-type interventions, with the support of this process by mental health professionals with appropriate expertise. This fits within the culture of the organization and can reinforce morale. As is also noted here, these workers had to continue with their tasks and a one-off intervention might be quite inappropriate in such circumstances. The chapter provides a further contribution to potential models for debriefing those affected by traumatic stresses, and for implementation in circumstances of ongoing stressor experience that must be managed.

Introduction

This chapter reports on the body-handling exercise following the Piper Alpha oil platform disaster. It contains six sections. The first describes the background to the exercise. The second addresses conceptual issues relating to the welfare provisions (including debriefing) made available to the personnel involved in the retrieval and identification of human remains after this disaster. The third section provides the empirical results of a three-year follow-up of these personnel. The fourth section offers some explanations for the interesting findings from this follow-up. The penultimate section represents a critical appraisal of the results, with particular reference to defusing and debriefing. The last section highlights the primary conclusions that this study appears to justify.

Background to the Piper Alpha oil platform disaster

A more detailed account of this major incident has been provided elsewhere (e.g. Alexander, 1991, 1993a). However, the circumstances of this disaster, the world's worst oil industry accident, are described in outline below.

The platform was sited about 200 kilometres off the north-east coast of Scotland; Aberdeen was the nearest city. The installation had housed an all-male crew of just over 200. At approximately 22:00 hours on Wednesday, 6 July 1988, an initial and relatively minor explosion set in motion a series of explosions, which culminated in a fireball, the core of which reached almost 2000°C. This engulfed the entire platform. One hundred and sixty-seven men died on site (only one died after being rescued). Despite the efforts of major fire expert Red Adair and his team, the fires were still not completely under control until 4 September 1988.

Several months after the disaster, 105 bodies were still missing, and it was established that most of them had been entombed in the accommodation module, which was lying in over 120 metres of water in the North Sea.

After three months of a particularly complicated technical operation this module was raised and towed on a giant barge to the remote island of Flotta, in the Orkney archipelago, where Occidental Petroleum (the oil company that owned the Piper Alpha) had an oil terminal. The latter provided good facilities for the police officers and other personnel who were required to search the module. Because of its isolated setting, an exclusion zone was able to be established around the island, with high levels of security, to deter the predatory and omnipresent media personnel.

The body handlers

The local police force (the Grampian Police) selected a team of officers to work with various personnel during the search of the module; these other individuals included divers, archivists, scaffolders, welders and photographers. In addition to the 23 officers (22 males and 1 female) at Flotta, there were 48 officers (41 males and 7 females) based at the temporary mortuary close to Aberdeen airport to where the bodies were taken by helicopter. The officers at Flotta were concerned largely with the retrieval and body bagging of the remains; the mortuary officers were responsible for the stripping, washing, photographing and identification thereof. Each body was allocated a mortuary officer, who was responsible for it while in the mortuary, and an enquiry officer who was responsible for its ultimate identification. Nineteen bodies were dissected daily by a team of local pathologists.

All the officers were volunteers but all had been invited to take part because they worked in departments that commonly dealt with sudden death. One officer declined this invitation. Only one officer had previously been involved in a large-scale disaster. The only other primary selection criteria were that preference was given to older officers and to those with a sense of humour! Generally, officers worked in pairs; an inexperienced officer was attached to a more experienced one. Three-quarters of all officers were police constables (the most basic rank).

Officers worked shifts of 8–14 hours depending on how many bodies had been found. At Flotta their duties were rotated regularly (if possible), and no officer was involved in these duties for more than seven days (apart from one senior operational officer).

Psychiatric involvement

Throughout the various stages of the disaster there was involved a small psychiatric team (comprising myself and five other senior clinicians). Their contribution was flexible, low key and accessible. It was agreed that I should be available on request at Flotta. My presence at the Flotta site caused no concern or surprise as I was known to most of the police officers, having been involved during most of the earlier stages of the disaster.

It was anticipated that the duties at Flotta might be the most stressful because the remains had been the victim of the effects of sea water, sea life, fire and explosion. The working environment was also physically unpleasant and occasionally dangerous.

Psychiatric opinion was sought on the content and nature of the induction that all personnel had to attend. Emphasis was placed on the need for physical safety (particularly in the module, which was upside down and its inside had been wrecked), hygiene, security and emotional and physical welfare. The normality of reactions, such as disgust and apprehensiveness, was strongly emphasized; no effort was made to foster a macho climate. Methods of coping with emotional reactions were openly discussed. My presence at Flotta was referred to in a low-key manner, and it was agreed that anybody could have access to me at any time for a chat. (Quite deliberately, the word 'counselling' was never used.)

Under Scot's Law a sudden death is a police responsibility, until the cause of death and the victim's identity have been established. Thus, the body-handling exercise was conducted under the aegis of the Chief Constable of Grampian Police. Ultimately, therefore, all executive decisions as to how the exercise should be carried out were left to the police. In an effort to be consistent with that policy and with the agreed philosophy of the psychiatric contribution, it was agreed that the daily defusings and subsequent debriefings should be conducted not by a mental health professional but by experienced police officers (in consultation with myself).

Conceptual issues relating to defusings and debriefing

First, it should be noted that the exercise does not entail a single traumatic or critical incident, as it took about three weeks for all the remains to be processed. It was decided that, at the end of each day, there was to be, for all those involved in the handling of human remains and/or working in the module at Flotta, a daily defusing with debriefings provided at the end of the whole exercise.

Defusings (Mitchell & Everly, 1995) were used at the end of daily duties in deference to the fact that the following day the personnel would still be required to deal with unpleasant matters until the exercise had been completed. With regard to the model of debriefing used it is impossible to be precise as it had been agreed (for the reasons outlined above) that I would not take part in the sessions.

However the model that would most comfortably fit what was aimed for is the multiple stressor model described by Armstrong et al. (1991) – a suitable one in view of the fact that personnel of different training, skills and background were faced with different needs and emotional demands.

The philosophy of prophylaxis permeated the entire proceedings. It has long been argued by, for example, Meichenbaum (1994) that stress inoculation training prior to potentially stressful encounters is helpful, and Mitchell & Dyregrov (1993) refer to the need to provide 'stress mitigation education'. The rationale, as well as the nature of the compulsory induction sessions, are consistent with their views.

Maslow (1971) referred to the need to address physical needs before emotional ones can be catered for. While no hierarchical approach was pursued here, the induction sessions were clearly aimed at addressing both physical and emotional needs. (In the section on the results of the follow-up an interesting observation is made regarding a problem that was encountered in relation to the catering arrangements for the police officers.)

Follow-up of the police officers

Further details of the outcome of a three-month and three-year follow-up of these police officers have been presented elsewhere (Alexander & Wells, 1991; Alexander, 1993b).

A key feature of the follow-up study was the opportunity to use predisaster baseline data on the police officers and a matched control group. This was made possible by the fortuitous circumstance that, only a few months before the disaster, I and two colleagues from the medical school had been commissioned to carry out an occupational health survey of the Grampian

Table 8.1. Response rates for Flotta/mortuary officers and matched control group

Group	Total no.	No. who had completed Occupational Health Project	No. who completed post-disaster questionnaires	No. who completed both Occupational Health Project and post-disaster questionnaires
Flotta	23	19	20	18
Mortuary	48	34	34	30
Controls	53	53	42	42

Adapted from Alexander & Wells (1991).

Police Force (Alexander et al., 1993). Thus, for most of the officers who worked at the mortuary and on Flotta, there were data available on their emotional state. Also, it was possible to derive a control group of officers who had not been involved in the disaster but who were matched for age, gender, seniority and scores on a measure of mental health.

Three-month follow-up

Subjects

The response rates for the Flotta and mortuary police officers and the control group are presented in Table 8.1, with the numbers thereof who contributed to the initial Occupational Health Survey.

Measures

Each police officer at Flotta and the mortuary was invited to complete the following measures.

Revised Impact of Event Scale (RIES) (Horowitz et al. 1979): Widely used after traumatic incidents, this 15-item scale measures subjective distress in terms of intrusive phenomena (such as nightmares and flashbacks) and avoidant behaviour in face of reminders of the traumatic event.

Hospital Anxiety and Depression Scale (HADS) (Zigmond & Snaith, 1983): This is a valid and reliable 14-item measure of anxiety and depression. It had also been used in the Occupational Health Survey conducted in the Grampian Police, and the control group in the follow-up study were also asked to complete it.

The Body Handling Questionnaire (BHQ): This 24-item questionnaire was designed specifically to assess the views of the officers on a series of matters relating to their duties at Flotta and at the mortuary.

Coping Strategy Questionnaire: Although there are many measures to assess coping style and strategy, for this study it was decided to use a measure that reflected my own observations and what officers reported to me about how they had coped. In the questionnaire, respondents had to indicate whether or not they had used a particular method of coping and to what extent it had been helpful.

Sick leave: Twelve months after the human remains had been retrieved, the sick leave records of the Grampian Police Force were made available to me to determine whether or not the records of the body handling officers differed from those of the control group. This objective measure also provided an opportunity to identify delayed psychopathological reactions.

Results

The personality profiles of the officers, as defined by the Eysenck Personality Questionnaire (EPQ) are comparable to the normative data provided by Eysenck & Eysenck (1975). Thus, these officers are not atypical in terms of their emotional make-up. Michaelis & Eysenck (1971) have demonstrated that, where subjects are motivated to present themselves in an unduly favourable way, the correlation between the EPQ Lie Scale and the Neuroticism Scale approaches or even exceeds -0.5.

Table 8.2. Responses of police officers to Body-Handling Questionnaire

	Question	Strongly agree (%)	Agree (%)	Undecided (%)	Disagree (%)	Strongly disagree (%)	Comparison Flotta and mortuary groups
1.	Adequate steps were taken to ensure my safety at work at Flotta/the mortuary	24	59	11	4	2	NS
2.	Standards of hygiene at work at Flotta/the mortuary were good	28	46	11	15	0	$p < 0.05$
3.	Morale among personnel at Flotta/the mortuary was high	41	42	9	4	4	NS
4.	I was not given a clear idea of my duties at Flotta/the mortuary	6	22	5	52	15	NS
5.	I was given regular feedback about my work at Flotta/the mortuary	6	48	11	26	9	NS
6.	I found work at Flotta/the mortuary more stressful than routine police work	20	41	11	26	2	NS
7.	I still feel under some stress due to my work at Flotta/the mortuary	0	2	15	55	28	NS
8.	There were good relationships among the police officers of all ranks at Flotta/the mortuary	33	48	7	8	4	NS
9.	Eating arrangements were inadequate at Flotta/the mortuary	11	28	4	35	22	$p < 0.01$
10.	The organization of the retrieval of the bodies was good	26	61	9	4	0	NS
11.	Overall, I felt I was doing a useful task at Flotta/the mortuary	32	61	5	2	0	NS
12.	I disliked the media's coverage of the retrieval of the bodies	7	13	52	26	2	NS
13.	There were good relationships among the various personnel at Flotta/the mortuary	44	50	2	4	0	NS
14.	I gained more support than usual from fellow police officers while *at work* at Flotta/the mortuary	9	37	35	19	0	NS
15.	I gained more support than usual from fellow police officers *outside work hours* at Flotta/the mortuary	7	28	32	33	0	$p < 0.01$
16.	I gained more emotional support than usual from the other professionals while *at work* at Flotta/the mortuary	7	45	28	20	0	$p < 0.01$
17.	I gained more support than usual from other professionals *outside work* at Flotta/the mortuary	7	45	24	24	0	$p < 0.02$
18.	There was little sense of team spirit at Flotta/the mortuary	0	9	0	33	58	NS

Table 8.2. (*cont.*)

	Question	Strongly agree (%)	Agree (%)	Undecided (%)	Disagree (%)	Strongly disagree (%)	Comparison Flotta and mortuary groups
19.	I thought the visits from the Chief Constable were helpful	7	28	39	19	7	NS
20.	I am glad I was a member of the police team at Flotta/the mortuary	26	48	17	9	0	NS
21.	I would not wish to be involved in similar work in the future	6	7	20	37	30	NS
22.	On balance, I do not think I coped well with my duties at Flotta/the mortuary	4	4	0	46	46	NS
23.	The anticipation of the actual work at Flotta/the mortuary was more stressful than the actual work itself.	7	44	19	26	4	NS
24.	The experience I gained from being involved with Piper Alpha will be of little benefit to me in future police work	4	7	2	48	39	NS

NS, not significant.

χ^2 analysis were carried out comparing the Flotta and the mortuary groups in terms of 'agreement' and 'disagreement' (irrespective of the strength). Where cell values fell below the level required for valid χ^2 analysis, Fisher's Exact test was used.

From Alexander & Wells (1991).

The figure for this sample was well below that pre-scribed figure.

Table 8.2 displays the police officers' replies to the Body Handling Questionnaire. There were 54 respondents for this measure, although the total number of officers involved in the whole exercise was 51; the disparity was because three officers worked at both sites. Overall, there is a similar pattern to the replies from the officers at the two sites. The last column of the table indicates the results of chi-squared analyses on the results of the two groups of officers. The officers at the mortuary were less impressed than their Flotta colleagues with the support from colleagues and other professionals and with their eating arrangements. (At one stage, staff at the airport objected to the officers sharing their canteen facilities because of the nature of their mortuary duties.)

For all officers it can be seen that good relationships are an important issue. Also, it is noteworthy that most officers viewed their duties as useful, most felt their anticipatory anxiety was worse than their anxiety dur-ing the body-handling exercise, most believed they had fulfilled their duties successfully, and almost all were glad to have been involved in this work. Finally, it should be noted that at three months only one officer claimed that he was suffering from stress associated with his Piper Alpha duties. The remainder of the replies demonstrate that most officers had a favourable view of the organization of this exercise.

How and with what success the officers had used various methods of coping can be seen in Table 8.3. From this table it can be seen how popular and how helpful humour was as a way of coping with the work. Similarly, talking to colleagues was a frequently used and successful coping strategy. Thinking about the positive benefits of what they were doing was also commonly and successfully used. By far the least successful and popular strategy was keeping thoughts to themselves.

A comparison of the HADS scores from the three-month follow-up with those derived from the Occupation Health Survey indicated that, in relation to their

Table 8.3. Responses of officers to Coping Strategy Questionnaire ($n = 54$)

Method of coping[a]	Did not use (%)	Very helpful (%)	Helpful (%)	Unhelpful (%)	Very unhelpful (%)
Humour	2	74	24	0	0
Talking to my colleagues	4	50	44	2	0
Looking forward to getting off duty	52	7	35	6	0
Keeping my thoughts to myself	41	4	23	28	4
Thinking about my family	54	11	24	7	4
Thinking of outside interests	46	9	39	6	0
Thinking about the positive benefits of this work	22	31	41	6	0
Avoiding thinking about what I was doing	46	11	24	17	2

[a] χ^2 analyses were calculated comparing the Flotta and mortuary groups in terms of 'used' and 'did not use' the method in question. When the cell values fell below the level for valid χ^2 analysis, Fisher's Exact test was used. None of the comparisons was statistically significant at the 5% level.
From Alexander & Wells (1991).

anxiety scores, 31 officers had fallen into the 'Normal' category in the earlier survey; 37 did so at the three-month follow-up. For depression, 45 officers were classified as 'Normal' at each of these two assessments. The number in the 'Borderline' anxiety category dropped from 11 officers to 6 over the Occupational Health Survey and the three-month follow-up, respectively; 'Pathological' scores for anxiety dropped from 6 to 5 respectively across these two assessments.

The results of a series of Wilcoxon paired signed ranks comparisons of the scores before and after the body handling study are described in Table 8.4. The comparisons confirm that there is no difference for the depression scores across the before and after assessments but there is a highly significant drop in the level of the officers' anxiety scores after the body-handling exercise.

Sick leave

An examination of the sick leave records of the body-handling officers and the control group over the 12 months after their Piper Alpha duties (by means of the Wilcoxon matched pairs signed ranks test) confirmed that there was no difference between the groups in

Table 8.4. Wilcoxon comparisons for the 'before' and 'after' anxiety and depression scores on the HAD Scale for officers at Flotta and the mortuary, and the control group

	Wilcoxon z	
	Anxiety	Depression
Combined (Flotta and mortuary)	−3.03*	−1.21
Control	−1.35	−0.72

*$p < 0.002$.
Adapted from Alexander & Wells (1991).

terms of the number of days of sick leave. The mean time off work for the Flotta mortuary group was 2.79 days, with a standard deviation of 4.28 days. The respective figures for the control group was 3.98 days and 7.03 days. For each group the median was one day of sick leave.

Three-year follow-up

At this stage officers in the body handling group and the control group were asked to complete the HADS, the

Table 8.5. Percentage response of police officers to the Body-Handling Questionnaire at three months (3M) and at three years (3Y)

Item	Strongly agree		Agree		Undecided		Disagree		Strongly disagree	
	3M	3Y	3M	3Y	3M	3Y	3M	3Y	3M	3Y
I still feel under some stress due to the body-handling exercise	0	6	3	3	14	8	55	43	28	40
I am glad I was a member of the police body-handling team	26	31	48	55	17	11	9	3	0	0
I would not wish to be involved in similar work in the future	6	6	6	6	20	17	37	40	31	31
On balance, I do not think I coped well with my duties during the body-handling exercise	3	3	3	6	0	3	47	46	47	42
The experience I gained from being involved with the police body-handling team will be of little benefit to me in future police work	3	6	6	6	3	0	49	40	39	48

From Alexander (1993b).

Table 8.6. Numbers of police officers classified according to the Hospital Anxiety and Depression Scale scores, predisaster (PD) at three months (3M) and at three years (3Y)

Category	Anxiety			Depression		
	PD	3M	3Y	PD	3M	3Y
Normal	24	30	26	33	32	31
Borderline	8	3	8	1	2	4
Pathological	3	2	1	1	1	0

From Alexander (1993b).

RIES and selected items from the BHQ. Of the original number of 48 officers who contributed to the initial follow-up, 46 were available for subsequent follow-up, and 35 agreed to contribute. For each of these officers there was a matched control.

A comparison by means of the Wilcoxon matched pairs signed ranks test established that there was no difference between the assessments for the avoidance scores on the RIES but there was a significant difference for the intrusion and the total scores (p 0.03; $p < 0.0001$, respectively). Thus the level of subjective distress in terms of experience of intrusive phenomena reduced significantly over the two assessments.

The officers' longer-term views on their duties after the disaster are summarized in Table 8.5. It can be seen that overall these officers showed even more positive attitudes towards their duties. In particular, it should be noted that most officers at three years would wish to be involved in similar work in the future; most felt they had gained from their experience, and only one officer regretted having been a member of the body-handling team. On the other hand, at three years, three officers claimed that they were still stressed by their body-handling duties. (However, an examination of their medical records confirmed that one of these officers had had substantial emotional problems before the Piper Alpha disaster.)

Table 8.6 above recorded the categorical distribution of the HADS scores at three years compared to that at three months. A series of Wilcoxon matched pairs signed ranks tests revealed that, for the anxiety and depression scores of the body handlers and their controls, the only statistically significant difference was that between the baseline anxiety scores and those at three months ($p < 0.01$) and at three years ($p < 0.05$).

Explanatory concepts

Despite some professional and lay expectations (the latter fuelled to some extent by doom-laden predictions from sections of the local media), the results of this study provide powerful evidence to confirm that body handling need not lead to post-traumatic psychopathology. Certainly, these officers found their work distasteful and distressing, but neither at three months nor at three years were there any signs of pathological levels of anxiety or depression. Similarly, a review of their sick leave records compared to those of a matched control group did not suggest that these officers had experienced any long-term health problems.

The officers emphasized the value of black humour. The protective value of this has been widely acknowledged; however, McCarroll et al. (1993) have reported that some individuals using such humour fear that this indicates that they have 'gone over the top' or have become insensitive. It may be helpful therefore (as was done here) to reassure individuals in advance that black humour is a perfectly normal and healthy method of coping.

Talking with colleagues was also regarded as very helpful, and it occurred spontaneously while they were conducting their duties and also at the defusing and debriefing sessions. (At their induction, officers were informed that talking openly was an effective way of coping with their demanding duties.) It is impossible to disentangle cause from effect. Did the formal sessions promote the on-site talking or vice versa? Perhaps the most likely possibility is that they were mutually facilitating. A similar observation has been made by Deahl et al. (1994) in relation to military body handling during the Gulf War.

The other principal method of coping endorsed by these police officers was that of being able to translate unpleasant (and at times physically dangerous) duties into valuable and meaningful ones. Again, at the induction, it was emphasized that for the sake of the families and for the sake of the legal enquiry the retrieval of the remains (and the archival material) was particularly worth while. Raphael (1986) and Durham et al. (1985) have also indicated how adversity can lead to positive gains. It is of note therefore that at three years nearly all

of the officers were glad to have taken part in the exercise and felt that they had gained from their experience. An interesting example of cognitive restructuring (Lazarus & Folkman, 1984) is to be found in an officer's reappraisal of what was facing him in order that he could cope with it, 'Sir, when I go in there [the accommodation module] as far as I am concerned I'm going to a spaceship looking for Martians'.

In addition to their own coping methods, it must be noted that these officers placed considerable weight on organizational and managerial factors. The essential ones seem to have been an attention to their needs (emotional and physical), good interpersonal relationships, and high team morale. Similar observations have been reported in a follow-up of a specialist group of body handlers (Thompson & Solomon, 1991). The value of *esprit de corps* has also been reported to have a protective role among aircrew following their ejection from their aircraft (Aveline & Fowlie, 1987). The emphasis on the value of mutual support derived from group cohesiveness is of course central to the traditional model of debriefing (Mitchell, 1983; Dyregrov, 1997).

An issue that evoked strong (and initially divergent) views was whether the bar in the living quarters at Flotta should be available to the body-handling personnel. (McCarroll et al. (1993) have already commented on how alcohol is used to cope with such work.) It was agreed, however, that the bar should be open for all personnel for two hours each evening. There was no evidence that this facility was abused, and it may have done much to normalize the experience of these personnel, to develop further social bonds and to encourage open discussion of feelings, etc. A particularly revealing finding from this study is that the police officers highlighted the psychoprophylactic value of the organizational and managerial features of the body-handling exercise. In the earlier occupational health survey it was the lack of these features in relation to routine police work that was found to be strongly correlated with stress, ill health and problems in the original Occupational Health Survey.

Previous experience of dealing with unpleasant events is purported by some (e.g. Grundy, 1990) to help the individual cope with subsequent events. There was, however, no evidence in this study that the more experienced officers coped better with their duties than their less experienced colleagues. It is possible that the pairing of more experienced and less experienced officers may have masked any possible differences. Modelling may also have featured at the defusing and debriefing sessions, as it was reported that the more senior and experienced officers were very willing to describe their own feelings and reactions to the more unpleasant aspects of their duties.

The duties of the personnel involved in this exercise did not constitute a homogeneous set of experiences, but there are two factors that should be addressed here. The first is gruesomeness, a dimension identified by McCarroll et al. (1995) to constitute a particularly potent source of distress for body handlers. Many of the bodies were most distasteful in appearance because of their prolonged exposure to the effects of the explosion, fire, sea water and sea life. However, some officers reported that the most disturbing occasions were when a body had a relatively normal external appearance, but on examination was found to have been eaten away from the inside by sea life (some specimens of which made their appearance when the bodies were being stripped and washed!).

'Emotional attachment' was also reported by McCarroll and his colleagues to be a factor that made it harder for body handlers to cope with their duties. No doubt this is why many coping strategies, including black humour, serve to dehumanize the deceased or to distance the handler from the humanness of the deceased. This was observed by myself, but another phenomenon was also noted. Some officers made a particular effort to personalize the bodies for which they had responsibility, even to the point of having mock conversations with them (e.g. 'Don't worry lad, I'll find out who you are and get you home'). This almost paradoxical attachment to the body may be linked to the point made earlier, namely, the importance and meaningfulness of the body recovery and identification procedures. It should also be borne in mind that common methods of distancing oneself from a dead body, e.g. by not looking at the face and hands, were not available to many of the police officers in view of the finger printing and

odontological procedures required for identification.

A particularly important finding from this longitudinal study is the durability of the changes observed in the scores from the measure of anxiety and depression. Why did the three-year level of anxiety settle between that recorded at the three-month follow-up and that recorded by the same officers during the Occupational Health Survey? The fact that the levels for the control group did not change indicates this finding could not be accounted for by any changes that took place in the Grampian Police Force over that period of time.

Several possibilities suggest themselves. First, having emotionally survived the exercise, and having completed it successfully, may have greatly enhanced these officers' self-confidence. Secondly, the sense of having been a member of an elite or at least a special group may have boosted their self-esteem. Thirdly, it would appear that these officers genuinely acquired new skills and coping strategies that may have been of value in subsequent duties. The fact that the officers who were the least satisfied with the exercise were those who had to guard the perimeter of the mortuary (the one duty that involved no exposure to human remains) may provide support for these suggested explanations.

Critical appraisal of the results

The value of the findings from this study is enhanced by relatively high response rates, before and after data and a matched control group.

Inevitably, however, the study had to be very reliant on self-report data (apart from the health records), and no effort has made to validate the HADS against a standardized clinical interview. For reasons to be discussed later, it was felt inappropriate to ask anything else of these officers.

The use of the personality measure offered some reassurance against any suggestion that the police officers were atypical in terms of their basic personality traits. Also, the data from the Lie and Neuroticism Scales provide no evidence that these officers had sought to present themselves in an unduly favourable light.

Obviously, in view of the circumstances in which this study had to be conducted, there was no opportunity to carry out a randomized controlled trial of defusing and debriefing; operational duties had to take priority. For similar reasons, these post-incident interventions could not have been conducted rigorously according to a predetermined theoretical model. Since the sessions were not recorded, one can judge from the self-reports of the participants only what were the general principles underlying the way they were conducted. Certainly, some flexibility was required in view of the different backgrounds, professions and duties of the personnel involved. Also, there was an important cultural dimension that had to be acknowledged. Unlike the majority of the other personnel, most of the police officers were locals. The north-east Scot usually displays a legendary stoicism and a profound dislike of emotional display (even *in extremis*). Thus, it was intended that the debriefings and defusings should be conducted in a fashion that could not be seen as emotionally threatening and confrontational. (The general issue of tailoring a psychological intervention to accommodate the personal style and values, etc., of those involved is of course not new.)

Another open question is to what extent the discreet psychiatric presence made any contribution to the outcome. Certainly, there was universal support for the fact that the author's presence was nonintrusive. However, the senior officers also appeared to welcome back-up and the opportunity to discuss management issues with me, and some of the junior officers commented that they were pleased that I was 'around in case there's any need'. Consistent with the philosophy of a low-key presence was the fact that none of the interventions was run by a mental health professional. There does seem to be implied a mixed message if such sessions are run by a psychologist or psychiatrist, while emphasizing that debriefing and defusing are not treatments and that the participants are displaying 'normal reactions to an abnormal event'. (More recently, Ørner (1997) also enunciated the value of the mental health specialist providing advice and support for managers rather than for front-line personnel.)

Certain authorities would have preferred a more detailed follow-up of the officers. Admittedly, the study leaves unanswered a number of important questions. For example, it is not clear what in particular the offi-

cers found distressing about their duties. Also, the issue of anticipatory anxiety (before such duties) needs further consideration because it can obviously have a deleterious effect, but it is likely also to have a motivating influence on how personnel respond and benefit from such matters as inductions and post-incident interventions. Another key question is what were the respective contributions of the different factors in this study, which might have had therapeutic and psychoprophylactic potential. More specifically, the particular contribution of the defusings and debriefings cannot be precisely measured because they were inextricably part of a wider welfare plan.

Naturally, some caution has to be exercised with regard to the generalizability of the findings, for a number of reasons. First, the human remains did not involve those of women or children. Secondly, the police had several months to prepare for this exercise. (This circumstance is in stark contrast to what prevailed, for example, following the crash of the Pan Am 103 flight at Lockerbie.) Thirdly, although only one officer had had personal experience of mass carnage, all these officers had had some experience of sudden death, and they were volunteers.

However, while it would have been ideal to have the opportunity to answer the questions above, the welfare and needs of the police officers had to be paramount. For several months they were the subject of media and other interest; they had a difficult job to do, and they had already completed a very lengthy and detailed set of questionnaires for the Occupational Health Survey. I therefore determined that, while scientific information would have to be sacrificed, these officers should not feel themselves to be psychological 'guinea pigs' and the subject of excessive scrutiny.

Conclusions

This longitudinal study of a group of police officers who had been engaged in the retrieval and identification of the victims of a major industrial calamity, demonstrates that psychiatric morbidity is not an inevitable consequence, despite the concerns generated by previous studies of body handling teams. The fortuitous availability of pre Piper Alpha data on the officers' mental health and of a matched control group reinforce the strength of the conclusions.

Certain personal coping strategies were reported by the officers to be particularly helpful. In particular, they referred to the use of black humour, talking with colleagues and their perception of their duties as meaningful and valuable. It is also clear that the manner in which the exercise was organized and managed reflected a considerable prophylactic potential. Particular reference was made to the value of an efficient organization, good interpersonal relationships and attention to physical and emotional needs.

With regard to the individual contribution of defusings and debriefings arguments have been adduced here as to why their specific contributions cannot be more precisely specified. They were elements within an overall strategy of welfare for the body-handling personnel. Such a strategy is of course entirely compatible with the views of those who have developed the concept of critical incident stress debriefing. Such authorities have consistently argued that such interventions should not be regarded as 'single-shot' responses to critical incidents, conducted in isolation from other measures provided for the welfare of personnel after critical incidents.

In view of the reports from these officers at three months and three years, it could be argued further that the outcome of interventions, such as debriefing, should not be confined to symptom reduction, rather they should also include such matters as enhanced self-confidence, the acquisition of new professional and coping skills, a more positive perspective on critical incidents, and enhanced group cohesiveness and support.

REFERENCES

Alexander, D. A. (1991). Psychiatric intervention after the Piper Alpha disaster. *Journal of the Royal College of Medicine*, **84**, 8–11.

Alexander, D. A. (1993a). The Piper Alpha oil platform disaster. In J. P. Wilson and B. Raphael (Eds.) *International Handbook of Traumatic Stress Syndromes* (pp. 461–70). New York: Plenum Press.

Alexander, D. A. (1993b). Stress among police body handlers. A long-term follow-up. *British Journal of Psychiatry*, **163**, 806–8.

Alexander, D. A. & Wells, A. (1991). Reactions of police officers to body-handling after a major disaster: a before-and-after comparison. *British Journal of Psychiatry*, **159**, 547–55.

Alexander, D. A., Walker, L. G., Innes, G. & Irving, B. L. (1993). *Police Stress at Work*. London: Police Foundation.

Armstrong, K., O'Callahan, W. & Marmar, C. R. (1991). Debriefing Red Cross disaster personnel: the multiple stressor debriefing model. *Journal of Traumatic Stress*, **4**, 581–93.

Aveline, M. O. & Fowlie, D. G. (1987). Surviving ejection from military aircraft: psychological reactions, modifying factors and intervention. *Stress Medicine*, **3**, 15–20.

Deahl, M. P., Gilham, A. B., Thomas, J., Searle, M. M. & Srinivasan, M. (1994). Psychological sequelae following Gulf War: factors associated with subsequent morbidity and the effectiveness of psychological debriefing. *British Journal of Psychiatry*, **165**, 60–5.

Durham, T. W., McCammon, S. L. & Allison, E. J. (1985). The psychological impact of disaster on research personnel. *Annals of Emergency Medicine*, **14**, 664–8.

Dyregrov, A. (1997). The process of psychological debriefing. *Journal of Traumatic Stress*, **10**, 589–605.

Eysenck, H. J. & Eysenck, S. B. G. (1975). *Manual of the Eysenck Personality Questionnaire*. London: Hodder & Stoughton.

Gibson, M. (1996). The Kegworth experience: influence in practice in Northern Ireland. In C. Mead (Ed.) *Journeys of Discovery* (pp. 47–57). London: National Institute for Social Work.

Grundy, S. (1990). After the disaster. *Police Review*, **98**, 234–6.

Horowitz, M. J., Wilner, N. & Alvarez, W. (1979). Impact of Event Scale: a measure of subjective stress. *Psychosomatic Medicine*, **41**, 209–18.

Lazarus, R. S. & Folkman, S. (1984). *Stress, Appraisal and Coping*. New York: Springer-Verlag.

Maslow, A. (1971). *The Further Reaches of Human Nature*. New York: Viking Press.

McCarroll, J. E., Ursano, R. J., Wright, K. M. & Fullerton, C. S. (1993). Handling bodies after violent death: strategies for coping. *American Journal of Orthopsychiatry*, **63**, 209–14.

McCarroll, J. E., Ursano, R. J., Fullerton, C. S., Oates, G. L., Ventis, W. L., Friedman, H., Shean, G. L. & Wright, K. M. (1995). Gruesomeness, emotional attachment and personal threat: dimensions of the anticipated stress of body recovery. *Journal of Traumatic Stress*, **8**, 343–9.

Meichenbaum, D. (1994). *A Clinical Handbook/Practical Therapist Manual*. Ontario: Institute Press.

Michaelis, W. & Eysenck, H. J. (1971). The determination of personality inventory factor patterns and inter-correlations by changes in real life motivation. *Journal of Genetic Psychology*, **118**, 223–4.

Mitchell, J. T. (1983). When disaster strikes … The critical incident stress debriefing. *Journal of Emergency Medical Services*, **8**, 36–9.

Mitchell, J. T. & Dyregrov, A. (1993). Traumatic stress in disaster workers and emergency personnel. In J. P. Wilson & B. Raphael (Eds.) *International Handbook of Traumatic Stress Syndromes (pp. 905–14)*. New York: Plenum Press.

Mitchell, J. T. & Everly, G. S. (1995). *Critical Incident Stress Debriefing*. Ellicott City, MD: Chevron Publishing.

Ørner, R. J. (1997). Triage for psychological debriefing: an evidence-based protocol for emergency responders. Paper presented at the 5th European Conference on Traumatic Stress, Maastricht, the Netherlands.

Raphael, B. (1986). *When Disaster Strikes: How Individuals and Communities Cope with Catastrophe*. New York: Basic Books.

Thompson, J. & Solomon, M. (1991). Body recovery teams at disasters: trauma or challenge? *Anxiety Research*, **4**, 235–44.

Zigmond, A. S. & Snaith, R. P. (1983). The Hospital Anxiety and Depression Scale. *Acta Psychiatrica Scandinavica*, **67**, 361–70.

9

Debriefing after massive road trauma: perceptions and outcomes

Rod Watts

EDITORIAL COMMENTS

Massive road trauma such as the crash of a tourist or school bus brings widespread physical and psychological trauma. These effects are experienced by survivors (injured and uninjured), bereaved family members of those who die, rescue and emergency personnel, and the communities in which they occur.

Watts reviews studies in this field, and describes his own research findings, which cover three major incidents of this kind in Australia. His and other findings are clear about the substantial and often long-lasting morbidity that may follow. With each of the groups involved there are identified needs for psychological assistance and Watts reviews what is known about debriefing, which has been the most frequently applied prevention and support measure. The findings of this work make clear that debriefing is not appropriate for survivors or the bereaved, as it may add to their distress. Nevertheless group-based support focussing on information and sharing of concern may be helpful. Such groups may arise naturally, or be drawn together and may represent the grouping of those affected who were a prior established group (e.g. class of school children, club group of the elderly). In any case this is not a traditional debriefing but may be classified, Watts suggests, as an 'adaptive' debriefing in that it has information, shared understandings of what has occurred and mutual support for planning and needs as its role.

With respect to emergency and rescue personnel, Watts' studies show, as does other research such as that described by Robinson (Chapter 6) and Mitchell and Everley (Chapter 5) in this book, that these interven-

tions are perceived to be helpful by those who received them and seen as an indication of their own and others' support. However, there was no relationship of perceived helpfulness to outcome. And in each instance those debriefed showed higher symptom levels than those who were not, with those multiply debriefed showing the highest levels. This must give rise to concern. Watts explores a number of possible explanations, such as that they were more distressed. Despite this finding, he believes that debriefing is inherently positive and should be provided and available. It cannot, however, be assumed to prevent the development of psychological morbidity post trauma, and a range of other interventions should be available to achieve this including specific counselling for those at high risk.

The author's approach is careful, bearing in mind the high level of demand, occupational health and safety implications, and perceived helpfulness. However, the potential for debriefing, as applied, to be potentially harmful, or to interfere with natural pathways of resolution, needs to be further considered, particularly in view of the research results reported.

Introduction

How best to pro-actively provide psychological support following massive road trauma is a pressing question due to the severity and persistence of psychological sequelae likely to be sustained by those involved. Safeguarding well-being and privacy while responding to the varying needs of those affected in a way that maximizes benefit are central issues to address. This includes when, how, for whom, and what to focus on when providing psychological intervention, including debriefing. The effects of massive road trauma are summarized in this chapter, evidence of the efficacy of psychological intervention examined, an outline of intervention strategies for survivors, bereaved, personnel and members of the community presented, and issues discussed and recommendations given in relation to debriefing.

The effects of massive road trauma

Road crashes that result in death, severe injury, or a narrow escape from either can be traumatic for those involved. Malt (1988), in Norway, in the first randomly assigned longitudinal study of the psychological effects of road crashes ($n = 107$), found 22% likely to have had a psychiatric disorder at some time during the first two years post injury, but only one case of post-traumatic stress disorder (PTSD). Two subsequent studies of consecutive admissions to hospital after car crashes, one in the UK (Mayou et al., 1993), the other in Australia (Green et al., 1993), found slightly fewer than 20% were severely affected in the short-term, with approximately 11% having PTSD. These and other research findings (Brom et al., 1993; Goldberg & Gara, 1990; Watts et al., 1996) indicate that road crashes cause persistent psychological sequelae of some severity for up to 20% of injured individuals.

Massive road trauma, on the basis of greater magnitude of trauma, such as the degree of exposure to death, dying and destruction, will generally result in higher incidence of persistent psychological sequelae among survivors than that after more typical car crashes. Hovens & van de Weerd (1998) found 18% of the 17 survivors assessed at six months after a multifatality coach crash in Germany had PTSD. Forty-one per cent of the 29 survivors assessed by the author 13 months after a Queensland coach crash, in which 11 people were killed, had PTSD; 79% were likely to have had a psychiatric disorder and 52% had high levels of intrusion or avoidance phenomena (Watts, 1995a). In this crash some of the elderly passengers were thrown from the coach as it skidded off a steep embankment, several were crushed as it rolled, with the remainder strewn within the wreckage. All survivors, including the driver, were admitted to hospital owing to injuries sustained. Seeing the bodies and/or death of one of the passengers were the predominant factors that caused severe distress, both at the time of the crash and in a recurring way over time. The period in hospital was a contributing factor for some. Reminders of the crash, recurrent or intrusive recollections, avoidance of thoughts and feelings associated with what occurred, poor concentration, being easily startled and difficulties with sleep were the most common persistent difficulties (Watts, 1995a).

Family members of people killed in large-scale road crashes are also at considerable risk of incurring psychological harm. Sudden and unexpected death can have a long-lasting effect on the bereaved (Parkes & Weiss, 1983; Lundin, 1984; Sanders, 1988), including deaths caused by road trauma (Lehman & Wortman, 1987). Multiple fatalities intensify the trauma and correspondingly increase the risk of psychological difficulties (Hodgkinson & Stewart, 1991). Griffiths & Watts (1992) found that family members of the people killed in two large-scale bus crashes were as severely psychologically affected (probable psychiatric disorder, intrusion and avoidance phenomena) at 12 months post trauma as the injured survivors. Similarly the parents of the 'seventh-grade' children killed in a school bus crash were as severely affected at one, three and five years post crash as parents of the injured children who were not killed (Winje, 1996). Winje (1996) found that while there was some reduction of trauma-specific sequelae over time among parents of the children involved, there was no significant reduction in general psychological distress. A small proportion showed improvement.

Emergency workers who respond to, or who subsequently become involved in either medical care or support may also be at risk of sustaining post-trauma sequelae in the short to long term. For example, body retrieval on a large-scale causes severe sequelae among even the most experienced personnel (Taylor & Frazer, 1982; Jones, 1985; Ursano & McCaroll, 1990). The magnitude of 'inescapable horror' (Burges Watson, 1987) is a distinguishing characteristic between massive road trauma and single-fatality crashes for personnel. Two hundred and eighty-eight emergency hospital and support workers involved in either the Grafton or Kempsey coach crashes were assessed 12 months post trauma

(Griffiths & Watts, 1992). Both massive road crashes occurred in the state of New South Wales, Australia, in 1989. Twenty-one people were killed and 23 injured in the Grafton crash, which occurred when a truck drove into the path of an interstate passenger coach. The force of the impact ripped open the right side of the coach. The Kempsey coach crash was caused by two interstate passenger coaches colliding head on, with the front sections of each coach concertinaed together. All of the seats were ripped from their moorings, leaving over one-third of the back of each coach completely empty.

Forty-seven per cent of personnel ($n = 288$) had at least moderate levels of intrusion or avoidance phenomena, including 13.5% who had high levels of either at 12 months post crash. A subgroup of 24 state emergency workers were assessed at 1, 3 and 12 months after their involvement in the Kempsey coach crash. Forty-three per cent were likely to have had a psychiatric disorder at 1 month, 18% at 3 months and 17% at 12 months. These findings indicate a high degree of persistent sequelae. The lack of reduction between 3 and 12 months is particularly significant. McFarlane (1989) found that psychological sequelae at 12 months post trauma among fire fighters involved in the Ash Wednesday Bush Fires in South Australia had not decreased at 24 months. If this finding can be extrapolated to massive road crashes, it would indicate that at least 14% of emergency workers would remain substantially negatively affected by their involvement in either the Grafton or Kempsey road crashes.

The fourth group of victims that can be negatively psychologically affected by large-scale road crashes are members of the community in which these disasters occur. There are limited research data to quantify or describe what these effects might be. However, observations of the Kempsey community (a rural area of the state of New South Wales) following the Kempsey coach crash, what remains as the largest road fatality in Australia, indicate effects do occur (Watts & Wilson, 1998). Whilst none of the passengers killed or injured lived in the Kempsey area, the impact was experienced in several ways by members of the community. In addition to the rescue, medical and support staff who lived in the community, those affected included the families of personnel involved and staff at the local airport and motels who met the bereaved and families of survivors as they converged on the town. Local ministers of religion and politicians, at the memorial service held in Kempsey during the first week post crash, expressed the 'state of despair and shock' in the town, whose 'heart' was torn by the disaster (*Macleay Argus*, 28 December 1989). Other indicators of community members being affected included:

1. The formation of a Community Action Force that sought the means of upgrading the highway, as they believed this would eradicate any risk of further crashes.
2. Fifty-four of the 156 publications of the local paper during the first year carried headlines and articles in its first five pages on the coach crash, or related issues.
3. The Kempsey Lions Group erected a memorial garden at the side of the road where the crash occurred. Club members raised the necessary funds by a well-publicised 400 kilometre walk.
4. Five hundred people attended the first anniversary commemorative service held at the memorial garden.

It should be noted that, while these factors indicate an impact on the community, there are many potentially positive aspects, highlighting the fact that disasters may strengthen and motivate communities as well as damage them. This of course also applies to the individual.

Available evidence indicates that survivors of large-scale road crashes, the families of those killed, emergency personnel including support workers, and members of any community within which these disasters occur can be detrimentally psychologically affected. These are, respectively, primary, secondary, tertiary and fourth-level victims according to Taylor & Frazer's (1981) victim classification. Survivors, bereaved and personnel are at high risk of sustaining moderate to severe and persistent psychological sequelae from this type of trauma. The high prevalence and associated detrimental affects warrant effective and systematic follow-up. This follow-up would aim primarily to promote recovery, including preventing the development of psychopathology and secondary difficulties whenever possible. Early detection of psychological sequelae and intervention, when warranted, is the optimum approach (Horowitz et al., 1980; Kuch et al., 1985; Burges Watson, 1987). Early intervention it is suggested can reduce the intensity of acute reactions, mitigate the development of secondary problems, and minimize the onset of long-term psychopathology.

Evidence of benefit from psychological intervention

Survivors

Examining research findings about the efficacy of psychological intervention indicates that there is a lack of demonstrated quantifiable benefit. For survivors, there are no research findings to support the idea that a particular type of psychological intervention will reduce post-trauma sequelae. Brom et al. (1993) found that psychotherapy for individuals injured in road crashes, despite the vast majority reporting it as helpful, did not contribute to the reduction of sequelae over time. A randomized controlled trial of psychological intervention for adults during 24–48 hours of admission after being injured in a road crash did not find it to be associated with a reduction of sequelae at four months post injury (Hobbs et al., 1996). Similarly, all of the 15 Queensland bus crash survivors who received psychological assistance at some time (range was from 2 to over 20 sessions) during the first 12 months reported being helped by it, but as a group had neither more nor less intrusion or avoidance phenomena than those who did not receive psychological assistance (Watts, 1995b). All of the 17 bus accident survivors who were assessed at six months post trauma received debriefing, social and psychological support; 18% had PTSD (Hovens & van de Weerd, 1998).

Sixty-six per cent of the Queensland bus crash survivors assessed at 13 months post trauma reported that they did not, or rarely wanted to, talk to hospital personnel about their ordeal. Seventy-six per cent reported that they did not, or rarely thought they needed, psychological assistance (Watts, 1995b). Several reported finding comfort from talking with fellow survivors while in hospital. The benefits of mutual support

were observed by Alexander (1990) among survivors of the Piper Alpha oil rig disaster. The commonality of experience, the closeness of bonds that can so quickly be established in the face of catastrophe and the opportunity to review what occurred with other survivors are reasons why this mutual support would be helpful at this time. From the reluctance of the majority of these elderly survivors to talk with hospital staff about their crash experience, or perceive that they needed psychological help, it would have at the least been an imposition, if not potentially harmful, to expect them to attend any group debriefing sessions. Gaining mastery and control over the situation and reactions being encountered are cornerstones to a victim's psychological recovery. The provision of any form of psychological intervention that impedes, or even threatens, the regaining of mastery and control would more than likely be detrimental to recovery.

The ambivalence of trauma victims in seeking help is a factor when providing psychological first aid (Raphael, 1986). This includes survivors of massive road crashes (Schwarz & Kowalski, 1992). Disclosing the trauma experience, even when doing so is perceived as helpful, evokes distress. There is a tendency to avoid becoming distressed – hence the ambivalence of seeking, or participating in, a process that encourages disclosure and being reminded of what occurred. Being in hospital is another factor to consider, as hospitalization can increase feelings of helplessness (Alexander, 1990). A higher degree of helplessness would increase the risk associated with disclosing in a group. Feelings of helplessness are not conducive to participating in a debriefing.

Methodological limitations preclude concluding that intervention for survivors is without benefit. In Brom et al.'s (1993) study the group who received the two to six sessions of psychotherapy had higher levels of intrusion and avoidance phenomena than did the control group (who did not receive any sessions of psychotherapy) prior to treatment. The author's investigations of survivors who received counselling (Watts, 1995a) and that of Hovens & van de Weerd (1998) were not controlled trials. Further, the controlled trial by Hobbs et al. (1996) found post-trauma sequelae had not significantly reduced at four months post crash for either the intervention group ($n = 54$) or the control group ($n = 52$). The natural course of recovery over time following massive trauma can entail persistent and distressing traumatic stress reactions over many years, if not life long (Solomon, 1989; Grace et al., 1993). Persistence of sequelae can be part of the legacy of the trauma itself, rather than indicate the lack of benefit of any particular psychological intervention, or other types of support received.

Shalev (1992) found assessments during the first week after a terrorist attack on a bus in Israel were not predictive of psychological outcome of survivors at 8 to 10 months post trauma. Perhaps any benefits gained by crisis intervention in general during the acute phase post trauma are not measurable over time, just as early reactions do not prescribe what will be experienced over time. Hobbs et al. (1996) concluded from their controlled trial of intervention that psychological follow-up might be more effective when designed to address specific emerging difficulties, rather than a generalized approach for all survivors. The benefits of debriefing and psychological intervention in general for survivors have not been established. There is therefore no guarantee that debriefing will contribute to recovery among survivors of massive road trauma. Further, implementing strategies may not be wanted by the survivors, risk worsening their plight (such as increasing feelings of helplessness, vulnerability and loss of control), and impede recovery.

Emergency workers

There is substantial evidence from the disaster literature that personnel, by becoming involved in what they regard as critical incidents, can become negatively affected. Consequently, effective strategies are required that will prepare them for such involvement, support them during the operation and assist personnel positively in dealing with any negative consequences encountered. Dunning (1988) categorized the range of strategies available to organizations into three types, these being pre-, trans-, and post-disaster stress management. The preinvolvement phase includes education about the typical effects of traumatic events, stress management techniques, and establishing a work cul-

ture where the need for support is not associated with an inability to cope. Strategies during the event that aim to protect and support personnel include establishing demobilization areas, assigning staff to provide support to their colleagues during a prolonged event, and varying deployment to minimize high exposure. Post-disaster strategies include defusing immediately after completion of duty, group and individual debriefings during the first two to three days, plus a range of other follow-up strategies in the short to long term, including family support. There are several types of group debriefings, such as:

1. *Operational debriefings*, which critically examine the response with the aim of improving performance and practices of personnel.
2. *Didactic debriefings*, which aim at informing personnel about psychological and behavioural reactions to the type of event in which they were involved.
3. *Psychological debriefings*, which include information about reactions, but encourage the ventilation of affect and the sharing of experiences among participants.

Critical Incident Stress Debriefing (CISD), as developed by Mitchell (1988), is the most widely used protocol for psychological debriefing. The CISD process has seven phases and aims to mitigate initial distress and promote recovery (Mitchell & Bray, 1990; Hodgkinson & Stewart, 1991; see Mitchell and Everley, Chapter 5). There are other models of psychological debriefing, such as that proposed by Bergman & Queen (1986a,b), where the primary focus is on enhancing coping skills and cognitive restructuring. The term debriefing used in this chapter, unless otherwise specified, refers to the Mitchell model.

All but two of the 30 state emergency service workers and ambulance officers involved in the Queensland coach crash (described previously), who attended a debriefing, reported their attendance as being helpful when interviewed 13 months post crash; 70% reported that the debriefing was very or extremely helpful (Watts, 1995b). This is consistent with the findings of other research (Burns & Hollins, 1991; Hytten & Hasle, 1989; Robinson, 1989; Robinson & Mitchell, 1993). However, the 59% who attended a CISD session following the Queensland coach crash were no differently affected than their colleagues who did not attend a debriefing. Thirty-nine per cent in the Griffiths & Watts (1992) study did not attend a debriefing after the Grafton or Kempsey coach crash but had lower levels of intrusion and avoidance phenomena at 12 months post crash than personnel who attended a debriefing. Further the 32% who attended more than one debriefing had the highest levels of intrusion and avoidance phenomena, significantly greater than the 31% who attended one session (Griffith & Watts, 1992). Other studies have failed to find a quantifiable difference in psychological sequelae among workers who attended a debriefing and those who did not (Hytten & Hastle, 1989; Kenardy et al., 1995).

As a proponent of debriefing and a trainer for over six years I find some difficulty in concluding that attending a debriefing will result in a reduction in the incidence or severity of psychological sequelae sustained when those who attend are assessed as a group. However, debriefings should not be discarded as they are perceived as beneficial by the majority of emergency workers who attend them. They are likely to have benefits other than reducing sequelae and preventing the onset of psychopathology. Perhaps similarly, general stress counselling for policemen, on the basis of this being valued by subjects, argues for it being of potential benefit. This was despite no quantifiable difference in psychological distress and sick leave found among the intervention and nonintervention group in a clinical trial examining the efficacy of brief psychotherapeutic intervention (Doctor et al., 1994). Tunnecliff & Roy (1993) argued that the benefits of debriefing include a reduction of distress, increased clarity and associated understanding of what occurred, realization of normality of reactions, increased knowledge of stress reactions and methods of coping, and the establishment of a self-support mechanism among those involved.

These comments reflect the perceived benefits described by emergency workers interviewed in the Queensland, Grafton and Kempsey coach crash studies (Griffiths & Watts, 1992; Watts & Walkden, 1994). Positive features of debriefing described in these studies included the sharing that occurred, the realization that their reactions were normal, not being the only member of the crew affected by the accident, obtaining a broader view of what occurred, gaining an understanding of how other personnel were coping, the common bond that developed, and achieving emotional relief. Research findings indicate that the majority of those who attend will report their attendance as being helpful (Griffiths & Watts, 1992; Robinson & Mitchell, 1993).

However, not all personnel report attending a debriefing as helpful; some will probably find attendance elevates their distress. In the Grafton and Kempsey study, 24% of emergency workers reported that attending a debriefing was not helpful, 31% reported that it was somewhat helpful, with 45% reporting that it was very or extremely helpful (Griffiths & Watts, 1992). Aspects of debriefing attendance that have been reported as being disliked, or distressing, include being disturbed by some of their colleagues' descriptions of what occurred, not knowing other participants, confused about their own reactions, the attendance of senior personnel, feeling pressured to have a particular reaction, and the group being too large and impersonal. Coping processes vary, as do defensive methods. A worker needing to avoid reminders of what occurred as part of his or her cognitive processing is unlikely to be assisted by being involved in a debriefing that actively encourages the opposite. In such cases attendance could compound reactions and/or jeopardize recovery. McFarlane (1988) examined the pattern of occurrence of psychiatric disorder (acute, chronic and delayed) among a cohort of firefighters with the factors of debriefing attendance and use of support from colleagues. The acute disorder group avoided debriefings and shunned the support of colleagues and, it appears, recovered after the acute episode.

A common concern among paid emergency workers, such as ambulance officers and police (state emergency service workers and some rural firefighters are volunteers in Australia) in the Grafton and Kempsey study was the potential negative consequences if they were perceived as not coping well with what occurred (Griffiths & Watts, 1992). Concerns were primarily about reduced promotional opportunities or not being assigned difficult but challenging tasks and responsibilities. These concerns were despite assurances of confidentiality given by the debriefers and at times related to whether or not senior personnel were among the participants. Notwithstanding some negative perceptions of attending debriefings, many emergency workers interviewed recommended additional sessions, opportunity to have one-to-one assistance, help for their partners/families, and routine assessments three or six months after major events (Griffiths & Watts, 1992).

What interventions to provide and to whom

Focussing on follow-up, thus not including pre- and trans-disaster phases of strategies, the following is offered as an outline of what to consider after massive road trauma. The specific strategies are best decided upon after assessing the situation, rather than prescribing a set response. Groups who would potentially benefit from intervention after massive road trauma include survivors, bereaved, personnel, and any identifiable local community in which the crash occurred. Actual strategies to consider include the following.

1. Survivors

Survivors of massive road trauma are likely to have sustained serious injury, will have witnessed the death of fellow passengers, who could include family members or close others, and narrowly escaped death. Individually based crisis intervention for this group would be the primary focus, where psychological assistance is practically oriented and supportive in nature. Placing injured survivors admitted to hospital in the same or nearby wards would assist them having the opportunity to informally support one another. Under certain conditions a group debriefing would be appropriate, taking a didactic rather than a psychological approach. When an established group is involved in a severe trauma, such as a massive road crash, those who survive will be faced with individual, family and group issues. Examples of common group issues include new arrangements for any immediate commitments or involvements, funerals to organize and attend if a member or members were killed, the practicalities about how the group can support its members in the days and weeks ahead, and the post-trauma affects as they ripple through the membership over time (Bartone & Wright, 1990; Watts & Wilson, 1998). The group is a community that will have traumatic stress reactions, something that individually based crisis intervention can help with only indirectly.

A number of group, family and individually based strategies were used following the 1988 Swedish school bus multifatality, for example, but none included a CISD type of debriefing (Winje & Ulvik, 1995). This massive crash killed 12 children and 4 parents. Initially the relatives of the children killed felt numb and unable to do much, but they did want to know details about the injuries of their respective child and the manner in which they had died quite early post crash (Winje & Ulvik, 1995). Assigning a support worker per family, helping families attend to the necessary practical details during the first week and a half post crash, supporting them in viewing the deceased, and providing detailed information about the accident site rescue work that occurred, as well as typical trauma reactions that can occur, were among the response strategies that were implemented. Organizing relatives as a group facilitated the provision of practical support and helped them to support one another (Wijne & Ulvik, 1995).

A different approach was taken by the coordinated crisis intervention that occurred after a school bus carrying seventh graders in Israel, the first of a convoy of four, collided with a train (Klingman, 1987). Twenty-two were killed (19 children, 1 parent, 1 teacher and the driver), 15 were critically injured. Group sessions of varying types were used. For example, on the third day small group meetings were held for teachers during which they were encouraged to 'air their feelings and share with one another the full range of their emotions' (Klingman, 1987, p.610). Further, a psychologist and school counsellor attempted to encourage ventilation of feelings among the children in the three buses in the convoy, other than the one hit by the train, as they returned to the school. These children were direct victims, having witnessed the trauma, as well as being among the bereaved. They had the multiplicity of traumatic loss and the trauma itself – reinforcing their high risk.

One of the difficulties in providing follow-up to survivors is how best to nonintrusively yet pro-actively provide a safety net of care. The complexity of this increases when the survivors are not members of the immediate community; thus the first hospital to which they are admitted will only see the beginning of their treatment and post-trauma psychological care. The more critically injured may even be air-lifted from the scene to a tertiary hospital at some distance from where the crash has occurred, increasing the logistic difficulties in spanning geographical areas, where even the health delivery systems and associated regulations may differ. Owing to the high risk of sustaining psychological harm, such as PTSD or other pathologies, a routine systematic review of each survivor involved in a massive road trauma is recommended.

2. Bereaved

Crisis intervention for the bereaved and then bereavement counselling when appropriate are the two approaches recommended. What typically occurs now is that the bereaved are supported by health service staff, such as counsellors, social workers, psychologists, or support workers attached to metropolitan forensic departments. The families of those killed in massive road crashes are at high risk and are at times considered as a suitable group that would benefit from debriefing. The intensity of traumatic loss reactions, the nature of grief and mourning, the vulnerability of those suffering the anguish of having a loved one killed in what can be horrific circumstances are reasons why debriefing for the bereaved following massive road trauma is not advised. Risks of doing so include provoking too many memories of what occurred, too much distress to successfully integrate within a group, particularly if participants are encouraged to express their feelings. Convening a group to disseminate and discuss pertinent information and ensuring that the bereaved have the means of supporting one another, if they so choose, would be useful to consider under some circumstances. The time course of reactions to loss also dictate the need for focussed counselling in the early weeks and months for those at high risk.

3. Personnel

One of the difficulties in the follow-up provided to personnel involved in the Kempsey and Grafton coach

crashes was that the ambulance, fire, police, state emergency and health services all arranged their own procedures, with no coordinated overall approach. Some of the debriefings were available to all personnel, but attendance was determined entirely by the workers themselves. As these crashes both occurred in the midst of rural communities it was possible that partners could belong to different services and many knew one another across service boundaries. There was no mechanism to identify those who were repeatedly seeking help by attending a number of different debriefings, for example. This group had significantly higher intrusion and avoidance phenomena than those who attended one debriefing and those who attended none, thus its members were possibly at greater risk (Griffiths & Watts, 1992).

Coordinating psychological intervention across the services involved in a particular massive road trauma is the preferred approach, particularly when the event occurs in rural communities. This will have the added advantage of sharing resources when possible and so gaining efficiencies, in addition to potentially being of greater benefit. A number of personnel interviewed in the Grafton and Kempsey coach crash study suggested that individual counselling and further follow-up would have been beneficial, such as a review at three or six months post crash (Griffiths & Watts, 1992). Several texts on disaster response (such as that by Hodgkinson & Stewart, 1991) describe general principles and procedures to follow, but components that particularly relate to massive road trauma include:

1. Defusing at the completion of duties.
2. Psychological debriefing 2-4 days post-crash.
3. Individual counselling and family support.
4. Possibility of a therapy group being formed.
5. Review of highly exposed personnel at three to four months post-crash.
6. Review in group format at 12 months post crash.

4. Community members

As previously described rural communities will be affected when a massive road trauma occurs within its midst, more so if passengers were community members. There is some evidence to suggest that engaging members of the community in any intervention will be difficult (Lindy et al., 1981). Other communities, such as schools, businesses, social organizations, can be affected when members are involved in major trauma. An underlying principle is to assist the community affected re-establish function and structured daily activities as quickly as possible. The nature of the community is a major factor when deciding which strategy or strategies to use and how.

When communities are likely to be negatively affected by a massive road crash, intervention during the immediate aftermath is advised. Strategies to consider include:

1. Establishing a 'community map', which lists structure and subgroups according to victim classification guidelines.
2. Convening a community meeting.
3. Publication of signs of distress and stress management suggestions.
4. Publicity about a help line that can be contacted or establishing one for the first month if one does not exist.
5. Identifying any high risk subgroups and convening a didactic debriefing.
6. For small communities in particular (e.g. schools), several meetings may be required during the first weeks as a means of communication and support.
7. Incorporating access to individual counselling and support.

Psychological debriefing for survivors

The increasing use of debriefing for people other than emergency services personnel after disasters in general, or large-scale events, warrants some specific comments about the use of this intervention strategy. While the lack of documented benefits should be acknowledged, there is a place for a type of debriefing for survivors on some occasions. Group intervention can be more effective than individually based assistance in:

1. ensuring that all group members have the same information;
2. clarifying how best to support one another;
3. assisting the development of confidence in planning

for any likely difficulties ahead in relation to group dynamics, commitments and general functioning (of the group); and
4. providing the opportunity for survivors to piece together what occurred in a mutually supportive and understanding context.

Many survivors of massive road trauma, but not all, will want to know what happened, what caused, or contributed to the crash (if known at an early stage), and details about the consequences, including learning who was killed and being kept informed of progress of other injured members. Individually based crisis intervention can meet these needs, but survivors collaboratively establishing an account of what occurred enhances their capacity to support one another and minimizes the likelihood of any particular member feeling isolated and alone.

The timing of when and the how this type of group-based intervention occurs is crucial, with some survivors likely never to want to learn any more than what they can recall. Some will want to avoid being distressed by hearing other survivors' accounts, or prefer not to learn of further details due to the anguish they fear such knowledge will cause. This avoidance is an integral and common feature of trauma response (Horowitz et al., 1979). Overexposure to the details of what occurred, or distress being exacerbated by witnessing the upset of others is a risk of group-based crisis intervention for survivors of major road trauma, if not all primary victims. If these risks are minimized by the way group interventions are organized and conducted, the survivors report (from my experience) benefiting from compiling a collective account of what occurred.

On the basis of these possible benefits I recommend an adaptation to the seven-phase debriefing process. This approach would warrant consideration only when: (a) survivors were part of a group pre crash; (b) the group dynamics were perceived by members as supportive and positive; and (c) there were sufficient levels of trust and friendship. Considerable caution in conducting a debriefing is required when a group member or members were killed in the crash, and debriefing of this type may be ill advised if members were not of an appropriate age (less than 15 or 16 years).

The aim of this adapted debriefing is to ensure that individual survivors have the information about their circumstances that they require and for the group to address constructively any immediate issues that it faces. Encouraging expression of reactions is ill advised in debriefings of this type, as the intensity of affect is too great, particularly when there has been traumatic loss. Additional group sessions to the initial adapted debriefing may be necessary to continue supporting the members and facilitating the process of group recovery. These subsequent sessions become group work in orientation, rather than debriefing as a crisis intervention strategy. They are specifically designed to cater for the unique dynamics and situation of each particular group. How best to establish a supportive process that helps traumatized groups, including conducting these ongoing groups is beyond the scope of this chapter.

The adapted debriefing would be held within the first week post trauma, but not necessarily within the 24–72-hour time frame advised for CISDs (Mitchell & Bray, 1990). People directly involved, or primary victims, may require more time to begin to regain control of their own personal circumstance before feeling able to participate in a group. Conversely, speaking with other survivors about what occurred may be warranted shortly after the crash. Forming subgroups rather than a single group of all survivors able to attend may also be a viable option. Each group is different, just as each massive road trauma is different – although there are similarities. Part of the initial assessment of the post-crash situation is to ascertain the needs of individual survivors, the needs of the group, and the most suited strategies. It cannot be assumed that a particular crisis intervention strategy, including debriefing, will apply to all situations. Strategies must be selected on the basis of identified need and requirements, rather than applying a set formula of response on the basis of the type of trauma that occurred.

It should be noted that groups such as these frequently develop spontaneously after a disaster, and should be supported to achieve similar ends if this is appropriate.

Best practice guidelines for conducting these adapted debriefings are required but have yet to be developed. In their absence the following structure is offered for consideration:

1. Generally, a debriefing for survivors of massive road trauma goes for at most 60 to 90 minutes and is led by two, if not three, health professionals, depending on the size of the group. These health professionals are experienced in both debriefing and group work.

2. Members of the group are encouraged to attend, with one of the debriefers making a commitment to report back, within the constraints of confidentiality, to the surviving members who preferred not to be involved.

3. The introduction is brief, the focus being on ensuring that the aim of the debriefing is understood, confidentiality is agreed to, and that everyone is comfortable (e.g. some of the injured present may be in pain).

4. The second phase of the debriefing is about establishing what occurred. Building a collaborative account can be achieved in several ways, such as: requiring everyone to describe what happened to them; asking for contributions to establish the sequence of events, with no expectation that all will contribute; or asking one person to provide the core account, one that is subsequently added to when he or she has finished.

5. Establishing the condition/health status of injured group members not present at the debriefing is part of the second phase, or if not introduced by a member of the group at this time, is posed as a question by one of the debriefers in the final phase. Not always but usually the group initiates listing the names of those killed in the crash. Alternatively, they are listed when funeral arrangements, including whether to attend or not, are discussed later in the debriefing.

6. The debriefers acknowledging the magnitude of what has occurred and describing some of the likely post-trauma effects is the next stage of this adapted debriefing. Information is not detailed. A summary of likely effects can reassure the normality of what survivors may encounter. Prescribing what survivors, or an individual survivor will experience is to be avoided. This stage is similar to the symptom phase

and incorporates the educative phase of a CISD procedure, except that it does not call upon survivors to describe their symptomatology and rather identifies responses as part of a normal positive process in such circumstances.

7. The last stage encompasses issues about 're-entry', and is similar to the last phase of CISD. The focus of this final stage is in identifying how the group can support itself and individual members and how best to address identified issues.

Issues that are usually pertinent to a group of survivors following massive road crashes include: funerals, if a member or members have been killed in the crash; what to say to the family members of those killed, or families of fellow survivors; how to continue the activities of the group, at least to some extent during the immediate aftermath of the crash; how best to support those seriously injured and disabled, or those who may still be critically ill; who is going to attend to any pressing important commitments and responsibilities and how. Information about police and coronial enquiries is useful, if not during this debriefing then soon after, as is information about the relevant legal and compensation system. The timing of giving this information, by whom, and the detail required are among the issues of crisis intervention that are best resolved as the response evolves, corresponding at all times to the assessments of the needs and state of those who are attempting to recover.

Psychological debriefing for personnel

The seeming reliance upon debriefing to assist personnel after disasters also requires further comment in relation to uncertainties about the efficacy of such an approach. It is evident from available evidence about the effects of massive road trauma, such as multifatality bus crashes, that a proportion of emergency workers involved will sustain persistent psychological sequelae, and debriefing will be perceived by some as not helpful, disturbing, or both. The majority who attend will likely report being helped by attending. No evidence, apart from self-reporting of perceived helpfulness, has indicated that debriefings reduce the prevalence, fre-

quency of occurrence, or duration of psychological sequelae. However, emergency workers now expect debriefings to occur and regard them as a means by which organizations, or employers, express support to staff. The lack of demonstrated benefit highlights the necessity of not relying upon them to ensure recovery post trauma. One danger of its popularity is that conducting of a debriefing will be regarded as sufficient after major trauma. Clearly it is not.

The following safeguards are suggested worthy of consideration when one is arranging debriefings for emergency workers involved in massive road trauma to reduce the risk that attendance will cause harm and increase the chance that it may be beneficial. These safeguards include:

Ensuring attendance is voluntary, never mandatory.

Taking added precautions when participants include both junior and senior members of the organization.

Checking whether there are organizational matters that are likely to impact negatively on the debriefing, such as conflict, structural changes and lack of trust.

Clarifying how those assessed by the debriefer(s) as not managing well, or of being at some risk of not doing so, can be identified and appropriately followed up without breaching confidentiality.

Altering the relative focus of each of the stages of the debriefing depending on the specifics of what occurred and the circumstances of those who are attending, particularly when there has been traumatic loss.

Arranging the availability of assistance over time when warranted (after major events).

Debriefings and other crisis intervention strategies are provided generally after massive road trauma for emergency workers. The persistence of clinically significant sequelae to such disasters highlight the importance of assistance being available beyond the first few weeks, or even first months post crash. Some workers will require support over a lengthy period of time; a small number will probably not fully recover or regain their preinvolvement psychological status (Watts & Walkden, 1994). Debriefing is not suited to all emergency workers; some will prefer individually based assistance. Debriefing cannot be relied upon to achieve its aims, those of mitigating initial distress and promoting recovery. The range and complexity of post-trauma sequelae should be sufficient indication not to expect one strategy to help all emergency workers who are involved and/or affected. Caution as to any potential to cause harm should also be borne in mind and closely monitored.

Summary and conclusions

Massive road trauma is on the higher end of severity of traumatic accidents, owing to the degree of exposure to death, destruction, injury and human suffering. Those affected, such as survivors, bereaved, emergency personnel and members of communities in which the events occur, are at considerable risk of sustaining moderate to severe and persistent sequelae. The severity and prevalence of these negative psychological effects demand strategies of response that effectively promote recovery, including prevention of the development of pathology and secondary difficulties.

Research findings have not thus far demonstrated that psychological interventions make any quantifiable difference to recovery. They are likely, however, to be perceived as helpful. One-to-one crisis intervention should be the primary strategy for survivors and bereaved. There are advantages of group-based intervention for some victim groups in certain circumstances. The necessity of being cautious when deciding to conduct a debriefing and what format it should take cannot be overemphasized. Unless indicated by assessments at the time, debriefing that encourages the ventilation of feelings has no place in the immediate response for survivors or bereaved. There are risks of compounding distress and interfering with recovery in conducting debriefing for these groups. The conditions under which group debriefing is used and suggested protocols to follow for survivors have been described in this chapter. Strategies of response for personnel and community members have also been outlined, and key issues about psychological debriefing discussed.   The popularity of debriefing and generally perceived benefit among emergency services

personnel warrants it remaining an integral part of the response strategy, following massive road crashes. However, attending a debriefing cannot be relied upon to help personnel to recover. Individually based intervention and assistance over time needs to be part of the agreed-upon procedures after such events, with attendance voluntary, not mandatory, for personnel. Further research is required to identify more clearly when debriefing is helpful and under what conditions. Until this has occurred, debriefing cannot be claimed to be evidence-based practice and if automatically applied to all individuals affected by massive road trauma it is likely to cause them undue distress and possibly compromise recovery.

REFERENCES

Alexander, D. A. (1990). Psychological intervention for victims and helpers after disasters. *British Journal of General Practice*, **40**, 345–8.

Bartone, P. T. & Wright, K. M. (1990). Grief and good recovery following a military air disaster. *Journal of Traumatic Stress*, **3**, 523–39.

Bergman, L. H., & Queen, T. (1986a). Critical incident stress. Part 1. *Fire Command*, May, 52–6.

Bergman, L. H. & Queen, T. (1986b). Critical incident stress: Part 2. *Fire Command*, June, 43–9.

Brom, D., Kleber, R. J. & Hofman, M. (1993). Victims of traffic accidents: incidence and prevention of post-traumatic stress disorder. *Journal of Clinical Psychology*, **49**, 131–40.

Burges Watson, P. (1987). Post-traumatic stress disorder in Australia and New Zealand: a clinical review of the consequences of inescapable horror. *Medical Journal of Australia*, **147**, 443–7.

Burns, T. P. & Hollins, S. C. (1991). Psychiatric response to the Clapham rail crash. *Journal of the Royal Society of Medicine*, **84**, 15–19.

Doctor, R. S., Curtis, D. & Isaacs, G. (1994). Psychiatric morbidity in policemen and the effect of brief psychotherapeutic intervention – a pilot study. *Stress Medicine*, **10**, 151–7.

Dunning, C. (1988). Intervention strategies for emergency workers. In M. Lystad (Ed.) *Mental Health Response to Mass Emergencies* (pp. 284–310). New York: Brunner/Mazel.

Goldberg, L. & Gara, M. (1990). A typology of psychiatric reactions to motor vehicle accidents. *Psychopathology*, **23**, 15–20.

Grace, M., Green, B., Lindy, J. H. & Leonard A. (1993). The

Buffalo Creek disaster: A 14-year follow-up. In J. P. Wilson & B. Raphael (Eds.) *The International Handbook of Traumatic Stress Syndromes* (pp. 441–9). New York: Plenum Press.

Green, M., McFarlane, C. A., Hunter, C. & Griggs, W. (1993). Undiagnosed post-traumatic stress disorder following motor vehicle accidents. *Medical Journal of Australia*, **159**, 529–34.

Griffiths, J. A. & Watts, R. (1992). *The Kempsey and Grafton Bus Crashes: The Aftermath*. Lismore, New South Wales: Instructional Design Solutions, UNE.

Hobbs, M., Mayou, R., Harrison, B. & Worlock, P. (1996). A randomised controlled trial of psychological debriefing for victims of road traffic accidents. *British Medical Journal*, **313**, 1438–9.

Hodgkinson, P. & Stewart, M. (1991). *Coping with Catastrophe: A Handbook of Disaster Management*. London: Routledge.

Horowitz, M., Wilner, N. & Alvarez, W. (1979). Impact of event scale: a measure of subjective stress. *Psychosomatic Medicine*, **41**, 209–18.

Horowitz, M., Wilner, N., Kaltreider, N. & Alvarez, W. (1980). Signs and symptoms of posttraumatic stress disorder. *Archives of General Psychiatry*, **37**, 85–92.

Hovens, J. E. & van de Weerd, M. (1998). Posttraumatic stress disorder in debriefed survivors of a bus accident. *Psychological Reports*, **82**, 1075–81.

Hytten, K. & Hasle, A. (1989). Fire fighters: a study of stress and coping. *Acta Psychiatrica Scandinavica*, **80**, Suppl. 355, 50–5.

Jones, D. R. (1985). Secondary disaster victims: the emotional effects of recovery and identifying human remains. *American Journal of Psychiatry*, **142**, 303–7.

Kenardy, J. A., Webster, R. A., Lewin, T. J., Carr, V. J., Hazell, P. L. & Carter, G. L. (1995). Stress debriefing and patterns of recovery following a natural disaster. *Journal of Traumatic Stress*, **9**, 37–49.

Klingman, A. (1987). A school-based emergency crisis intervention in a mass school disaster. *Professional Psychology – Research and Practice*, **18**, 604–12.

Kuch, K., Swinson, R. P. & Kirby, M. (1985). Post-traumatic stress disorder after car accidents. *Canadian Journal of Psychiatry*, **30**, 426–7.

Lehman, D. R. & Wortman, C. B. (1987). Long-term effects of losing a spouse or child in a motor vehicle crash. *Journal of Personality and Social Psychology*, **52**, 218–31.

Lindy, J. D., Grace, M. & Green, B. L. (1981). Survivors: outreach to a reluctant population. *American Journal Orthopsychiatry*, **51**, 468–78.

Lundin, T. (1984). Morbidity following sudden and unexpected bereavement. *British Journal Psychiatry*, **144**, 84–8.

Malt, U. F. (1988). The long-term psychiatric consequences of accidental injury – a longitudinal study of 107 adults. *British Journal of Psychiatry*, **153**, 810–18.

Mayou, R., Bryant, B., & Duthie, R. (1993). Psychiatric consequences of road traffic accidents. *British Medical Journal*, **307**, 647–51.

McFarlane, A. C. (1988). The longitudinal course of posttraumatic morbidity: the range of outcomes and their predictors. *Journal of Nervous and Mental Disease*, **176**, 30–40.

McFarlane, A. C. (1989). The aetiology of post-traumatic morbidity: predisposing, precipitating and perpetuating factors. *British Journal of Psychiatry*, **154**, 221–8.

Mitchell, J. (1988). Development and functions of a critical incident stress debriefing team. *Journal of Emergency Medical Services*, **12**, 43–6.

Mitchell, J. & Bray, G. (1990). *Emergency Services Stress*. Englewood Cliffs, NJ: Prentice-Hall.

Parkes, C. M. & Weiss, R. S. (1983). *Recovery from Bereavement*. New York: Basic Books.

Raphael, B. (1986). *When Disaster Strikes: How Individuals and Communities Cope with Catastrophe*. New York: Basic Books.

Robinson, R. (1989). Critical incident stress and psychological debriefing in emergency services. *Social Biology Resources Centre Review*, **3**, 1–4.

Robinson, C. & Mitchell, J. T. (1993). Evaluation of psychological debriefings. *Journal of Traumatic Stress*, **6**, 367–82.

Sanders, C. M. (1988). Risk factors in bereavement outcome. *Journal of Social Issues*, **44**, 97–111.

Schwarz, E. D. & Kowalski, J. M. (1992). Malignant memories: reluctance to utilise mental health services after a disaster. *Journal of Nervous and Mental Disease*, **180**, 767–72.

Shalev, A. Y. (1992). Posttraumatic stress disorder among injured survivors of a terrorist attack. *Journal of Nervous and Mental Disease*, **180**, 505–9.

Solomon, Z. (1989). A three-year prospective study of PTSD in Israeli combat veterans. *Journal of Traumatic Stress*, **2**, 59–73.

Taylor, A. J. & Frazer, A. G. (1981). *Psychological Sequelae of Operation Overdue following the DC-10 Air Crash in Antarctica*. Victoria University of Wellington Publications in Psychology, no. 27. Wellington: Victoria University.

Taylor, A. J. & Frazer, A. G. (1982). The stress of post-disaster body handling and victim identification work. *Journal of Human Stress*, **8**, 4–12.

Tunnecliffe, M. & Roy, O. (1993). *Emergency Support: A Handbook for Peer Supporters*. Palmyra, Western Australia: Bayside Books.

Ursano, R. J. & McCarroll, J. E. (1990). The nature of a traumatic stressor: handling dead bodies. *Journal of Nervous and Mental Disease*, **178**, 390–1.

Watts R. (1995a). Posttraumatic stress disorder after a bus

accident. *Australia and New Zealand Journal of Psychiatry*, **29**, 75–83.

Watts, R. (1995b). The reactions and follow-up after large-scale road accidents. PhD thesis, University of Queensland, Brisbane.

Watts, R. & Walkden, R. (1994). Trauma: the initial impact and consequences for rescue personnel. *Journal of Mental Health*, **3**, 123–9.

Watts, R. & Wilson, M. (1998). The Kempsey Bus disaster: the effects on Australian community rescuers. In E. Zinner & M. Williams (Eds.) *When a Community Weeps: Case Studies in Group Survivorship*. New York: Taylor & Francis Publishers.

Watts, R., Horne, D., Sandells, J. & Petrie, M. (1996). The need for acute hospitals to provide counselling following motor vehicle accidents. *Australian Health Review*, **19**(3), 93–103.

Winje, D. (1996). Long-term outcome of trauma in adults: the psychological impact of a fatal bus accident. *Journal of Consulting and Clinical Psychology*, **64**, 1037–43.

Winje, D. & Ulvik, A. (1995). Confrontations with reality: crisis intervention services for traumatised families after a school accident in Norway. *Journal of Traumatic Stress*, **8**, 429–44.

10

Debriefing and motor vehicle accidents: interventions and outcomes

Michael Hobbs and Richard Mayou

EDITORIAL COMMENTS

This carefully focussed review of psychological traumatization after motor vehicle accidents shows that such consequences are not uncommon. Hobbs and Mayou review those studies that have provided any sort of intervention of the debriefing kind after motor vehicle accidents, considering five studies including one of their own.

None of these studies showed benefits for a brief one-off intervention. Their own careful and manualized, controlled trial of a debriefing intervention showed that there might well be an increase in psychological symptoms in the group who received intervention. The authors hypothesize that it may be that early psychological/debriefing interventions interfere with the progressive and titrated processing of the experience. Or they may reinforce dissociation by exposure/re-exposure to the trauma. The authors conclude by concurring with Ørner's finding that debriefing should not be routinely applied after critical incidents of this kind in view of the lack of scientific evidence regarding its effectiveness.

It may indeed be that a single, active, debriefing session re-exposes without a real opportunity for cognitive processing of the experience. Immediate emotional support, information and practical help, with perhaps later individual crisis intervention are seen as appropriate, as is cognitive behaviour therapy.

These findings are clearly similar to the large-scale studies of Watts (Chapter 9), particularly with respect to his findings concerning survivors. They constitute a further cause for concern about the widespread use of psychological debriefing techniques in such settings, particularly as they may be seen to obviate the need for appropriate follow-up interventions more tailored to individual need for those who are at risk of post-trauma morbidity.

Introduction

Motor vehicle accidents (MVA) are common and a major cause of physical injury, permanent disability and death. Only in the last few years, however, has attention been given to the widespread adverse psychological consequences of road accidents.

Epidemiological data confirms that MVAs are more common than is generally appreciated. From a community survey in the USA, Norris (1992) demonstrated that the annual risk of being involved in a road accident sufficiently serious to cause injury or death to one or more persons is 2.6%, and the lifetime risk is 23.4%. Her demonstration of an associated high incidence (12%) of post traumatic stress disorder (PTSD) in the survivors of serious road accidents led Norris to conclude that MVAs are 'perhaps the single most traumatic event' to which humans are exposed.

From data collected by the WHO, Murray & Lopez (1997) established that road accidents were the ninth commonest cause of death in 1990, accounting for 990 000 deaths worldwide. Within the countries of the European Union (EU), it has been estimated that 50 000 people die and 1.5 million are injured each year; this death toll was equated by the Director General of the EU's Transport Division to the loss, without survivors, of one full jumbo jet every 70 hours (Gloag, 1993).

Table 10.1. Psychiatric disorders following road accident injury

- Cognitive disorders: delirium, dementia, organic personality disorder, focal syndrome, post-concussional syndrome
- Acute stress disorder
- Emotional distress: anxiety, depression
- Post-traumatic syndromes: post-traumatic stress disorder, phobic travel anxiety
- Alcohol and substance abuse

Although technological advances in vehicle and road engineering have led to recent modest reductions in fatalities from road accidents in some countries, these have not been achieved worldwide and lag behind reductions in other causes of death. Consequently it is predicted that, by the year 2000, road accidents will be the sixth most common cause of death (Editorial, 1997).

Shocking though these statistics are, they give no indication of the psychological and social impact of MVAs on those who survive them, and on those who witness them, who are bereaved by them, or whose jobs involve responding to them. Surprisingly, it is only recently that the psychiatric effects of road accidents have been studied systematically (Mayou, 1992). It is recognized (Di Gallo & Parry-Jones, 1996; Schnyder & Buddeberg, 1996) that there is an unequivocal need for more research into the psychiatric effects of road accidents, and how best to manage them.

This chapter summarizes the available data about the psychiatric impact of MVAs, examines the aetiology of these effects, reports on the few studies of debriefing interventions designed to "prevent" the adverse effects, and explores further the question about how these may be limited or treated.

Pre-accident psychiatric problems

Psychiatric disorders and their treatment predispose to trauma (McDonald & Davey, 1996), and, in particular, problem drinking and other substance abuse (Cherpitel, 1993). Other causes include dementia, schizophrenia, affective disorder, prescribed psychotropic drugs, suicidal and risk-taking behaviour, sleep disorders and the whole range of personality and behavioural factors included in accident neurosis. Such long-standing problems increase vulnerability to the

whole range of post-traumatic complications described below. They may well require treatment in their own right. Where previously recognized, this treatment should be by those already involved in care. However, it is not uncommon for chronic psychological problems to be diagnosed after an accident and in such cases psychiatric referral may be required.

Psychiatric consequences of motor vehicle accidents

The psychiatric consequences of MVAs (see Table 10.1) are in many ways similar to those described for acute illnesses and events but, in addition, a small proportion of victims suffer cognitive and other disorders due to head injury and brain damage and many suffer from post-traumatic syndromes. A tendency in the literature and also in clinical practice to focus discussion of assessment and services on PTSD should not obscure the clinical significance of a wider range of consequences and also the importance of subthreshold distress.

Until recently, there have been few systematic reports of the psychiatric consequences of motor vehicle accidents but there have now been a number of reviews (Blanchard et al., 1995a; Taylor & Koch, 1995; Blanchard & Hickling, 1997; Mayou, 1997) and prospective studies, several of which relate to representative samples of hospital attenders (Yule & Carr, 1987; Rothbaum et al., 1992; Murray, 1997; Ehlers et al., 1998). Evidence that psychiatric consequences are considerable in uninjured hospital attenders indicates that there may be substantial psychiatric morbidity amongst people who have not sought medical care for physical injuries.

A recent large study of consecutive emergency department attenders (Ehlers et al., 1998) has shown that, although more than half of MVA victims have a good psychological outcome, a large minority suffer from psychiatric consequences. Overlap and comorbidity of the three main types of psychiatric consequence are common but there is a considerable variety of patterns. Psychological consequences were not related to the type of accident – motor vehicle, motor cycle, pedal cycle and pedestrian – and were generally not related to the type or severity of the injuries or to admission to hospital. Patients with minor injuries, or indeed no injuries, were just as likely to suffer post-traumatic symptoms and disorders as those with severe injuries.

Acute responses

Psychological studies show that dissociation is an important and conspicuous component of acute reaction to trauma. Dissociation is not a unitary or well-defined concept, having complex historical origins. It would seem that it has several components and that the most widely used measures cover rather different aspects of the whole overall concept. Trait and state dissociation predict the development and maintenance of post-traumatic symptoms as do phenomena associated with dissociation, such as evidence of fragmented memories of the event (Murray, 1997).

Atchison & McFarlane (1997) suggested that it is possible to identify five patterns of immediate response:

  absence of distress,
  good recall of the accident,
  hyperamnesia (vivid memories without affective disturbance),
  intense intrusive thoughts, mild anxiety,
  overt distress with many intrusions and avoidance.

Acute stress disorder

Despite the general lay acceptance that emotional shock is a common and entirely appropriate response to a frightening accident, the acute impact of MVAs has received little research attention. However, syndromes of acute stress disorder (ASD) introduced in *The Diagnostic and Statistical Manual of Mental Disorders* IV (DSM-IV; American Psychiatric association, 1994) and

International Classification of Diseases (ICD) 10 and derived from experience relating to other types of trauma appear to be common in many MVA victims. There is an important difficulty in diagnosis in that the ICD and DSM classifications are quite different, the former relating to a much briefer period after the trauma. Most published evidence relates to the DSM formulation, which derives from criteria for PTSD but with a greater emphasis on dissociation (Bryant & Harvey, 1997).

Estimates of ASD following MVAs indicate that it is common. Harvey & Bryant (1998) report 13% ($n = 92$). Murray (1997) found it to be 28.5% ($n = 117$) immediately after the accident and 10.3% at four weeks, with 33.5% satisfying criteria at some time during the first four weeks. The main distinction from the symptom patterns in PTSD appeared to be the higher levels of dissociation in ASD. Beyond the initial week, ASD was predicted by high trait dissociation. There is a strong correlation with later PTSD. Murray (1997) found that 45% of those who had suffered ASD had PTSD at 24 weeks. However 15% of those without ASD also had PTSD at 24 weeks. Acute problems are not a good clinical indicator of later outcome.

Anxiety and depression

The course, determinants and characteristics of anxiety and depression are similar for all types of trauma. All cause acute emotional distress in a high proportion of subjects and up to a quarter may describe persistent mood and anxiety disorders. Continuing psychiatric complications are likely in those who are psychologically vulnerable, in those who have difficult social circumstances and where there is evidence of continuing or relapsing physical problems. We have found emotional disorders to be more common than population expectation throughout the year after being injured in a road accident (Mayou et al., 1993).

Post-traumatic stress disorder

PTSD is very frequent following MVAs (Blanchard et al., 1995a; Ehlers et al., 1998). Prevalence estimates have varied between 1% and 42%, but best estimates using

Table 10.2. Predictors of post-traumatic stress disorder

- Female sex
- Conscious and therefore no amnesia of accident
- Previous emotional problems
- Previous motor vehicle accidents and other major trauma
- Perceived threat of injury or death in the accident
- Dissociation at the time of accident
- Maintaining psychological factors:
    negative interpretation of intrusions
    rumination
    anger
- Other maintaining factors:
    adverse social consequences
    long-term physical problems
    long-term financial problems
    litigation

standard measures suggest that it is something like 20% at three months and 15% at one year (Ehlers et al., 1998). There is marked improvement between three months and one year and it is also evident that there may be new cases later than three months and indeed perhaps up to years after a road accident (Ehlers et al., 1998). A proportion of cases appear to be prolonged (Mayou et al., 1997). In addition, there is considerable subthreshold post-traumatic distress, which fails to meet the diagnostic criteria but may, none the less, be clinically significant.

In the recent large Oxford study (Ehlers et al., 1998), the prevalence of PTSD at three months was 23% and 17% at one year. Those with PTSD at three months had a 50% chance of still suffering from the disorder at one year. Of those who did not have PTSD at three months 6.2% satisfied criteria at one year (Blanchard et al., 1995a,b; Blanchard & Hickling, 1997). The predictors of the onset and early maintenance of PTSD in MVAs (Blanchard et al., 1995a,b; Ehlers et al., 1998) are numerous but they do not include measures of initial injury severity or type of accident (see Table 10.2). It would seem that over a longer period of several years, PTSD is especially common in those in which there are conspicuous reminders of the accident and its consequences, such as continuing physical problems, financial difficulties and litigation (Mayou et al., 1997).

Table 10.3. Effects on travel

Driver
Giving up car or motorcycle
Changes to safer vehicle
More cautious
Phobic travel anxiety
Limitation of extent of travel
Specific anxiety about place of accident and similar situations
Avoidance

Passenger
Avoidance of travel
Phobic anxiety

Travel anxiety

The clinical significance of phobic anxiety about travel has not been recognized until recently (Radanov et al., 1993; Mayou & Bryant, 1994). It was formerly seen as an occasional neurotic and maladaptive response. It is now apparent that many victims behave more cautiously in a generally sensible and appropriate way but that a sizeable minority suffer marked anxiety about travel and also avoidance, which may be limiting (Table 10.3).

Phobic travel anxiety overlaps with PTSD but is probably more common and perhaps more disabling. Around one-fifth of victims describe significant and disabling effects on travel that satisfy diagnostic criteria for phobic anxiety.

Phobic anxiety is usually most severe for forms of travel similar to those of the accident, i.e. those who were passengers are most concerned about being passengers, pedestrians worry about walking on pavements and crossing roads. However, there is marked generalization in many subjects.

Effects of head injury

A small minority of victims suffer severe brain damage with significant neuropsychiatric consequences that may be persistent (Lishman, 1998). A much greater number suffer head injuries that may be associated with mild degrees of cognitive impairment (King, 1997). The course of these disorders remains uncertain.

PTSD is uncommon in those who have been unconscious and have amnesia of the accident. When it does occur, the intrusive memories are related to events following the accident, including those in hospital.

Post-concussional disorder in those suffering head injury has attracted considerable interest. While there has been much dispute about physical as opposed to psychological causes, it seems reasonable to conclude that there is an interaction between the physical and the psychological, and that psychological factors become relatively more important the more persistent the syndrome (Jacobson, 1995; Lishman, 1998).

Road accident victims who have suffered significant head injury appear to be somewhat less likely to suffer specific post-traumatic problems but may well suffer significant psychiatric difficulties associated with brain damage. Specialist assessment and access to neurological rehabilitation are required.

Other psychological consequences

Other conspicuous features in road accident victims are anger about being an innocent victim and suffering physical injury, financial loss, the irritations of litigation and a lack of recognition of their suffering.

A small proportion of patients suffer conspicuous disfigurement or the prospect of long-term arthritis or other complications and these are a source of significant distress and social avoidance.

Alcohol problems appear to continue relatively unchanged after road accidents, and changes to drinking in relation to driving are modest (Mayou & Bryant, 1995). Changes are, in fact, more common in those without drinking problems than in those in whom alcohol may well have contributed to the cause of the accident.

The role of compensation

It has frequently been alleged that compensation is a major determinant of psychological status and disability after road accidents. However, it would seem that this has been an erroneous conclusion based on highly selected clinical experience in assessing those in disputed litigation. Evidence from less selected series and comparison of subjects before and after settlement consistently suggest that outcome for those involved in litigation is generally similar to those who are not seeking compensation. In these series relatively few subjects have seemed to be preoccupied with compensation settlements with any possibility of exaggeration or simulation (Mendelson, 1995; Mayou, 1996; Bryant et al., 1997).

Although the evidence suggests that compensation is not a major factor, it is likely that it is one of a number of social variables that do affect longer-term outcome. It is not unreasonable that financial worry and uncertainty, the frustrating and slow progress of most litigation and the associated anger about the lack of recognition of suffering should have some influence on mental state and social adjustment.

Social consequences

The social consequences of road accident injury can be very considerable and are due not only to the physical injury itself and the disability it causes, to financial problems that may result from increased expenses, inability to work and loss of a vehicle, but also to the occurrence of psychiatric complications. While those with more severe injuries are likely to suffer the greatest social difficulty, even those who do not suffer physical injury may report considerable social problems arising from financial losses and post-traumatic psychiatric complications.

The size and nature of the clinical problem

Published evidence and clinical experience suggest that MVAs cause immediate distress and other psychological consequences for many people. Most of these consequences are transient. In the early months, distress, PTSD and travel anxiety are frequently described but all may improve over a period of months. Even so, a year or more after an accident, psychiatric complications are apparent and associated with substantial disability. These problems are not closely related to any physical injury or to the type of accident (Table 10.4).

Analysis of predictors has suggested that numerous medical, psychological and social variables are

Table 10.4. Long-term outcome

- Anxiety
- Depression
- Persistent travel anxiety
    driver
    passenger
    other travel
- Post-traumatic stress disorder
- Subclinical post-traumatic stress disorder
- Concern re disfigurement
- Concern re future disability
- Dissatisfaction/anger
- Cognitive disorder

statistically significant predictors of later problems. However, many patients with early difficulties rapidly improve and others develop substantial complications only months after the accident. This would suggest that offering immediate psychological, social and practical help after the accident to those who have clear problems and needs, and subsequently concentrating on the early recognition of further problems during convalescence, would be more effective than unproven, routine, early psychological intervention.

Debriefing after MVAs: conceptual basis and rationale

In view of the high incidence of psychiatric problems associated with MVAs, and their substantial cost to society, it is self-evident that strategies that could reduce their psychosocial impact would be widely welcomed and of significant economic benefit.

Psychological models of trauma recognize that the perceived threat challenges, impairs or overwhelms the person's coping resources. As a consequence, the traumatic experience is not fully processed emotionally and cognitively, or thereby integrated into the individual's or family/social group's mental functioning.

Psychological debriefing has been conceptualized as an intervention that promotes adaptive adjustment to traumatic events, in part through facilitating emotional and cognitive processing of the experience. It has been suggested that psychological debriefing can prevent psychiatric problems after traumatic events, although

the aims specified by those who have done most to promulgate the provision of psychological debriefing are more circumspect.

Mitchell & Bray (1990, p. 143), writing about the origins and management of stress in emergency services personnel, specified that the 'two major goals of debriefings are to reduce the impact of a critical event and to accelerate the normal recovery of normal people who are suffering through normal but painful reactions to abnormal events'. Furthermore Critical Incident Stress Debriefing (CISD) developed and described by Mitchell & Bray is a group intervention for teams of emergency services staff for whom the group's cohesion and support is of central importance. They assert that 'debriefings are considered a good *stress* prevention method' (present authors' italics), but do not claim that CISD prevents later psychiatric complications.

Parkinson (1997) makes clear that psychological debriefing 'is not a cure for post-traumatic stress or an injection against the development of post-traumatic stress disorder'. Instead 'it is a method of intervention that attempts to reduce the degree of traumatic reactions... It assumes that after traumatic incidents most people will cope, but that they will recover more quickly if they have a structured procedure to follow which enables them to talk through what has happened and how they have reacted'. Parkinson makes clear, as do other authors, that debriefing is not counselling or therapy but 'a cognitively based model which aims to help those involved to integrate the incident into their experience and into their lives'. Parkinson has adapted the debriefing model for use with individuals, couples and both small and large groups of people, after a wide range of short-lived and prolonged traumatic experiences, including traffic accidents.

Dyregrov (1997, pp. 589–90) identified the aims of psychological debriefing as follows: 'to prevent unnecessary after-effects, accelerate normal recovery, stimulate group cohesion (in work groups or natural groups), normalise reactions, stimulate emotional ventilation, and promote a cognitive "grip" on the situation'. He proposed that more emphasis should be given to the study and use of group processes in debriefing.

Joseph et al. (1997, p. 118) noted that, in common with current treatments for PTSD, psychological debriefing involves re-exposure to the traumatic incident, but debriefing 'is concerned with prevention rather than the amelioration of symptoms'. As they observe, 'many workers in the field of disaster research are agreed that group debriefing sessions are desirable, and that they reduce later morbidity' (Joseph et al., 1997, p. 128). Their own studies of children involved in a maritime disaster confirmed that group meetings were welcomed by survivors, and showed that the children who participated after rescue in group debriefing and subsequent problem-solving sessions were less troubled by intrusive symptomatology than survivors who received no help (Yule, 1992).

A number of authors refer to the value of a crisis intervention approach after traumatic events (Raphael, 1986; Hodgkinson & Stewart, 1991; Joseph et al., 1997), including road accidents (Bordow & Porritt, 1979; Brom et al., 1993; Schnyder, 1997). Crisis intervention (Hobbs, 1984) differs from psychological debriefing, especially Mitchell's CISD (Mitchell & Bray, 1983), in several significant ways. Crisis intervention is undertaken with individuals, families and groups. It requires a detailed initial analysis of the developments that generated the crisis, in order to define the problem to be addressed, but would not usually involve a step-by-step reconstruction of the traumatic event. Catharsis is encouraged, but more emphasis would be given to the mobilization of coping resources in the individual and his or her social network. Like debriefing, crisis intervention would be initiated soon after the traumatic event. Unlike debriefing, where the emphasis is on the initial highly structured session, crisis intervention is less prescriptive and would usually involve several sessions of work over a few days or weeks.

Debriefing aims to encourage "normalization" of the reactions to trauma; that is, for participants to recognize that their reactions are part of a normal and natural psychophysiological response, and to enable them to make sense of and thereby integrate their traumatic experience. Crisis intervention may include this cognitive work, but places emphasis also on the mobilization of social support. This has been shown to contribute to recovery following trauma. Neither debriefing nor crisis intervention is a method of treatment, but a means for promoting adaptation to critical experiences.

Framework for intervention following MVA

The psychological victims of MVAs, in common with many other traumatic events, are widely dispersed. Those who are not injured will leave the site of the accident, possibly in a state of shock, their identities known, if at all, only to the police.

Those who are significantly injured in the accident will be taken to hospital, often (by virtue of where the accident occurred) many kilometres from their home, family and friends. The majority will be discharged from hospital within a day or two, however, reducing the time frame in which interview or intervention may be achieved in this setting. The severely injured may be too ill for early access to be possible, perhaps for weeks after the accident, by which time the traumatic impact of the accident itself has been compounded by successive medical and surgical interventions. In psychological terms, a simple (single-incident, or type 1) trauma may have become a complex (type 2) trauma (Terr, 1991).

MVAs impact on a range of people in addition to those directly involved in the accident. Witnesses to the accident may be traumatized by what they see, including the impact itself, mutilating injury, death and dying. They may be involved in attempts at rescue and resuscitation of the primary victims. Again, they may leave the scene without trace. Relatives and friends of the primary victims may be affected emotionally, especially, but not only, if bereaved. Only the minority of these people will be offered or seek help.

The provision of support or other intervention is more likely after road accidents in which a number of people are killed and injured, as in a coach crash, particularly if the victims are known to each other and are children. Such events usually now attract an organized psychosocial response and media attention. The victims of the everyday small-scale MVA, although perhaps equally traumatized, obtain little support and no public sympathy. Written and oral information about the common psychological consequences of MVAs can be given to patients who are admitted and those who attend hospital follow-up, but it is likely to be more effective to publicize the importance of assessment and treatment to general practitioners and other staff in primary care, and to lawyers and motoring organizations. Better care will depend not only on much greater medical awareness, but also on public awareness that suffering anything more than immediate, moderate distress after a road accident is an appropriate reason for medical consultation. However, active encouragement to seek help would be required for the numerous traumatized MVA victims who display significant degrees of avoidance, specifically avoidance of the distressing recall of their traumatic experience.

Logistically, because of their dispersal, it would be extremely difficult to deliver an early psychological intervention to even the primary victims of road accidents. The population for whom this is most feasible will be those who are hospitalized. They represent a captive audience, although mostly for a short period of only one or two days. For this reason there has been interest in the delivery of an early debriefing session within 24–72 hours of the accident. The authors' study of debriefing for MVA victims, summarized below, aimed to deliver the intervention in this time scale, which is consistent with the recommendations of authorities in the debriefing field (Dyregrov, 1989; Mitchell & Everly, 1995; Parkinson, 1997). For pragmatic reasons, this single session is unlikely to be followed in most areas by further sessions.

The provision of debriefing or other psychological interventions for people in the community would require sophisticated tracing and outreach services, which, in the economic climates prevailing in most countries, are likely to be seen as prohibitively expensive. Outcome and cost-offset studies are needed to establish whether such intervention programmes might prove cheaper than the substantial costs of psychological disability and later treatment.

An additional problem for the delivery of early psychological interventions, even for hospitalized MVA victims, concerns who would provide them. Ideally dedicated staff, trained in the practice of the chosen intervention, would be employed for this work. In practice, even in large acute hospitals, this work would be combined, and therefore would compete, with other responsibilities. Because accidents occur at unpredictable intervals, staff will find it difficult to deliver debriefing within the necessary time scale unless it is accorded the highest priority. Follow-up appointments

at the hospital may prove impossible for the majority of patients, in some cases because of the restricted mobility associated with their injuries.

The last, but probably most important, service issue is what form of intervention should be provided, and for whom. Where debriefing has been available, it has been offered generally to whole populations, without selection. This is the basis on which the few intervention studies to date have been undertaken, including that reported below by the present authors. There is enough evidence for risk factors now, however, to select more specifically those individuals most vulnerable to psychiatric complications. Future research may be able to target those most at risk, but it is not yet clear what intervention should be delivered to them.

Research evidence

Although there have been descriptive accounts of psychological interventions for road accident victims (Horowitz, 1986; Schnyder, 1997), there is relatively little research evidence relevant to debriefing after MVAs. Methodological differences make it difficult to compare the few published studies. Nevertheless some preliminary conclusions may be drawn, and some hypotheses generated for future research.

Analogue studies

Laboratory studies of psychological debriefing would be difficult to envisage or organize. However, analogue studies may help us to understand the effects of the early re-exposure to distressing images of road accidents that is fundamental to psychological debriefing.

Ehlers and Steil (1995) sought evidence for the hypothesis that exposure aids, and avoidance or dissociation obstructs, psychological recovery (assimilation and acceptance) after traumatic experiences. Healthy volunteers were randomized to two groups. In all subjects, intrusive recollections of traumatic scenes were induced experimentally by exposing them to ambulance service video recordings, taken at the scene of road accidents, of severely injured, dying and mutilated dead people. Each subject was asked to maintain a daily diary of intrusive recollections, their quality, the distress generated, and how they coped with them. The video was shown again one week later.

One group of subjects was instructed to do all they could to avoid recollection of the video material (avoidance group). The other was instructed to relive the scenes in their imagination, think and talk about the material (exposure group). Diary measures in the first week showed that the exposure group recorded higher distress in relation to recollections of the accident material. The distress experienced during the second showing of the video was higher for the exposure group. Increase in skin conductance was also higher in the exposure group during subsequent tests in which subjects were asked to imagine the worst scene from the video film.

Ehlers & Steil observed that instruction to expose oneself to, think and talk about traumatic images increases rather than extinguishes distress, and speculate that this may be due to visual rehearsal. They conclude that early re-exposure to traumatic experience may not be the best strategy, and suggest that their results may help to explain the lack of efficacy of debriefing after trauma.

Studies of early psychological intervention

Five published studies of psychological intervention for road accident victims have been identified. Three of these were included in a *Cochrane Review* of debriefing (Wessely et al., 1998).

1. Canberra, Australia

Bordow & Porritt (1979) reported an experimental evaluation of crisis intervention, using subjects who had been injured in road accidents.

Selection

The subjects were 70 of the first 73 males who were hospitalized in the study period following injury in road accidents, and who stayed in hospital for at least one week.

Group allocation

The first 30 patients received no intervention, but were contacted three to four months after injury (delayed contact group, DC). The next 10 patients (immediate review group, IR) were seen once during the first week

after their accident, a structured interview being used to elicit information about accident and hospitalization; but this afforded only minimal emotional, and no social, support. The remaining 30 patients were interviewed similarly, but then offered by one of three social workers a crisis intervention incorporating emotional, practical and social support (full intervention group, FI).

Intervention

The emotional support included exploration of the subject's emotional reactions to the traumatic event, and promotion of constructive, nonblaming, problem-solving behaviours. Social support was fostered by encouraging family and friends to be accepting, and receptive to the patient's concerns. Limited to a maximum of 10 hours, the crisis interventions ranged from 2 to 10 hours in total.

Measures

A range of instruments was used, including measures of psychiatric symptomatology, social and work readjustment, health deterioration, and social support.

Findings

The three study groups displayed similar sociodemographic profiles, except that fewer subjects in the DC group were married; but this was shown not to account for the outcome results. No differences between groups were found for the extent and severity of injuries, and no subjects suffered permanent physical disability. All subjects reported intense emotional reactions to injury and hospitalization, suggesting that the experience represented a crisis for all. The main outcome findings were as follows:

1. The outcome at three to four months post injury was most favourable for the FI group on all but one measure. The only exception was a nonsignificant trend for more DC subjects to have returned to work, and the authors discussed the significance of this finding.
2. The outcome data from one symptom checklist suggested that the FI group were no more symptomatic than normal young males in the study area, whereas the DC group were comparable to psychiatric outpatients.

3. There was a significant tendency for subjects who reported more supportive social environments to have better relative outcomes, regardless of their group.

Conclusions

The authors concluded that:

1. Road accident injury and hospitalization is a highly stressful crisis experience that, without intervention, leaves the victim as distressed as typical psychiatric outpatients.
2. 'A single session within a few days of the experience to review the events and the individual's reactions might be sufficient to allow some people to mobilise support and return to normal functioning 3–4 months after injury. For others, this intervention is not enough' (Bordow & Porritt, 1979, p. 255).
3. An active, time-limited intervention providing emotional and practical support, and mobilizing social support, can enable the recipient to retrieve pre-accident levels of functioning.
4. Mobilization of genuine concern and understanding from people important to the patient 'plays a causal role in determining outcome' (ibid., p. 255).
5. Bordow & Porritt suggested that hospitalized patients could be interviewed routinely to identify those who require more support, and to whom crisis intervention could be offered. They argued for an active outreach programme to diminish the long-term psychiatric morbidity after road accidents.

2. Utrecht, the Netherlands

Brom et al. (1993) reported the outcome of an outreach intervention programme for survivors of serious road accidents.

Selection

Subjects were identified prospectively for one year from a police register of road accidents, and selected if involved in a moderately severe to severe accident. The police invited 738 persons to participate in the study, either in 'a research project' (monitoring, or control, group) or a 'secondary prevention programme' (the intervention group) by randomization.

Groups

Eighty-three subjects (response rate 36%) were recruited to the 'monitoring' group, and 68 (response rate 13%) to the intervention group. Apart from the element of self-selection, there were significant differences between the groups: fewer subjects were married and income was lower in the intervention group, both factors representing higher risk for development of psychiatric complications. Men were overrepresented in those who dropped out (24% of monitoring group, 16% of intervention group), and their accidents were slightly less severe, but the authors concluded that this did not have a large impact on their data.

Intervention

Two experienced psychotherapists delivered the interventions according to a written protocol, the programme comprising three sessions that could be extended to a maximum of six. The intervention included:

1. information about psychological reactions to serious life events;
2. practical information about medical procedures and sources of specialized advice;
3. support (a safe, quiet environment; opportunity to explore the traumatic experience; identifying emotions; encouragement for the victim's mobilization of their own social network); and
4. confronting and 'reality testing', in order to integrate the traumatic experience into the individual's belief structure.

The sessions were spaced over two or three months after the accident, in order to follow the course of working through the experience and discourage denial and other maladaptive solutions. This extended contact facilitated early detection and response to severe emotional reactions, which are risk factors for psychiatric disorder.

Findings

The main findings were as follows:

1. The intervention group showed higher initial scores on the Impact of Event Scale (IES) (Horowitz et al., 1979) and other measures than the monitoring group.

2. In both groups, there were significant reductions in intrusion and avoidance scores between initial testing and follow-up at six months post accident (three months after conclusion of contact in intervention group), but there was no significant difference between groups in symptom reduction.

3. More than 90% of the participants were satisfied with the intervention.

Conclusions

The authors conclude that they were unable to show that the intervention programme was more effective in reducing symptoms than the passage of time. They speculate that this may have been because, for organizational reasons, the interventions were not initiated until one month or more after the accident. This delay before commencing the intervention is typical neither of psychological debriefing nor of crisis intervention.

3. Bath, England

Stallard & Law (1993) reported the outcome of a late group debriefing for seven adolescents who, six months earlier, had been involved in a minibus accident but not seriously injured. All subjects reported intrusive symptoms, travel anxiety and impaired concentration.

Intervention

Two three-hour debriefing sessions were held at an interval of one week, conducted by a senior clinical psychologist and a trainee in psychiatry. The debriefing sessions were designed to encourage sharing of thoughts, feelings and understanding of the traumatic experience, and to promote adaptive coping.

Measures and control comparison

All participants completed a PTSD screening battery (Yule & Udwin, 1991), which included the IES (Horowitz et al., 1979) prior to the first group session and three months later. Obviously there was no control group, but the authors showed their data to be closely comparable with that reported by Yule & Udwin (1991) for groups of adolescent survivors following two maritime diasters, one of which received a psychological intervention, the other providing a control population.

Findings

Follow-up findings confirmed that there was a significant reduction in the group scores on the IES and a depression scale. The reduction in IES scores was attributable entirely to a reduced score on the intrusion scale; the avoidance score had increased slightly. These findings are similar to those reported by Yule (1992), who showed that adolescent survivors of maritime disasters who received an early psychological intervention scored significantly lower on the IES at follow-up than a nonintervention control group, the strongest effect being shown on the intrusion subscale.

Conclusions

The authors concluded that group psychological debriefing, even when relatively late after the traumatic incident, can be effective in reducing intrusive thoughts, possibly by allowing reattribution and emotional discharge.

4. London, England

Stevens and Adshead (Hobbs & Adshead, 1997) undertook a study of 'counselling' for injured victims of road accidents, assault by strangers or dog bites.

Selection

Subjects were recruited from patients who attended a hospital accident department with minor injuries (i.e. not necessitating admission to hospital) from road accidents, stranger assault, or dog bites. The number of refusals is not identified. Recruits were allocated randomly to intervention or control conditions.

Intervention and follow-up

Those randomized to the intervention group were offered a single standardized one-hour session within 24 hours of injury, with an experienced counsellor. They were asked to recount their experience in detail and encouraged to express their feelings. Surprisingly, those who became 'unusually distressed' during the interview were excluded from the study. Both counselled and control groups were assessed at interview at one week, one month and three months after the index trauma, using standardized measures including the IES.

Findings

Sixty-three subjects entered the study, 44 males and 19 females. The 21 who were lost to follow-up did not differ significantly on sociodemographic and clinical parameters from those who completed the study. Randomization generated skewing, the intervention group being older and showing higher depression and trait anxiety scores; but the two groups did not differ on IES scores. Overall, 38% of the study sample developed PTSD as diagnosed by selected questionnaire items, and 12% developed clinical anxiety or depression. Of the patients who entered the study with high depression and/or trait anxiety scores, 65% developed PTSD and 60% developed clinical depression or anxiety.

Outcome

There were no significant differences between the intervention and control groups in symptom scores or development of PTSD. However, in those with high depression or trait anxiety scores at entry, the counselled group showed a significantly greater reduction than controls in depression and anxiety at three months. Sixty-six per cent of respondents stated that they had found the counselling session useful, and the rest said that they had not. Some of the latter indicated that the intervention had been too early, others that they had not needed it.

Conclusion

Although there was no discernible impact on specific post-traumatic symptomatology, the authors noted the trend towards more rapid resolution of anxiety and depressive symptoms in those who participated in a single early session of counselling.

5. Oxford, England

This study, undertaken by Hobbs and Mayou (Hobbs et al., 1996; Hobbs & Adshead, 1997; Mayou et al., 2000), was designed to test the hypothesis that a feasible early psychological debriefing for road accident victims would reduce later psychiatric morbidity.

Selection

The subjects were road accident victims whose injuries necessitated immediate admission to hospital. Consecutive admissions aged 18–65 years were identified, but patients were excluded from the study if they had suffered significant head injury, were intoxicated at the time of the accident, had no memory for the accident, lived too far away to permit follow-up, or were unavailable for interview. Eight patients refused to participate.

Allocation and screening

Those who agreed to participate were randomized to intervention or control conditions. All subjects were screened by a research assistant who used a semistructured interview and two standardized questionnaires, the IES and Brief Symptom Inventory (BSI; Derogatis & Melisaratos, 1983). These measures were repeated at interview four months and three years after the accident, except in a few cases where postal follow-up proved necessary.

Intervention

The intervention was designed on the lines of psychological debriefing. It was undertaken within 24–48 hours of the patient's admission to hospital in most cases, for a high proportion of subjects were discharged from hospital after only one or two days. Initially the interventions were conducted by experienced psychiatric nurse specialists or social workers, who had had a brief preparatory training for this task. Unfortunately the primary clinical responsibilities of these staff prevented their interviewing most potential subjects before their discharge from hospital; so, regrettably, after the first 10 interventions, the psychological debriefing was conducted immediately following the screening interview by the research assistant, who was an experienced occupational therapist. This compromised both 'blindness' and the integrity of the debriefing, but reflected all too accurately the difficulties inherent in delivering an early intervention.

The psychological debriefing, of around one hour's duration, followed a standard format. The aim of the intervention was to promote emotional and cognitive processing of the traumatic experience. The patients were encouraged (a) to recount their involvement in the accident in detail, (b) to express associated emotions, and (c) to review their thoughts and feelings about the experience. The intervention was concluded by the interviewer giving information about common psychological reactions to traumatic experiences. She emphasized the value of expressing rather than suppressing thoughts and feelings about the accident, and the importance of early return to road travel. Each subject in the intervention group received a leaflet that consolidated the information and advice given, encouraged the support of family and friends, and advised consultation with the family doctor if problems persisted.

Findings

One hundred and fourteen patients were recruited to the study, and allocated randomly to intervention ($n = 59$) or control ($n = 55$) groups. The intervention group exhibited a higher mean injury severity score (6.04 versus 4.19) and mean duration of hospital stay (7.7 days versus 3.7 days) than the control group, indicating problematic skewing of the samples. There was no significant difference between intervention and control groups with regard to psychiatric symptomatology, including specific post-traumatic symptomatology, at entry to the study. Nor were there any significant differences in interview reports of travel anxiety (31% intervention group versus 29% controls) or distressing recollections of the accident (34% versus 38%). Significantly fewer of the intervention group (71%) than controls (91%) responded to four-month follow-up appointment or postal contact.

Outcome

At four-month follow-up neither group showed significant reduction in mean scores for specific post-traumatic symptomatology, depression, or travel anxiety. There were no differences between the groups in the main outcome measures (IES scores or the global General Severity Index generated by the BSI), or in the interview ratings of intrusive or avoidance symptomatology. However, subscales of the BSI demonstrated a significant reduction ($p < 0.01$) in somatization, and a trend ($p < 0.05$) towards reduction in anxiety, in the control group. In contrast, there were trends towards increased depression ($p < 0.01$), hostility/irritability ($p < 0.05$), and psychoticism/alienation ($p < 0.05$) in the intervention group. Irritability and alienation (interpersonal detachment or distancing) are characteristic of PTSD.

Despite one of the specific aims of the psychological debriefing, the intervention group were somewhat less likely than controls ($p < 0.05$) to talk to family or friends about their traumatic experience.

At the three-year follow-up, the intervention group had significantly worse outcome than controls, in terms of general psychiatric symptoms, travel anxiety as passengers, physical pain and overall level of functioning. Subjects who initially had high intrusion and avoidance symptoms (on the IES) remained symptomatic if they had received intervention, but recovered if they did not receive debriefing. For those with low initial scores, there were no differences in IES scores at three years between the intervention and control groups.

Conclusion

This study provided no evidence that an early psychological debriefing could reduce psychiatric symptomatology after injury in a road accident. Indeed, there was evidence of a worse outcome for subjects who had high initial post-traumatic symptoms and received psychological debriefing than for controls.

The studies cited here fail to demonstrate any preventive effect from early psychological debriefing. The only study to show benefit is one in which a supportive, relatively nonexposing intervention is initiated early but extended up to 10 sessions over several weeks (Bordow & Porritt, 1979). The obvious conclusion is that a crisis intervention approach is more likely to benefit the victims of road accidents than an early, exposure-based psychological debriefing. Similar positive findings were found in a controlled study of early brief cognitive-behavioural therapy for patients with acute stress disorder after accidents, mostly MVAs (Bryant et al., 1999).

Basis for possible adverse effects of debriefing

In psychodynamic terms, mental defence mechanisms are seen as necessary unconscious strategies for protecting oneself against fear and distress. Too much distress overwhelms coping resources, and thereby obstructs emotional and cognitive processing. The numbness that is so common in the immediate aftermath of traumatic events, including road accidents, can be thought of as an adaptive defence, which, as the frightening reality of what has been survived gradually breaks through, perhaps enables the victim to come to terms progressively with the experience. This may be a natural means of titrating review and processing of the trauma: exposure in small doses. Early psychological debriefing, particularly if it is undertaken within the first 24 or 48 hours after the event, may disrupt this natural defensive function.

On the other hand, more extreme degrees of dissociation preclude the progressive re-exposure from which processing and integration of the trauma follows, and must be regarded as maladaptive. Psychological debriefing may have no impact exactly because of the strength of the defence, or may prove deleterious if the dissociation is reinforced by a powerful exposure of the subject's underlying trauma.

In a well-conducted group debriefing, group cohesion may protect the individual to some degree from destructive re-exposure to the horror of the traumatic event. Because the narrative recounting is shared, the individual may not feel on his or her own with the horror and helplessness of the traumatic situation. It is salutary to remember that psychological debriefing was introduced as a group intervention for professional staff (emergency services and military personnel) whose work exposed them to traumatic events, and who were trained to some extent for this eventuality.

Nevertheless, there is still no scientific evidence that even group debriefing for professional workers is effective in reducing psychosocial problems after traumatic incidents. Ørner (1997) has reported that emergency services in Lincolnshire, England, have abandoned routine post-incident debriefing because, although participants reported high levels of satisfaction with the meetings, the rated helpfulness of the debriefing was inversely proportional to the severity and reported impact of the incident on the workers.

Conclusions

The evidence cited here suggests that psychological debriefing for individuals after road accidents does not reduce later psychiatric problems, particularly specific post-traumatic symptoms. There is possibly an adverse effect when a single, active debriefing session re-exposes more seriously injured victims to the horror of the accident without a real opportunity for cognitive processing of the experience, and without active follow-up.

There is growing evidence that cognitive-behavioural therapy is an effective later treatment for PTSD. The question here still is, 'Can PTSD be prevented?'.

Immediate emotional support, information and practical help may be of more value to trauma victims than an active, directive psychological debriefing. A crisis intervention programme, individualized for each patient and incorporating practical, emotional and social support, also may be more effective in promoting longer-term adjustment and minimizing later psychosocial problems. This necessitates several sessions over the 8–12 weeks after the accident, however, and may not be feasible for the large numbers of people affected by road accidents. With the increasing tendency towards personal injury compensation claims though, plaintiffs may seek to recover the cost of both physical and psychological care from insurance providers. Although this would inevitably push up premiums, it would have the advantage of placing the financial burden of road accidents increasingly where it belongs, with those who cause 'accidents'.

It is clear that most road traffic accident victims recover psychologically from their traumatic experience without professional intervention, but with the support of family and friends. Others do not recover and, in some of these, risk factors may be identifiable after the accident if routine screening were feasible. Those at risk include people with pre-existing psychiatric problems (depression, alcohol dependence, etc.), who may be in contact already with medical services, and also those with major social or economic difficulties. Family doctors, but also drivers' organizations, solicitors and others could do much more to encourage those who need early help or later treatment to seek it.

Resource constraints are such that psychological interventions after a common but potent trauma like a road accident must be targeted at those most at risk of developing psychiatric problems. The evidence suggests that universal psychological debriefing is neither warranted nor effective in preventing psychiatric morbidity. Individualized crisis intervention programmes for those at risk may have more validity, and further research is needed to determine whether such interventions are clinically effective and cost effective.

REFERENCES

American Psychiatric Association (1994). *Diagnostic and Statistical Manual of Mental Disorders*, 4th edn. Washington, DC: American Psychiatric Press.

Atchison, M. & McFarlane, A. (1997). Clinical patterns of acute psychological response to trauma. In M. Mitchell (Ed.) *The Aftermath of Road Accidents: Psychological, Social and Legal Consequences of an Everyday Trauma* (pp. 49–58). London: Routledge.

Blanchard, E. B. & Hickling, E. J. (1997). *After the Crash: Assessment and Treatment of Motor Vehicle Accident Survivors*. Washington, DC: American Psychological Association.

Blanchard, E. B., Hickling, E. J., Taylor, A. E. & Loos, W. (1995a). Psychiatric morbidity associated with motor vehicle accidents. *Journal of Nervous and Mental Disease*, **183**, 495–504.

Blanchard, E. B., Hickling, E. J., Taylor, A. E., Loos, W. R., Forneris, C. A. & Jaccard, J. (1995b). Who develops PTSD from motor vehicle accidents? *Behavioural Research Therapy* **34**, 1–10.

Bordow, S. & Porritt, D. (1979). An experimental evaluation of crisis intervention. *Social Science and Medicine*, **13**, 251–6.

Brom, D., Kleber, R. J. & Hofman, M. C. (1993). Victims of traffic accidents: incidence and prevention of post-traumatic stress disorder. *Journal of Clinical Psychology*, **49**, 131–9.

Bryant, R. A. & Harvey, A. G. (1997). Acute stress disorder: a critical review of diagnostic issues. *Clinical Psychology Review*, **17**, 757–73.

Bryant, B., Mayou, R. & Lloyd-Bostock, S. (1997). Compensation claims following road accidents: a six-year follow-up study. *Medicine Science and Law* **37**, 326–36.

Bryant, R. A., Harvey, A. G., Dang, S. T., Sackville, T. & Basten, C. (1999). Treatment of acute stress disorder: a comparison of cognitive behavioural therapy and supportive counselling.

Journal of Consulting and Clinical Psychology, in press.

Cherpitel, C. J. (1993). Alcohol and injuries: a review of international emergency room studies. *Addiction*, **88**, 923–37.

Derogatis, L. R. & Melisaratos, N. (1983). The brief symptom inventory: an introductory report. *Psychological Medicine*, **13**, 595–605.

Di Gallo, A. & Parry-Jones, W. L. (1996). Psychological sequelae of road traffic accidents: an inadequately addressed problem. *British Journal of Psychiatry*, **169**, 405–7.

Dyregrov, A. (1989). Caring for helpers in disaster situations: psychological debriefing. *Disaster Management*, **2**, 25–30.

Dyregrov, A. (1997). The process in psychological debriefings. *Journal of Traumatic Stress*, **10**, 589–605.

Editorial (1997). From what will we die in 2020? *Lancet*, **349**, 1263.

Ehlers, A. & Steil, R. (1995). An experimental study of intrusive memories. A paper presented to the World Congress of Behavioural and Cognitive Psychotherapy, Copenhagen.

Ehlers, A., Mayou, R. & Bryant, B. (1998). Psychological predictors of chronic PTSD after motor vehicle accidents. *Journal of Abnormal Psychology*, **107**, 508–19.

Gloag, D. (1993). Europe needs more road safety. *British Medical Journal*, **306**, 165.

Harvey, A. G. & Bryant, R. A. (1998). The relationship between acute stress disorder and posttraumatic stress disorder: a prospective evaluation of motor vehicle accident survivors. *Journal of Consultancy Clinical Psychology*, **66**, 507–12.

Hobbs, M. (1984). Crisis intervention in theory and practice: a selective review. *British Journal of Medical Psychology*, **57**, 23–34.

Hobbs, M. & Adshead, G. (1997). Preventive psychological intervention for road crash survivors. In Mitchell, M. (Ed.) *The Aftermath of Road Accidents: Psychological, Social and Legal Consequences of an Everyday Trauma* (pp. 159–71). London: Routledge.

Hobbs, M., Mayou, R., Harrison, B. & Worlock, P. (1996). A randomised controlled trial of psychological debriefing for victims of road traffic accidents. *British Medical Journal*, **313**, 1438–9.

Hodgkinson, P. E. & Stewart, M. (1991). *Coping with Catastrophe: A Handbook of Disaster Management*. London: Routledge.

Horowitz, H., Wilner, N. & Alvarez, W. (1979). Impact of Event Scale. A measure of subjective stress. *Psychological Medicine*, **41**, 209–12.

Horowitz, M. J. (1986). *Stress Response Syndromes*, 2nd edn. Northvale, NJ: Aronson.

Jacobson, R. R. (1995). The post-concussional syndrome: physiogenesis, psychogenesis and malingering: an integrative model. *Journal of Psychosomatic Research*, **39**, 675–93.

Joseph, S., Williams, R. & Yule, W. (1997). *Understanding Post-Traumatic Stress: A Psychosocial Perspective on PTSD and Treatment*. Chichester: Wiley.

King, N. (1997). Literature review. Mild head injury: neuropathology, sequelae, measurement and recovery. *British Journal of Clinical Psychology*, **36**, 161–84.

Lishman, W. A. (1998). *Organic Psychiatry. The Psychological Consequences of Cerebral Disorder*, 3rd edn. Oxford: Blackwell Science.

Mayou, R. A. (1992). Psychiatric aspects of road traffic accidents. *International Review of Psychiatry*, **4**, 45–54.

Mayou, R. (1996). Accident neurosis revisited. *British Journal of Psychiatry*, **168**, 399–403.

Mayou, R. (1997). The psychiatry of road traffic accidents. In M. Mitchell (Ed.) *The Aftermath of Road Accidents: Psychological, Social and Legal Consequences of an Everyday Trauma* (pp. 33–48). London: Routledge.

Mayou, R. A. & Bryant, B. M. (1994). Effects of road accidents on travel. *Injury*, **25**, 457–60.

Mayou, R. & Bryant, B. (1995). Alcohol and road traffic accidents. *Alcohol and Alcoholism*, **30**, 709–11.

Mayou, R., Bryant, B. & Duthie, R. (1993). Psychiatric consequences of road traffic accidents. *British Medical Journal*, **307**, 647–51.

Mayou, R., Tyndel, S. and Bryant, B. (1997). Long-term outcome of motor vehicle accident injury. *Psychosom Med* 59, 578–584.

Mayou, R., Ehlers, A. & Hobbs, M. (2000). A three year follow-up of a randomised controlled trial of psychological debriefing for road traffic accident victims. *British Journal of Psychiatry*, in press.

McDonald, A. S. & Davey, G. C. L. (1996). Psychiatric disorders and accidental injury. *Clinical Psychological Review*, **16**, 105–27.

Mendelson, G. (1995). 'Compensation neurosis' revisited: outcome studies of the effects of litigation. *Journal of Psychosomatic Research*, **39**, 695–706.

Mitchell, J. T. & Bray, G. (1983). When disaster strikes: the critical incident debriefing process. *Journal of the Emergency Medical Services*, **8**, 36–9.

Mitchell, J. T. & Bray, G. (1990). *Emergency Services Stress: Guidelines for Preserving the Health and Careers of Emergency Services Personnel*. Englewood Cliffs, NJ: Prentice Hall.

Mitchell, J. T. & Everly, G. S. (1995) *Critical Incident Stress Debriefing: An Operations Manual for the Prevention of Traumatic Stress Among Emergency Services and Disaster Workers*. Ellicott City, MD: Chevron Publishing.

Murray, J. (1997). Trauma and dissociation. D.Phil. thesis. University of Oxford.

Murray, C. J. L. & Lopez, A. D. (1997). Mortality by cause for eight regions of the world: Global Burden of Disease study. *Lancet*, **348**, 1269–76.

Norris, F. H. (1992). Epidemiology of trauma: frequency and impact of different potentially traumatic events on different demographic groups. *Journal of Consulting and Clinical Psychology*, **60**, 409–18.

Ørner, R. (1997). Emergency service may abandon critical incident stress debriefing. *Traumatic Stress Points*, International Society of Traumatic Stress Studies, Winter, 5.

Parkinson, F. (1997). *Critical Incident Debriefing: Understanding and Dealing with Trauma*. London: Souvenir Press.

Radanov, B. P., Sturzenegger, M., Schnidrig, A., DiStefano, G. & Aljinovic, M. (1993). Factors influencing recovery from headache after common whiplash. *British Medical Journal*, **307**, 652–5.

Raphael, B. (1986). *When Disaster Strikes: How Individuals and Communities Cope with Catastrophe*. London: Unwin Hyman.

Rothbaum, B. O., Foa, E. B., Riggs, D. S., Murdock, T. & Walsh, W. (1992). A prospective examination of posttraumatic stress disorder in rape victims. *Journal of Traumatic Stress*, **5**, 455–75.

Schnyder, U. (1997). Crisis intervention in psychiatric outpatients. *International Medical Journal*, **4**, 11–17.

Schnyder, U. & Buddeberg, C. (1996). Psychosocial aspects of accidental injuries: an overview. *Langenbecks Archiv für Chirurgie*, **381**, 125–31.

Stallard, P. & Law, F. (1993). Screening and psychological debriefing of adolescent survivors of life-threatening events. *British Journal of Psychiatry*, **163**, 660–5.

Taylor, S. & Koch, W. J. (1995). Anxiety disorders due to motor vehicle accidents: nature and treatment. *Clinical Psychology Review*, **15**, 721–38.

Terr, L. C. (1991). Childhood traumas: an outline and overview. *American Journal of Psychiatry*, **148**, 10–20.

Wessely, S., Rose, S. & Bisson, J. (1998). A systematic review of brief psychological interventions ('debriefing') for the treatment of immediate trauma related symptoms and the prevention of post traumatic stress disorder. *The Cochrane Library*, **3**.

Yule, W. (1992). Post traumatic stress disorder in child survivors of shipping disasters: the sinking of the 'Jupiter'. *Journal of Psychotherapy and Psychosomatics*, **57**, 200–5.

Yule, W. & Carr, J. (1987). *Behaviour Modification for People with Mental Handicaps*, 2nd edn. New York: Croom Helm.

Yule, W. & Udwin, O. (1991). Screening child survivors for post-traumatic stress disorders: experience from the 'Jupiter' sinking. *British Journal of Clinical Psychology*, **30**, 131–8.

11

Debriefing with service personnel in war and peace roles: experience and outcomes

Zahava Solomon, Yuval Neria and Eliezer Witztum

EDITORIAL COMMENTS

This overview of debriefing theory and practice shows that there is still a need for further work to be done in establishing what may be effective and for whom. While the historical context is set, it is clear from the review that models used, for instance in the military setting, cannot be guaranteed to achieve the goals that are hoped for, namely the prevention of post-traumatic stress disorder. Solomon et al. contrast instrumental and psychological debriefing and explore the theoretical rationale for debriefing, as well as some of the models that have been developed.

In their review of effectiveness, they examine studies involving both controlled trials, including the military, and non-controlled trials. The limitations of the few controlled trials that do exist are noted: for instance the fact that in many instances the groups are not well matched and that the debriefed group may start off with a higher level of distress and symptoms, or be self-selected. However, even with these provisions they note grounds for caution with a significant number of studies showing negative results. Solomon et al. hypothesize on possible causes for this: does debriefing actually permit the interaction and working through that are believed to be helpful? The failure to do so may be related to excessive structuring, inadequate time, or even perhaps inappropriate timing. Furthermore, debriefing may be inappropriate or potentially harmful for some, for instance depressive individuals with a tendency to negative ruminations. These could be reinforced by debriefing. People whose successful coping relies on avoidance may not be helped and may be overwhelmed. Persons with previous traumatic experience may be 'poor candidates for debriefing' because of the potential to reactivate prior trauma that cannot be worked through in the debriefing context. The authors also point out that soldiers suffering combat stress reactions or acute stress disorder could be harmed by debriefing as they may have their already powerful anxieties further heightened and little opportunity to deal with them. The skills and expertise of those who provide debriefing are also very relevant.

Solomon et al. conclude by suggesting formats for further research and, in the combat context, perhaps building on the positive outcomes of front-line psychological treatment. Further research and evaluation are necessary to determine the future directions of debriefing. The authors conclude that 'only rigorous research will shed more light on the effectiveness of debriefing' and that there is a 'moral obligation to deepen our knowledge of prevention strategies'.

Introduction

The stress of combat is notoriously pathogenic. Soldiers exposed to the imminent threat of injury and death, witness to the deaths of friends and enemy soldiers, and participants in the killing frequently fall prey to both short- and long-term psychological disorders. Between 20% and 30% of all injured combatants suffer from an acute psychological breakdown, today termed a combat stress reaction (CSR), on or near the battlefield (e.g. Solomon, 1993). In some cases, the CSR is a transient crisis with spontaneous remission. In other cases it develops directly into chronic post-traumatic stress disorder (PTSD), the most common long-term response to the stress of combat. PTSD can also develop without any overt signs of CSR, while transient CSR often produces a latent vulnerability that may be readily reactivated into full-blown PTSD years later.

PTSD is a debilitating psychological disorder that can produce tremendous emotional suffering and wreak havoc in every area of the individual's life: the intimacies of the family, the pleasures of company and friendship, the daily routines of work, and the person's physical health (American Psychiatric Association, 1994). A persistent anxiety disorder, it is very difficult to treat (e.g. Johnson et al., 1996), and periods of apparent recovery can be interspersed with sudden flare-ups. Its costs to society are high, as alienated, angry, withdrawn, and inwardly tormented PTSD veterans are often unable to fulfil their responsibilities at home and at work; they draw heavily on rehabilitation, health, and welfare services and they often merit years of regular compensation payments.

Needless to say, the prevention of combat-induced PTSD is a top priority both within and outside the military. Debriefing, which can be carried out in group fashion shortly after battle with entire units, takes little time, is at relatively low cost, and is well anchored in various psychological theories; thus it has natural appeal. Its effectiveness, however, is unproven, and it may even be damaging to certain individuals (Neria & Solomon, 1999).

This chapter presents the theory and development of psychological debriefing, looks at its outcomes, discusses the difference between theory and practice, and presents an alternative suggestion for the prevention of combat-related PTSD.

Debriefing and the philosophy of prevention

Traditionally trauma-induced disorders are treated by clinicians, in their offices or clinics, after the emergence of symptoms. In recent years, greater awareness of the importance of prevention has led to the search for ways of reducing the risk of long-term disorders by intervening soon after the exposure to traumatic stress, before symptoms become apparent (e.g. Brom & Kleber, 1989; Neria & Solomon, 1999).

Prevention is the inhibition of disease before it develops. Three basic types of prevention of stress reactions have been conceptualized (Caplan, 1964). Primary prevention involves preparing the individual or the community to cope with an expected traumatic event before it occurs. Secondary prevention refers to early intervention, right after the exposure to the stressful event, in order to limit its long-term damage. Tertiary prevention entails efforts to reduce the virulence and chronicity of psychological disturbance reactions among those who suffer from them.

In the field of trauma, secondary prevention (Freedy & Donkervoet, 1995; Norris & Thompson, 1995) has involved efforts to keep people who were exposed to traumatic stress from developing long-term disorders (Armfield, 1994; Lundin, 1994; McCarroll et al., 1995). Debriefing is proposed as one form of secondary prevention, administered shortly after exposure and before the appearance of symptoms. According to the theory, the earlier the debriefing occurs, the less the opportunity for maladaptive cognitive and behavioural patterns to become established (Neria & Solomon, 1999). Not a form of therapy, debriefing is aimed at helping all persons exposed to a traumatic event regardless of their immediate emotional response. It has been used to try to attenuate the detrimental impact of traumatic stress among a variety of groups, including emergency workers, rescue teams, accident victims and hostages, and combat soldiers (Dunning & Silva, 1980; Mitchell, 1981, 1982, 1983, 1986; Raphael et al., 1983; Jones, 1985; Melton, 1985; Shalev, 1994).

Instrumental and psychological debriefing

Preventive debriefing falls under the heading of what is known as 'psychological' or 'psychosocial' debriefing. Psychological debriefing has its roots in various forms of instrumental debriefing designed for the purpose of gathering information about, and drawing lessons from, a variety of tasks. Instrumental debriefing is aimed, first and foremost, at improving future task performance through a combination of analyses of how the task had been performed and the enhancement of group cohesion that comes from the joint review and clarification of the event. Instrumental debriefing is used in a variety of institutions, such as firefighting and rescue organizations. A type of instrumental debriefing in current use in both military and nonmilitary settings is task-oriented debriefing. For example, the Israel Defence Force routinely and systematically debriefs soldiers and commanders after every mission (Gal, 1986).

Needless to say, cognitive and educational elements take precedence over emotional and expressive ones in this type of debriefing. At the same time, the discussion of the event by the participants may bring a good deal of emotion to the surface, give order and meaning to what was probably a rather chaotic experience, and help individuals to integrate the experience into more stable frameworks, both their own and that of the institution to which they belong.

Like instrumental debriefing, psychological debriefing is a group-oriented intervention in which the participants examine the major elements of the stressful event shortly after their exposure. All those who were exposed to the event participate in the debriefing, whatever their immediate psychological response to it. There is great variety in what is actually done in debriefing sessions, but they generally combine elements of emotional expression with cognitive appraisal, and counselling with instruction.

One of the major assumptions behind this method is that peers can assist the individual's healing and that a person's traumatic experiences are better worked through with others who shared them. The model for debriefing is humanistic rather than psychiatric. That is, all the reactions to the event are considered normal responses to traumatic stress, and no reaction, however bizarre, is labelled deviant, abnormal or pathological. Among the reasons for this is that spontaneous recovery has been observed in many individuals who suffer from quite severe immediate reactions (Solomon, 1993; Shalev, 1996).

Theoretical rationale for psychological debriefing

The three basic elements of psychological debriefing are emotional abreaction or ventilation, cognitive processing of the traumatic material, and social support. Abreaction and cognitive processing have been linked

to recovery from trauma by a long line of theoreticians, from Freud (e.g. 1937) through Horowitz (e.g. 1986). Theories of traumatization provide reason to believe that abreaction helps the individual to discharge the emotional overload experienced in traumatic events, facilitates the working through of the traumatic event, and helps to release susceptible individuals from the freezing of affect and surrender to the threat that may follow upon their exposure. Theories of cognitive processing emphasize the role of cognitive schemata in modulating stress reactions (Janoff-Bulman, 1985). Horowitz (1986) pointed to the critical role of the dialectic process of denial and mental occupation with the traumatic experience in the working-through process. Danielli (1985), combining the two approaches, suggested that abreaction and the adoption of a new perspective on the traumatic event and acceptance of it as part of one's personal history are essential to the restoration of the trauma-shattered personality. In apparent confirmation of the use of the combination of abreaction and cognitive processing, Pennebaker (e.g. 1990) and his colleagues presented evidence from an impressive series of empirical studies that demonstrated the psychological and physiological benefits of talking about traumatic experiences shortly after they occur, and the negative effects of not talking about them.

Similarly, there is considerable evidence that social support – which may be obtained from the debriefing group – both buffers stress and moderates its pathological impact (Turner, 1981; Green et al., 1985; Fullerton et al., 1992).

The development of debriefing

Marshall's historical group debriefing

Perhaps one of the things that contribute to the appeal of debriefing in the military is that this is where the first documented use of debriefing is found. As far as we know, the method was first developed by Brigadier General S. L. A. Marshall, Chief Historian of the US Army during World War II (Marshall, 1944, 1956; Spiller, 1980; Shalev, 1994). Marshall developed a form of instrumental briefing which he termed 'historical group debriefing'. This form of instrumental debriefing consisted of a highly detailed, comprehensive reconstruction of the battle by the surviving soldiers carried out in its immediate wake (see Shalev, Chapter 1).

Marshall's historical group debriefing is an important precursor of current psychological debriefing. Indeed, it included many elements that are familiar to psychotherapy. The data that were gathered included the soldiers' thoughts and feelings as they engaged in the fighting, so that the process involved reliving the experience. Premature closure was avoided, high levels of ambiguity tolerated and contradictory renditions accepted until the information permitted a conclusion. Attention was paid to acknowledging the contributions of the soldiers who had been killed, and the leaders of the debriefing sessions, who were military men, were instructed to be uncritical and encouraging and not to pull rank.

Psychological group debriefing

Modern psychological debriefing was developed in the 1980s to help rescue workers and other persons in high-risk occupations deal with the inevitable stresses of their jobs so as to avoid the development of stress reactions in the future. In keeping with this aim, the balance of cognitive and emotional elements in Marshall's historical briefing is reversed, with the latter now taking precedence.

The two main developers of the psychological debriefing are Beverley Raphael and Jeffrey Mitchell. Raphael (1986) formulated guidelines for helping teams of rescue workers and helpers in the Granville rail disaster (see also Raphael et al., 1983). She recommended formal group sessions in which 'the experience is given a cognitive structure and the emotional release of reviewing helps the worker to a sense of achievement and distancing' (Raphael, 1986, p. 255). Great weight is placed on the workers' expression of their feelings, ranging from the helplessness and frustration they felt during their work, through their nightmares, intrusive images, and fear of dying afterwards. Also discussed are the workers' relationships with the families of the disaster victims and their relations with one another.

Mitchell (1981, 1982, 1986) devised for the emergency services a method that he termed Critical Incident Stress Debriefing (CISD), to be carried out by teams consisting of specially trained professional peers (e.g. fire personnel, police personnel) with the support of mental health professionals. The idea is that the people involved in a potentially traumatogenic event be given the opportunity to discuss their experiences in a rational, structured manner, to diffuse their emotions, and to see that they are not alone. The CISD is carried out in a series of stages: to begin with there is a factual discussion of each participant's role in the event and an exploration of their thoughts about their experience; then there is a discussion of his or her emotional reactions; and then moving back to the cognitive plane, with a discussion of the participant's stress symptoms and instruction on the normality of the symptoms and ways of managing them. For mass disasters, Mitchell modified the model somewhat, so as to include a reframing stage and conclude with a summary emphasizing the lessons learned and the positive things the participants can take away from the disaster. In both cases, the solicitation of the participants' emotional reactions is carefully enclosed in a cognitive framework, presumably to keep them from getting out of hand.

Raphael's and Mitchell's work was rapidly followed by the development of a variety of debriefing approaches, each with its own name and permutations. They employ a variety of procedures: cognitive rehearsal, ventilation, and 'resource mobilization' (Mitchell, 1983), sharing and education (Raphael, 1986), active counselling and teaching (e.g. Wagner, 1979), and resource mobilization (e.g. Bergman & Queen, 1986).

Today, what goes by the name of debriefing is actually a variety of interventions, some of them in groups and some of them as individuals or couples, administered anywhere from days to months after the critical event, ranging anywhere from a single hour to several sessions spread over a few weeks, which have in common their brevity, a predetermined structure, and a melange of education, ventilation, and social support, in different proportions and emphases.

Effectiveness of debriefing

Despite the intuitive soundness and theoretical grounding of debriefing, its effectiveness is far from clear. There are relatively few studies of the impact of debriefing and a good many of them do not use controls. Comparison and evaluation are hampered by the variety of the groups studied, the variety of measures and time frames used, the diversity of techniques of intervention, the failure of most writers to describe how the debriefing they evaluated was conducted, and the inevitable inconsistency in the skill of the persons who carry out the debriefing.

Strikingly, in both the civilian and military spheres, there is a fairly consistent difference in the findings of the studies that use control groups and those that do not. Most of studies without control groups report findings that point to the effectiveness of debriefing, while those with control groups show either no effect or a worrisome negative impact.

Civilian studies

Non-controlled

Raphael et al. (1983) stated that debriefed rescue workers reported being able to assimilate their stressful experience. Mitchell & Bray (1990) concluded that emergency personnel who underwent CISD debriefing showed diminishing job turnover, less early retirement and fewer mental health problems. Robinson & Mitchell (1993) showed similarly a reduction of stress symptoms following debriefing among 172 debriefed emergency service, welfare and hospital personnel.

In a repeated measures study, Stallard & Law (1993) found that a group of seven adolescent survivors of a minibus accident who were screened three months after the event, then debriefed, and screened again three months later had significantly lower anxiety, depression, and intrusion in the second screening. In another repeated measures study, Chemtob et al. (1997) report reduced Impact of Event Scale (IES) scores among two groups of helpers who were debriefed six and nine months after a hurricane in Hawaii. More recently, however, Amir et al. (1998), also using a repeated measures design, found that Israeli women who had been exposed to a terrorist attack on the bus they took to work obtained no substantial relief of their stress symptoms at both three and six months after having been debriefed.

Controlled

On the whole, the studies using control groups encourage scepticism about the claimed benefits of debriefing. At best they show no improvement. Hytten & Hasle (1989) found that firefighters who had undergone formal psychological debriefing after a hotel fire scored the same on the IES as those who had talked informally among themselves. This finding suggests that the value of debriefing may lie not in its technique or content but in the opportunity it affords for expression and review, which can occur in any number of settings, but often does not.

At worst, the controlled studies reveal the possibility of higher vulnerability and more severe psychopathology among the debriefed subjects. Griffiths & Watts (1992) found that at a 12-month follow-up emergency personnel in bus crashes who attended stress debriefings had higher IES scores than those who did not attend. Similarly, the debriefed police officers studied by Carlier et al. (1994) reported more PTSD symptoms, depression, agoraphobia, and anger than their nondebriefed counterparts. Kenardy et al. (1996) similarly found that policemen, emergency workers, welfare volunteers and counsellors who received CISD following the Newcastle earthquake in Australia showed greater general psychological morbidity and more intrusion and avoidance than those who were not debriefed. Bisson et al. (1997) found that, at a 13-month follow-up, burn victims who underwent individual or couple debriefing while still in hospital suffered from significantly greater anxiety and depression than those in the control group and three times the PTSD rate. A rare exception to this trend among the controlled studies is Jenkins' (1996) investigation of 36 emergency workers, fairly evenly divided between those who underwent voluntary debriefing and those who did not. This study found evidence that those who underwent CISD in the aftermath of working a mass shooting incident suffered less depression and anxiety in the subsequent month. But the small sample size and lack of longer-term follow-up make the results less than conclusive.

Military studies

There are very few published reports of debriefing in the military. We found three, all of them involving debriefing of Gulf War veterans. Like the studies in the civilian sector, these too yield mixed results.

The first, by Fitzgerald et al. (1993), does not purport to be an empirical study. It rather describes a two-phased debriefing process carried out on physically injured male soldiers at Walter Reed Army Medical Center. The first stage consisted of four hours of individual debriefing by a specially trained 'clinical nurse specialist'. This stage combined discussion of the soldier's fears and experiences (especially those involving the injury event and evacuation process) with information aimed at encouraging the soldier to seek social support, talk about the experience, and mobilize effective coping mechanisms. It also included information about normal stress responses following injury events and the suggestion that such responses would pass in a few weeks. The second stage harks back to Marshall's historical debriefing. It consisted of a support group designed to provide a safe environment that would afford the opportunity for abreaction and catharsis and enable the soldiers to reframe the meaning of their experience.

The authors contend that the debriefings facilitated integration and decreased emotional reactivation. Their article, however, contains no measures to support the claim, no comparison with nonbriefed soldiers, and no effort to control for the effects of time. The only evidence that the authors provide is one very brief case description of a soldier who told of finally getting a full night's sleep after talking in the debriefing about his prior experience in Vietnam.

The second study, by Ford et al. (1993), combined a description of what the authors term 'family psychosocial debriefing' for Operation Desert Storm couples with efforts to measure its effect. The process was quite different from that described in other models of debriefing. It entailed two to six sessions with veterans and their spouses held between two and six months after deactivation. The persons who received the intervention were a small, self-selected group of volunteers (7.5% of those approached ($n = 1000$)), who sought treatment for marital problems subsequent to their service. The intervention itself consisted of a combination of strategies from Mitchell's critical incident debriefing and a variety of family therapy approaches.

Ford and his colleagues used both a repeated measures design and a control group. But although they claim that the veterans and their spouses who underwent the debriefing were able to resolve the symptoms of psychosocial malfunctioning prevalent among returning soldiers and their families, the evidence does not support this. Retesting a year or so after the war revealed an improvement in most measures; but the authors themselves noted that there is no way of knowing whether the source of the improvement was any (or which) of the treatment paradigms or the passage of time. Moreover the improvement that was shown was no greater than that found in the control group that did not seek or receive treatment. Nor did the intervention reduce the symptoms of the treated group to the lower level of the controls.

The third investigation, by Deahl et al. (1994), is a well-designed study of two groups of British soldiers who had served in the Army War Graves Service during the Gulf War. All the soldiers had worked closely together and handled dead bodies. Most of the soldiers received debriefing. For operational reasons, one group did not, and served as a natural control group.

The intervention included an educational session, in which PTSD symptoms were explained as a normal human reaction to abnormal stress and a small group debriefing session with two welfare workers, using the Dyregrov (1989) model, there was advice about where to get help. The emphasis was on the frequency and normality of any disturbing symptoms, in an attempt to destigmatize the distress and facilitate help-seeking.

Testing nine months later showed no difference in the two groups either on the General Health Questionnaire or on the IES. The factors found to be associated with outcome were prior psychological problems and the veteran's belief that his life had been in danger.

The overall disparity in the findings of the controlled

and uncontrolled studies in different populations, over different types of traumatic encounter, and in both the civilian and military sectors makes it very difficult to determine how effective debriefing is or is not as a preventive instrument. The uncontrolled studies, by their very nature, cannot provide sufficient evidence for the effectiveness of debriefing. On the one hand, various of the uncontrolled studies reported that a good portion of the participants found the debriefing 'helpful' (Hytten & Hasle, 1989; Robinson & Mitchell, 1993; Turner et al., 1993) or were otherwise satisfied with it (Flannery et al., 1991). If these are not socially desirable responses, they suggest that the debriefing made at least some people feel better and answered needs that they had. On the other hand, there is no necessary connection between satisfaction and mental health; in fact, some of the controlled studies (Griffiths & Watts, 1992; Bisson et al., 1997) that investigated the possibility of a link found none. Moreover, it is impossible to know whether the symptom reduction that some of these studies reported is the outcome of the debriefing or of spontaneous recovery over time. None of the studies, even the more rigorous ones, adequately controlled for the impact of time.

The findings of the controlled studies showing that debriefed groups suffer from more PTSD, more anxiety, and more depression are also ambiguous. Although they seem damning, they do not necessarily mean that debriefing is in fact damaging.

For one thing, the negative effects may be as much the result of reporting bias as of real damage. Because debriefing raises negative emotions and stress symptoms to awareness, debriefed subjects may simply be more prone to report the symptoms than subjects who have not been debriefed and who might also suffer from them (Bleich et al., 1992a). These possibilities point to the need for clinical assessment, including physiological measures (Orr & Kaloupek, 1997), to supplement the self-reporting measures used.

The negative findings may also stem from the possibility that the debriefed groups were, to begin with, more distressed than their nondebriefed counterparts. In most of the studies reported (with the notable exception of that by Deahl et al., 1994), the people undergoing debriefing were self-selected, and tended to be

more distressed than those who did not attend. The debriefed subjects in Ford et al.'s (1993) and Griffiths & Watts' (1992) studies had higher levels of distress symptoms to begin with than the controls.

Even where efforts were made to obtain randomized groupings, the debriefed and control groups were not necessarily evenly matched. Bisson's groups are a particular example. The controls, it turned out, had less severe burns than the debriefed subjects, shorter hospital stays, a lower rate of experience with previous traumas, significantly less likelihood that others were involved, and less severe initial symptomatology than the debriefed group. Although most of these differences did not reach significance, the findings showed that poorer outcome was associated more with the severity of the burn and initial intrusion and avoidance than with the debriefing or lack thereof.

Practice versus theory

The ambiguities of the research findings reveal a marked gap between the convincing theory behind debriefing and the empirical evidence, which leaves many questions as to its effectiveness. Yet there is a certain reluctance to abandon a measure that seems to have such strong underpinning from so many theoretical perspectives. It is tempting to suggest this or that modification, with the expectation that, if some small change were made, the debriefing would fulfil its promise. Deahl and his colleagues (1994), for example, whose own findings showed that debriefing did not alleviate the sufferings of the Gulf War body handlers, reaffirmed their commitment to debriefing, with the proviso that it be conducted by lay rather than professional helpers. Chemtob et al. (1997) tried to save the procedure by suggesting that it would be more effective if carried out some months after the traumatic event, when the extreme sensitivity that characterizes the individual in the immediate wake of such events has subsided somewhat.

But the empirical findings raise a more fundamental question about the relation between theory and practice: does debriefing actually permit the abreaction and genuine cognitive reframing that is necessary to working through the trauma?

Psychological debriefing, as practised today, is a very short and highly structured process. While Marshall's historical group debriefings allotted four to five whole days to intensive, continuous discussion and did not end until the entire reconstruction of the event was completed, the debriefings described in most of the research cited above lasted only a few hours, some as little as one hour. Moreover, that short time tended to be rather rigidly divided up into separate sections variously focussed on emotions and cognitions, expression and instruction. One may wonder what kind of abreaction and reframing are actually possible in such a setting.

Critics of debriefing charge that it raises emotions without enabling the participants to work them through. Bisson et al. (1997), for example suggested that debriefing brings to the surface distressing feelings, images and recollections without providing enough time for habituation or desensitization.

It stands to reason that the brevity and structure of debriefing could combine, on the one hand, to prevent adequate emotional expression and, on the other, to prevent closure. We can take Mitchell's CISD as a paradigmatic case in point. The discussion of the participants' emotional reactions – their grief, fear, anger, guilt, confusion, and shame – is sandwiched between fact finding and cognitive reframing. It is unlikely that sufficient attention can be paid to the tumultuous and scary feelings aroused by traumatic exposure. Worse, it is quite likely that people who begin to express themselves are soon cut off for lack of time for them to expand. With their feelings thus aroused but not properly dealt with, the distressed individuals who attend debriefings may be left anxious, depressed and overwhelmed.

It is also unlikely that genuine cognitive reframing can take place within the time frame and structure of debriefing. Debriefing may be an adequate vehicle for the transmission of knowledge, which may help some people to place their own stress responses in perspective and thereby comfort and reassure them. But without sound emotional grounding, knowledge is sterile and does not lead to reframing.

The possibility of harm

One of the advantages touted for debriefing is its applicability to all those who are exposed to a particular traumatic event. But there is a real question as to whether it is in fact suitable for everyone. Although the findings of increased distress among debriefed individuals can be accounted for by reporting bias and preselection, the possibility that debriefing can be harmful cannot be ruled out.

The literature provides indications of types of people who may be harmed by debriefing and should not participate in it. The literature on mood suggests that depressive and dysphoric individuals are probably best not encouraged to ruminate on distressing experiences, since that has been found to perpetuate their negative mood and result in less effective functioning (Lyubomirsky & Nolen-Hoeksema, 1993, 1995). Moreover, while debriefing may benefit people who rely on active coping strategies and information seeking, those who rely on the coping mechanisms of denial, avoidance and repression may be overwhelmed by their feelings when these defences are not permitted to work in debriefing.

People who suffered from prior traumatic experiences are also probably poor candidates for debriefing. The literature on trauma documents the risk of reactivation of former traumatic reactions upon exposure to experiences that recall the initial trauma. Debriefing of combat soldiers who had fought in previous campaigns may thus open up old emotional wounds and trigger reactivation (see e.g. Solomon, 1993). Above all, persons showing signs of acute stress disorder (ASD) may be harmed by debriefing. Soldiers with combat stress reaction (CSR) run the risk of having their already powerful anxieties stirred up by debriefing, and are likely to be inundated by their feelings in a situation that provides inadequate means for alleviating them.

The importance of debriefers being capable of identifying participants who are at risk for psychological morbidity has been stressed. Yet the very format of debriefing – its group nature, prescribed format, short time, overseeing by persons who are not trained professionals, and the built-in refusal to label any symptom as pathological – impedes the identification of persons who are symptomatic or otherwise at risk.

Instead of debriefing, what?

The lack of convincing evidence that psychological debriefing prevents the development of PTSD and the possibility that it may further traumatize some of those who undergo it argue against its routine use in the military, or in any other setting for that matter. Although disappointing, this conclusion does not necessarily mean, however, that we must abandon all hope of prevention.

The obstacle, at this point, is that we still have a very limited understanding of the aetiology of PTSD, which makes it difficult to know where and how to intervene in its progression. We do, however, have some potentially useful knowledge: although PTSD can develop without any prior signs (Ingraham & Manning, 1986; Kulka et al., 1990), the existence of an acute stress reaction (ASD or CSR) is a good predictor (Bleich et al., 1992b; Solomon, 1993); and the likelihood that CSR will develop into long-term PTSD seems to be tempered by the application of what is termed front-line treatment. Although what determines whether or not an ASD or CSR will abate and become a passing event or, alternatively, develop into long-term psychopathology is little understood, the link between PTSD and severe symptomatology at the time of the traumatic event and the apparent ability of front-line treatment to affect this link can serve as a starting point for an experimental treatment and research programme.

Front-line treatment

Before proceeding with the suggestions, a few lines about front-line treatment are in order (for more details, see Neria & Solomon, 1999). Front-line treatment is today the accepted treatment for battlefield CSR in most Western armies (see e.g. Johnson et al., 1992; Solomon, 1993). First formulated by the military psychiatrist T. W. Salmon (1919) on the basis of the experience of the British and the French armies during World War I and later developed by Artiss (1963), front-line treatment is aimed at helping a soldier weather the

crisis of CSR and return to military functioning. It has three basic principles:

1. Proximity: treatment should be administered close to the traumatic incident.
2. Immediacy: treatment must be given as close as possible to the time of the onset of the symptoms.
3. Expectancy: the victim must understand that the crisis is transient, and that he or she is to return to the unit immediately after the short intervention.

Building on these principles, modern front-line treatment, conducted on the front but removed from the fire, proceeds from meeting the casualty's physiological needs for food, drink and sleep to preventing him or her from becoming isolated, lonely and detached. The treatment generally lasts from three to five days, during which time the military atmosphere is carefully maintained. It combines group and individual therapy carried out by mental health professionals, activities such as relaxation and physical fitness, and the performance of noncombat tasks. Although the activities vary from programme to programme, as do the aim and orientation of the therapy itself, it is generally agreed that the therapy emphasizes the soldiers' experiences in the battle and their current emotions and avoids delving into their personal histories.

Most of the evidence for the effectiveness of front-line treatment is based on clinical impressions in various wars. World War I (Hausman & Rioch, 1967; Panagapoulos, 1980), World War II (Artiss, 1963; Hausman & Rioch, 1967), the Korean War (Hausman & Rioch, 1967) and the Vietnam War (Bloch, 1969; Pettera et al., 1969). However, a quasi-experimental study carried out by the Israel Defence Forces on the treatment outcomes of CSR casualties in the Lebanon War provided convincing empirical evidence of front-line treatment's potential. The findings showed that the more front-line treatment principles that a soldier's treatment incorporated, the more likely he was to return to his unit and the less likely to develop PTSD a year later (Solomon & Benbenishty, 1986).

In its relative immediacy and brevity, focus on the here and now, encouragement of ventilation, and provision of social support, front-line treatment has certain similarities to debriefing. Its apparently greater effectiveness may derive from two advantages: the fact that front-line treatment is given only to identified casualties means that vulnerable persons are not placed at risk of further traumatization; and the employment of trained mental health professionals in front-line treatment in comparison with debriefing may better allow for the abreaction and reframing necessary to working through the traumatic experience, as may the longer duration of this type of intervention.

Post-combat intervention and research

What we suggest is that at the wake of combat, combatants be assessed and divided into three groups:

1. Asymptomatic soldiers.
2. Symptomatic soldiers without major problems in functioning.
3. Symptomatic soldiers with major problems in functioning.

The asymptomatic soldiers should include those who show no overt signs of distress. They should be sent home and followed up periodically for delayed onset of stress reactions. Efficient, economical follow-up procedures that do not encourage faking of stress reactions should be devised, and the soldiers who show delayed onset should be treated. Nonintervention in the case of asymptomatic soldiers permits them to mobilize their own coping resources and avoids inadvertent harm to soldiers whose vulnerabilities may be hidden or latent.

The two groups of symptomatic soldiers should be given a version of front-line treatment. The reason for separating symptomatic soldiers on the basis of their functioning lies in the fact that CSR and ASD are diagnosed functionally rather than clinically. For a diagnosis of CSR soldiers must cease to function militarily and act in a manner that may endanger themselves and/or their fellow combatants (Kormos, 1978). For a diagnosis of ASD, the individual must show not only a clinical level of distress but the inability to function normally and to carry out necessary tasks (American Psychiatric Association, 1994).

The division of soldiers who show signs of CSR from those whose psychiatric status is less severe enables tailoring the intervention to their different needs. Intervention for soldiers who have major problems in functioning might focus first on facilitating a return to functioning, while that for symptomatic soldiers who function could focus on the amelioration of symptoms and the working through of the trauma.

Certainly, the suggested screening is far from foolproof. Difficulties in distinguishing the normal stress after combat from pathological responses and the subjectiveness and situation dependency inherent in judging functioning mean that mistakes will be made (Solomon, 1993). The professionals who carry out the front-line intervention should be on guard for that possibility and ready to change any soldier's treatment modality as required.

Research should be carried out on the three groups in the following order. After the initial assessment, the soldiers from the three groups should be matched for sociodemographic, military and health backgrounds, and then random samples should be drawn from among the matched triplets. Next, the three groups should be evaluated by blind assessors at selected intervals for a period of several years. This will yield a controlled, longitudinal study, which avoids the problem of self-selection that casts doubt on the outcomes of the debriefing studies.

The psychological price that many soldiers pay for the proclivity of the human race for war is enormous. Not only are millions of veterans around the globe severely afflicted, many of them suffer from chronic detrimental sequelae for the rest of their lives. Armies in many parts of the world recognize their responsibilities for their veterans' plight. Tremendous economic resources are invested in treatment of chronic PTSD, with relatively limited success. Therefore, the notion of prevention is most compelling. If successful, it may minimize the suffering and result in considerable saving of resources. Unfortunately, as noted in this chapter, close scrutiny of the debriefing literature reveals that, despite the appeal of this method, in its present form it does not yield the desired results. The literature review clearly demonstrates many questions remain unanswered. To mention only a few:

What constitutes a debriefing intervention?

Which forms of debriefing are, or may prove useful for, which types of survivors?

Who is the individuals most likely to benefit from such intervention?

What is called for are controlled, randomized trials of various debriefing protocols in various populations. Only rigorous research will shed more light on the effectiveness of debriefing.

In light of the significance of the task of helping the traumatized survivors, it is our moral obligation to deepen our knowledge of prevention strategies. This is clearly a challenge that should be addressed by mental health professionals.

REFERENCES

American Psychiatric Association (1994). *Diagnostic and Statistical Manual of Mental Disorders*, 4th eds. Washington, DC: American Psychiatric Press.

Amir, M., Weil, G., Kaplan, Z., Tocker, T. & Wiztum, E. (1998). Debriefing with brief group psychotherapy in an homogeneous group of non-injured victims of terrorist attack: a prospective study. *Acta Psychiatrica Scandinavica*, **98**, 237–42.

Armfield, F. (1994). Preventing post traumatic stress disorder resulting from military operations. *Military Medicine*, **159**, 739–46.

Artiss, K. L. (1963). Human behaviour under stress: from combat to social psychiatry. *Military Medicine*, **128**, 1011–15.

Bergman, L. H. & Queen, T. (1986). Critical incident stress: Part 1. *Fire Command* May, 52–6.

Bisson, J. I., Jenkins, P. L., Alexander, J. & Bannister,C. (1997). Randomised controlled trial of psychological debriefing for victims of acute burn trauma. *British Journal of Psychiatry*, **171**, 78–81.

Bleich, A., Shalev, A., Shoham, S., Solomon, Z. & Kotler, M. (1992a). PTSD: theoretical and practical considerations as reflected through Koach-An innovative treatment project. *Journal of Traumatic Stress*, **5**, 265–71.

Bleich, A., Dycian, A., Koslowsky, M., Solomon, Z. & Wiener, M. (1992b). Psychiatric implications of missile attack on civilian population. *Journal of the American Medical Association*, **268**, 613–15.

Bloch, H. S. (1969). Army clinical psychiatry in the combat zone. *American Journal of psychiatry*, **126**, 289–98.

Brom D. & Kleber, R. J. (1989). Prevention of posttraumatic stress disorders. *Journal of Traumatic Stress*, **2**, 335–51.

Caplan, G. (1964). *Principles of Preventive Psychiatry*. New York: Basic Books.

Carlier, I. V. E., van Uchelen, J. J., Lamberts, R. D. & Gersons, B. P. R. (1994). The effect of debriefing. A study at the Amsterdam police after the Bijlmer plane-crash. Internal report, Academic Medical Center at the University of Amsterdam.

Chemtob, M. C., Tomas, S., Law, W. & Cremniter, D. (1997). Post-disaster psychosocial intervention: a field study of debriefing on psychological distress. *American Journal of Psychiatry*, **154**, 415–17.

Danielli, Y. (1985). The treatment and the prevention of long term effects of intergenerational transmission of victimization: a lesson from Holocaust survivors and their children. In C. R. Figley (Ed.) *Trauma and its Wake* (pp. 278–94). New York: Brunner/Mazel.

Deahl, M. P., Gillham, A. B., Thomas, J., Searle, M. M. & Srinivasan, M. (1994). Psychological sequelae following the Gulf War: factors associated with subsequent morbidity and the effectiveness of psychological debriefing. *British Journal of Psychiatry*, **165**, 60–5.

Dunning, C. & Silva, M. (1980). Disaster-induced trauma in rescue workers. *Victimology*, **5**, 287–97.

Dyregov, A. (1989). Caring for helpers in disaster situations: psychological debriefing. *Disaster Management*, **2**, 25–30.

Fitzgerald, M. L., Braudway, C. A., Leeks, D., Padgett, M. B., Swartz, A. L., Samter, J., Gary-Stephens, M. & Dellinger, N. (1993). Debriefing: a therapeutic intervention. *Military Medicine*, **158**, 542–5.

Flannery, R. B., Fulton, P., Tausch, J. & Deloffi, A. Y. (1991). A program to help staff cope with psychological sequelae of assaults by patients. *Hospital and Community Psychiatry*, **42**, 935–8.

Ford, J., Shaw, D., Sennhauser, S., Greaves, D., Thacker, B., Chandler, P., Schwartz, L. & McClain, V. (1993). Psychological debriefing after Operation Desert Storm: marital and family assessment and intervention. *Journal of Social Issues*, **49**, 73–102.

Freedy, J. F. & Donkervoet, J. C. (1995). Traumatic stress: an overview of the field. In J. R. Freedy & S. E. Hobfull (Eds.) *Traumatic Stress: From Theory to Practice* (pp. 3–28). New York: Plenum Press.

Freud, S. (1937). Construction in analysis. In *The Complete Psychological Works of Sigmund Freud*, standard edn, vol. 25, pp. 255–69. London: Hogarth Press, (Reprinted 1964).

Fullerton, C. S., Ursano, R.J., Kao, T. & Bhartiya, V. (1992). The chemical and biological warfare environment: psychological responses and social support in a high stress environment.

Journal of Applied Social Psychology, **22**, 1608–23.

Gal, R. (1986). *A Portrait of an Israeli Soldier*. Westport, CT: Greenwood Press.

Green, B. L., Grace, M. C. & Gleser, G. C. (1985). Identifying survivors at risk: long term impairment following the Beverly Hills Supper Club fire. *Journal of Consulting and Clinical Psychology*, **53**, 672–8.

Griffiths, J. & Watts, R. (1992). *The Kempsey and Grafton Bus Crashes: The Aftermath*. East Lismore, New South Wales: Instructional Design Solutions.

Hausman, W. & Rioch, D. (1967). Military psychiatry. *Archives of General Psychiatry*, **16**, 727–39.

Horowitz, M. J. (1986). *Stress Response Syndromes*. London: Jason Aronson Inc.

Hytten, L. & Hasle, A. (1989). Firefighters: a study of stress and coping. *Acta Psychiatrica Scandinavica*, **80**, Suppl. 355, 50–5.

Ingraham, L. & Manning, F. (1986). American military psychiatry. In R. A. Gabriel (Ed.) *Military Psychiatry* (pp. 25–65). New York: Greenwood Press.

Janoff-Bulman, R. (1985). The aftermath of victimisation: rebuilding shattered assumptions. In C. R. Figley (Ed.), *Trauma and its Wake: The Study and Treatment of Post-traumatic Stress Disorder* (pp. 15–35). New York: Brunner/Mazel.

Jenkins S. H. (1996). Social support and debriefing efficacy among medical workers after a mass shooting incident. *Journal of Social Behaviour and Personality*, **11**, 477–92.

Johnson, D. R., Rosenheck, R., Fontana, A., Lubin, H., Charney, D. & Southwick, S. (1996). Outcome of intensive treatment for combat-related posttraumatic stress disorder. *American Journal of Psychiatry*, **153**, 771–7.

Johnson, L. B., Cline, D. W., Marcum, J. M. & Intress, J. L. (1992). Effectiveness of a stress recovery unit during the Persian Gulf War. *Hospital and Community Psychiatry*, **43**, 829–31.

Jones, D. R. (1985). Secondary disaster victims: the emotional impact of recovering and identifying human remains. *American Journal of Psychiatry*, **142**, 303–7.

Kenardy, J. A., Webster, R. A., Lewin, T. J., Carr, V. J., Hazell, P. L. & Carter, G. L. (1996). Stress debriefing and patterns of recovery following a natural disaster. *Journal of Traumatic Stress*, **9**, 37–49.

Kormos, H. R. (1978). The nature of combat stress. In C. R. Figley (Ed.) *Stress Disorders among Vietnam Veterans*. New York: Brunner/Mazel.

Kulka, R. A., Schlenger, W. E., Fairbank, J. A., Hough, R. L., Jordan, B. K., Marmar, C. R. & Weiss, D.A. (1990). *Trauma and the Vietnam War Generation*. New York: Brunner/Mazel.

Lundin, T. (1994). The treatment of acute trauma: posttraumatic stress disorder prevention. *Psychiatric Clinics of North America*, **17**, 385–91.

Lyubomirsky, S. & Nolen-Hoeksema, S. (1993). Self-perpetuating properties of dysphoric rumination. *Journal of Personality and Social Psychology*, **65**, 339–49.

Lyubomirsky, S. & Nolen-Hoeksema, S. (1995). Effects of self-focussed rumination on negative thinking interpersonal problem solving. *Journal of Personality and Social Psychology*, **69**, 176–90.

Marshall, S. L. A. (1944). *Island victory*. New York: Penguin Books.

Marshall, S. L. A. (1956). *Pork Chop Hill*. New York: William Morrow & Co.

McCarroll, J. E., James, E., Ursano, R. J., Fullerton, C. S. & Lundy, A. C. (1995). Anticipatory stress of handling human remains from the Persian Gulf War: Predictors of intrusion and avoidance. *Journal of Nervous and Mental Disease*, **183**, 698–703.

Melton, C. (1985). The days after: coping with after effects of the Delta 1–1022 crash. *Firehouse*, December, 49–50.

Mitchell, J. T. (1981). *Emergency Response to Crisis: A Crisis Intervention Guidebook of Emergency Service Personnel*. Bowie, MD: Brady Co.

Mitchell, J. T. (1982). Recovery from rescue. *Response Magazine*, Fall, 7–10.

Mitchell, J. T. (1983). When disaster strikes. *Journal of Emergency Medical Services*, **8**, 36–9.

Mitchell, J. T. (1986). Critical incident stress management. *Response*, **5**, 24–5.

Mitchell, J. & Bray, G. (1990). *Emergency Services Stress*. Englewood Cliffs, NJ: Prentice Hall.

Neria, Y. & Solomon, Z. (1999). Prevention of posttraumatic reactions: debriefing and frontline treatment. In P. Saigh & J. D. Bremner (Eds.) *Posttraumatic Stress Disorder: A Comprehensive Text* (pp. 309–26). Boston, MA: Allyn & Bacon, Inc.

Norris, F. H. & Thompson, M. P. (1995). Applying community psychology to the prevention of trauma and traumatic life events. In J. R. Freedy & S. E. Hobfull (Eds.) *Traumatic Stress: From Theory to Practice* (pp. 3–28). New York: Plenum Press.

Orr, S. P. & Kaloupek, D. G. (1997). Psychophysiological assessment of posttraumatic stress disorder. In J. P. Wilson & T. M. Keane (Eds.). *Assessing Psychological Trauma and PTSD* (pp. 69–97). New York: Guilford Press.

Panagapoulos, M. C. (1980). Psychiatric casualties in battle. Lecture delivered at the 9th International Advanced Course for Young Medical Officers, Athens, Greece.

Pennebaker, J. W. (1990). *Opening Up: The Healing Power of Confiding in Others*. New York: William Morrow.

Pettera, R. L., Johnson, B. M. & Zimmer, R. (1969). Psychiatric management of combat reactions with emphasis on a reaction unique to Vietnam. *Military Medicine*, **134**, 673–8.

Raphael, B. (1986). *When Disaster Strikes: How Individuals and Communities Cope with Catastrophe*. New York: Basic Books.

Raphael, B., Singh, B., Bradbury, L. & Lambert, F. (1983). Who helps the helpers? The effects of disaster on rescue workers. *Omega*, **14**, 9–20.

Robinson, R. & Mitchell, J. (1993). Evaluation of psychological debriefings. *Journal of Traumatic Stress*, **6**, 367–82.

Salmon, T. W. (1919). War neuroses and their lesson. *New York Medical Journal*, **109**, 993–4.

Shalev, A. Y. (1994). Debriefing following traumatic exposure. In R. J. Ursano, B. G. McCaughey & C. S. Fullerton (Eds.) *Individual and Community Responses to Trauma and Disaster: The Structure of Human Chaos* (pp. 201–19). Cambridge: Cambridge University Press.

Shalev, A. Y. (1996). Stress versus traumatic stress: from acute homeostatic reactions to chronic psychopathology. In B. A. van der Kolk, A. C. McFarlane & L. Weisæth (Eds.) *Traumatic Stress: The Effects of Overwhelming Experience on Mind, Body, and Society* (pp. 77–101). New York: Guilford Press.

Solomon, Z. (1993). *Combat Stress Reaction: The Enduring Toll of War*. New York: Plenum Press.

Solomon, Z. & Benbenishty, R. (1986). The role of proximity, immediacy, and expectancy in frontline treatment of combat stress reaction among Israelis in the Lebanon War. *American Journal of Psychiatry*, **143**, 613–17.

Spiller, R. J. (1980). S. L. A. Marshall and the ratio of fire. *Royal United Service Institute for Defence Studies Journal*, **133**, 63–71.

Stallard, P. & Law, F. (1993). Screening and psychological debriefing of adolescent survivors of life-threatening events. *British Journal of Psychiatry*, **163**, 660–5.

Turner, R. J. (1981). Social support as a contingency in psychological well being. *Journal of Health and Social Behaviour*, **22**, 357–67.

Turner, S. W., Thompson, J. & Rosser, R. M. (1993). The Kings Cross fire: early psychological reactions and implications for organizing a 'phase-two' response. In J. P. Wilson & B. Raphael (Eds.) *International Handbook of Traumatic Stress Syndromes* (pp. 451–9). New York: Plenum Press.

Wagner, M. (1979). Airline disaster: a stress debrief program for police. *Police Stress*, **2**, 16–20.

12

Debriefing post disaster: follow-up after a major earthquake

Justin A. Kenardy and Vaughan J. Carr

EDITORIAL COMMENTS

Kenardy and Carr review experience of debriefing as reported by participants in a community-based study following an earthquake in Newcastle, New South Wales. They also review other work such as that of Mitchell's group, Watt's studies and other research. They note that the perceptions of helpfulness as described in Watt's work are nevertheless frequently uncorrelated with outcome – or, as Ørner has more recently reported, debriefing appears to be perceived as helpful by those who seem to need it least.

The issue of expectancy that debriefing will be beneficial is important, and needs to be addressed in any critical review of debriefing and its potential effectiveness. The authors note that their study was not originally designed as an empirical test of debriefing, but rather was a naturalistic opportunity to incorporate systematic questions into their investigation of the consequences of the earthquake and to explore specifically issues for professional and volunteer disaster workers. Their study evaluated and compared individuals (helpers) who reported having been debriefed with those helpers who did not experience debriefing but were equivalent in terms of personal threat experience and levels of stress in 'helping' roles, as well as working in dangerous settings. The debriefed group was composed of more 'counsellors' and more women. Their findings report that 80% found debriefing helpful, but outcomes (measured by the Impact of Event Scale and the General Health Questionnaires) were no different, nor was rate of recovery. In fact they found a reduced rate of recovery in those who were debriefed.

Kenardy and Carr critically appraise the broad use of debriefing, and state that many studies, like their own, question the usefulness of the technique in preventing adverse psychological outcomes; indeed they discuss the possibilities of debriefing contributing to adverse outcomes. They also note the importance of personal sources of support, such as the family, in talking through and sharing the emotional experience of disasters. Many of the criticisms they raise, including those of lack of evaluation and overrapid development of new models, could equally be applied to many psychological interventions in the real world as opposed to the research trial setting.

Useful insights are offered into the lack of a model informing much debriefing either as a form of brief therapy (which it cannot be) or a preventive intervention. The 'dose' may be too little, too soon, inappropriate for such goals, and may even contribute negatively by influencing those for whom it is provided into taking symptom pathways instead of coming to resolution. Positive evaluations may reflect cycles of mutual reinforcement between debriefers and those debriefed.

Quite rightly the authors conclude that debriefing, as provided broadly, requires extensive further and detailed scientific evaluation, and at this stage should be seen as an experimental intervention. They, like many others, consider that debriefing should never be compulsory and that its use must be very carefully questioned.

This chapter is a useful systematic naturalistic study, with acknowledged limitations. It provides further caution about the broadly based and extensive use of debriefing in communities affected by disasters.

Introduction

Psychological (or stress) debriefing is an intervention intended to facilitate the prevention of, or recovery from, the adverse psychological sequelae of traumatic events. This is said to be achieved by the provision of information regarding the expected reactions to such events, disclosing one's experience of, and emotional reactions to, the event, and being given preparation for managing future experiences arising in relation to the event. It has become very popular owing to increased recognition of adverse psychological effects post trauma. Over its history, debriefing has tended to move from being a 'natural' response in the aftermath of a traumatic event to become an obligatory service to be provided for those suffering from, or deemed to be at risk of, post-traumatic stress. However, this has occurred without adequate empirical evaluations of its effectiveness. Instead, its reputed effectiveness has been based largely on its perceived or face validity. Until recently most helping professionals involved in its application would probably have assumed that evidence of its efficacy had been documented. In fact, there have been many anecdotal reports of the effectiveness of stress debriefing, but only a handful of systematic evaluations of its effectiveness or efficacy (see Wessely et al., 1998).

Evidence supporting debriefing

Robinson & Mitchell (1995) claimed that there is overwhelming anecdotal evidence for the effectiveness of debriefing. This, the authors say, is based on the widespread and continued use of debriefing, the 'Why would so many people use it if it did not work?' argument. In fact, the evidence from evaluations of debriefing indicate that reported perceptions of debriefing helpfulness by recipients are generally positive, and that there is a general improvement in psychological and other functioning over time. However, there are significant problems with this supportive evidence. We will use an example to illustrate. Robinson & Mitchell (1993) reported on a series of 31 debriefings of 288 emergency and welfare workers. Participants were asked to rate whether they felt that the debriefing was

valuable. They were also asked to evaluate whether their distress following the debriefing had changed and, if so, whether it was attributable to the debriefing. Most participants reported that debriefing was helpful, a finding which has been replicated many times in the literature (e.g. Hytten & Hasle, 1989; Shapiro & Kunkler, 1990; Griffiths & Watts, 1992). Unfortunately, the validity of self-reported helpfulness of debriefing is in doubt as it is uncorrelated with psychological outcomes (Griffiths & Watts, 1992; Kenardy et al., 1996). There is, moreover, the problem of the validity of attributed cause of change as a measure of outcome. In other words, the expectation that debriefing will occur and the anticipated benefit associated with debriefing will bias the individual's evaluation of the relationship between the debriefing and subsequent perceptions of improvement in well-being irrespective of the cause of that improvement. This is particularly relevant as there is a normal course of recovery following most traumatic events (see e.g. Carr et al., 1997a) that may further confirm such subjective judgements of the helpfulness of debriefing. In short, evidence from anecdotal or uncontrolled studies of debriefing outcome is likely to support debriefing because of their methodological flaws rather than in spite of them.

In contrast, we now report on a naturalistic evaluation of debriefing in which a control was available.

The Newcastle earthquake (New South Wales, Australia)

Description

The data collected in our investigation of the psychosocial sequelae of the 1989 Newcastle earthquake provided an opportunity to examine the effectiveness of psychological debriefing. Although this study was not originally designed as an empirical test of debriefing, some data were obtained that permitted an examination of the issue. Before giving an account of this naturalistic investigation of psychological debriefing, a brief description of the Newcastle earthquake study is outlined in order to provide some understanding of the context within which the debriefing study was undertaken.

Soon after the earthquake, staff from the University of Newcastle commenced a prospective study of the psychosocial impact of this large-scale trauma on the community. It took the form of a longitudinal study of a community sample of Newcastle adults who were assessed on four occasions by postal questionnaire over two years (for an overview of the study, see Carr et al., 1997c). As part of that study a supplementary sample of professional and volunteer disaster workers was identified through various agencies for the purpose of documenting the recovery patterns of this at-risk group and contrasting their responses to the disaster against other at-risk groups (see Carr et al., 1997b). Thus the longitudinal methodology for the disaster workers was the same as that used in the larger community sample. In addition, a small proportion of the community sample had acted in the role of disaster workers, but had not been specifically identified through the agencies used to recruit the supplementary sample. Of 845 subjects who were assessed initially and completed one or more of the three follow-up surveys, 195 professional and volunteer emergency service and welfare workers (the 'helpers') were identified and similarly followed-up at approximately six-monthly intervals over more than two years following the earthquake. Questions about psychological debriefing had been included in the questionnaires administered in the first follow-up survey. Thus we could directly compare the long-term patterns of recovery of the 62 individuals in our sample of helpers who reported having been debriefed against 133 who were not debriefed. The two groups of helpers had had similar degrees of exposure to threat-related experience, similar levels of perceived stress in relation to their helping role, and were equally likely to have worked in threatening (i.e. dangerous) situations. There were slightly more individuals who acted as counsellors within the debriefed group, and there was also a greater proportion of women who were debriefed.

Results

The findings of this study, which have been published by Kenardy et al., (1996), were unexpected. Although debriefing was generally reported by its recipients as helpful, with 80% (50 of 62) reporting it as at least somewhat helpful, no relationship was found between the reported degree of helpfulness of debriefing and psychological outcome. The latter was measured in terms of symptoms of post-traumatic stress and other psychological distress using standardized measures, the Impact of Event Scale (IES) and the General Health Questionnaire-12 (GHQ-12). Surprisingly, there was also no relationship found between being debriefed and rate of recovery. That is, if a person had been debriefed he or she was no more likely to have a better rate of recovery than someone who had not been debriefed. In fact, there was even a trend for a reduced rate of recovery amongst debriefed helpers who showed less improvement in symptoms (IES and GHQ-12) than those who were not debriefed.

Methodological issues

As already stated, our study was not originally designed as an empirical test of the efficacy of debriefing. In fact, it would have been very difficult under the circumstances of the disaster to conduct a randomized controlled trial in which debriefing was withheld from a subgroup of emergency service workers. Voluntary participation rates for such a study would have been very low, not to mention the apparent ethical problems of withholding an intervention that was then generally believed to be necessary and useful. Furthermore, the actual debriefing protocols used were not constrained. Some professional organizations would have had debriefing as an integral component of their usual procedures while other individuals would have received debriefing organized on an ad hoc basis. The absence of standardization of debriefing procedures meant that the content, quality and appropriateness of the debriefing were all unknown. Even if an empirical evaluation of debriefing had been incorporated into the study design, it would have been logistically very difficult to ensure control of the conduct of the debriefing under the circumstances of the disaster aftermath. Nevertheless, at the time of the disaster, the dominant debriefing model was that of Mitchell (1983), and it was assumed that this model was applied in line with usual practice. Thus the conduct of debriefing was probably valid in the sense that it was more representative of actual practice than would have been the case if the debriefing had been subjected to a research protocol.

Notwithstanding the failure to randomize to debriefing versus no-debriefing control conditions, we did control for factors that might have influenced differences between the debriefed versus not debriefed groups by statistically adjusting for precursors such as degree of exposure to danger and loss, and self-reported distress. However, statistically controlling for these potentially confounding factors did not alter the findings summarized above. While a randomized, controlled trial is the 'gold standard' for evaluation of treatment effectiveness, it can be argued, in defence of the study's methodology, that random assignment in controlled trials may not necessarily provide the strongest support for causal inferences (Rubin, 1991). A naturalistic study can potentially be as powerful if the factors that predispose selection to one or another condition can be adjusted for (cf. Rosenbaum & Rubin, 1983). As previously indicated, in the case of the Newcastle earthquake, a randomized trial might have created such a biassed sample, through participant self-selection, as to render the study invalid.

At the time of publishing our debriefing data we were circumspect about the implications of our findings (Kenardy et al., 1996). In particular, we did not want to make recommendations that indicated that debriefing was ineffective or, indeed, potentially harmful. In retrospect, we were probably too conservative. The pattern of other findings using a nonrandomized design suggests that our results were valid (e.g. McFarlane, 1988; Hytten and Hasle, 1989; Deahl et al., 1994; Carlier et al., 1998) and studies employing randomized design methods have since then not contradicted our original findings (Hobbs et al., 1996; Lee et al., 1996; Bisson et al., 1997).

In summary, the naturalistic study design used in our investigation, together with an approach to data analysis that controlled for potential confounds, supports the validity of our results, which, in turn, concur with those of other naturalistic studies of debriefing as well as those employing a randomized controlled design.

The current state of knowledge

Our study of debriefing allowed us to draw three conclusions. First, there is no relationship between perceived helpfulness of debriefing and psychological outcome measured in terms of psychological distress. Secondly, debriefing is not associated with a greater degree of recovery in psychological morbidity compared with those who are not debriefed. Thirdly, those who are debriefed show less improvement in psychological symptoms than those who are not debriefed. As already outlined, these conclusions are consistent with the results of other published studies of debriefing (Wessley et al., 1998).

One of the criticisms levelled against these conclusions is that the debriefing that took place may have been conducted inadequately. The reasoning behind this charge is faulty, since it is predicated on the belief that there exists a form of debriefing that is effective if applied correctly. However, since there is no valid database of evidence to support this belief, there is no standard against which a particular (mis-)application of debriefing can be compared.

A principal tenet of psychological debriefing as it is currently practised is the usefulness of providing information. However, since this proposition has not been tested empirically, we do not know whether giving information is actually useful. In particular, we do not know what information may be useful to give or for whom it will be useful, when information of what type is best given, how and by whom (see e.g. Watts, Chapter 9; Soloman et al., Chapter 11). For example, some information may trigger a heightened sense of distress in certain individuals and, conceivably, thereby compound psychological morbidity rather than prevent or relieve it. Again, if information is needed should it be presented by a 'trained' debriefer or would a simple brochure be sufficient?

Another foundation of debriefing is that emotional self-disclosure, the articulation of a personal narrative of one's experience of the traumatic event and related feelings, is beneficial. This is simply a version of the ancient belief in the therapeutic value of catharsis, which is often associated with a sense of immediate subjective relief. There are data to support self-disclosure as beneficial under post-trauma circumstances (Greenberg & Stone, 1992). However, it is still unclear when, for whom, and in what way such self-disclosure might be beneficial. For example, it has been suggested (Eysenck, 1968) that incomplete exposure and associated sensitization due to the abbreviated nature of a debriefing might account for a lack of positive outcome among some individuals under some circumstances. While it is commonly reported that talking about a traumatic event is a widely felt need among survivors, this impression may have been created by those who indeed feel such a need, whereas those who do not may have kept even that to themselves. It is not known whether those who wish to talk about their experience benefit from doing so, nor whether those who do not wish to talk should, but these are the expectations of current debriefing practice. If self-disclosure is beneficial, at least for some, does it matter who listens? The effectiveness of the written disclosure paradigm employed by Pennebaker and colleagues (Esterling et al., 1999) suggests that it does not.

It has been said that debriefing sessions may be useful to screen for those likely to develop problems subsequently. Perhaps not talking about the event is an indication of the introverted avoidance coper at risk of significant psychological morbidity at a later date. Notwithstanding some of the findings in our earthquake study (Carr et al., 1997a,b), we still do not know what to look for: 'early warning signs' (if any, what are they, when and how can they best be detected?), 'predisposed' or 'vulnerable' individuals (if any, how are they defined and reliably identified, and what forms of intervention are suited to which vulnerability characteristics?) or pattern of 'exposure' (if any, how is the degree of exposure to be efficiently gauged in relation to different events and, aside from the question of level of exposure, what role is played by the meaning or significance of the event?).

Who debriefs and how?

Much has been said about who should provide debriefing services (Berah et al., 1984; Everstine & Everstine, 1993; Paton, 1995). Given the absence of evidence for the effectiveness of psychological debriefing and the

many unknowns listed above, is there a legitimate role for professional debriefers and, if so, what should comprise their training? Any need that survivors may have for empathic understanding by others of the personal impact of the trauma would support the notion that peers may be the preferred debriefers. Peers may also be more likely than outsiders to comprehend operational and organizational factors as well as the particular social circumstances of the participants. In the Newcastle earthquake study (Carr et al., 1997c), the most commonly used source of support for dealing with the emotional effects of the earthquake comprised family members, friends and neighbours. If the immediate need is one of consolation, soothing and sympathy – and, on the face of it, these are the decent, compassionate responses to those under extreme stress – who better than members of the individual's immediate social network to respond in these ways?

On the other hand, if the debriefing is to be considered part of an overall debriefing management process whose boundaries stretch beyond the actual debriefing, then it could be argued that someone detached from the organization may be more appropriate in order to prevent possible conflicts of interest. The professional qualifications of such a person may be generic (e.g. counsellor) or specific (e.g. mental health professional, clinical psychologist, clinical social worker).

If debriefing is to be provided, and there are substantial medico-legal pressures to do so in spite of the lack of demonstrable effectiveness, how is it to be provided? There are a number of debriefing methods (e.g. Dyregrov, 1989; Mitchell, 1983; Armstrong et al., 1991) with their own protocols. Given their heterogeneity, it is not possible to determine clearly the adequacy or otherwise of one compared with another. In fact, there seems to be an almost organic quality in the ongoing development of debriefing. Newer protocols emerge from older ones without systematic evaluation of either. The new developments seem to be unrelated to empirically based decision-making processes, but rather to clinical experience. One example is how decisions are made in guiding the choice of most appropriate time for the provision of debriefing. There is a commonly held point of view that debriefing should be held as close as possible in time and space to the actual trauma. A time of 72 hours has been identified as the most desirable upper limit. How was this decided and on the basis of what evidence? There is a *prima facie* case, at least, to examine the impact of information provision and emotional self-disclosure at varying times after trauma.

Why debrief?

Psychological debriefing may need to clarify its purpose. If it is indeed to be a preventive intervention in terms of psychological morbidity, then that should guide associated activities such as identification of at-risk participants, follow-up and outcome evaluation. If, on the other hand, its purpose is to bond participants, then that would lead to a very different set of desirable outcomes that could be measured. If it is simply to acquire useful information, then that too should be associated with a particular set of measurable outcomes. Thus one of the key concerns about debriefing is that the intervention is either not having an impact on any factor that is relevant to recovery, or that it is focussing on the wrong target.

There has been concern raised that debriefing is attempting to impact on too broad a range of issues and factors. Debriefing is a very short, circumscribed intervention, and while it is not seen as a form of psychotherapy, it is still remarkably brief as a preventive procedure. As such, it would be hard pressed to produce any significant impact on a vulnerable or at-risk individual or group. Therefore, the failure of debriefing may lie in the low 'dosage' applied. From this, the argument would follow that a larger, more comprehensive approach to post-traumatic stress should be applied. Such has evolved from Mitchell's earlier model, the expanded Critical Incident Stress Management package (Robinson & Mitchell, 1995). The breadth and complexity of this package is intended to provide a more comprehensive stress management approach, but does not easily lend itself to empirical testing.

The other possibility is that debriefing targets the wrong aspects of the immediate post-trauma response, and that it is this error that produces few, no or possibly even adverse effects. This issue is currently being examined in a parallel field of study, the primary pre-

vention of eating disorders. As with traumatic stress, it is quite compelling to intervene at the stage of vulnerability to the development of later problems. Thus many researchers have applied 'preventive' programmes to school-age girls in an attempt to derail the development of pathological eating and weight loss behaviours (Paxton, 1993; Killen et al., 1993; Carter et al., 1997). What is remarkable about these studies is that none has produced any effect on later eating attitudes and behaviours, and in some cases may have produced adverse effects (Carter et al., 1997). Carter and colleagues found a short-term reduction in dysfunctional eating attitudes and behaviours followed by a longer-term increase to higher levels than baseline. One possible explanation for these failures might be that the preventive programmes target knowledge about disordered eating and dieting and, in so doing, facilitate the development of disordered eating attitudes and behaviours. The conceptualization of the problem as a function of lack of awareness of disordered eating issues may have inadvertently led, through mechanisms yet to be identified, to more disordered eating. Another possibility is that information about disordered eating practices and their consequences may simply have no impact on subsequent behaviours. What might have been considered as appropriate targets for change may not have been so. Alternatively, these programmes could have focussed on general preventive strategies that provide the person with skills to deal with overall threats to self-esteem.

Some parallels with debriefing can be drawn. Debriefing identifies the lack of awareness of post-trauma stress responses as a target for change for which information is the putative change agent. Debriefing may lack effectiveness as a preventive strategy because of this. Increased awareness of post-trauma stress responses may actually facilitate these responses in at-risk individuals (Dunning, 1995). At the very least, awareness raising may not be sufficient to prevent these responses.

If debriefing does not work as therapy and is not in fact viewed as a short-term therapy by its proponents, and if it is a very meagre preventive programme, what is its purpose? Part of the answer to this question may lie in the positive evaluation of the debriefing process by participants. That is, the recipients of debriefing often regard it as having been helpful. In our study, as with others mentioned previously (e.g. Griffiths & Watts, 1992), there was a strong endorsement of the debriefing process by participants. This could have an indirect perpetuating effect on the ongoing provision of debriefing. Since there is a positive feedback to debriefers from participants about the process, this is likely to lead to positive feelings amongst the debriefers concerning their impact on the problem and their own self-efficacy as debriefers. This will mean that debriefers will approach future debriefing sessions with an expectation of a positive evaluation of the process. Perhaps, in part, debriefing functions to meet the needs of the debriefer by helping to validate the debriefer's view of the process as helpful and therefore confirms a view of himself or herself as an effective debriefer.

It may also be that debriefing is helpful in unintended ways less accessible through measurements. For instance, it may simply function as a medium for the recognition of the individual's experiences and trauma. However admirable, there may be more parsimonious ways to achieve this.

Conclusions

The great attraction of debriefing is that it has excellent face validity in the eyes of its practitioners and those of many members of the public. It appears to be a humane response to the psychological distress experienced following a trauma. There is even an influential view that psychological debriefing ought to be routinely prescribed after all traumatic events. If there were compelling evidence that debriefing contributes to the recovery of an individual this position might be defensible. But this is not the case. There is now evidence from randomized controlled studies to show that psychological debriefing is not an effective intervention in terms of preventing post-trauma psychological morbidity in victims of trauma and may even have an adverse impact for some participants. Both increased awareness through the provision of information and inappropriate self-disclosure may be the means by which harmful effects are produced. As helping profes-

sionals we must continue to bear in mind the dictum 'above all else do no harm'.

One of the factors contributing to the growth of the psychological debriefing movement may be the effect it has on the debriefers themselves. Positive feedback from the recipients of debriefing is likely to be rewarding for the debriefers and thereby provide a source of validation of their efforts, with attendant enhancement of their sense of professional efficacy, not to mention self-esteem, as well as the need to assuage the very frequent feelings of helplessness experienced in the case of disaster. If there is a role for debriefing, it may be better left with the peer group or the individual's immediate social support network, since there is limited evidence that professional debriefing has more to offer.

Despite the fact that the debriefing movement has flourished in recent times, the application of psychological debriefing must be regarded as an experimental intervention. As such, it should be subjected to the same constraints on its implementation as any other experimental intervention. In this context, the procedures of the empirical trial, or at least those of the naturalistic study, should be employed in association with any implementation of debriefing in the field. The onus is on the advocates and practitioners of debriefing to provide what is, so far, resoundingly lacking, namely evidence for the effectiveness of what they purport. If this is not forthcoming, it is time for the movement to move on.

REFERENCES

Armstrong, K., O'Callahan, W. & Marmar, C. R. (1991). Debriefing Red Cross disaster personnel: the multiple stressor debriefing model. *Journal of Traumatic Stress*, **4**, 481–93.

Berah, E. F., Jones, H. J. & Valent, P. (1984). The experience of a mental health team involved in the early phase of a disaster. *Australian and New Zealand Journal of Psychiatry*, **18**, 354–8.

Bisson, J., Jenkins, P., Alexander, J. & Bannister, C. (1997). Randomised controlled trial of psychological debriefing for victims of acute burn trauma. *British Journal of Psychiatry*, **171**, 78–81.

Carlier, I. V. E., Lamberts, R. D., van Uchelen, A. J. & Gersons, P. R. (1998). Effectiveness of psychological debriefing: a controlled study of traumatised police officers. *Stress Medicine*, **14**, 143–8.

Carr, V. J., Lewin, T. J., Kenardy, J., Webster, R. A., Hazell, P. L. & Carter, G. L. (1997a). Psychosocial sequelae of the 1989 Newcastle earthquake. III. Role of vulnerability factors in post-disaster morbidity. *Psychological Medicine*, **27**, 179–90.

Carr, V. J., Lewin, T. J., Webster, R. A., Kenardy, J., Hazell, P. L. & Carter, G. L. (1997b). Psychosocial sequelae of the 1989 Newcastle earthquake. II. Exposure and morbidity profiles during the first two years post-disaster. *Psychological Medicine*, **27**, 167–78.

Carr, V. J., Lewin, T. J., Webster, R. A. & Kenardy, J. (1997c). A synthesis of the findings from the Quake Impact Study: a two-year investigation of the psychosocial sequelae of the 1989 Newcastle earthquake. *International Journal of Social Psychiatry and Psychiatric Epidemiology*, **32**, 123–36.

Carter, J. C., Stewart, D. A., Dunn, V. J. & Fairburn, C. G. (1997). Primary prevention of eating disorders: might it do more harm than good? *International Journal of Eating Disorders*, **22**, 167–72.

Deahl, M. P., Gillham, A. B., Thomas, J., Searle, M. M. & Srinivasan, M. (1994). Psychological sequelae following the Gulf War: factors associated with subsequent morbidity and the effectiveness of psychological debriefing. *British Journal of Psychiatry*, **265**, 60–5.

Dunning, C. (1995). Risk management in the emergency services. Keynote paper presented at the National Conference of the Australian Society for Traumatic Stress Studies, March, Hobart.

Dyregrov, A. (1989). Caring for helpers in disaster situations: psychological debriefing. *Disaster Management*, **2**, 25–30.

Esterling, B. A., L'Abate, L., Murray, E. J. & Pennebaker, J. W. (1999). Empirical foundations for writing in prevention and psychotherapy: mental and physical health outcomes. *Clinical Psychology Review*, **19**, 79–96.

Everstine, D. & Everstine, L. (1993). *The Trauma Response: Treatment for Emotional Injury*. New York: W. W. Norton.

Eysenck, H. J. (1968). A theory of incubation of anxiety/fear responses. *Behaviour Research and Therapy*, **6**, 309–22.

Greenberg, M. A. & Stone, A. A. (1992). Emotional disclosure about traumas and its relation to health: effects of previous disclosure and trauma severity. *Journal of Personality and Social Psychology*, **63**, 75–84.

Griffiths, J. & Watts, T. (1992). *The Kempsey and Grafton Bus Crashes: The Aftermath*. Lismore, New South Wales: Instructional Design Solutions, University of New England.

Hobbs, M., Mayou, R., Harrison, B. & Worlock, P. (1996). A randomised controlled trial of psychological debriefing for victims of road traffic accidents. *British Medical Journal*, **313**, 1438–9.

Hytten, K. & Hasle, A. (1989). Firefighters: a study of stress and coping. *Acta Psychiatrica Scandinavica*, **80**, Suppl. 355, 50–5.

Kenardy, J. A., Webster, R. A., Lewin, T. J., Carr, V. J., Hazell, P. L. & Carter, G. L. (1996). Stress debriefing and patterns of recovery following a natural disaster. *Journal of Traumatic Stress*, **9**, 37–49.

Killen, J. D., Taylor, C. B., Hammer, L. D., Litt, I., Wilson, D. M., Rich, T., Hayward, C., Simmonds, B., Kraemer, H. & Varady, A. (1993). An attempt to modify unhealthy eating attitudes and weight regulation practices of young adolescent girls. *International Journal of Eating Disorders*, **13**, 369–84.

Lee, C., Slade, P. & Lygo, V. (1996). The influence of psychological debriefing on emotional adaptation in women following early miscarriage: a preliminary study. *British Journal of Medical Psychology*, **69**, 47–58.

McFarlane, A. C. (1988). The longitudinal course of posttraumatic morbidity: the range of outcomes and their predictors. *Journal of Nervous and Mental Disease*, **176**, 30–9.

Mitchell, J. T. (1983). When disaster strikes. The critical incident stress debriefing process. *Journal of Emergency Medical Services*, **8**, 36–9.

Paton, D. (1995). Debriefing and recovery from work-related trauma: the relationship between process, environment and counselling intervention. *Australian Counselling Psychologist*, **11**, 39–44.

Paxton, S. J. (1993). A prevention program for disturbed eating and body dissatisfaction in adolescent girls: a 1-year follow-up. *Health Education Research*, **8**, 43–51.

Robinson, R. C. & Mitchell, J. T. (1993). Evaluation of psychological debriefing. *Journal of Traumatic Stress*, **6**, 367–82.

Robinson, R. C. & Mitchell, J. T. (1995). Getting some balance back into the debriefing debate. *Bulletin of the Australian Psychological Society*, **17**, 5–10.

Rosenbaum, P. R. & Rubin, D. B. (1983). The central role of the propensity score in observational studies for causal effects. *Biometrika*, **70**, 41–55.

Rubin, D. (1991). Practical implications of modes of statistical inference for causal effects and the critical role of the assignment mechanism. *Biometrics*, **47**, 1213–34.

Shapiro, D. & Kunkler, J. (1990). *Psychological Support for Hospital Staff Initiated by Clinical Psychologists in the Aftermath of the Hillsborough Disaster*. Sheffield: Sheffield Health Authority Mental Health Services Unit.

Wessely, S., Rose, S. & Bisson, J. (1998). A systematic review of brief psychological interventions ('debriefing') for the treatment of immediate trauma related symptoms and the prevention of posttraumatic stress disorder (Cochrane Review). *The Cochrane Library*, **3**. Oxford: Update Software.

Debriefing after disaster

Tom Lundin

Lundin reviews some of the studies that show the potential impact of disaster stress on disaster workers, rescue workers and others. These lead to conclusions about the need to try to address or mitigate any such effects. 'Debriefing' has been widely applied but rarely researched or examined systematically in terms of the changes that such an intervention might induce in populations of rescuers to whom it is provided.

In examining research studies from widely differing disasters such as the Armenian earthquake, the *Estonia* ferry disaster, and of Swedish NATO soldiers in Bosnia, the author shows that traumatic stress symptoms decrease over time, but that this may not be able to be related to debriefing. Degrees of preparation, training and previous experience may be more significant, as may 'professional' as compared with 'non-professional' roles. The enormous difficulties in identifying the influence of particular factors, including specific interventions, is highlighted in this research. However, it is of interest to note that with the largest number of subjects (Swedish NATO soldiers), peer support plus post-incident defusing had the most positive effect on mental health whereas peer support alone, or peer support followed by defusing and debriefing, had no better effect than no support at all, another finding indicating caution about debriefing. The author also comments on the importance of interventions being 'owned' by the system and suggests that the research questions and evaluation framework should be set up as a 'we' project, as should be debriefing. If this occurs, the research itself may also serve therapeutic or debriefing ends.

This chapter highlights both the importance of research in this field, particularly in disaster contexts, and how difficult it is to research the important questions in ways that meet rigid methodological criteria. Importantly, however, it shows the need for common core methodologies and measures, and the building of a knowledge base by critically 'pooling' findings from diverse sources.

Different types of disaster

After a disaster, different groups of people are affected in different ways. Disaster workers, like rescue and health care personnel, may well be directly or indirectly affected, according to the circumstances. There are considerable differences between military (Lundin & Otto, 1989; Lundin & Eriksson, 1997) and civilian disasters in the ways in which they affect the psyche, which might also influence the individual reactions. In a military setting, those directly affected and rescue workers will usually be the same people. Personnel on the battlefield are expected to risk their health and even their lives. This fact will influence strongly the ways in which they react. Among the civilian disasters there is an important difference between natural and human-engendered disaster and it is also necessary to distinguish between accidental and intentional disasters that lead to somatic injuries or death.

The impact of the disaster event on rescue workers will depend on several factors. First, it is necessary to consider whether there is the possibility of carrying out an effective rescue operation. This will depend amongst other things on: climate or weather; how far away from emergency care the incident has occurred; whether or not there are any survivors; and whether the incident has occurred in the air, ashore or at sea. It is also important to consider the distance between the epicentre of the disaster and the homes of survivors and relatives. An accident with no survivors and a large number of more or less mutilated dead bodies will imply particularly severe psychological stress. Even when the dead bodies have been taken away, visiting the disaster area may have a strong impact (Lindstrom & Lundin, 1982; Alexander & Wells, 1991; Fullerton et al., 1993).

Another aspect that influences the possibility of performing good rescue work is the demography of the directly affected group, e.g. whether they:

have the same language, ethnic or cultural background;
are living in the same area;
have come from the same place of work or school class;
have the same interests, or;
are members of an occasional group, as in most train accidents and aeroplane crashes.

All these and many other factors including personal maturity, education, training and earlier experiences strongly influence the reactions amongst rescue workers and their future needs for support (Hytten & Hasle, 1989), counselling and sometimes psychological treatment. Some examples of post-traumatic morbidity in disaster workers (McFarlane, 1987, 1988a,b, 1989) and their variable experiences are outlined below.

Nine months post disaster, 134 rescuers involved in an off-shore oil rig disaster were investigated (Ersland et al., 1989) by using a structured self-report questionnaire to chart their experiences of coping with disaster impact stressors and their mental and physical health nine months after the disaster. Seventy-six per cent of the rescuers reported that they had been exposed to danger during the rescue operation, and 62% found the experience to be their worst ever. The stressors inherent in this type of disaster seem to satisfy the *Diagnostic and Statistical Manual of Mental Disorders* (DSM-III–IV; American Psychiatric Association, 1980, 1994) stressor criterion for post-traumatic stress disorder (PTSD). Nine months after the disaster, 24% reported their mental health to be poor owing to the disaster impact, and only the most experienced rescuers had a low health risk compared with the others. The Impact of Event Scale (IES), measuring post-traumatic morbidity, was completed by 119 rescue workers as a measure of disaster impact.

Police officers who were involved in body-handling duties following the Piper Alpha disaster and for whom there were available data from predisaster assessments, have been studied (Alexander et al., 1991; see also Chapter 8, this volume). The results have been interpreted in terms of issues such as the officers' own coping strategies, and major organizational and managerial factors influencing positive outcomes. There were no high levels of post-traumatic distress or psychiatric morbidity. Ursano et al. (1995; see also Chapter 2, this volume) have examined acute and long-term intrusive and avoidance symptoms, depression, and PTSD, in disaster workers exposed to traumatic death after the *USS Iowa* gun turret explosion. Fifty-four volunteer body handlers were assessed at 1, 4 and 13 months. The IES was used. Intrusive and avoidance symptoms were elevated at 1, 4 and 13 months, and decreased over time. Body handler disaster workers who were single reported more avoidance than those who were married. These results indicate that exposure to traumatic death increases intrusive and avoidance symptoms and that symptoms can persist for many months.

Peritraumatic emotional distress and post-traumatic stress reactions among rescue workers after an earthquake freeway collapse were studied by Marmar et al. (1996). Nine per cent of the samples were characterized as having symptom levels typical of psychiatric outpatients. Compared with lower distress responders, those with greater distress reported greater exposure, greater peritraumatic emotional distress, greater peritraumatic dissociation, greater perceived threat, and less preparation for the critical incident.

Forty-three rescuers responding to a bus crash accident answered questionnaires at 1 and 13 months after the crash (Dyregrov et al., 1996). Voluntary and professional helpers were compared, using the IES. For all helpers taken together, the decline in IES intrusion and

IES total scores was significant between 1 and 13 months. The voluntary helpers reported significantly more intrusion and avoidance on the IES at 1 month than did professional helpers, and for avoidance the voluntary helpers still evidenced a significantly higher score than did professional helpers at 13 months.

Disasters and rescue workers

The Borås fire and its aftermath

On 9 June 1978 the spring term of all Swedish schools ended and around the country thousands of young people of between 18 and 22 years were celebrating their graduation. This was also the case in Borås, a town of just over 100 000 inhabitants in the centre of the textile industry area, 60 kilometres east of Gothenburg. On this evening one of the main hotels in Borås, the City Hotel, had over 500 young guests in the two restaurants, the nightclub and the disco. In the early morning of 10 June, at 2.35 a.m., during the last dance, a disastrous fire broke out. It started like an explosion on the first floor. Within a few minutes the whole place was like an inferno, with black smoke, heat and chaos. When the fire started about 175 people were still in the restaurants. Twenty of them were killed. Fifty-six close relatives were bereaved (Table 13.1).

The rescue and health care personnel (Table 13.1) were studied using questionnaires and personal interviews 10 months after the disaster. The response rate to the questionnaires was high, 93.5% ($n = 144$) (Figure 13.1).

This high rate of response was seen as evidence that such an investigation was of great interest to rescue workers and might perhaps meet a need. It was found that 50% had close contacts with the injured and about the same with relatives of the fire victims. Fifty-four persons were involved in transporting the dead bodies and 17 in identification. It was possible to identify some reactions that might be associated with PTSD (Table 13.2).

Eighty-three people had some education and training in disaster reactions, but most of these found their education inadequate. The psychological reactions started for around 50% of the rescue personnel in the

Table 13.1. Affected persons in the Borås fire disaster 1978

	Number
Directly affected	
Close relatives	
Parents	30
Siblings	26
Injured	49
Uninjured in the hotel	61
Uninjured outside the hotel	24
Hotel staff	17
Indirectly affected	154

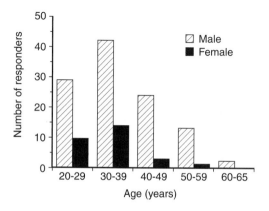

Figure 13.1. Health care and rescue personnel: responders.

early stage of the rescue operation – for some virtually directly when they were confronted with the disaster. Three types of reaction were found:

1. Those with a profound initial experience of chaos and shock.
2. Those with no such experiences but who described a gradually increasing awareness that this situation was a tragedy, which caused various emotional reactions later during the acute phase.
3. A third, small group described neither feelings of chaos nor any evident reactions later.

Some rescue workers developed a so-called 'Superman' reaction, which meant that they functioned effectively and without emotional reactions while wearing their uniforms. They developed symptoms and reactions later.

Table 13.2. PTSD symptoms among rescue and health care personnel ($n = 144$)

	Recurrent and intrusive thoughts (%)	Repetitive nightmares (%)	Sleep disturbance (%)
Often	66	3	8
Sometimes	30	19	28
Seldom	4	58	64

Table 13.3. Groups of disaster workers in terms of appearance on the scene of the disaster

On duty	Reserve	Voluntary	Additional
Fire fighters	Civil defence	Red Cross	Industrial civil defence
Police	Rescue centre	Dog handlers	Press
Health care ambulance staff	Social services	Clergy	Home defence
	Emergency telephone operators		Military forces
	Some groups of health care personnel		

Questions for the follow-up of disaster workers

There seems to be a consensus that rescue personnel might develop psychological reactions during and after rescue work. These reactions might be in accordance with the DSM-IV criteria for PTSD. The reactions seem to be more salient when the possibilities of rescuing survivors have been reduced.

Disasters are very different. It is therefore difficult to compile a standardized, fixed questionnaire, except for certain dependent variables. It is, however, important that specific areas are covered. Psychological and psychiatric effects can then be measured in a similar way across disasters. Such systematic measurement is important, not only for delineating those at high risk or decompensating, but also for addressing the extent of needs, outcomes and longer-term evaluation.

Main questions

Some of the principal questions that need to be addressed in studying the effects of disaster stress on workers, and the effectiveness of interventions in mitigating these include the following:

1. *Coping with disaster stress.* How do different groups of rescue workers cope with specific stressors? What are the importance of education, training and vaccination against stress, and the influence of the ability to rescue or carry out the tasks for which the rescuer is trained?
   A. Which groups can be identified (Table 13.3)?
   B. Who can be selected as having earlier experienced personal vulnerability?
   C. Who are the key players in organization and leadership?
2. *Post-traumatic stress problems.* How to identify psychosocial problems after rescue work: type and extent, duration and progress.
3. *Risk factors.*
4. *Debriefing*: What are the indications and effects of debriefing as intervention? When is it ultimately necessary: for whom, by whom and how?

Professionals versus nonprofessionals

In the most acute phase of a disaster, there will be mainly nonprofessional rescuers. The onlookers can be classified as helpless helpers if they are unable to act. It is of great importance to also follow up nonprofessionals, since they often present a lower degree of stress tolerance in combination with a high stress load.

Methodology

There will always be shortage of time when planning the research design for a group of rescue workers (Sund

Table 13.4. Procedure chart for studying rescue personnel

	Time 1	Time 2	Time 3
Type of survey	Primary survey	Main survey	Follow-up
When?	Within the first week	After one month	Between 6 and 12 months
Content	A few relevant questions	Complete questionnaire	Repeated questions + follow-up
Scales	IES-15	IES-15	IES-15
		GHQ-28	GHQ-28
		PTSS-10	
		Life events	

IES, Impact of Event Scale; GHQ, General Health Questionnaire; PTSS, Post-traumatic Symptom Scale.

et al., 1983; Raphael et al., 1983–4). It is preferable to start with a personal close and accurate interview with the leaders of the rescue team. The rationale for this is to obtain a detailed description of the preparedness, the situation, the equipment and the individual efforts: who did what? It will then be possible to choose a more appropriate formulation for the questions.

1. It is highly desirable that the research project will be perceived as a 'we' project, i.e. a collaboration that will probably result in a low frequency of dropouts. Establishing a 'we' project is to create a partner-like relationship with some of the organizations that have been directly affected by the disaster.
2. The next step is to distribute a short and nonintrusive questionnaire (Time 1) to all rescue workers (Table 13.4). This should be part of the early debriefing activities. Ideally the questionnaire is also therapeutic in some way.
3. The first follow-up (Time 2) will be the main questionnaire completed with self-rating scales and screening of risk groups.
4. In the follow-up survey (Time 3) some questions will be repeated; the main purposes of the follow-up are to identify cases of PTSD, to confirm findings from the second survey and to obtain information that might provide improvements in selection, education and training and may demonstrate effects of any interventions and what further interventions may be needed.

The first area to cover in a questionnaire should be a description of stressors experienced in the disaster

situation. It is important to make clear whether the respondents were working alone or as a part of a team, whether the equipment was sufficient or not, whether the leaders adequately fulfilled their duties, whether the respondents had served as leaders for others. It is also very important to investigate feelings of sufficiency or insufficiency in the very first phase of the rescue work. The following areas must also be included in the first part of a questionnaire:

experienced degree of threat or danger,
conflict: fear of doing wrong things,
the degree to which the task was clear,
competition for different tasks,
diversion of attention due to other impressions, and
capacity to endure inactivity.

This should be followed by questions concerning reactions experienced during the rescue work, such as feelings of hopelessness, frustration, helplessness and difficulties in concentration. What was most stressful?

Areas of content can be divided into separate items for the three questionnaires (Times 1, 2 and 3) and specific questions and questionnaires or scales are presented in Table 13.4.

A study like this cannot be performed anonymously, since the need for follow up is crucial. It is important to distribute the questionnaires via the leaders of the rescue work as well as to share the results with those who have taken part in the study. There should be questions on psychological experiences concerning somatic injuries, being witness to other people's deaths, danger to one's own life and experience of conflict trauma.

It is important to try to estimate personal coping strategies during rescue work, as well as what kind of formal and informal debriefing activities having been carried through and the personally experienced effects of these interventions.

The questionnaire should be completed with at least two open-ended questions:

1. What was the most stressing situation for you?
2. What was the most important factor that contributed to the opportunity to manage well?

If questionnaires have been compiled in accordance with these recommendations, they may also constitute part of the debriefing activities and are not likely to be intrusive for most of the respondents. They then form a database for defining problems, needs and outcomes.

The demographic background data can be queried in the second or third questionnaire.

Debriefing activities

Rescue workers who have been under extreme psychological stress with traumatic experiences or an overwhelming personal threat may be at risk of developing PTSDs. Such experiences may need to be psychologically worked through. It is important to talk about one's experiences – about what has been done as well as about feelings of insufficiency and guilt. It is important to be observed. The expectations from the public on rescue personnel are great, but the demands from oneself are generally still greater. After most disasters it appears likely that rescue personnel will demonstrate a need for debriefing. This includes three key elements.

1. On a structural level the rescue work should be recognized, confirmed and rewarded by significant leaders from official authorities.
2. It is important that the rescue personnel are informed in groups by representatives of authorities and their own group about normal psychological reactions after extreme stress.
3. On an individual level the personal emotional working through for the rescue workers should be facilitated.

The Armenian experience

On 7 December 1988, a disastrous earthquake occurred in southern Russia. It had its epicentre in the cities of Leninakan and Spitak in Armenia.

An official request for help was sent out from the Soviet authorities to the Western world. Two groups of rescue workers departed from Sweden in two flights on the 10th and 12th. After four days of rescue work, almost 24-hour working days and living in the centre of the disaster area, the Swedish group went back home; they had 24 hours' stay and rest in Jerevan and arrived in Stockholm on 17 December.

The members of the Swedish group had only two hours to consider whether they wanted to participate before departure to Armenia. Only some of them knew each other in advance, some of the firefighters had been trained together, but only very few had earlier experiences of really heavy disaster work. During the stay in the disaster area, the Swedish group had their campus on one side of a main street – opposite a collapsed factory and a collection area for dead bodies and a stock of coffins. During the four days of rescue work in Leninakan, there were no possibilities of getting in contact with their families at home. Almost all telephone wires were broken.

The Swedish group of rescue workers had the following structure:

Teachers from rescue services schools	10
Firefighters	17
Dog handlers (and their search dogs)	16 (+16)
Interpreters	3
Others (surgeon, nurse, journalist, operator)	4

The group consisted of two subgroups: professional and nonprofessional rescue workers (Table 13.5). Professionals were those who had been educated and trained for rescue work and who had experienced mass casualties or disaster. The firefighters might have had a long professional career, but ordinarily they had had no or very little education in psychological effects of the trauma of disaster on different affected groups. Before the Swedish rescue team returned from the mission in Armenia in December 1988, it was decided to provide a systematic debriefing. It was, however, difficult to plan this in detail, since very little was known about what the rescue workers had gone through during the week in Leninakan.

The debriefing of the Swedish group was performed as a joint activity between the occupational health-service and disaster psychiatry groups, together with leaders from National Rescue Services Board, which, by order of the Swedish government, organized the Swedish response team.

Debriefing performance

It was decided that no relatives should be at the airport to meet the rescue workers. Immediately after arrival, 17 December at 10.00 p.m., the whole group was brought to a special arrival hall apart from the public. The Minister of Defence made a short speech to the group on behalf of the government. After this the whole group was informed about normal reactions and symptoms under and after an extremely stressful situation. This information focussed on personal feelings and attitudes towards the environment. These two first parts of the structural debriefing lasted about 15 minutes and included a short leaflet with information about normal reactions and a very brief and nonintrusive questionnaire about the actual situation.

For practical reasons it was then decided to have group sessions during the first week so that everyone could be debriefed before Christmas. Interventions, group sessions, meetings and questionnaires are presented in Table 13.6.

The emotional debriefing was carried through with groups of people with the same occupational background. It would, however, probably have been better with debriefing of the rescue teams, for example those who had been working together – one or two dog handlers, two firemen and an interpreter.

The follow-up studies

The rescue work in Armenia was a very special experience for all groups of rescue workers. It was therefore considered to be of great importance to perform a systematic follow-up during the first year (Table 13.5) (Lundin & Bodegård, 1993). The questionnaires were

Table 13.5. Subgroups of rescue workers in the three follow-up studies after Armenia

Professionals (n = 20)
Fire fighters	(n = 17)
Teachers	(n = 2)
Surgeon ('Others')	(n = 1)

Nonprofessionals (n = 29)
Dog handlers	(n = 16)
Teachers	(n = 7)
Others	(n = 3)
Interpreters	(n = 3)

Table 13.6. Interventions with the Swedish group of disaster workers in Armenia

Date/time		Intervention
1988		
17 Dec.	22.00	Information for the whole group
18 Dec.	08.30	Rescue teachers (n = 4)
18 Dec.	10.00	Dog handlers, two parallel groups (2 × n = 8)
21 Dec.	08.00	Rescue teachers (n = 6)
	20.00	Interpreters (n = 2)
22 Dec.	11.00	Fire fighters (n = 17)
23 Dec.		Two telephone calls
1989		
12 Jan.		Second questionnaire (main survey)
21 Jan.	11.00–23.00	General meeting for the whole group (48 participants from the Swedish group)
22 Sept.		Third questionnaire (follow-up)

compiled following the guidelines given by Raphael et al. (1989).

Results

Only one person did not return any of the three questionnaires. The rescue workers were between 22 and 55 years of age, most of them were 30 to 49 years old.

When analysing the data with respect to background variables and variables of reaction it was of interest to compare rescue workers who had had experiences

Table 13.7. Swedish rescue workers in Armenia after the earthquake, 1988

	Professionals (%) ($n = 20$)	Nonprofessionals (%) ($n = 29$)	Total (%) ($n = 49$)
Frequency of returned questionnaires			
1	80	72	76
2	80	86	84
3	95	76	84
Major losses during the last three years	41	59	41
Education in disaster behaviour	100	52	71
Education judged as sufficient	27	23	25

from earlier missions of work in a disaster area or rescuing victims of big accidents (professionals) with those who had had no such experiences (nonprofessionals).

In the nine-month follow-up questionnaire there was a clear difference in frequency of returned questionnaires between professionals and nonprofessionals (Table 13.7). Both groups had experienced major personal losses (death of a close relative or divorce) during the last three years. It was interesting to note that both groups were unsatisfied with their training in disaster behaviour.

There was a marked and significant difference between professionals and nonprofessionals concerning unpleasant feelings both during the first week and in the long-term follow-up: professionals experienced unpleasant feelings to a significantly higher degree during the first week; after nine months the difference was the opposite, i.e. nonprofessionals were higher. This might be explained by a tendency among professionals to allow themselves to react in the acute phase and difficulties for nonprofessionals that led to working through their emotional feelings later during the first year.

Further training in rescue technique was judged as highly important for the training of disaster workers. Theoretical knowledge and practical skills in emergency care as well as disaster psychiatry were also judged to be important.

Those who were well prepared to meet a disaster like this had, during the first week after returning home as well as nine months later, reported significantly better ($p < 0.05$) feelings of having managed well.

Professionals and nonprofessionals did not differ significantly, in the GHQ-28 scoring nine months later or in the IES-15, in total or in subsets concerning intrusion and avoidance. There were no differences between professionals and nonprofessionals concerning depressive feelings, nightmares, or sleep disturbances.

The *Estonia* disaster and the rescue

In the middle of the night, 28 September 1994, the ferry *Estonia* capsized with 1000 people on board. The weather was very bad with a windspeed of around 30 metres per second. The bowgates broke and the ferry sank within half an hour. The ferry had left Tallin a few hours before the accident and was bound for Stockholm. The site of the accident was close to the Finnish coast. Due to the darkness and the weather, rescue operations were almost impossible during the first hours.

The rescue operations were under Finnish command. The rescue work during the first days after the *Estonia* disaster included nine helicopters from the Swedish Navy, four from the Swedish Air Force, two from Denmark and four from Finland. Fourteen survivors were rescued from the sea by the Swedish helicopter teams. They were also engaged in secondary transport of 22 survivors. Twenty-four dead bodies were winched from the sea.

During the first week 93 dead bodies were found and identified (38 Swedish passengers and 55 crew members). Almost 800 people are still missing; and have been declared dead. On 15 December, it was decided by the Swedish government not to raise the wreck or

Table 13.8. Self-evaluation of defusing and debriefing sessions ($n = 17$)

	Very good (%)	Good (%)	Less good (%)	Bad (%)
Defusing sessions	35	59	6	0
Debriefing session	41	47	6	6

Table 13.9. The *Estonia* Ferry Disaster: rescuers, distribution by age and sex

	n	Mean	S.D.	Range
Women	2	26.5	3.5	24–29
Men	14	29.9	3.3	26–37
Total	16	29.2	3.4	24–37

the dead bodies still on board. The ferry and the wreck site were declared to be a memorial and grave.

Psychological support

Immediately after landing, all naval helicopters' crews were taken care of and defusing sessions were carried out. A formal four-hour debriefing session was performed with the 19 rescue personnel after the first self-rating for post-traumatic stress symptoms, 12 days post disaster.

At the two-month follow-up interview, nobody reported any need for more psychosocial support or debriefing (Table 13.8).

Method

A group of young naval officers (Table 13.9), sonar operators ($n = 19$) served as rescuers in the nine naval helicopters (Boeing Vertol 107) especially equipped for rescue operations at sea.

They were followed up at 12 days, 2 and 14 months after the ferry disaster using questionnaires (Lundin & Eriksson, 1997). The frequency of stress symptoms was measured on the Post-Traumatic Symptom Scale, PTSS-10 ($n = 3$). All respondents completed the IES-15 ($n = 4$), the Sense of Coherence (12-item version) and questions on peritraumatic dissociation. There were no personal interviews.

Table 13.10. Post-traumatic stress symptoms (single items from the PTSS-10) as percentage, among rescuers ($n = 15$) from the Swedish Navy

Stress symptoms	Frequency after			
	12 days	2 months	14 months	sig.
Sleep disorders	20	7	7	NS
Nightmares	20	7	7	NS
Depression	53	13	20	$p < 0.05$
Startle reactions	7	7	0	NS
Withdrawal	20	13	0	NS
Irritability	20	7	13	NS
Affective instability	40	0	7	$p < 0.01$
Guilt feelings	27	0	7	$p = 0.07$
Fear of reminders	13	7	0	NS
Muscular tension	40	7	13	$p < 0.05$

Sig., significance; NS, not significant.

This method had earlier been used in a follow-up study of the crews of two missile carrier vessels after a collision at sea that resulted in one death (Lundin, 1995).

Results

Stress reactions

Twelve days after the disaster eight respondents reported symptoms of depression; three reported sleeping problems and nightmares. Six men reported affective instability and muscular tension. Withdrawal and irritability were reported by three men, while four reported feelings of guilt. Fear of reminders was reported by two people and a startle response was reported by one person. At the follow-ups, 2 and 14 months after the disaster, there was a significant decrease in reported stress symptoms, such as depression, affective instability, guilt feelings and muscular tension (Table 13.10).

The scored mean value for the PTSS-10 self-assessment scale was 2.60 12 days post disaster. There was a significant decrease after 2 months (0.67) and 14 months (0.73). The mean value for IES was 23.3, which reflects a moderate reaction. The mean values at the

Table 13.11. Rescuers ($n = 16$): post-traumatic stress symptoms and reactions as measured by the post-traumatic Symptoms Scale (PTSS-10) and the Impact of Event Scale (IES-15)

Stress symptoms	Frequency after			
	12 days	2 months	14 months	Sig.
PTSS-10 (range 0–10)	2.60	0.67	0.73	$p < 0.0001$
IES-15 (range 0–75)	23.3	10.1	12.0	$p < 0.0001$
IES-1	15.3	7.3	8.8	$p < 0.001$
IES-a	7.9	2.8	3.2	$p < 0.001$

Sig., significance.

follow-ups were 10.1 and 12.0, respectively (Tables 13.10 and 13.11).

Dissociation

Peritraumatic dissociative reactions were measured with questions according to the five DSM-IV criteria for acute stress disorder: emotional numbing, which was reported by six persons; reduction of awareness ($n = 3$); derealization ($n = 9$); depersonalization ($n = 4$); and dissociative amnesia ($n = 1$). Five persons reported no peritraumatic dissociative symptoms at all.

Swedish peace-keeping soldiers in Bosnia

Different forms of support (peer support, ventilation or defusing, and more formal debriefing sessions) follow-ing traumatic experiences have been evaluated, using a prospective study design (Larsson et al., 1997). The sample consisted of a Swedish battalion ($n = 510$), which was part of the North Atlantic Treaty Organization's (NATO) implementation force in Bosnia in 1996. Preservice assessment was made of personality, sense of coherence, and mental health. One-third of the soldiers experienced traumatic situations during their service. Poor mental health after service was more related to preservice mental health and sense of coherence than to trauma exposure and post-trauma support. Peer support followed by a defusing session had a positive effect on post-service mental health. Peer support alone, or peer support and defusing followed by a debriefing session, did not lead to a more favourable result than no support at all (Table 13.12).

Training programmes

Groups of rescue workers in Sweden are usually dominated by firemen. The first basic education and training (A, below) for these persons is provided by the local authorities for the fire brigades, the higher courses (B–D) are governmental responsibilities and run by the National Rescue Services Schools.

A. Introductory course following appointment as fireman, five weeks.
B. After the first year of service there is a course on professional competence, 15 weeks.
C. After five years of service, there is a selection,

Table 13.12. Mental health after service in Bosnia – comparison of different kinds of support

	No support $n = 56$	Peer, only $n = 29$	Peer + defusing $n = 60$	Peer + defusing + debriefing $n = 36$	Sig.
GHQ-28	15.1	14.2	11.8	14.6	$p < 0.05$
Somatic	3.9	3.3	2.7	3.9	NS
Anxiety	3.6	3.2	2.7	3.3	NS
Social	6.5	7.0	5.9	6.6	$p < 0.05$
Depression	1.2	0.4	0.4	0.9	$p < 0.05$
IES-15	8.7	11.4	9.0	10.8	NS
Intrusion	3.0	5.3	4.2	5.1	NS
Avoidance	5.7	6.1	4.9	5.7	NS

Sig., significance; NS, not significant.

around 20%, for education leading to appointment as fire foreman, 10 weeks.

D. Around 50% of the fire foremen will after *x* years be selected for a higher education, leading to a fire-master's certificate, 14 weeks.

E. A small number of fire-masters will continue with university studies for 3.5 years (2.5 years theoretical studies and 1 year practical training) leading to fire-engineer. This course is run at only one Swedish university.

In the schedules for the basic training courses there has earlier been no or very little education on disaster behaviour or psychological and psychiatric aspects of disaster as well as a systematic training of personal reactions. During the last decade this has improved very much. Following the last few years' experiences the education and training programmes for rescue workers now include also the psychological aspects of disaster.

Discussion and conclusions

Armenia

From a theoretical point of view it seemed of interest to compare the disaster experiences, both emotional and other psychological, of the rescue workers who could be defined as professionals and those who were non-professionals. A greater proportion of the professionals as compared with of the nonprofessionals seemed to have a better occupational situation and better support from the social network, and hence greater possibilities of psychologically working through their traumatic experiences. Only one quarter of all the rescue workers found their education and training sufficient for this mission. Rescue technique was considered by the group to be the most important area for education and training.

The feeling of preparedness was, not surprisingly, rated higher among non-professionals and also seemed to be a discriminating factor for the self-evaluation of the rescue workers' own rescue achievement. The mean IES-15 score was 20.5 for the whole group, which is somewhat higher than that of 18.2 reported by McFarlane (1988a) from a questionnaire study on 469

firefighters four months after a disastrous bush fire in Australia. Education and training seemed to be favourable factors for good coping strategies, including less preoccupation by unpleasant thoughts.

Most likely, however, professionals seem to allow themselves to react and give words to their feelings immediately after the traumatic event, which might also explain the decrease over time (working through). On the other hand, the nonprofessionals, perhaps as an effect of a lack of earlier disaster experiences, reported fewer unpleasant feelings in the beginning and did not show any change over time. The professionals also used a great many cognitive defences. They were highly resistant to describing 'feelings', because they ordinarily work in groups with the same personnel. In these fire station teams people might be reluctant to disclose inner feelings. Firefighters have learned to suppress their feelings until they are sure the mission is over. Then they may disclose slowly and to well-known and trusted people.

This group of rescue workers was recruited without any opportunity for providing specialized education and training to meet the special stress of working far away without any regular support from the social network. None of them had previously worked in an earthquake area. The proportions of different types of rescue workers in the group, however, seemed to be important.

Rescue workers who are to be exposed to extremely stressful situations with mass deaths and widespread destruction should not be too young (not below the age of 25 years). They should also be well experienced in rescue work with preferably more than three years of professional work as a background.

It would seem appropriate to provide specialised education and training for rescue teams that are to be sent on extremely stressful missions. All rescue workers reported a need for further education and training, especially in rescue technique. It seems reasonable that prior professional skills will make rescue workers more confident and thus better prepared to cope with the traumatic stress involved in disaster rescue operations.

Estonia

All helicopter crews were immediately offered defusing sessions. It was seen as important to keep the crew members together. They also all knew each other from previous work together. They were young full-time employed naval officers and had had earlier experiences of this type of rescue activity – although on a minor scale. Most rescuers found the formal debriefing activities, 12 days post disaster, very helpful for working through their emotional experiences. There seemed to be no risk for developing PTSD. This might be an effect of several concurrent factors: they were not too young, with a mean age of 29.2 years (range 24–37); they were well trained and had good routines for peer support. They rescued both survivors and dead bodies. Their efforts were very well recognized by the government and official authorities.

Bosnia

For the Swedish peace-keeping soldiers, the post-trauma support was of limited favourable effect. It was found, however, that the combination of peer support and an initial defusing session led by the platoon commander (or similar) had a positive effect on the post-service mental health of the participants. Peer support alone, or peer support and defusing followed by a debriefing session, did not lead to a more favourable result than no support at all.

Poor mental health after NATO service seemed to be more related to mental health and sense of coherence before service than to trauma exposure and post-trauma support. In the longer term, the effects of peer support plus a defusing session thus seemed to be of marginal value.

For nonprofessional and professional rescue workers, in both civilian and military settings, more effort should be put into the selection process, education and training, and not least into finding good leaders for the mission or the rescue work.

REFERENCES

Alexander, D. A. & Wells, A. (1991). Reactions of police officers to body-handling after a major disaster. a before-and-after comparison. *British Journal of Psychiatry*, **159**, 547–55.

American Psychiatric Association (1980). *Diagnostic and Statistical Manual of Mental Disorders*, 3rd edn. Washington, DC: American Psychiatric Press.

American Psychiatric Association (1994). *Diagnostic and Statistical Manual of Mental Disorders*, 4th edn. Washington, DC: American Psychiatric Press.

Dyregrov, A., Kristoffersen, J. I. & Gjestad, R. (1996). Voluntary and professional disaster-workers: similarities and differences in reactions. *Journal of Traumatic Stress*, **9**, 541–55.

Ersland, S., Weisæth, L. & Sund, A. (1989). The stress upon rescuers involved in an oil rig disaster. 'Alexander L. Kielland,' 1980. *Acta Psychiatrica Scandinavica*, **80**, Suppl. 355, 38–49.

Fullerton, C. S., Wright, K. M., Ursano, R. J. & McCarroll, J. E. (1993). Social support for disaster workers after a mass-casualty: effects on the support provider. *Journal of Psychiatry*, **47**, 315–24.

Hytten, K. & Hasle, A. (1989) Fire fighters: a study of stress and coping. *Acta Psychiatrica Scandinavica*, **80**, Suppl. 355, 50–5.

Larsson, G., Michel, P. O. & Lundin. T. (1997). Systematic assessment of mental health following psychological debriefing. *Military Psychology*, in press.

Lindström, B. & Lundin, T. (1982). Stress reactions among rescue and health care personnel after a major fire disaster (Swedish text). *Nordic Psychiatric Journal*, **36**, Suppl. 6.

Lundin, T. (1995). Collision at sea between two Navy vessels. *Military Medicine*, **160**, 323–5.

Lundin, T. & Bodegård, M. (1993). The psychological impact of an earthquake on rescue workers: a follow-up study of the Swedish group of rescue workers in Armenia, 1988. *Journal of Traumatic Stress*, **6**, 129–39.

Lundin, T. & Eriksson, N. G. (1997). Post-traumatic stress reactions among 19 rescue men from the Swedish Navy after the Estonia Ferry disaster. Unpublished report.

Lundin, T. & Otto, U. (1989). Stress reactions among Swedish health care personnel in UNIFIL, South Lebanon 1982–1984. *Stress Medicine*, **5**, 237–46.

Marmar, C. H. R., Weiss, D. S., Metzler, T. J., Ronfeldt, H. M. & Foreman, C. (1996). Stress responses of emergency services personnel to the Loma Prieta earthquake Interstate 880 freeway collapse and control traumatic incidents. *Journal of Traumatic Stress*, **9**, 63–85.

McFarlane, A. C. (1987). Life events and psychiatric disorder: the role of a natural disaster. *British Journal of Psychiatry*, **151**, 362–7.

McFarlane, A. C. (1988a). Relationship between psychiatric impairment and a natural disaster: the role of distress. *Psychological Medicine*, **18**, 129–39.

McFarlane, A. C. (1988b). The longitudinal course of post-traumatic morbidity. The range of outcomes and their predictors. *Journal of Nervous and Mental Disease*, **176**, 30–9.

McFarlane, A. C. (1989). The aetiology of post-traumatic morbidity: predisposing, precipitating and perpetuating factors. *British Journal of Psychiatry*, **154**, 221–8.

Raphael, B., Singh, B., Bradbury, L. & Lambert, F. (1983–4). Who helps the helpers? The effects of a disaster on the rescue workers. *Omega*, **14**, 9–20.

Raphael, B., Lundin, T. & Weisæth, L. (1989). A research method for the study of psychological and psychiatric aspects of disaster. *Acta Psychiatrica Scandinavica*, **80**, Suppl. 353, 1–75.

Sund, A., Ersland, S. & Weisæth, L. (1983). *Alexander L. Kielland katastrofen, 27 mars 1980. Rednings personellets erfaringer. En forelöpig forskningsrapport.* Oslo.

Ursano, R. J., Fullerton, C. S., Kao, T. C. & Bhartiya, V. R. (1995). Longitudinal assessment of post-traumatic stress disorder and depression after exposure to traumatic death. *Journal of Nervous and Mental Disease*, **183**, 36–42.

14

Children and debriefing: theory, interventions and outcomes

Ruth Wraith

EDITORIAL COMMENTS

This overview of the conceptualization of the debriefing model and its application to children and adolescents reflects a strong clinical basis and understanding of the developmental issues relevant to the impact of critical incidents in this age range. Wraith draws a distinction, as is common in the Critical Incident Stress Debriefing/debriefing field, between stress and trauma and emphasizes that, as with adults, the debriefing model is intended to assist with stress but that traumatized children require a specially focussed and individualized approach. There is strong emphasis on the need to assess children before they are provided with a group debriefing process. The model suggested is composed of two parts: psychological first aid and clinical debriefing. However, there is a need to address further the spectrum of preventive, as compared with clinical, interventions, and the sanctions that must apply if an intervention is to be provided at all: i.e. do no harm; consider the ethics, appropriateness and propriety of providing such an intervention; and, if it is to be provided, consider the skills and knowledge necessary for the task.

Wraith questions the appropriateness of debriefing for children and emphasizes the vital role of parents, their needs and responses, particularly for younger children. However, it may be that debriefing is not an appropriate model and it is critical that assumptions of benefit and social demand that are so powerfully driving the debriefing movement are challenged in this context. Because children usually have so little previous experience of critical incidents and coping with these it is even more important that no harm is done – either by interventions that may override natural healing and recovery processes, or by the introduction of a clinical framework that thereafter dominates the response to the inevitable challenges of life. Wraith's skills suggest this is unlikely to be the case in her hands, but may well be in those of others.

Again, the model suggested in this chapter throws into sharp relief the clinical skills and knowledge that should inform even the possibility of such interventions with children. Despite the vital importance of working through traumatic experiences in childhood for the child's development and mental health, there is a gross lack of empirical data to underpin a prevention model in this area.

Introduction

When reading or talking to people about the psychological debriefing of children a confused understanding becomes apparent. It is not always clear whether the basis of the discussion is a particular technique used within a group or individual session, a concept that illuminates and expands management options, or a process that may be developed in a range of circumstances within individual, family or group settings over a period of time. There may not be clear differentiation of the ages of the children under discussion – preschool (3–5 years), primary school (5–11 years) or early (12–15 years) or late adolescence.

Used loosely, the term debriefing may include talking with children about an unpleasant experience in an open and responsive way. In its more technical application the term is used to describe a circumscribed group intervention conducted by a trained leader following a stressful experience such as an accident or the death of a loved person. Herman (1992), with reference to adults, distinguished between debriefing and other group events that focus on safety, remembrance, and mourning and reconnection. Talking about debriefing, she said,

Debriefings must observe the fundamental rules of safety. Just as it is never safe to assume that a traumatized individual's family will be supportive, it is never safe to assume that a group of people will be able to rally and cohere simply because all of its members have suffered from the same terrible event. Underlying conflicts of interest may actually be exacerbated rather than overridden by the event. (Herman, 1992, p. 219)

The intervention was originally designed as a defined language-based group technique to facilitate the management of undue stress in adult emergency service workers in the days following a critical incident (Mitchell, 1983) and has been adapted to particular populations such as defence personnel, industry employees, human service workers and, less frequently, for application to adults in disaster, war, medical and other similar contexts. Mitchell & Everly (1995, p. 8) described Critical Incident Stress Debriefing (CISD) as 'a group meeting or discussion about a distressing critical incident. Based upon core principles of education and crisis intervention … [debriefing] is designed to mitigate the impact of a critical incident and to assist the personnel in recovering as quickly as possible from the stress associated with the event'. They warned of a number of common problems with CISD, including overly rigid adherence to CISD guidelines, over zealous applications, failure to be subtle in the transition of stages within a session, dysfunctional countertransference and failure to comply with the basic principles and techniques (Mitchell & Everly, 1995). The historical and theoretical underpinning of current practice was elucidated in depth by Shalev (1994), who also explored common elements and goals of debriefing methods for adults.

Most of the debriefing practices currently provided for children are replications or derivatives of the adult

models and are given a range of names, including creative debriefing (Eriksson, 1996), group treatments (Stallard & Law, 1993; Monahan, 1995), classroom interventions (Johnson, 1989) and CISD. 'Although CISD is a technique which was developed specifically for emergency personnel, it has been applied with great success … to school children' (Mitchell & Everly, 1995, p. 15). Mitchell & Everly cited its use following the *Jupiter* ferry sinking, and the Armenian earthquake, and for children of surviving emergency personnel after duty death in an organization.

The aims of debriefing of children include providing 'understanding and increased feelings of personal control … [they] are an attempt to salvage group cohesiveness from the disintegrating effects of a crisis' (Johnson, 1989, p. 74), 'to normalize responses and aid recovery through the child's expression of emotions and reactions' (Brooks & Siegel, 1996, p. 21), and 'facilitate the recovery process rather than treat presenting symptoms' (Yule & Canterbury, 1994, p. 145).

Debriefing models described include a variety of individual formats, group interventions, classroom activities or family engagement (Pynoos & Nader, 1988; Johnson, 1989; Dyregrov, 1991; Denholm, 1995; Monahan, 1995). It would seem that often the strategies and programmes developed do not arise out of assessment of the individual child's needs, but out of the adult's anxiety and countertransference, including the desire/need to be protective or healing, and not infrequently in response to the impact of the event on themselves being displaced onto the child (Dyregrov, 1991; Gillis, 1993). The group debriefing interventions may be prescriptive and related to the nature of the external events (Brooks & Siegel, 1996), and not necessarily cognisant of and responsive to the child's subjective state. While protocols may provide direction and comfort for the uncertain teacher or clinician, they may fail to meet the individual child's needs.

On the occasion of the first anniversary of the 1996 Port Arthur massacre in Tasmania, one primary school district in another state quite removed from any direct connection with the event decided on a debriefing event for all children. It is reported that for many children, teachers and parents the degree of arousal engendered by the systemic approach resulted in incidents of acute stress, distress and for a few children secondary traumatization through the artificially introduced interface with other issues in their lives.

Literature directly addressing children and group debriefing is less comprehensive than the adult literature (see Johnson, 1989; Dyregrov, 1991; Yule & Udwin, 1991; Stallard & Law, 1993; Yule & Canterbury, 1994; Brooks & Siegel, 1996. There are references to debriefing children within other topics; for example, Hendricks et al. (1993) focussed on children who had seen their father kill their mother and Gillis (1993) considered debriefing in the context of individual and group psychotherapy for children involved in trauma and disaster.

The more evaluative critiques of child debriefing are those of Yule & Udwin (1991), Yule (1992), Joseph et al. (1993), Stallard & Law (1993) and Yule & Canterbury (1994). In the context of a lack of adequate evaluative data, Hendricks and colleagues (1993) recommended a pragmatic approach.

The appropriateness of debriefing as a specific intervention for children is often assumed (O'Hara et al., 1994; Brooks & Siegel, 1996), as is the relevance of adult CISD models. There is a need for careful examination of child-specific issues and the development of models of debriefing that are appropriate for children. There is also a need for consideration of the subjective nature of the experience requiring debriefing and how it intersects with other elements in the child's life.

Debriefing has been described as being conducted by parents (Sheridan et al., 1996) as well as by a range of professional groups, including teachers, counsellors, psychologists and welfare workers. Leadership training and skills may or may not be seen as requisites. Debriefing may be provided in response to specific requests (O'Hara et al., 1994) but the quality of the assessment is not always clear.

Evaluation outcomes of the efficacy of adult group models is a subject of energetic debate (Raphael et al., 1995; Robinson & Mitchell, 1995). While adults report that debriefing assists them, what this describes is yet to be clarified. However, even this degree of evaluation and monitoring is not a component of regular appraisal with children. Children's capacity to conceptualize and articulate what assists them and what is not helpful needs elucidation before this stage can proceed.

There are times when group debriefing appears to be the 'right' intervention for the 'right' child at the 'right' time (Stallard & Law, 1993; Yule & Canterbury, 1994). But there are also some very concerning stories about the use of the group debriefing technique with children. As part of a debriefing programme in a school after the death of three 11-year-old pupils in a transport accident off the school grounds, children aged 5–7 years who did not know the children involved nor were witness to the incident were debriefed in a class event. Some of these children were reported by their parents to have emerged from the debriefing frightened and clingy, and to have developed nightmares and reactive bedtime separation problems. The parents would not let their children return to school until the school 'had settled itself down'. From this anecdotal report it appears that there was a relationship between the debriefing experience and the development of reactive stress behaviours in the children.

Models of group debriefing that are appropriate to children and their various developmental stages, encompass individual nuances and vulnerabilities and take into account the quality of the experience have not been developed, tested or evaluated. None the less, the provision of group debriefing to children in all age groups from school entry onwards, in all variety of circumstances, grows exponentially.

Group debriefing is conceptually different from small-group psychotherapy provided for children following major events in their lives (Galante & Foa, 1986; Yule & Williams, 1990; Gillis, 1993; Monahan, 1995). In group psychotherapy, the focus is on integration of the ramifications of the experience into the various parameters of the child's life, including external, internal and existential domains, whereas group debriefing is focussed on the incident.

Children's responses to significant events

Children may experience a range of phenomena following a major event on a continuum from stress to post-traumatic stress disorder (PTSD) and other psy-chopathologies. Their reactions are similar to those experienced by adults but with important developmental differences in presentation and progression of symptoms (Gordon & Wraith, 1993; Pynoos, 1993; Pynoos & Nader, 1993; Pynoos et al., 1995).

These may include a range of regressions, re-experiencing phenomena, psychological numbing, avoidance, increased arousal behaviours, fears and feelings of helplessness. Any of these responses may appear in a child of any age at any time, from the moment of the incident and may last indefinitely. Nader (1995) made a clear distinction between the impact on, and the needs of, children who have experienced trauma, grief or traumatic grief. When a child experiences loss there may be yearning and reunion wishes, disbelief, searching and reminiscing, sadness, anger and irritability. Traumatic grief involves a complex interaction of trauma and grief responses.

It is important to differentiate stress reactions from traumatic reactions. Trauma reactions require specific clinical interventions as their impact can lead to damage to psychic functions by breaking past established coping and defensive operations. Debriefing practitioners indicate that stress reactions may be ameliorated within a debriefing context (Duckworth, 1986; Yule, 1992; Robinson & Mitchell, 1993; Stallard & Law, 1993; Brooks & Siegel, 1996) and it is these reactions, i.e. stress reactions as opposed to trauma reactions, which are considered within this discussion.

There are some age-specific stress responses that must also be taken into account when one is developing group debriefing programmes for children. Pre-school children (under 5 years) may exhibit increased attachment behaviours, a regressive return to less mature behaviours, decreased verbalization and capacity to play, and cognitive confusion as a response to stress (Eth & Pynoos, 1985; Terr, 1985). School-age children may respond with any of these and may also exhibit their distress through behavioural changes of aggression, withdrawal, inconsistent behaviour and school difficulties. With increased verbal capacities, they may also need to continually retell their story rather than replay it as in earlier years (Pynoos, 1990; Gordon & Wraith, 1993).

Adolescents may also respond with any of the above behavioural changes. The peer group is of central significance for the early adolescent who processes and validates much of their subjective experience through it. Mid to late adolescents are likely to catapult into premature adult-type behaviours that may appear to indicate increased maturity, but in fact mask depression and other regressive changes. Pseudo-maturity and disguised dependence can be expressed by a premature closing of education, early marriage or inappropriate dedication to the family of origin or other cause. The affront to the idealization of adolescents, in combination with their vulnerability, may lead them to respond with acting out of behaviours of aggression, violence to self or others, substance abuse, delinquency and precocious sexual activity (Pynoos, 1990). The importance of the peer group as a reference point decreases with proximity to adulthood.

Debriefing: a concept, a process, a technique?

At the time of writing there is no clearly elaborated conceptual basis for understanding the requirements and the processes for the debriefing of children after stressful experiences. Consequently, the adult-derivative techniques that are used with children, particularly within the group context, may not be appropriate to the incident-generated requirements of children, and cognisant of their functional, as distinct from their chronological developmental levels.

The following discussion introduces a framework for differentiation of the concept of debriefing from the group-based technique or format and the processes engaged within a well conducted debriefing (Figure 14.1).

Debriefing, as a concept, provides the opportunity, frequently but not exclusively in a group context, for the development of an accurate cognitive framework of the experience, the recognition and validation of incident-related experiences and feelings, reassurance of the appropriateness of these and information about their management.

The process of debriefing provides the opportunity for reduction of isolation, engagement of the experience within a relationship, facilitation of symbolic rep-

---

```
CONCEPT OF DEBRIEFING

PROCESS OF DEBRIEFING

TECHNIQUE OF DEBRIEFING
```

Figure 14.1. Parameters of debriefing.

resentation of internal and external manifestations of the experience and the integration of the incident and its sequelae into the social, cognitive, psychodynamic and existential frames of the individual. The process may be experienced in an individual, family or group setting. Dyregrov (1997) emphasised the importance of exploration and discussion of process issues within CISD. The meeting of higher-order needs of children after a disaster – described by Boatright (1985) as belonging, love, information and understanding – are contingent upon due attention to the notion of the process as described here. If the process is not properly engaged, the goals within the concept and the technique to achieve them will not be attainable.

The specific technique or the format known as debriefing has been developed to facilitate the execution of the concept and provide a basis for the fulfilment of the process in an individual, family or group setting. The technique, when applied within a group, includes defined rules about leadership and leadership training, venue, timing, confidentiality and the progression of stages within a completed session. These have usually been modelled on the principles developed by Mitchell (1983), although, as noted above, there is no evidence or evaluation to confirm the appropriateness of this model for children.

The group application of debriefing in a circumscribed context following a critical incident is the focus of this discussion.

Aims of critical incident stress debriefing that are relevant for children

There are a number of aims within the CISD model (Mitchell & Everly, 1995) that have the potential to assist children in their recovery from untoward experiences. Children as well as adults may need the oppor-

tunity for emotional relief via discharge of intense experiences and feelings. They may need the opportunity to have their feelings recognized, named, validated and held by another through sharing (Gillis, 1993; Yule & Canterbury, 1994). They may need reassurance about the appropriateness of their responses and the opportunity to learn about the reasons for the emergence of these responses, the management of them and their progression in the future. Children need to understand the reality of the situation in which they were engaged and to gain previously unknown but relevant information about the incident as is appropriate for them. They may also require identification and amelioration of myths and fantasies surrounding the event. Maintenance of cohesiveness of the incident group (Dyregrov, 1997) can also assist children with the processing and amelioration of their experience. However, whether or not such aims are best achieved through the debriefing model remains to be established.

Debriefing and children – differential factors

If it is accepted that debriefing as a concept, a process and a technique is appropriate for children in certain circumstances, there are some issues that require further examination to ensure that children's needs are properly met.

The CISD model was developed for workers to follow an incident in which they were professionally engaged and therefore had obligations and responsibilities for the conduct of the incident. This factor immediately differentiates the needs, requirements and processes of CISD from the debriefing process that may be required by children (Stallard & Law, 1993). Only exceptionally rarely would children be workers, and these probably would be adolescents. Children very occasionally may have some responsibility within an incident in relation to the activities in which they are engaged, such as patrol leader on a scout camp or a form captain in a school incident. Within an incident, children may assume a responsibility for tasks or actions. They may not be able to conceptualize, recognize or communicate this shift. Therefore the resulting sense of responsibility may not be available to be worked with in the overt sense that it is for adults who have a responsibility as a

Table 14.1. Issues in debriefing children

- Involvement of parents
- Developmental issues in child
- Role of peer group
- Modalities for expression and conversation
- Level of engagement
- Self-disclosure/confidentiality
- Limited coping skills
- Retraumatization/secondary traumatization
- Trained leadership

defined part of their role and function. The key point is that children are participant victims, observers or associates of victims or the impacted environment, rather than being in roles such as workers who have defined responsibilities with respect to an incident.

Adult debriefing aims to identify, articulate and integrate personal experiences and responses in relation to assigned tasks or engagement in an incident. Often the experiences and consequent responses are the result of a preincident contract in a prescribed area of life, for instance employment, or tasks that are self-assigned or imposed by the nature of the incident. Children do not have an identified operational function to provide a context and boundaries for location and containment of the experience and the consequent sequelae.

In response to a critical incident, adults make a shift from the objective domain of the external context of the experience to the personal and subjective domain. The debriefing technique and process supports the understanding of these domains, the movements and interactions between them, and provides the opportunity for re-establishment of the balance of the objective/subjective dimensions within the individual. When children experience a critical incident, the impact is likely to be global and diffuse; more so the younger the child. Developmental factors limit children's capacity to identify and objectify external and subjective elements.

The post-incident process needs to counteract the sense of vulnerability, provide containment and an experience of internal and external safety. It needs to provide differentiation of the objective and subjective dimensions and provide understanding for the child of the reality of their internal and external domains. Support is required for the vulnerable ego, owing to the developmentally weaker skills and defence mechanisms (Gillis, 1993).

Because children are developmentally immature there are a number of factors to be considered regarding the appropriateness of group debriefing, particularly when derivatives of adult models are used (Table 14.1). The younger the child the greater the potential for the critical incident to compromise the vital sense of safety. The developmentally determined incomplete internalization of significant caring others generates this age-specific vulnerability. Damage to the interactive process of internalization by the child of his or her primary caregivers is a foundation for future attachment disorders and their sequelae. After a critical incident, the sense of safety is re-established for a child through the act of re-engagement of the *protective cocoon provided primarily by parents and family* or significant other and also by their community. When the sense of safety is engaged, physiological and psychological reactions can begin to abate and the child's own developmentally appropriate coping skills can begin to emerge. It is only at this point that the debriefing technique may be considered, if required at all.

The role of parents and significant others as the core reference point for framing and processing unusual experiences and providing information and a sense of safety and containment is crucial (Raphael, 1986; McFarlane, 1987; Yule & Williams, 1990; Yule, 1991; Gillis, 1993; James, 1996) and must be supported to ensure that any engagement in a group does not undermine the child–parent relationship. The primary requirement for children of all ages is to experience safety (Herman, 1992) in the physical environment and also in the physiological and psychological domains. Following a critical incident, a sense of safety generally will not re-emerge until a child is psychologically reunited and engaged with their parents or their significant other. To assist the process of reduction of stress, psychological as well as physical safety issues must be addressed.

As the child matures, the peer group or surrogate parent such as a school teacher begins to form an increasingly significant part of the cocoon of safety.

Towards puberty and adolescence, the well-grounded child is more able to be sustained by their own internalized representation of caring others in moments of crisis until the external world is able to provide the required net of safety to counteract the vulnerability introduced by the incident.

The younger the child the more the parents automatically and appropriately regard themselves as integral to the life experiences, survival, health and welfare of their child. Management strategies must take the parental role into account. The findings of Milgrom & Toubiana (1996) from data collected from 675 school children following death and injury of fellow students in a bus accident showed that the children found their parents to be the most helpful to them, more than teachers and other support people. Debriefing of children in group situations needs to be integrated into the contexts of their families' reactions, understandings and processing, and should not aim to supplant these.

Developmental imperatives require support for the child–parent bond, elucidation of the child's experience in fact and in fantasy, the development of a range of modalities to express the experience, validation of the experience, opportunities for emotional relief and for expression of thoughts, ideas and questions. These need to be engaged in the realm of the shared common experience with the parents. The child requires simple, age-appropriate but accurate and pertinent facts about the event and what is to happen in the immediate future. Parents also need the facts of the events, information about their child's and their own reactions and management strategies in the present and the future.

The involvement of their child in a major event is always of high significance and extraordinarily demanding for a parent. There is the basic immutable parental protective concern for their child. There may be guilt because they have failed to provide this protective function and their child was exposed to the incident or they perceive that they have failed in this function. Parents may be experiencing horror of what their child has gone through. They may have had previous experiences of their own aroused. They may have been involved in the incident themselves. The 'child in the parent' may be painfully or frighteningly awakened.

Therefore parents need to be engaged independently to support reconciliation of their own issues and to help them understand their own and each others' responses. Parent parallel groups and parent information sessions provide these opportunities (Pynoos & Nader, 1988; Monahan, 1995). Only then will they be able to engage appropriately in their parental role and be available to be 'psychologically present' with their child as individuals and as a parental dyad in these circumstances.

Preschool children need to be managed within their relationship with their parents and primary school-aged children, as they mature from 'beginner' grades at age 5 to Grade 6 level at around 11 or 12 years, will require a combination of interventions within their relationship with their parents and perhaps their family, and potentially with their incident group (Stallard & Law, 1993).

Parents and family have a central function in the process of debriefing, with the second core dimension being the developmental context of childhood. In relation to debriefing, readiness of children for a group experience of this nature must be evaluated. The group technique of debriefing requires maturation in conceptual, communication and social skills, self-awareness and self-regulation. It cannot be assumed that all children, particularly after a difficult experience, are functioning at the required level in each area to enable them to engage productively in a language-based group debriefing event. Resolution may be achieved within the metaphor through play, drawing, drama or music, all outside the realm of verbal communication (MacLean, 1977; Terr, 1989; Gillis, 1993).

What elements of the debriefing process maybe relevant for younger children remains to be established. The child who is functioning below four years of age is not readily able to symbolize and engage in representational thought, nor maintain memory of interactions, and thus is not able to reflect and re-examine self and general knowledge. These attributes are requisites for group debriefing. Babies and toddlers have different requirements for facilitation of integration and processing of untoward events from group debriefing as described in this chapter.

The technique and the processes of debriefing have

to occur within the context of the age-appropriate developmental tasks, needs and capacities of the child and recognize and respond to regressive shifts generated by the experience, cognitively, behaviourally and psychodynamically. A preschool child has very different tasks, needs and capabilities from those of an adolescent.

The third dimension is the role of the peer group which will be of greater significance for the preadolescent and adolescent than the younger child. Identification with the experience of peers in the context of an immaturely established sense of self may lead to contagious engagement with the experience within the group setting and possibly secondary traumatization by it (Terr, 1985).

The fourth dimension arises because immaturity means the child has a weaker ego structure than an adult and also less consolidated defence mechanisms. The limited repertoire of established successful coping skills, and the wide range of immature coping skills and defence mechanisms in children need to be taken into account when one considers the appropriateness of group debriefing for an individual child in a specific set of circumstances. These factors mean that any intervention such as debriefing has the potential to maintain the trajectory of stress in which the child is engaged and lead to traumatization of the child. It may be more appropriate for children to experience, in an individual context, the kind of support that debriefing is assumed to provide for adults.

The fifth dimension for consideration, as regards children of different ages, is the positive or negative impact of self-disclosure amongst peers. The capacity to maintain confidentiality needs consideration according to the age of the group. It is against the age-appropriate needs of a young child to withhold into themselves information, reactions and experiences that need to be shared and held in a context of a trusting relationship with a parent or other adult. It is only when children move into late adolescence that they have the psychological maturity to maintain confidentiality of emotionally and psychologically significant issues without it causing further stress or traumatization.

Self-disclosure within peer groups may not be appropriate or advisable for an individual child. Engagement in the group process may unwittingly draw a child into a level of disclosure that is beyond their best interests. Owing to developmental immaturity and inexperience it may be difficult or impossible for a child to determine and maintain a level of involvement appropriate to the circumstances. This also applies to the capacity of a child to maintain a position of confidentiality in relation to what they observe and hear from other children.

It may be difficult for a child to disengage from active participation in a debriefing exercise in the way an adult is able to via silence, because of the importance of compliance to adult authority in the child–adult relationship. Depending on the format and modality of the debrief a child may or may not be able to find the opportunity for the level and style of engagement appropriate to them at that time.

Other differences requiring consideration are the time a child is able to concentrate and attend to the matter at hand, the availability of sufficiently skilled staff to monitor the levels of engagement and distress in the children, and the range of modalities of expression and communication that may be required and therefore need to be available.

Finally, children are likely to have available to them a limited repertoire of experiences successfully coped with, and therefore of the skills that develop as a result.

Debriefing: as a process for children

The process of managing the psychological impact of critical incidents begins for children in the immediate moments following a crisis. Important child-related differences require that models appropriate for children of different ages are developed. The preceding identification of the underpinnings of the concept and also of the outcomes required of the debriefing process leads to clarification of the techniques required.

The technique and the process of debriefing may be conducted within the group, family or individual contexts depending on the age of the child, the needs of the child and the particular set of circumstances present at the time. Each require specific consideration but there is also considerable overlap.

If debriefing is considered as a process it can be

Table 14.2. Psychological first aid for children who have shared a common experience

	Age		
	Under 7 years	7–11 years	11–13 years
Strategy	Work through parents (if possible)	Work through 'trusted' others	Work through 'trusted' others
	Engage 'trusted' others	Engage parents	Support and work with peer or incident group
	Re-engage peer group	Support 'incident' group or peer group as appropriate	Engage parents
Peer/incident group involvement	Secondary to parents and 'trusted' others	Central	Central
Parent involvement	Essential	Essential	Active support
Modalities (in order of priority)	Child/parent dyad	Child	Child
	Parent parallel work	Child/parent dyad	Parent parallel work or parent information
	Child – individually		
	Physical contact	Incident/peer group	Language
	Language	Language	
		Physical contact	

seen to have two principal steps. Stage 1 constitutes psychological first aid, and stage 2 is clinical group debriefing. Beyond this, children and their families may require treatment interventions if reactions are severe or entrenched or other vulnerabilities are present.

Psychological first aid

As with physical assault and damage, psychological first aid provides immediate first-line care through short-term measures that aim to contain any damaging impacts and also to prevent secondary damage. It is provided in the moments and immediate hours following the focus incident and is directed to addressing the sequelae of that incident. For the child it has the primary requirement to establish a general experience of safety and containment, orientation to the event and the opportunity for emotional release. Reunion and engagement with significant others is imperative and needs to be addressed and managed sensitively (Yule & Canterbury, 1994). The opportunity exists to screen children and identify those who may be in need of

immediate and more comprehensive attention (Yule & Udwin, 1991; Yule & Canterbury, 1994). While the goals are the same for the different age groups, the strategies, involvement of parents, peer/incident group and the modalities selected to operationalize the procedure differ. Table 14.2 provides a structure according to three age groups, under 7 years, 7 to 11 years and 11 to 13 years. Because of the regressive pull generated by frightening and overwhelming experiences these age-based categories must be used in the context of functional levels at the time of the engagement and not as definitive chronological categorizations. The table identifies the subtle shifts in emphasis between the age groups.

This stage needs to be overseen by sensitive, clear-headed and responsible leaders who are able to observe the multiplicity of needs of the children and parents and facilitate the meeting of them in what is often a chaotic and personally challenging context. It is important that homeostasis is attained through psychological first aid before formal group debriefing is embarked upon.

The following vignette describes the application of

psychological first aid principles during and immediately after a siege in a kindergarten where four four-year-old children were held hostage for seven hours during a cold winter day.

'Escapees'

The seventeen children who had escaped had been cared for by their teachers who told stories and entertained them while awaiting their parents' arrival. The children then went home. The consultants who arrived at the scene a short time later arranged to meet with the parents (predominantly mothers) and children of this group during the afternoon to provide the parents with an opportunity to identify their own feelings and reactions, and contain and support their engagement with their child's experience and reactions. The children were observed, listened to and responded to as they played and made comments about their experience in the morning. A working alliance was thus established and a more extensive meeting was arranged for the next evening, when there was an opportunity for fathers and other family members to be present, and a wider-ranging and more detailed discussion could occur.

'Kindergarten teachers and pre-school system'

While the siege was in progress, the consultants met briefly with the kindergarten teachers, the district preschool adviser, the regional director and relevant staff of Community Services, Victoria, to provide them with some orienting information on reactions that could be expected in the children and their families and to consider the future management of the children and the kindergarten.

'Parents of the hostage children'

During the afternoon of the siege, the consultants also met a number of times with the parents of the four children who were held hostage. Initially they were introduced to the rescue procedures through the Commander of Police Operations as the Medical Displan mental health coordinators. Opportunities were provided for the parents to orient themselves to the new and alien circumstances into which they had been catapulted, to consider the possible reactions that their children might have experienced and to consider how these could be managed with the child and within the family. Throughout the afternoon the police provided update reports on the strategies being employed, progress in the negotiations, and as far as could be anticipated, potential outcomes. With the passage of time, the situation became more intense and hope for an 'easy' resolution and release diminished. Eventually circumstances required the police to prepare the parents for the possibility that their children might at best sustain injuries. During this phase the parents were gradually, as a group and as couples, introduced to the structure of the recovery system, the services that would be available to them and to the role and function of the author as a coordinator of it. They were prepared for the release of the children and their reunion with them through consideration of what they thought would be helpful, including greetings, physical contact, expression of feelings and words of comfort and reassurance. They were also encouraged to connect with their own personal support networks and to spend time alone or with each other as they needed. During the hours of waiting much time was spent walking in the surrounding garden or sitting quietly in a room.

'Release and reunion'

News that the children had been released was disseminated chaotically with a rippling call through the siege precinct, 'they're out!'. The parents had to struggle though the mêlée to find their children. The cordoned medical emergency centre was lit by blazing arc lights glaring in the falling night. It was the central focus of the scores of emergency services personnel who, with concerned curiosity, witnessed this final phase of a tense and demanding day in which they had been engaged.

The children were placed on prepared treatment areas on the ground and attended to by medical personnel. The parents were brought into the emergency area and encouraged by the consultants to place themselves to one side of their child where the child could see them, remaining as close as procedures would permit, and to speak to and touch their child using familiar greetings, words of comfort and comment even though the children were in varying states of consciousness as a result of inhalation of the fumes from petrol with which the assailant had doused the children some hours earlier. The parents in turn were supported and consoled by the now familiar mental health coordinators, and questions about their child's condition addressed.

Arrangements to transport the children to hospital included (apart from one critically ill child) that at least one parent travelling in the ambulance with the child, accompanied by a mental health worker to support the parent and facilitate their parenting function in relation to the child.

Hospitalization

To prevent further separation of the children from their parents and to protect the bonds of reunion the consultants arranged for the parents to remain with their children through triage and stabilization in the emergency department, transfer to the ward and admission and subsequent medical procedures. The children sustained significant chemical burns to various parts of their bodies from petrol immersion, which required often painful treatment.

The children were placed in an area that provided some separation from general ward activities while not isolating them. The aim was to provide the children with constant contact with familiar people from their normal world, support cohesion of their group, facilitate opportunities for communication about their experience in the siege and provide a shared experience for post discharge. A parallel aim was to provide similar opportunities for the parents.

Ward staff responded readily to the request to

nurture and care for the parents as well as for the children. Day-beds were provided for the arents at the children's bedsides throughout the five- to six-day admission to hospital.

The decision was made not to 'debrief', 'treat' or engage in direct therapeutic contact with the children but to work through the parents. Assessments were made and reviewed through observations of the children and families, discussion with the parents and ward staff and minimal contact with the children. The first priorities were to address any fracturing of the bonds in the parent–child relationship and compromises in the child's trust in the parents' capacity to respond to them, and the parents' capacity to trust their own parenting capabilities and the world's predictability.

The parents were engaged by the consultants individually, as parenting couples, and also as a parent group, where particular issues could be raised in the appropriate context and worked with. Parents were assisted to understand their child's reactive behaviours, fragments of communication, and to place these in the context of the total experience, and of the child's developmental stage and personality. The parents were supported to fulfil an active therapeutic role in relation to their children.

Pynoos & Nader (1988) also described a model of psychological first aid for children which, on a continuum, is between the model described and the traditional debriefing model. They focussed on the reactions of a school-based population after community violence. A strength of their model is the consideration given to children according to age, from (according to their report) preschool through second grade, third grade through fifth grade and adolescents from sixth grade onwards. They identified a range of symptomatic responses, and recommended appropriate first aid activities, for example if the preschool child experiences generalized fear the adult protective sheath needs to be re-established. Some of the responses and activities identified in this model would fit into formal group debriefing after the incident has subsided, for instance it is recommended that the adolescent's symptomatic responses of sense of shame, detachment and guilt are addressed by encouraging discussion of the event, feelings about it and realistic expectations of what could have been done.

Clinical group debriefing

As stated previously, the term debriefing covers a range of styles of interventions and is one of the options available to address the reactions and needs of children after the initial crisis has subsided.

Debriefing, by definition (Mitchell & Everly, 1995), is a stress management technique and should therefore be used only with children who have been assessed as 'stressed', with those screened as traumatized excluded from a group debriefing event and managed according to their particular needs. It is important that the application of group debriefing strategies as a tool for expedient management be avoided when it is appropriate for individually focussed interventions to be applied.

This more formalized second stage of the process has different aims from stage 1. It is a more focussed cognitive format where increased understanding of factual data of the common experience is possible, with illumination and understanding of one's own and others' issues and reactions. The child can be assisted to identify management options in the present and for the near future. It also provides the opportunity for the engagement of coping strategies within the child and for the child via the group process. Triage may take place and the leader can use the process to assist with consolidation of the group. This stage more resembles the model of adult CISD. It is complex and requires careful prior assessment of the child (Monahan, 1995) as well as skilled leadership encompassing psychodymanic, developmental and group leadership knowledge and skills. It is these factors that demand the nomenclature of 'clinical'. For a clinical debriefing to be constructive it has to be conducted with a sound awareness of the general and developmental capabilities and issues for each child within the group.

Practitioners of formal debriefing note that the appropriate timing for an adult group debriefing session is in the time between the emergence from the state of shock and numbing and before consolidation of the

experience becomes established (Yule & Gold, 1993; Mitchell & Everly, 1995). Experience indicates that this is likely to be similar for children.

Johnson (1989), Dyregrov (1991) and Yule & Canterbury (1994) described a procedure with close affinity to the Mitchell (1983) model. Brooks & Siegel (1996) described a four-step model that includes preparation of the leaders as step 1, having the children tell the story and share reactions as steps 2 and 3, and survival and recovery as the final step. A time frame is outlined for each stage.

Hendricks and colleagues (1993) have developed a framework for individual intervention in which the child tells his or her story through language or play. The story is then explored in detail including associated fantasies and feelings and is followed by closure, which includes the child's transition back into school and everyday life.

Pynoos (1990) has elucidated the aims of debriefing of children, extending these within the CISD model. They are: dispelling cognitive confusions and encouraging active coping through: bolstering the child's observing ego and reality-testing functions; assisting children to anticipate, understand and manage everyday reminders; assisting children to distinguish between current life stressors and past trauma, and decrease the impact of the trauma on the present experience; legitimizing children's feelings and reactions and assisting in the maintenance of self-esteem; preparing children to deal with the intermittent return of unresolved feelings; and providing the opportunity both to monitor responses and coping skills and to triage.

There may be a need for issues addressed in the psychological first aid stage to be readdressed depending on the circumstances of the incident and ongoing information. As the emotional meaning of the event is embedded in details of the experience as well as the personal and subjective impact, children may need to use a range of modalities to recreate the original context, which for adults is more readily recalled and communicated through language.

Children use play, drawing, dramatization and relationships with others, as well as language, to communicate their experiences. They may use any number of these modalities to express segments of the event, and skill is required to work with the child to piece together

Table 14.3. Clinical group debriefing for children who have shared a common experience

	Age		
	Under 7 years	7–11 years	11–13 years
Strategy	Work through parents	Engage parents	Work through 'trusted' others
	Engage peer/incident group	Work through 'trusted' others	Work with incident/peer group
		Work with incident/peer group	Engage parents
Peer incident group involvement	Central	Central	Central
Parent involvement	Essential	Essential	Active support
Modalities	Child – individually	Child group	Child group
	Parents	Parent parallel work	Parent parallel or parent information sessions
	Peer/incident group	Support the child's network	Support child's network
Techniques	Drawing	Play	Language
	Play	Language	Conversations, stories, poems, drawing, drama
	Language	Conversations	
		Stories	
		Drawing	
		Drama – puppets	

the fragments communicated within the different modalities into a correct and coherent whole.

The format may be variable depending on the age of the child and the level at which the regressive pull has settled. Therefore a debrief for a child may be facilitated through discussion and the verbal medium, through play, drawing, drama or a combination of the modalities. The modalities in combination with other considerations will dictate the venue, the time allocated and the format of the session. Considerable adaptability and ingenuity may be required on behalf of the leaders.

In some circumstances, the work of debriefing the child, especially the young child, may be achieved within the child–parent relationship if appropriate support and debriefing opportunities are made available to the parents.

Group debriefings of children need to be conducted with ground rules similar to those used for adults, but adapted to the maturational level of the children. A group clinical debriefing according to the format and modality identified as appropriate for a particular group of children should follow the phases of: introduction; establishment of facts; identification of thoughts, feelings, fantasies and mythology; reactions; symptoms; a teaching phase appropriate to the preceding content; and a re-entry phase (Dyregrov, 1991). This may need to be repeated in one or more subsequent sessions and provision made for post-debriefing follow-up according to individual or group needs. Depending on individual or small-subgroup needs, other strategies may need to be put into place to meet the needs of individual children and families and to support the debriefing process.

A representation of the issues is given in Table 14.3. As with the representation of psychological first aid in

Table 14.2, there are subtle shifts in tasks and focus as the child functions at developmentally more mature levels.

The aims and the content of the debriefing have significant variation depending on the psychological impact of the incident on the child. When the incident has primarily been about loss, grief is the principal psychological component. A personal experience of violence and life threat generates issues of safety, guilt and possible death, while an environmental disaster has possibly involved an experience of overwhelming natural and perceptually primitive forces and probable massive destruction of the personal environment and also community and natural environments. Very frequently each of these components are present in any one of a number of combinations with varying degrees of significance for each child and the process and technique need to be responsive to these individual nuances.

Ongoing Critical Incident Stress Management

Following the debriefing process of psychological first aid and clinical debriefing there is a need to monitor children both individually and as a group for ongoing reactions, many of which may subsequently present as symptoms of PTSD. Children, their family and incident group also need to be monitored for the emergence of new reactions and for vulnerabilities that may subsequently arise because of ongoing life issues or newly emergent life issues months to years later. A range of management and treatment options may need to be available to meet individual requirements in the short, medium and long term.

Leadership of the debriefing process for children

Usually discussions in the literature on group debriefing of children do not consider the training and skills required of the person providing this arguably clinical service. Dyregrov (1997) and Mitchell & Everly (1995) drew attention to the importance of training for adult debriefing workers in group and debriefing skills. Dyregrov (1997) noted the influence of personal skills in the successful conduct of a group debriefing process. He identified the need for research to identify the required leadership skills for adults and also discusses training leaders as a resource group to assist children to deal with the death of peers within a school or playgroup (Dyregrov, 1991).

The team conducting psychological first aid and clinical debriefing for children needs to meet a number of criteria (Table 14.4). First, to respond to the requirement for the establishment and maintenance of safety, the anchor person, who would be seen by the children as being the person in control, must be someone known and trusted by the child. This person may be the schoolteacher, scout leader or similar (Dyregrov, 1991). As this person is likely also to be a participant in the incident themselves, care must be taken to provide them with the appropriate support, debriefing and clinical services they require. Secondly, there needs to be an adult in the team who knows each child well from the developmental perspective, and understands their preferred modes of expression, signs of distress and nuances of behaviour and other issues the child might be engaged in prior to the incident or running parallel with it.

The third requirement for a clinical debrief is skills that include a thorough grounding in normal psychological and emotional development in children, childhood responses to stress and the indications of traumatization, including the presentation of traumatic responses, fantasies of reversal, redoing and the need to change the outcome. There needs to be a capacity within the leaders to be alert to the subtlety of the presentation of psychological issues in children and to recognize unconscious processes and meanings. Finally the clinical debriefing must be conducted by a person trained, experienced and skilled in childhood critical stress and debriefing, childhood psychopathology and family and group work.

The requirements of those conducting the stages of the debriefing process for children are therefore different from those requirements for people conducting adult CISD. It can be helpful if the person providing the clinical aspect within the debriefing team is available to provide the follow-up services of supervision of programmes provided to the children, families and school or group that may have been engaged in the incident.

Table 14.4. Leadership of debriefing process

- Known and trusted by child
- Knows each child developmentally and functionally
- Understanding
    Child development
    Childhood trauma reactions
    Childhood psychopathology
    Family and group processes
- Trained in childhood debriefing

This provides continuity, knowledge and experience, which is an important factor for children in the re-establishment of the cocoon of safety. It also provides a support and monitoring facility for staff engaged in the incident with the children and the debriefing process, and assistance to the school or the organization.

Because the debriefing process can be professionally demanding and personally challenging, leaders require a forum where countertransference issues can be identified, skill and process supervision provided and support received (Cohen, 1988).

Issues, questions, risks

A careful consideration of debriefing for children raises some questions. Should children experience a group debriefing technique? If so, what are the goals, what are the techniques? What are the dynamics at play within a group of children who have experienced a debriefing? Should children be mandated to participate? With whose authority should a child debriefing be conducted – parents, school, other? Who has ultimate responsibility for the children within, and following, a debriefing group? What are the legal implications of exposure to and participation in the technique and process? Are we overservicing children with broad-brush programmes not based on careful assessment of need?

Yule & Udwin (1991) noted the dearth of psychological triage methodologies for children in the early hours and days following a disaster – the time when debriefing is most likely to take place. Current practice is usually based on replicative or derivative models of the Mitchell model. Are these appropriate? Helpful? Harmful? Do we know how to achieve the aims of debriefing

that are appropriate for children and ensure that they are in the best interest of the child? If not, should the practice continue? What might serve as alternative and more appropriate ways to meet children's needs? Where is the evaluative data? What are the accountability processes – to the client group and professionally?

There are risks involved in applying adult group debriefing models and techniques to children. Unless a sensitive individual evaluation of each child is made at the time of the debriefing, the child may be exposed to information and emotions beyond his or her capacity to process and integrate, adaptive mechanisms may be destabilized, defence mechanisms challenged and overridden, fantasy engaged or stimulated and pre-existing vulnerabilities aroused. There may be inhibition of appropriate closure processes already engaged, secondary or vicarious traumatization, retraumatization and contagion as a result of participating in a debriefing.

An additional consideration when planning a debriefing process is the ethical/legal issue of the receipt or not of parental permission for involvement of the child in what is a powerful psychological intervention modality. There could be issues of legal accountability and perhaps liability for debriefing staff and their organizations in the absence of such permission. Technical issues arise if parents decide that their child is not to participate in the debriefing process with their incident/peer group.

Discussion

This chapter has considered the topic of debriefing as it relates to groups of children who, together, have experienced critical incidents arising from unexpected, challenging, overwhelming or calamitous events in their environment. Understanding the subject of debriefing may be facilitated when it is considered from the three parameters of the concept, the process and the technique.

There are major differences in the context in which debriefing is to be used with children in comparison with adults. These include the increased compromised sense of safety, more so in the younger child, the inherent immaturity and the unfolding developmental process with a gradual attainment of skills as the child matures, and the central role of parents and peers in the social context. These differences demand that techniques appropriate to the requirements of children at various stages of development be devised, implemented and evaluated.

Debriefing as a technique must be adapted to the developmental needs of each child individually, taking into account psychological, cognitive, emotional, social, family and vulnerability factors. As well as having the potential to support children in their recovery from untoward experiences, debriefing also holds the potential for harm and serious damage to children through ill-considered and managed application of the concept using a technique developed for adults. It needs to be used with utmost discretion after a careful assessment process. Group debriefing may or may not be in a particular child's best interests but the debriefing process may have efficacy when adapted to the developmental stages and in response to the individual child. It needs to be placed in the context of overall management and treatment.

Prior to engaging a child in any response or management activity, including group debriefing, it is essential to identify, for each child, the quality of the impact of the event and the life context in which it has occurred for that child. A state of stress, crisis, critical incident stress, trauma or traumatic grief may be present. Each is different in genesis, response, process and outcome. Each of these states requires specific management and care must be exercised to avoid maintaining or escalating the response.

The suggested model is one of psychological first aid within the immediate response phase of an incident followed by a clinical debriefing exercise. Together they combine to provide the debriefing process. The model is responsive to variations in the different age groups and may, for some children, be sufficient to meet their needs. Other children, families and groups may need other services to meet ongoing or emergent requirements.

The role of leaders within the debriefing process is as significant as it is for adult debriefing. However the role, functions and criteria for suitability for leadership

are different. The principal difference is the replacement of peer support debriefing personnel with a person who is able to provide for the child an experience of safety and continuity. The second difference is the importance of the leader having skills in child development, in childhood reactions to traumatization, childhood psychopathology, family dynamics and peer group processes in children.

Evaluative mechanisms for child debriefing models need to be established. Group debriefing may meet a child's needs. If so, at this stage, we do not fully understand how or why. It may work counter to the child's needs. Again we need to know more.

REFERENCES

Boatright, C. (1985). Children as victims of disaster. In J. Laube & S. Murphy (Ed.) *Perspectives on Disaster Recovery* (pp. 131–49). East Norwalk, CT: Appleton-Century-Crofts.

Brooks, B. & Siegel, P. (1996). *The Scared Child: Helping Kids Overcome Traumatic Events*. New York: John Wiley and Sons Inc.

Cohen, R. (1988). Intervention programs for children. In M. Lystad (Ed.) *Mental Health Response to Mass Emergencies*, (pp. 262–83). New York: Brunner/Mazel.

Denholm, C. (1995). Survival from a wild attack: a case study of analysis of adolescent coping. *Maternal–Child Nursing Journal*, **23**, 26–34.

Duckworth, D. (1986). Psychological problems arising from disaster work. *Stress Medicine*, **2**, 315–23.

Dyregrov, A. (1991). *Grief in Children*. Guildford: Biddles Ltd.

Dyregrov, A. (1997). The process in psychological debriefing. *Journal of Traumatic Stress*, **10**, 589–605.

Eriksson, M. (1996). The trauma/refugee project of the County Council of Stockholm: 'Bosnienprojektet', at the Karolinska Hospital. *Traumatic Stress Points*, **10**(1), 4.

Eth, S. & Pynoos, R. (1985). Developmental perspective on psychic trauma in children. In C. R. Figley (Ed.) *Trauma and its Wake*, (pp. 36–52). New York: Brunner/Mazel.

Galante, R. & Foa, D. (1986). An epidemiological study of psychic trauma and treatment effectiveness for children after a natural disaster. *Journal of the American Academy of Child Psychiatry*, **25**, 357–63.

Gillis, H. (1993). Individual and small-group psychotherapy for children involved in trauma and disaster. In C. Saylor (Ed.)

Children and Disaster (pp. 165–86). New York: Plenum Press.

Gordon, R. & Wraith, R. (1993). Responses of children and adolescents to disaster. In J. P. Wilson & B. Raphael (Eds.) *International Handbook of Traumatic Stress Syndromes* (pp. 561–75). New York: Plenum Press.

Hendricks, J., Black, P. & Kaplan, T. (1993). *When Father Kills Mother*. London: Routledge.

Herman, J. (1992). *Trauma and Recovery*. New York: Basic Books.

James, B. (1996). *Treating Traumatized Children*. New York: Free Press.

Johnson, K. (1989). *Trauma in the Lives of Children*. Claremont, CA: Hunter House.

Joseph, S., Brown, C.R. & Yule, W. (1993). Causal attributing and post-traumatic stress in adolescents. *Journal of Child Psychology and Psychiatry*, **34**, 247–53.

MacLean, G. (1977). Psychic trauma and traumatic neurosis: play therapy with a four year-old boy. *Canadian Psychiatric Association Journal*, **22**, 71–6.

McFarlane, A. C. (1987). Posttraumatic phenomena in a longitudinal study of children following a natural disaster. *Journal of the American Academy of Child and Adolescent Psychiatry*, **26**, 764–9.

Milgrom, M. & Toubiana, Y. (1996). Children's selective coping after a bus disaster: confronting behaviour and perceived support. *Journal of Traumatic Stress*, **9**, 687–702.

Mitchell, J. T. (1983). When disaster strikes: the critical incident stress debriefing process. *Journal of Emergency Medical Services*, **8**, 36–8.

Mitchell, J. T. & Everly, G. S. (1995) *Critical incident Stress Debriefing: An Operations Manual for the Prevention of Traumatic Stress Among Emergency Services and Disaster Workers*. Ellicott City, MD: Chevron Publishing.

Monahan, C. (1995). *Children and Trauma: A Parent's Guide to Helping Children Heal*. New York: Lexington Books.

Nader, K. (1995). *Psychological First Aid for Trauma, Grief and Traumatic Grief*. Laguna Hills, CA: The author.

O'Hara, D., Taylor, R. & Simpson, K. (1994). Critical incident stress debriefing: bereavement support in schools – developing a role for an LEA educational psychology service. *Educational Psychology in Practice*, **10**, 27–34.

Pynoos, R. (1990). Post-traumatic stress disorder in children and adolescents. In B. Garfunkel, G. Carlson & E. Weller (Eds.) *Psychiatric Disorders in Children and Adolescents* (pp. 48–63). Philadelphia: W. B. Saunders Co.

Pynoos, R. (1993). Traumatic stress and developmental psychopathology in children and adolescents. In J. Oldham, M. Riba & A. Tasman (Eds.) *American Psychiatric Press Review of*

Psychiatry, vol. 12 (pp. 205–38). Washington, DC: American Psychiatric Press.

Pynoos, R. & Nader, K. (1988). Psychological first aid and treatment approach to children exposed to community violence: research implications. *Journal of Traumatic Stress*, **1**, 445–73.

Pynoos, R. & Nader, K. (1993). Issues in the treatment of post-traumatic stress in children and adolescents. In J. P. Wilson & B. Raphael (Eds.) *International Handbook of Traumatic Stress Syndromes* (pp. 535–49). New York: Plenum Press.

Pynoos, R., Steinberg, A. & Wraith, R. (1995). Developmental model of childhood traumatic stress. In *Developmental Psychopathology*, vol. 2, I. Cicchetti & I. Cohen (Eds.) *Risk, Disorder and Adaptation* (pp. 72–95). New York: John Wiley and Sons Inc.

Raphael, B. (1986). *When Disaster Strikes: How Individuals and Communities Cope with Disaster*. New York: Basic Books.

Raphael, B., Meldrum, L. & McFarlane, A. (1995). Does debriefing after psychological trauma work? *British Medical Journal*, **310**, 1479–80.

Robinson, R. & Mitchell, J. (1993). Evaluation of psychological debriefing. *Journal of Traumatic Stress*, **6**, 367–82.

Robinson, R. & Mitchell, J. (1995). Getting some balance back into the debriefing debate. *Bulletin of the Australian Psychological Society*, **17**, 5–10.

Shalev, A. (1994). Debriefing following traumatic exposure. In R. J. Ursano, B. G. McCaughey & C. S. Fullerton (Eds.) *Individual and Community Responses to Trauma and Disaster – The Structure of Chaos* (pp. 201–19). Cambridge: Cambridge University Press.

Sheridan, S., Dee, C., Morgan, J., McCormack, M. & Walker, D. (1996). A multimethod intervention for social skills deficits in children with ADHD and their parents. *School Psychology Review*, **25**, 57–76.

Stallard, P. & Law, F. (1993). Screening and psychological debriefing of adolescent survivors of life-threatening events. *British Journal of Psychiatry*, **163**, 660–5.

Terr, L. (1985). Psychic trauma in children and adolescents. *Psychiatric Clinics of North America*, **8**, 815–35.

Terr, L. (1989). Treating psychic trauma in children: a preliminary discussion. *Journal of Traumatic Stress*, **2**, 3–20.

Yule, W. (1991). Work with children following disasters. In M. Herbert (Ed.) *Clinical Psychology: Social Learning Development and Behaviour* (pp. 349–63). Chichester: John Wiley.

Yule, W. (1992). Post-traumatic stress disorder in child survivors of shipping disasters: the sinking of the 'Jupiter'. *Journal of Psychotherapy and Psychosomatics*, **57**, 200–5.

Yule, W. & Canterbury, R. (1994). The treatment of posttraumatic stress disorder in children and adolescents.

International Review of Psychiatry, **6**, 141–51.

Yule, W. & Gold, A. (1993). *Wise Before the Event*. London: Turnaround Distribution Ltd.

Yule, W. & Udwin, O. (1991). Screening child survivors for post-traumatic stress disorders: experiences from the 'Jupiter' sinking. *British Journal of Clinical Psychology*, **30**, 131–8.

Yule, W. & Williams, R. (1990). Post-traumatic stress reactions in children. *Journal of Traumatic Stress*, **3**, 279–95.

15

Debriefing adolescents after critical life events

Paul Stallard

EDITORIAL COMMENTS

This chapter describes a background of development and its implications for debriefing children and specifically adolescents, after a traumatic event. Studies relevant to this age group are reviewed, but are small in number.

The concepts of group debriefing and individual debriefing through a child interview technique are also discussed. Many of the reports reviewed provide few systematic data, although one study showed no positive benefits for the adolescent girls, for whom debriefing was provided either with or without group counselling sessions. Indeed their scores, on measures of anxiety and depression had significantly increased, and their scores on the Impact of Event Scale (IES) remained high. Another similar study with controls did however show some reduction on intrusion scores on the IES but no differences in depression or anxiety.

Stallard's own work was with debriefing provided more than three months later for seven survivors of a school minibus accident. Three months after the start of debriefing these young people showed positive changes (ie. a reduction of symptoms) on the IES, the whole being due to changes on the intrusion scale.

The author explores some important questions about debriefing: its conceptualization and what it is intended to achieve for adolescent groups; issues of the optimum time for intervention for children and adolescents; and whether, if provided after the first few weeks it can it be seen to have a preventive role. He discusses: who should be drawn together in groups for debriefing (issues of development, responsibility, gender);

whether debriefing with adolescents is preventive (little evidence supports this); whether debriefing with adolescents is effective (he suggests it may be so only for those with high levels of post-traumatic stress, e.g. high IES scores).

The importance of tailoring any such intervention to both the levels of development and the particular needs of the child is noted. Stallard also emphasizes the need for much further work in this field, and for randomized controlled trials using standardised interventions. These studies should also identify for whom debriefing may be of benefit, the optimal timing and the relative contributions of different components in terms of a developmental perspective.

This chapter contributes by suggesting the effectiveness of a delayed intervention – which may perhaps be more appropriate because it is provided at a time of greater sense of security for the young person. The need for systematic research in the whole field of psychological trauma and its effects on children and adolescents is highlighted as is the need for empirical research into interventions and their effectiveness.

Introduction

There is now acceptance that children and young people (under 18 years), like adults, suffer significant and long-lasting psychological distress following critical life events (Yule, 1994). A number of studies have detailed the effects upon children and young people of natural disasters such as flooding (Newman, 1976; Green et al., 1991), fire (McFarlane et al., 1987), lightning strikes (Dollinger et al., 1984), gale damage (Parker et al., 1995), hurricanes (Lonigan et al., 1991), landslide (Lacey, 1972) and earthquakes (Pynoos et al., 1993). Transport accidents have been studied, particularly shipping disasters (Yule et al., 1990; Yule & Williams, 1990), traffic accidents (DiGallo et al., 1997; Mirza et al., 1998) and coach crashes (Curle & Williams, 1996; Casswell, 1997). Finally the negative effects of human-engendered traumas such as kidnapping (Terr, 1983), bombing (Curran et al., 1990) and playground sniper attacks (Pynoos et al., 1987) have been reported.

Trauma reactions

The psychological reactions of children and young people after such events are varied but often include a number of core features (Terr, 1991; Vogel & Vernberg, 1993; Yule, 1994). Persistent re-experiencing of the critical event either in the form of repetitive intrusive thoughts, flashbacks, nightmares or trauma-related play are often reported. These may be triggered by reminders of the incident or occur at times when the child is unoccupied. High levels of anxiety and the development of trauma-related fears are described, resulting in children and young people avoiding places or events associated with the incident. Depression, feeling numb, unresponsive, lethargic and uninterested in previously enjoyable activities are common feelings. Unhappiness and regular bouts of tearfulness, often triggered by recollections of the trauma, are frequently described. This may have an effect upon the children's relationships and they may socially withdraw and isolate themselves from their friends or appear irritable, touchy and angry with their parents. Finally, children have been found to display high levels of arousal following traumatic events and sleeping problems in the form of either difficulty in getting off to sleep or early morning waking are common. Problems in focussing attention and sustaining concentration on school work have also been described and children may appear hypervigilant and generally alert to any potential forms of danger.

Developmental perspective

While children and young people are equally affected by traumatic events, the specific manifestations of their symptomatology occurs along a developmental perspective. The cognitive development of preschool children (under 5 years) is more limited. Their thinking is concrete and egotistical and they are unable to imagine ways in which the trauma could be prevented or altered. They may appear withdrawn or subdued and re-enact the trauma in a very factual and descriptive way through their play. Parents may notice the loss of previously acquired developmental skills, particularly toileting, resulting in soiling and wetting accidents. Disturbed sleep is common and young children may be troubled by recurrent and distressing dreams or appear fearful about going to bed. Finally they may become very clingy, refusing to be left alone at playgroup or nursery, wanting instead to sit with their parents during the day and to sleep with them at night.

The school-age child (over 5 years) has a larger repertoire of cognitive responses and can imagine the traumatic event, having a range of possible outcomes. Rather than re-enacting the trauma, school-age children may talk about or act out different endings in which they may fantasize about executing revenge or prevent fatal or serious injury. Like younger children, their emotions are often reflected in their behaviour and they can present with a wide range of reactions from apparent indifference to extreme irritability, anger and defiance. Their physical and verbal anger is often projected onto their parents or friends, which in turn may have a detrimental effect upon these important relationships.

Young people reach a stage of cognitive maturity in which they are able to understand and conceptualize more abstract issues such as accountability, survivor guilt and alternative action. They are able to create and explore a range of possible trauma scenarios that may emphasize and be critical of, their own action or inaction. Young people are very aware of their own limitations and highly sensitive to the views of others. Often these critical thoughts remain private and are seldom shared, although their anger is expressed in more extreme and noticeable ways. This may be directed outwards in the form of truancy, substance abuse, rebelliousness or delinquency, or inwardly as manifest by deliberate self-harm, eating disorders or depression.

Post-traumatic stress disorder

A number of studies have demonstrated that children and young people present with multiple symptoms that often cluster together to form anxiety and depressive and post-traumatic stress disorders (PTSD). These disorders are not always clearly distinct and there is often considerable overlap between them (Davidson & Foa, 1991; Yule, 1994).

PTSD is the more widely researched and for diagnosis requires fulfilment of the following criteria. The individual has first to experience an event that is outside the range of usual human experience. This must result in persistent re-experiencing of the trauma, avoidance of stimuli associated with it and increased rates of arousal. These symptoms have to persist for longer than one month and cause clinically significant distress or impairment in social, occupational or other areas of functioning (American Psychiatric Association, 1994).

Estimates of PTSD in children and young people involved in critical life-threatening events vary enormously from 10% to 100% (Yule, 1994). PTSD has been found in children exposed to a wide range of incidents when assessed at varying times ranging from a few days to over a year after the event, using a variety of different assessment measures (Vogel & Vernberg, 1993). While these studies often confirm the presence of PTSD in children and young people exposed to critical life-threatening events major methodological problems limit the conclusions that can be made. Variable response rates lead to questions regarding the representativeness of the subjects studied. The absence of appropriate comparison groups and use of different rates and methods of assessment limit the general applicability of study findings. The variable times of assessment after the trauma limit conclusions regarding the prevalence and natural course of PTSD. Finally the adequacy of applying the diagnostic criteria of PTSD developed on the basis of work with adults to children has been questioned, since the criteria do not adequately describe the wide range of symptoms presented by children (Vogel & Vernberg, 1993; Yule, 1994; Street & Sibert, 1998).

Risk factors

Not all children and young people present with PTSD or other disorders. Children and young people respond differently to critical life events, although comparatively little is known about significant risk or protective factors (Udwin, 1993; Yule & Canterbury, 1994). Risk factors found to increase the likelihood of psychological problems include disaster characteristics such as the degree of exposure to a critical event (Pynoos et al., 1987; Lonigan et al., 1991), individual characteristics such as gender (Green et al., 1991), level of predisaster functioning (Earls et al., 1988), and family characteristics such as parental reactions (McFarlane et al., 1987). Children of all ages seem vulnerable to the psychological effects of critical life-threatening incidents. Comparatively little research has focussed upon the role of the young person's cognitive appraisal of the event in relation to the development of PTSD. Studies examining the causal attributions of adolescent survivors of a cruise ship sinking found greater post-traumatic stress one year after the accident in those young people with more internal negative causal attributions (Joseph et al., 1993).

Psychological interventions

Much of the early work examining the effects of critical life-threatening events on children and young people was descriptive and concerned with identifying and detailing symptomatology. Researchers have now turned their attention to prevention and treatment and a range of disaster-related psychological interventions have been described (Vernberg & Vogel, 1993). These include: predisaster interventions such as preparing a major disaster plan; impact phase interventions such as psychological first aid that are provided in the immediate period following the trauma; short-term adaptation phase interventions provided in the three months preceding the trauma and including small-group and family interventions; and long-term adjustment phase interventions such as individual cognitive-behavioural interventions delivered three months or more after the critical event. Vernberg & Vogel concluded that 'so little treatment outcome research exists in the disaster literature that there is little solid evidence to support (or question) the different treatment recommendations in terms of efficacy, or even to demonstrate that any of the interventions have any important effects upon child and adolescent adjustment' (ibid., p. 496). Despite the lack of substantive evidence, psychological interventions are now widely viewed as an integral part of a comprehensive response to critical life-threatening events. In particular front-line interventions such as psychological debriefing have gained much popularity and are often seen as essential for both trauma survivors and rescuers, although this has been questioned (Bisson & Deahl, 1994; Raphael et al., 1995).

Psychological debriefing

Critical Incident Stress Debriefing (CISD) originated in the work of Mitchell (1983) as a form of crisis intervention designed to help ambulance personnel cope with the emotional consequences of their work. The process has been modified, termed psychological debriefing, and been widely used with disaster survivors and those who help, such as rescuers, emergency service personnel and the providers of psychological support (Dyregrov, 1989). It has also been adapted to be used with children within a classroom setting to talk about death and other critical life-threatening events (Dyregrov, 1991).

Psychological debriefing aims to prevent the development of future psychological problems by providing a structure in which the trauma can be discussed in depth. The debriefing attempts to meet the individuals' need to understand what has happened and how the critical event has affected them emotionally. During the meeting the child is encouraged to describe the critical life event within a safe holding environment that is designed to promote his or her cognitive and emotional processing of the trauma.

The group debriefing process

For children and young people the debriefing session typically adopts a standard structure (Dyregrov, 1991). The suggested format can be used individually but is designed primarily for groups.

The debriefing starts with an introduction, during which the purpose and format of the meeting is explained. The children are encouraged to talk about the critical life event in order to understand what happened and how they and others feel and might react. The rules of the session are highlighted during this stage. What occurs within the session is private and is not to be shared with others who did not attend the meeting. Nobody should be teased or criticized for what they say or how they react. No one has to talk if they do not want to but if they do each child is to talk for him or her self, not for others.

The second stage of the meeting is the fact phase in which the facilitator helps to build up a picture of what actually happened. The event is reconstructed from beginning to end, thereby enabling all involved to gain a common understanding and to correct any misunderstandings. Dyregrov (1991) emphasized the importance for children of concrete information and facts and suggested that the facilitator gathers as much relevant information as possible from different sources prior to the meeting.

The factual discussion leads into the third stage of the debriefing, which is concerned with the children's thoughts about the trauma. They are encouraged to describe their initial thoughts about the event at the time when they realized that something was wrong. This subjective appraisal is fairly soon followed by a discussion about the emotional impact of the trauma both during and immediately after the event and how the children are currently feeling. Dyregrov (1991) suggested that direct attempts to elicit feelings should be avoided but that indirect methods should be used to encourage the children to talk. They could be asked to talk about the worst thing that happened during the event, encouraged to draw pictures or complete unfinished sentences. The facilitator can help the children to explore a range of sensory impressions, such as smell, sound and visual images, that may stir strong emotions. Once these have been described, the facilitator encourages others to join in and share their experience, thereby helping the children to recognize that others have similar feelings. The thought and reaction stage will occupy the majority of the debriefing. The emotional release and opportunity for children to discuss thoughts of blame, guilt, helplessness and anger are seen as a major part of the process.

The fifth stage is the information phase, during which the facilitator attempts to draw out similarities between the children's thoughts and feelings. These are clearly explained as normal reactions to a highly unusual event. The normalization of these reactions helps the children to recognize that they are neither unusual nor going out of their minds, but that their emotional reaction is both expected and understandable. Information is provided about the range of possible reactions that follow such critical life events and the children are warned that these may persist for some weeks. General advice as to how they can cope with their thoughts and feelings such as encouraging them to talk, write them down, etc., is provided.

During the ending phase, the facilitator summarizes the meeting, attempts to help the children plan what to do next and addresses any unanswered questions. The children are informed about what they should do if their distress persists and the facilitator follows up any who appear particularly affected.

Individual debriefing – the child interview

A technique of interviewing individual children who have been exposed to extreme acts of violence has been described (Pynoos & Eth, 1986). The authors reported that the interview technique has been used extensively with children aged 3 to 16 years who have witnessed a variety of trauma, including homicide, suicide, rape and kidnapping. The interview is usually conducted shortly after the trauma and some have been interviewed only a few hours after the critical event. Although the technique is not described specifically as psychological debriefing, the interview does have a preventative aim and shares a similar structure and content.

The interview is designed to be used with children fairly soon after a trauma and aims to help them to understand what has happened and how they are feeling. The first stage is the opening, during which the child is informed that the facilitator has met many children who have 'gone through what you have gone through'. The young person is encouraged to draw a picture about anything they like as long as they can tell a story about it. The facilitator probes the child's drawing and story and starts to identify the traumatic references. These are used to lead into the second stage of the interview, which is concerned with relieving the traumatic experience by systematically reconstructing events. Within a supportive holding relationship, the child is encouraged to describe what they saw. Actual events are discussed in detail, the accompanying sensory experience described, and the worst moment for the child explored. Common feelings and emotional reactions including guilt, accountability and anger are discussed. The interview then moves into the final stage of closure, during which the facilitator reviews and summarizes the session. Children are reassured that feelings of helplessness and fear are common and alerted to the possible future course of their reactions. Finally, the child is invited to contact the facilitator if they wish to talk again. The interview is used by the facilitator as a way of screening the child to identify whether any further intervention is required.

Debriefing adolescents

Reports of debriefing adolescents after critical life events are notably lacking from the literature. This may in part be due to the comparatively recent acceptance that children and young people suffer significant psychological distress after critical life-threatening incidents. Until relatively recently the majority of studies have therefore been concerned with describing symptomatology rather than evaluating interventions.

Pynoos & Eth (1986) provided a detailed account of using the child interview with an 11-year-old girl five days after her mother was shot by an estranged boyfriend. The account graphically highlights the key stages of the interview and ends with the girl reporting that the interview 'made me feel hurt and stuff, but it also made me feel good'.

Interventions that have reported using group debriefing or have incorporated the core aims and structure of this process have typically been described in relation to transport disasters. Klingman (1987) described a range of crisis interventions that were provided to 675 13-year-old children after a disaster in which a school bus was struck by a passing train. The disaster, in which 19 children died and 15 were critically injured, was witnessed by many children in the following coaches. Within hours of the accident as they returned to school to be reunited with their parents the children in the following coaches participated in group meetings. These were designed to be preventative and focussed upon expression and acknowledgement of feelings in order to reduce anxiety and so prevent disorientation. Children were given factual information and those at risk of potentially developing severe reactions were identified. A range of other interventions were provided at various times after the disaster and so it is not possible to ascertain whether debriefing per se had any positive effect upon the prevention of future difficulties.

Casswell (1997) described the response of a mental health team to a school bus crash involving 59 young people aged 11 to 18 years. The double-decker school bus was hit head-on while carrying the pupils home from school, resulting in the death of the bus driver and one pupil. Counsellors sat with parents during the six hours after the accident until the children were reunited with their parents. In the subsequent days the team talked with teaching staff about the effects of trauma and how they could help distressed pupils. Preparations were made to provide psychological debriefing for all the bus victims and other school children who were travelling behind the bus at the time of the accident. A total of 46 survivors attended one of the debriefing groups that took place away from the school premises approximately two weeks after the accident. Children were grouped according to age and siblings split into separate groups in order to prevent any inhibitory influences. The session followed the format of the CISD (Mitchell, 1983) process and a follow-up debriefing was arranged six weeks later. Unfortunately the children were not assessed prior to the debriefing and so it is not possible to determine whether the intervention had any positive effects on the prevention of future psychopathology.

Yule & Udwin (1991) conducted psychological debriefing with 24 girls aged 14–16 years 10 days after the school cruise ship *Jupiter* collided with an oil tanker and sank. Approximately 400 British school children

and 60 teachers were aboard the ship, although amazingly only two seamen and two passengers died in the disaster. The authors conducted a group debriefing with all the girls from one of the schools who were abroad the ship. The meeting aimed to help the girls understand what had happen and allowed them to share their feelings about the tragedy. The girls were prepared for some of the normal reactions that follow such abnormal events and completed a PTSD screening battery consisting of the Impact of Event Scale IES, (Horowitz et al., 1979), Revised Children's Manifest Anxiety Scale (Reynolds & Richmond, 1978) and the Birleson Depression Inventory (Birleson, 1981). A series of voluntary school-based group counselling sessions were provided and after five months the children were reassessed using the same screening battery. The study failed to demonstrate any positive benefits of psychological debriefing with or without group counselling sessions. The children's scores on the anxiety and depression scales had significantly increased and they continued to score highly on the IES.

In a subsequent study *Jupiter* survivors who received debriefing and the opportunity to participate in group counselling sessions were compared with 15 girls who had received no such intervention until one year after the accident (Yule, 1992). Once again the groups did not differ on either the anxiety or depression scales, although there were significant differences on the IES. The intervention group had significantly lower scores and this difference was particularly noted on the intrusion rather than avoidance subscale.

The strongest evidence suggesting the value of psychological debriefing comes from a study of seven survivors of a school minibus accident (Stallard & Law, 1993). The pupils were on a school trip when the bus veered off the road and rolled over three times before coming to rest in the middle of a field. The accident resulted in no fatalities or serious physical injuries, although all the children were taken to hospital and it took several hours before they were reunited with their families. Three months later one of the children was referred to the authors by her general practitioner, suffering from intrusive thoughts and extreme anxiety. It emerged that none of the young people involved in the accident had received any help and so the authors arranged provision of two debriefing sessions at their school, following the standard format suggested by Dyregrov (1991). At the start of the first session the young people were asked to complete the PTSD screening battery suggested by Yule & Udwin (1991). This was posted to them again three months later and significant reductions were found on all measures. Interestingly the whole of the reduction of the IES was attributable to changes on the intrusion scale, a finding similar to that reported by Yule (1992).

These studies that have used psychological debriefing with adolescent survivors of critical events highlight a number of issues that have not been previously systematically explored or evaluated.

What is psychological debriefing?

There is considerable confusion and variation in the literature on children and adolescents as to what constitutes psychological debriefing. The term is used interchangeably to describe interventions with various objectives such as emotional unloading, prevention of future distress and a reduction in present symptomatology.

The content and structure of psychological debriefing overlaps considerably with other post-disaster interventions. The Task Force Report of the American Psychological Association into interventions with children after disasters described interventions provided during the impact phase, i.e. the first 24 hours after the trauma (Vernberg & Vogel, 1993). The intervention reported by Klingman (1987) was provided during this stage and, although Vernberg & Vogel (1993) argue, that these meetings were different from debriefing interviews, which involve a more detailed retelling of events, the similarities are none the less considerable. The Task Force Report similarly details various short-term (i.e. up to three months post disaster) adaptation phase interventions. Psychological debriefings are described as well as small-group interventions, although once again it is difficult to distinguish the difference between them. Small-group interventions (or group therapy) are described by Terr (1989) as a preventative intervention. The intervention aims to encourage children to express their thoughts and feel-

ings about a shared critical event within a safe environment. Reassurance and normalization of their emotional and cognitive reactions is a key aim as the group is helped to develop coping skills. Although the structure of the sessions may be different it remains unclear whether their content is substantially different from that of psychological debriefing.

What is the optimum time to provide debriefing?

There are temporal variations in the way debriefing is provided. Casswell (1997) provided one debriefing session and a six-week follow-up, Stallard & Law (1993) two debriefing sessions one week apart, while Yule & Udwin (1991) provided one debriefing session, although they offered subsequent monthly group sessions. With regard to timing, psychological debriefing was originally conceived of as a form of crisis intervention to occur within two to three days of a traumatic event (Mitchell, 1983). Others argue that children and young people may be too numbed to benefit from a debriefing so soon and suggest an optimal post-disaster time of 7 to 14 days (Yule, 1994). The issue of psychological readiness is important in determining the optimum time for conducting debriefing (Chemtob et al., 1997). At present there are wide variations regarding the time at which debriefing is provided with some counsellors undertaking interviews within hours (Pynoos & Eth, 1986; Klingman, 1987), while others have conducted debriefing several months after the critical incident (Stallard & Law 1993). The optimum time for debriefing children and adolescents remains to be established. It is, however, questionable whether psychological debriefing provided more than four weeks after a critical event can be conceived of as a crisis or preventative intervention.

Should membership of adolescent debriefing groups be selective?

The composition of psychological debriefing groups has received minimal attention. It has been recommended that in terms of small-group interventions, young people should be grouped by age and degree of exposure to the traumatic event (Terr, 1989). Older children (16 to 18 years) have been reported to be particularly interested in metaphysical issues such as the role of fate, whereas younger children (11 to 13 years) were keen to learn that their reactions were normal (Casswell, 1997). Grouping by gender has received little attention, even though there is evidence to suggest that girls are more at risk of suffering from significant psychological trauma and cope with traumatic events differently from boys (Curle & Williams, 1996). Stallard & Law (1993) recommend that the level of responsibility of the trauma group be determined, since in their report of minibus survivors both the adolescents and the teacher who was driving attended the first debriefing session. Whether psychological debriefing should be targeted upon high-risk groups, occur in groups structured along identified variables or provided collectively to all involved in the critical event has not been systematically explored or evaluated.

Is psychological debriefing with adolescents preventative?

Of the studies describing psychological debriefing most are descriptive and anecdotal, the efficacy of the debriefing is rarely evaluated and the longer-term benefits in terms of preventing future psychopathology remain unproven. Furthermore, the specific contribution of debriefing to overall outcome is often difficult to ascertain, since it is often provided as one component of an on-going trauma intervention programme.

In terms of outcome, Pynoos & Eth (1986) 'hesitate to predict that our interview technique will be proven to be preventative'. Casswell (1997) did not report any pre- and post-debriefing comparisons, although when she assessed 34 survivors for legal purposes between 9 and 15 months after the school bus crash only six pupils had high scores on the IES. Whether debriefing prevented the remaining 28 pupils developing significant psychological distress or whether they were only mildly affected by the accident remains unknown. These data and those provided by Yule and his colleagues reported earlier provide no clear evidence to support the preventative role of psychological debriefing.

Is debriefing with adolescents effective?

While the preventative role remains unproven there is evidence from two studies with young people to suggest that psychological debriefing has a positive effect in terms of reducing intrusive thoughts. Yule (1992) and Stallard & Law (1993) both found significant reductions on the intrusion subscale of the IES, following debriefing. This is consistent with the results of a partially controlled study of adult hurricane survivors where debriefing was found to significantly reduce total and subscale scores on the IES (Chemtob et al., 1997). It has been suggested that intrusive thoughts may reflect specific cognitive distortions such as negative automatic thinking or guilt-provoking causal attributions (Joseph et al., 1995). If this proves to be the case then the results of these studies would suggest that a key function of debriefing is externally to validate and challenge the individual's perceived experience. Doubts, worries, negative thoughts and questions about the accident can be shared and addressed rather than internally rehearsed and thereby remaining unanswered. The debriefing process aims to clarify what actually happened, thereby allowing a reinterpretation of attributions, particularly those related to guilt, blame and responsibility. In turn, this external public clarification and validation may reduce the need for repeated cognitive rehearsal and the generation of associated intrusive negative thoughts.

Theoretically these results are consistent with cognitive theories of PTSD. Rachman's (1980) cognitive theory of emotional processing assumes that the emotional impact of traumatic events needs to be cognitively absorbed so that other experiences can proceed without disruption. Failure to absorb the emotional consequences of the critical event results in repetitive and intrusive re-experiencing of the trauma. Horowitz (1986) proposed a similar model, arguing that traumatic events provide information that is inconsistent with an individual's internal cognitive schema. This generates distress and a need to revise existing cognitive schema in order to accommodate the new experience. During this process, incoming information is kept at a tolerable level by an internal control system utilizing strategies of trauma intrusion and avoidance. Both theoretical models therefore view intrusive thoughts as evidence of poor adjustment. Consistent with these theoretical models psychological debriefing may provide the individual with an opportunity to emotionally process the experience and to assimilate the event into their cognitive schema. Debriefing may provide an opportunity for cognitive attributions and negative intrusive thoughts to be reappraised within a framework that acknowledges, encourages and normalizes emotional expression.

The literature in this area is not, however, consistent and reductions on the IES have not always been found with adults. A number of better-designed studies have reported no significant differences between individuals who received debriefing and those who did not (Deahl et al., 1994; Hobbs et al., 1996; Kenardy et al., 1996). These conflicting results may be due to methodological variations, differences in the content of the debriefing sessions or the post-disaster time at which debriefing was provided. There may be differences in the nature of the critical events, in terms of single versus repeated trauma, level of exposure or the nature and severity of physical injuries. Alternatively the difference in results may be due to subject variables such as perceived life threat or degree of post-trauma pathology. In terms of initial distress, both Yule (1992) and Stallard & Law (1993) reported average IES scores of slightly above 35, the recommended cut-off to identify clinical levels of distress. The average preintervention IES scores in the studies with adults reported above, which failed to demonstrate the effectiveness of debriefing, were below 20. Whether these individuals were suffering significant clinical distress that either required or was sufficient to be moderated by debriefing is therefore questionable.

Developmental considerations

According to Piaget (1950), conceptual development progresses through a number of key stages during which the child's thinking is qualitatively different. Older children aged 11 to 14 years are able to handle more abstract concepts and will be more aware of hypothetical issues surrounding the critical event, such as potential danger, threat to life, the role of fate and survivor guilt. Children aged 7 to 11 years are more concerned with factual information and observable behaviour. They find it difficult to conceptualize and explore abstract issues but can begin to consider alternative scenarios and understand the irreversibility of death. Younger children aged 2 to 7 years function at the preoperational stage and have an egotistical magical belief that they are somehow responsible for what occurs. The developmental nature of conceptual thinking may therefore have an effect upon the content, formation and/or perpetuation of intrusive traumatic thoughts, which in turn may influence the overall effectiveness and individual value of the specific components of psychological debriefing.

In terms of content, traumatic imagery can take many forms. The imagery could be factually descriptive or result in the generation of alternative scenarios in which the survivor imagines and cognitively rehearses other courses of action or outcomes to the trauma. The conceptual development of children would suggest that the traumatic imagery of adolescents and young children may be different. Younger children have a more limited comprehension and it is probable that they experience more factual and descriptive imagery. Adolescents are able to undertake a more abstract and complex exploration of the trauma and are able to imagine alternative actions and other possible outcomes. Tentative support for this possibility was found by Schwarz & Kowalski (1991), who reported on the effects of a school shooting. They found that older children experienced more anger than younger children and suggested that this was due to an increased cognitive ability to understand the wider context and potential implications of the shooting. Debriefing may therefore need to focus upon describing the actual traumatic event for younger children, while a fuller exploration of alternative scenarios and the perceived consequences of their action or inaction may be indicated for adolescents.

The traumatic images will be accompanied by a range of attributions as the individual attempts to explain why the trauma occurred. These vary along a developmental perspective and evolve from the magical and egocentric to more concrete factual explanations until multiple and more abstract concepts can be considered (Schwarz & Perry, 1994). The importance of these causal attributions in the development and maintenance of PTSD has been highlighted, one of the dimensions receiving most attention being that of internal–external controllability (Joseph et al., 1997). Adolescent survivors of a cruise ship disaster with more internal causal attributions for disaster-related events were found to have more intrusive thoughts and higher levels of depression (Joseph et al., 1993). If these findings were substantiated it would suggest a central role of causal attributions in the development and maintenance of chronic traumatic reactions. In turn this would indicate that debriefing with adolescents should focus more upon their causal attributions about the event and issues of self-blame, survivor guilt, and accountability should be fully explored. Younger children have a more self-centred approach and debriefing with this group should focus clearly upon the removal of responsibility for the trauma from the child.

Considering traumatic reactions within a developmental perspective would suggest that psychological debriefing should be more closely tailored to the developmental level of the child. A greater emphasis upon the factual stage of the debriefing may be particularly helpful for younger children. This would enable them to realize that they had not caused the critical event and would correct any factual misunderstandings that had occurred. Older children, as reported by Casswell (1997) may be more interested in exploring abstract issues that challenge their internal cognitive schema and causal attributions. Debriefing with this age group may need to focus more upon the cognitive and emotional stages thereby allowing causal attributions to be reappraised.

Conclusion

There is considerable confusion within the literature on children and adolescents regarding what constitutes psychological debriefing and the time at which it should be provided. Comparatively few studies have been reported and most have failed to evaluate the effectiveness of the intervention. There is no evidence to suggest that debriefing adolescents is effective in preventing future psychopathology, although some studies have reported reductions in intrusive negative cognitions.

Randomized controlled trials using standardized interventions are needed to evaluate the effectiveness of psychological debriefing with adolescents. The trials should attempt to identify for whom it may be of benefit, the optimum post-disaster time at which it should be undertaken, and the value of the individual components of the debriefing process along a developmental perspective.

REFERENCES

American Psychiatric Association (1994). *Diagnostic and Statistical Manual of Mental Dis◆ders*, 4th edn. Washington, DC: American Psychiatric Press.

Birleson, P. (1981). The validity of depressive disorder in childhood and the development of a self rating scale. *Journal of Child Psychology and Psychiatry*, **22**, 73–88.

Bisson, J. I. & Deahl, M. P. (1994). Psychological debriefing and prevention of post traumatic stress. More research is needed. *British Journal of Psychiatry*, **165**, 717–20.

Casswell, G. (1997). Learning from the aftermath: the response of mental health workers to a school bus crash. *Clinical Child Psychology and Psychiatry*, **2**, 517–23.

Chemtob, C. M., Thomas, S., Law, W. & Cremniter, D. (1997). Post-disaster psychological intervention: a field study of the impact of debriefing on psychological distress. *American Journal of Psychiatry*, **154**, 415–17.

Curle, C. E. & Williams, C. (1996). Post traumatic stress reactions in children: gender differences in the incidence of trauma reactions at two years and examination of factors influencing adjustment. *British Journal of Clinical Psychology*, **35**, 297–309.

Curran, P. S., Bell, P., Murray, A., Loughrey, G., Roddy, R. & Rocke, L. G. (1990). Psychological consequences of the Enniskillen bombing. *British Journal of Psychiatry*, **156**, 479–82.

Davidson, J. R. T. & Foa, E. (1991). Diagnostic issues in post-traumatic stress disorder: Considerations for the DSM-IV. *Journal of Abnormal Psychology*, **100**, 346–55.

Deahl, M. P., Gillham, A. B., Thomas, J., Searle, M. M. & Srinivasan, M. (1994). Psychological sequelae following the Gulf War. Factors associated with subsequent morbidity and the effectiveness of psychological debriefing. *British Journal of Psychiatry*, **165**, 60–5.

DiGallo, A., Barton, J. & Parry-Jones, W. L. I. (1997). Road traffic accidents: early psychological consequences in children and adolescents. *British Journal of Psychiatry*, **170**, 358–62.

Dollinger, S. J., O'Donnell, J. P. & Staley, A. A. (1984). Lightening-strike disaster: effects on children's fears and worries. *Journal of Consulting and Clinical Psychology*, **52**, 1028–38.

Dyregrov, A. (1989). Caring for helpers in disaster situations: psychological debriefing. *Disaster Management*, **2**, 25–30.

Dyregrov, A. (1991). *Grief in Children: a Handbook for Adults*. London: Jessica Kingsley.

Earls, F., Smith, E., Reich, W. & Jung, K. G. (1988). Investigating psychopathological consequences of disaster in children: a pilot study incorporating a structured diagnostic approach. *Journal of the American Academy of Child and Adolescent Psychiatry*, **27**, 90–5.

Green, B. L., Korol, M., Grace, M. C., Leonard, A. C., Gleser, G. C. & Smitson-Cohen, S. (1991). Children and disaster: age, gender and parental effects on PTSD symptoms. *Journal of the American Academy of Child and Adolescent Psychiatry*, **30**, 945–51.

Hobbs, M., Mayou, R., Harrison, B. & Worlock, P. (1996). A randomised controlled trial of psychological debriefing for victims of road traffic accidents. *British Medical Journal*, **313**, 1438–9.

Horowitz, M. J. (1986). Stress-response syndromes. A review of posttraumatic and adjustment disorders. *Hospital and Community Psychiatry*, **37**, 241–9.

Horowitz, M.J., Wilner, N. & Alvarez, W. (1979). Impact of Event Scale: a measure of subjective stress. *Psychosomatic Medicine*, **41**, 209–18.

Joseph, S., Brewin, C., Yule, W. & Williams, R. (1993). Causal attributions and Post traumatic stress in adolescents. *Journal of Child Psychology and Psychiatry*, **34**, 247–53.

Joseph, S., Yule, W. & Williams, R. (1995). Emotional processing in survivors of the Jupiter cruise ship disaster. *Behaviour Research and Therapy*, **33**, 187–92.

Joseph, S., Williams, R. & Yule, W. (1997). *Understanding Post-traumatic Stress: A Psychological Perspective on PTSD and Treatment*. Chichester: Wiley.

Kenardy, J. A., Webster, R. A., Lewin, T. J., Carr, V. J., Hazell, P. L. & Carter, G. L. (1996). Stress debriefing and patterns of recovery following a natural disaster. *Journal of Traumatic Stress*, **9**, 37–49.

Klingman, A. (1987). A school-based emergency crisis intervention in a mass school disaster. *Professional Psychology: Research and Practice*, **18**, 604–12.

Lacey, G. N. (1972). Observations of Aberfan. *Journal of Psychosomatic Research*, **16**, 257–60.

Lonigan, C. J., Shannon, M. P., Finch, A. J., Daugherty, T. K. &

Taylor, C. M. (1991). Children's reaction to a natural disaster: symptom severity and degree of exposure. *Advances in Behaviour Research Therapy*, **13**, 135–54.

McFarlane, A. C., Policansky, S. & Irwin, C. P. (1987). A longitudinal study of the psychological morbidity in children due to a natural disaster. *Psychological Medicine*, **17**, 727–38.

Mirza, K. A., Bhadrinath, B. R., Goodyer, I. M. & Gilmour, C (1998). Post-traumatic stress disorder in children and adolescents following road traffic accidents. *British Journal of Psychiatry*, **172**, 443–7.

Mitchell, J. I. (1983). When disaster strikes... The critical incident stress debriefing process. *Journal of Emergency Medical Services*, **8**, 36–8.

Newman, C. J. (1976). Children of disaster: clinical observations at Buffalo Creek. *American Journal of Psychiatry*, **133**, 306–12.

Parker, J., Watts, H. & Allsopp, M. R. (1995). Post-traumatic stress symptoms in children and parents following a school-based fatality. *Child Care, Health and Development*, **21**, 183–9.

Piaget, J. (1950). *The Psychology of Intelligence*. New York: Harcourt.

Pynoos, R. S. & Eth, S. (1986). Witness to violence : the child interview. *Journal of the American Academy of Child Psychiatry*, **25**, 306–19.

Pynoos, R. S., Fredrick, C., Nader, K., Arroyo, W., Steinberg, A., Eth, S., Nunez, F. & Fairbanks, L. (1987). Life threat and post traumatic stress in school-age children. *Archives of General Psychiatry*, **44**, 1057–63.

Pynoos, R. S., Goenjian, A., Tashjian, M., Karakashian, M., Manjikian, R., Manoukian, G., Steinberg, A. M. & Fairbanks, L. A. (1993). Post-traumatic stress reactions in children after the 1988 Armenian earthquake. *British Journal of Psychiatry*, **163**, 239–47.

Rachman, S. (1980). Emotional processing. *Behaviour Research and Therapy*, **18**, 51–60.

Raphael, B., Meldrum, L. & McFarlane, A. C. (1995). Does debriefing after psychological trauma work? *British Medical Journal*, **310**, 1479–80.

Reynolds, C. R. & Richmond, B. O. (1978). What I think and feel: a revised measure of children's manifest anxiety. *Journal of Abnormal Child Psychology*, **6**, 271–80.

Schwarz, E. D. & Kowalski, J. M. (1991). Malignant memories: PTSD in children and adults after a school shooting. *Journal of the American Academy of Child & Adolescent Psychiatry*, **30**, 936–44.

Schwarz, E & Perry, B. D. (1994). The post-traumatic response in children and adolescents. *Psychiatric Clinics of North America*, **17**, 311–26.

Stallard, P. & Law, T. (1993). Screening and psychological

debriefing of adolescent survivors of life threatening events. *British Journal of Psychiatry*, **163**, 660–5.

Street, E. & Sibert, J. (1998). Post-traumatic stress reactions in children. *Clinical Child Psychology and Psychiatry*, **4**, 553–60.

Terr, L. C. (1983). Chowchilla revisited: the effects of psychic trauma four years after a school bus kidnapping. *American Journal of Psychiatry*, **140**, 1543–50.

Terr, L. C. (1989). Treating psychic trauma in children: a preliminary discussion. *Journal of Traumatic Stress*, **2**, 3–20.

Terr, L. C. (1991). Childhood traumas – an outline and overview. *American Journal of Psychiatry*, **148**, 10–20.

Udwin, O. (1993). Children's reactions to traumatic events. *Journal of Child Psychology and Psychiatry*, **34**, 115–27.

Vernberg, E. M. & Vogel, J. M. (1993). Task Force Report Part 2. Interventions with children after disasters. *Journal of Clinical Child Psychology*, **22**, 485–98.

Vogel, J. M. & Vernberg, E. M. (1993). Task Force Report Part 1. Children's psychological responses to disasters. *Journal of Clinical Child Psychology*, **22**, 464–84.

Yule, W. (1992). Post traumatic stress disorders in child survivors of shipping disasters: the sinking of the 'Jupiter'. *Psychotherapy and Psychosomatics*, **57**, 200–5.

Yule, W. (1994). Posttraumatic stress disorders. In M. Rutter, E. Taylor & L. Hersov (Eds.) *Child and Adolescent Psychiatry: Modern Approaches*, 3rd edn (pp. 392–4060). Oxford: Blackwell Scientific Publications.

Yule, W. & Canterbury, R. (1994). The treatment of post traumatic stress disorder in children and adolescents. *International Review of Psychiatry*, **6**, 141–51.

Yule, W. & Udwin, O. (1991). Screening child survivors for post-traumatic stress disorders: experiences from the 'Jupiter' sinking. *British Journal of Clinical Psychology*, **30**, 131–8.

Yule, W. & Williams, R. (1990). Posttraumatic stress reactions in children. *Journal of Traumatic Stress*, **3**, 279–95.

Yule, W., Udwin, O. & Murdoch, K. (1990). The 'Jupiter' sinking: effects on children's fears, depression and anxiety. *Journal of Child Psychology and Psychiatry*, **31**, 1051–61.

PART III

Adaptations of debriefing models

16

Delayed debriefing: after a disaster

Claude M. Chemtob

This chapter challenges the conventions of psychological debriefing as an intervention that is only applicable in the earliest period post disaster. After dissecting debriefing as a trauma prevention strategy, Chemtob highlights the need to examine the traditional elements that have been seen to potentially prevent morbid outcomes. These include prevention aims, supporting processing of the emotions, dealing with the cognitive distortion produced by the event, providing systematic information about the course of recovery over time so as to counter perceptions generated by cognitive disturbances, social support, public health screening and monitoring function. Three additional 'propositions' are added to this list as a result of the author's clinical observations and research: adaptation to the cultural environment, debriefing specific to the psychological tasks of the particular phase of recovery, taking into account individually specific ways of responding to life events. The last of these the author has described further in terms of 'survival-mode' psychological distortions that people use for necessary adaptation. He considers that understanding of these through education is likely to assist the recovery process.

Chemtob makes a strong case for the 'clear specification of procedural steps' involved in debriefing before it can be appropriately evaluated for intervention integrity and fidelity and for effectiveness as a preventive approach to post-trauma morbidity. Debriefing research is limited and findings difficult to appraise because procedures and aims have seldom been defined or measured.

Qualitative and quantitative assessment of the use of broadly based debriefing models of this kind some months after a disaster, and positive outcomes achieved are also presented, with descriptions of work with helpers, children and teachers and school environments. This is an innovative approach, and its conceptualizations are of interest. It is likely to contribute further findings if the research presented is extended. Nevertheless it rests on an acceptance of traditional wisdom about the need to work through the experience in this talking or narrative manner. These concepts need to be further challenged and researched. The author does not discuss the possibility that the extensive debriefing intervention provided in the early phase of the disaster that he describes appeared to have had little long-term benefit, or possibly negative effects, thus leaving this population in need of further intervention. Nevertheless, the model he puts forward is more normalizing in that it does not appear to educate to pathology, but rather to a recovery ethos, and survival models. This more positive, less pathology-oriented basis may contribute to the improved outcomes found in the studies presented. The conceptualization overlaps somewhat with others in this volume (e.g. Stallard, Chapter 15), but provides additional insights and a model for further evaluation.

Introduction

Psychological debriefing is a specific procedural intervention designed for use in a well-defined context with specific populations. However, recently psychological debriefing has also increasingly been viewed as a broad approach to the application of trauma prevention principles. This definitional confusion can interfere with undertaking appropriate efficacy research on specific psychological debriefing procedures. It may also impede the clear formulation of trauma prevention principles applicable beyond the immediate aftermath of stressful events.

Well-defined prevention principles can guide the design of interventions to support trauma recovery processes across the entire recovery cycle, starting with the immediate after effects of a potentially traumatic event and extending in time until recovery is complete. Thus clear formulation of such prevention principles would facilitate the design of trauma prevention procedures, which are appropriate for the recovery needs of people at different points in the trauma recovery cycle. Moreover, disentangling conceptual and procedural aspects of psychological debriefing should support the clearer specification of specific procedural interventions. In turn, this would serve to increase the internal and external validity of debriefing research.

This chapter presents a brief description of the conceptual origins of psychological debriefing. Then, specific trauma prevention principles embedded in psychological debriefing are described. Some extensions of these principles used by the author are also given. Case examples of extended applications of psychological debriefing are then presented to illustrate broader application of these principles. Well-controlled additional research on trauma prevention that capitalizes on advances in field and naturalistic research is called for in the conclusion of the chapter.

Conceptual origins of psychological debriefing

Psychological debriefing originally was defined as an intervention to ameliorate the immediate after effects of potentially traumatic stressors among emergency services workers. Its early formulation and dissemination can be credited largely to Mitchell's (1983) work with emergency responders and to Raphael's (1986) work with disaster rescue workers. Dunning (1988) has pointed out that other contributors participated in the early formulation of acute post-trauma interventions. Currently, psychological debriefing is often used as a generic term to describe any procedure that purports to support the recovery of normal people exposed to potentially traumatic stressors. Thus psychological debriefing has been used to describe activities as diverse as meeting with hundreds of people in a psycho-educational context (Young, 1988) and holding a single-session individual intervention with severely burned patients (Bisson et al., 1997).

Some psychological debriefing procedures, such as Critical Incident Stress Debriefing, have well-delineated treatment manuals (Mitchell & Everly, 1996). However, most debriefing procedures do not have treatment manuals. This has made critical evaluation of research on debriefing interventions difficult, since it is not always clear what is being evaluated.

Psychological debriefing was named by reference to the after-action review process (debriefing) routinely used by military forces, emergency responders, and police forces (amongst others) to review operational matters and lessons learned from a specific mission. Using the familiar term 'debriefing' and adapting elements of a familiar after-action process helped to facilitate the acceptance of the principal innovation promoted by psychological debriefing, namely the systematic review and processing of the emotional impact of the work mission at issue.

Psychological debriefing was originally conceptualized as a highly focussed intervention intended to support the resolution of discrete stressful events encountered as a routine part of work, e.g. by an emergency responder, a disaster worker, or a police officer. Perhaps in part because these stressful events tend to compel attention, a disproportionate amount of attention has been directed on uses of psychological debriefing immediately after a stressful event.

Implicit in the early development of psychological debriefing was the proposition that the work cultures of first-line responders (at least in the USA) put a premium on the suppression rather than the expression of emotion, and that this conspired to interfere with the resolution of horrific and stressful work experiences. The failure to achieve such resolution was seen as generating substantial human and economic costs to the individual and to the organization. Thus psychological debriefing has been promoted as an occupational health innovation intended to support psychological health and safety and to facilitate the retention of effective workers.

Consequently, most specific debriefing protocols put an emphasis on initiating psychological debriefing within narrow windows of opportunity defined by temporal proximity to the stressful work event. In this respect, psychological debriefing implicitly incorporates the military psychiatry doctrine of 'proximity, immediacy and expectancy' which has governed combat-related interventions and the associated military purpose of preserving the fighting force. In the context of debriefing, preserving the response capacity represented by first-line responders faced with the sometimes overwhelming physical and psychological demands of their work has been considered analogous to maintaining soldiers on the front line.

In recent years, the use of psychological debriefing has become extremely widespread. It is increasingly viewed by first-line response organizations, such as emergency medical services, fire departments, and police departments, as a standard of responsible personnel management. The US Occupational Safety Health Administration has recently promulgated a requirement for employers to provide post-event stress management support. A recent legal decision in the USA held an employer potentially liable for failing to provide such post-event psychological intervention. Where it used to be an uphill battle to convince employers to use post-event debriefing interventions, the weight of regulatory and legal opinion have increasingly solidified the place of psychological support in the workplace after traumatic events. This is so whether the events are experienced as part of the occupational hazards associated with a given occupation, or are due to catastrophic events such as workplace violence.

Thus the rise of psychological debriefing has both supported and been abetted by a change in cultural mores about the managing of painful life experiences. If the prevailing cultural norm in the past might be described as 'maintaining a stiff upper-lip' in the face of adverse life experiences, the emerging cultural prescription seems to be to express one's feelings in a supportive social context in the face of adversity (e.g. note the extraordinary popularity of various self-help affinity groups).

As psychological debriefing has become more widely accepted, its original highly specific workplace focus has been broadened. For example, psychological debriefing has been applied to the resolution of the emotional after effects of aircraft disasters for both affected passengers and for the employees of the airlines involved (Butcher & Hatcher, 1988). It has also been used to assist both victims and responders in the aftermath of natural disasters, hostage-taking, armed hold-ups (Grainger, 1995), and following staff assaults in hospitals (Flannery et al., 1996). Unfortunately, despite its rapid dissemination, psychological debriefing lacks an empirical research base that establishes its efficacy or a well-developed theoretical framework to guide its use (Raphael et al., 1995).

Moreover, perhaps reflecting relatively short training periods that do not usually incorporate clear proficiency markers, or continued training to criterion to ensure treatment integrity, there has been some increasing confusion about what actual therapeutic operations are enacted when psychological debriefing is described. This has led to some substantial controversy regarding the efficacy of debriefing and the aptness of some research that purports to evaluate debriefing. Research on the efficacy of psychological debriefing has suffered from clarity as to what constitutes a debriefing intervention. Reflecting this, efficacy research has encompassed a range of definitions from a single-session intervention directed at inpatient burn victims (Bisson et al., 1997) to accident victims (Hobbs et al., 1996), and providing debriefing several months after a natural disaster (Chemtob et al., 1997).

In one instance, research on debriefing addressed the efficacy of a debriefing intervention delivered several months after the index event and thus well outside the 72-hour window that is traditionally prescribed for some debriefing interventions (Chemtob et al., 1997). While that study made use of classical debriefing procedures, simply applied later in time, some might ask whether late application of debriefing procedures is not better defined as psychotherapy. This example highlights the sometimes conceptually unclear demarcation between psychological debriefing procedures and other types of psychosocial treatments.

The context in which psychological debriefing generally occurs, that is to say shortly after a potentially traumatic event or after a disaster, itself militates against easily undertaking psychological debriefing efficacy research. There are a number of barriers to intervention research in post-disaster environments. These include a sensitivity of people post disaster to being exploited and thus experiencing research as a kind of voyeurism directed to their misfortune. There are also ethical constraints that make the randomization of people to a treatment or no-treatment group difficult. In addition, there has been a notable lack of commitment in debriefing research to modern concepts of treatment integrity and to fidelity controls.

Finally, the use of psychological debriefing procedures has tended to be limited to close proximity to the event. This limitation seems more to reflect the specific conceptual origin of debriefing than limitations inherent in the presumed effective ingredients of it as an intervention. Indeed, it might be argued that trauma prevention procedures should be applied later, when a person has begun to recover from the immediate aftershock of a traumatic event. In any event, the legitimate question of when psychological debriefing interventions would be best undertaken has not been empirically studied.

The usual application of debriefing to the immediate post-disaster period may reflect its military and emergency services origins. There is no empirical evidence to direct such time-bound applications. This application may also reflect the financial and political context of psychological support following disasters. Such psychological support usually follows immediately after a disaster, reflecting genuine humanitarian concern as well as the availability of formal emergency political and financial infrastructures. In addition, its purposes at this stage are to ensure the maintenance, through return to action, of an optimal fighting or operational force.

However, typically within weeks or months, responder attention diminishes greatly. By the end of a year, most psychological support has tapered off. Despite this time-limited horizon of response, there is an emerging recognition that major disasters may have substantial long-term consequences that extend well beyond a year (Green, 1995). Thus the tendency to limit the use of psychological debriefing to the immediate aftermath of a potentially traumatogenic event may be driven more by practical than by theoretical concerns. Also, despite an avowed commitment to screening and

monitoring as part of psychological debriefing, in practice this is rarely undertaken systematically. In summary, it is increasingly evident that psychological debriefing has come to denote both a specific though often unspecified procedure and a broad approach to preventing stress disorders. As a result, there appears to be some definitional confusion as to how to conceptualize debriefing. Is it a specific preventive intervention procedure, a general approach to trauma prevention, or, even as has been suggested, a kind of social movement (Gist et al., 1998)?

An expanded conception of psychological debriefing

In this chapter, it is proposed that it is useful to disentangle the underlying conceptual assumptions involved in psychological debriefing in order to inform an expanded use of the psychological principles that debriefing must be utilized to be effective. It is argued that psychological debriefing as a specific procedure and the conceptual advances that it implicitly incorporates have not been clearly distinguished.

It is possible to separate the conceptual advances incorporated into psychological debriefing, and popularized by it, from the specific procedures that purport to incorporate them. Doing so has at least three benefits: (1) conceptually derived accounts of purported effective ingredients permit more effective research, (2) distinguishing conceptual propositions from their specific procedural implementation in given special-purpose interventions gives designers of trauma services greater conceptual freedom to adapt trauma intervention design principles to particular needs, and (3) an improved conceptual structure facilitates engaging in research and training on specific trauma-related interventions by improving clarity about each intervention.

Psychological debriefing incorporates a number of generally accepted conceptual principles (although not necessarily directly research tested) about how to prevent stressful events from becoming traumatic. A number of these principles are reviewed briefly in this section. Then additional trauma prevention concepts are proposed as being necessary to provide for a fuller conceptual armamentarium needed for an expanded definition of psychological debriefing. This expanded set of principles is necessary to enable the design of a wider set of debriefing procedures, suitable for a broader range of post-disaster needs. There are eight dynamic conceptual propositions that, it is proposed, are implicitly incorporated into psychological debriefing. These are described below.

1. Psychological debriefing is one of a growing number of treatments aimed at the primary prevention of behavioural disorders

It is based on the broad recognition that exposure to life-threatening or horrific events increases the probability of subsequent trauma-related symptoms and distress. Like other preventive treatments, psychological debriefing incorporates an optimistic world view. In this case, that the consequences of exposure to highly stressful events can be managed and reduced. They need not be accepted simply as part of the cost of being alive and therefore to be endured without choice. Rather, exposure to a life threat or horrifying event is recognized as a specific risk factor that serves to increase the probability of psychologically deleterious consequences. Psychological debriefing calls for undertaking a set of psychologically informed activities to reduce the negative consequences of such harmful life events. While it might be argued that psychological debriefing, given appropriate technical modification, may have a role to play in secondary prevention, clearly it does not have a role (as presently conceived) to play in tertiary prevention. Once a person has a disorder sufficiently established to merit diagnosis as a stable and chronic condition, debriefing is replaced by more conventional treatment approaches. Note, however, that the demarcation between debriefing and conventional treatment is not always completely clear because preventive psychological treatments share a number of common elements with palliative treatments.

2. Supporting the processing of emotions and cognitive distortions provoked by exposure to stressful events is salutogenic

Psychological debriefing emphasizes supporting natural processes of recovery and removing barriers to resolution of the emotional impact of life-threatening events. The natural process of psychological assimilation following exposure to traumatizing events has been described by Horowitz (1976), who was the first to emphasize that interruption of effective emotional processing is a key factor in the development of trauma-related symptoms. There are two subpropositions which have now been recruited in support of this: (a) expressing oneself through narrative disclosure is salutary and ameliorates the consequences of stress exposure (see e.g. Pennebaker, 1993), and (b) exposure to traumatic memories promotes effective resolution of such memories (Foa et al., 1995).

3. Predictable cognitive distortions have been identified through clinical experience that constitute psychological risks for the development of symptoms

These include: (a) a fragmented representation of the trauma event, which is often incomplete and frequently distorted because of the subject having a limited grasp of all the aspects of the incident; (b) an inaccurate evaluation of one's influence in the outcome, which can perpetuate a sense of helplessness or provoke guilt; (c) a foreshortening of the future; (d) a lack of knowledge about normative emotional responses to catastrophic stressors that can lead to misattribution about one's functionality and even sanity; (e) a tendency to overestimate the likelihood of future threats; and (f) for some, increased psychological salience of pre-existing concerns (e.g. a pre-existing tendency to social isolation becoming intensified because of experiencing a disaster alone).

To counter these normative distortions, psychological debriefing calls for systematically providing information about the expected course of response and recovery associated with a particular traumatogenic event. This includes putting cognitive and emotional distortions in a context of normal response to unfamiliar and rare events. Such normalization serves the purpose of reassuring the exposed person that what he or she is experiencing is not 'crazy', although it may feel quite unusual. Normalization also serves to define the outer limits of what is normal. Affected participants are told to seek help if the reactions exceed the normative definition by virtue of exceeding normative intensity or persistence thresholds.

4. Social support is a major moderator of exposure to traumatic stress

Debriefing is generally conceived of as a group process. This reflects a conviction that social support moderates the impact of trauma exposure (Flannery, 1990). It is also based on observation of naturalistic processes of recovery. People tend to gather together to review and process stressful events. Some cultures institutionalize processes of group narrative construction following stressful experience. Examples include the Kava Ceremony in Fiji during the course of which a mildly intoxicating drink is shared and people describe their experiences with an eye to resolving any emotional disharmony. Similarly, in Hawaii, a process known as H'oponpono is used to resolve disharmony among members of a kin group. That process involves each person expressing their perception of the events, their feelings, and the spiritual consequences for them of the disharmony.

5. Psychological debriefing incorporates a public health-derived screening and monitoring function

Intervening to prevent symptoms also provides an opportunity to identify persons whose responses exceed normative levels. Once identified, these persons become candidates for more intensive support. The monitoring component of this aspect of debriefing refers to the need to follow up systematically with the participants to ascertain the trauma status of people some months after the exposure. In this view, debriefing influences a systematic and principled approach to designing an appropriate response to the extended support of people exposed to catastrophic stressors. There has been a tendency to neglect this component of psychological debriefing, which has been reflected in identifying psychological debriefing as a one-off intervention. However, recent trends in the psychological debriefing community (see Chapter 5, this volume) have been to reaffirm the need to see psychological debriefing in the framework of a more systematic time-extended approach.

Three additional propositions have been central to the debriefing work undertaken by our laboratory and are presented here as extensions of psychological debriefing principles.

6. Psychological debriefing must be adapted to the cultural circumstances of the environment in which it is deployed

Communities (whether they are defined in terms of a police department, a neighbourhood, or a county) have specific cultural histories. Any effort at providing trauma prevention must incorporate an understanding of community concerns that are culture bound. For example, following Hurricane Iniki, a catastrophic disaster affecting the Hawaiian island of Kauai, factors became very salient that had previously been in the background. This issue had to do with concerns about the large numbers of newcomers who had been moving to the island. For some time, long-term residents had been concerned that newcomers did not completely understand the nature of community membership on the island. A few months after the hurricane, this concern became widespread and tended to provoke pronounced community divisions that interfered with recovery. In this instance, issues of community membership overlapped with ethnocultural identity. These concerns were evident in psychological debriefing meetings held shortly after the hurricane. Part of the task of the psychological debriefing necessarily included addressing such issues. Failure to recognize and address these community cultural concerns would have meant that the debriefing groups were not culturally responsive. Psychological debriefing requires cultural specificity and adaptation to be effective.

A related issue is that the person in charge of the psychological debriefing process will probably be an outsider. Therefore it becomes essential to establish cultural credibility. This is best accomplished, in the experience of our group, through establishing a close working partnership with a representative of the affected group who is willing to use his or her personal credibility to vouch for the trauma expert, thus permitting acceptance within the community in the faster time frame required in a disaster environment. Recognizing this dynamic, we have developed the concept of pairing a local culture expert and a trauma expert as a functioning team. We define a culture expert as a person who is a member of the local culture and therefore understands and participates in the culture's norms. This person serves both to vouch for the trauma expert and to provide a culture-specific translation of trauma principles that facilitates the absorption of the trauma-related information. The trauma expert is defined as a person with substantial expertise and experience with normal and pathological trauma response. It is our experience that culturally appropriate trauma responses require such pairings to be effective. Mitchell's use of peer interveners in partnership with mental health clinicians appears to have intuitively recognized the need to pair members of a specific responding entity with a mental health professional. Unfortunately, in our view, true trauma expertise is difficult to develop, and the Critical Incident Stress Debriefing training process paired with standard mental health preparation is probably not sufficient to develop sufficient trauma response expertise.

It is also important to recognize that the role of the outside intervener is self-limiting. Communities will use the trauma expert up to a point but eventually the trauma expert will become an unwelcome reminder of unpleasant experiences. Therefore the trauma expert must plan an exit strategy from first entering the community. Part of the sensitivity to cultural issues in trauma response that we advocate calls for recognizing the difference between a culture of disaster recovery and ongoing community functioning, which can become in part defined by the exit of the trauma interveners.

7. Different phases of recovery are associated with distinct psychological tasks and require psychological debriefing procedures specific to those tasks

It is now known that disasters and other traumatic events have long-term consequences. In our view, it is no longer sufficient to provide psychological support to address the immediate aftermath of a disaster. There are psychological risks associated with different phases of trauma recovery. A systematic approach to supporting trauma recovery therefore requires the application of trauma prevention principles to the different phases of trauma recovery. Also, different phases of recovery are associated with different levels of readiness to engage explicitly defined disaster recovery activities. Early on in a major disaster nearly all people appreciate the need for psychological support. However, as time passes most people recover and as part of that recovery have strong desires to put the disaster event behind them. For those for whom recovery is not proceeding apace, it quickly becomes apparent that it is no longer socially normative to experience distress. Such people tend to mask their symptoms and become considerably more difficult to reach and help. Supporting psychological recovery in that kind of a post-recovery environment is substantially different from immediate post-disaster efforts. It requires the development of screening methods to identify those people who are still experiencing distress. Moreover, phase-specific debriefing procedures are required.

Also, in the instance of large-scale disasters there are often occasions where decisions made in the process of recovery have left substantial negative after effects that continue to affect the functioning of the work group or community. The extended effects of disaster require adaptation of the debriefing intervention to the phase of psychological response to trauma to which the intervention is directed. For example, the leader of a large work group on Kauai called for early return of workers to their tasks despite their homes being damaged. This was done because the workers' tasks were critical to support community recovery. Nevertheless substantial dissension arose because some of the workers and the state had not recognized their role as essential for disaster recovery in the past. Nearly two years later, factions that had formed regarding the decision continued to divide the work group and required intervention. Much of the intervention involved the use of education about the conflicts that people experience between personal and work roles. Also, making reference to similar conflicts experienced in other disasters normalized these conflicts. Finally, through recognition of the very real achievements of this work group, support was provided to all factions. This proved to be extremely helpful in initiating a process of reconciliation that had not started on its own and required an outsider's assessment and intervention.

8. People respond in highly specific ways to life-threatening events

Our laboratory has been engaged in developing a theory of trauma that we now describe as the survival-mode theory of post-traumatic stress disorder (PTSD) (Chemtob et al., 1988). Briefly, we have proposed that people respond to life-threatening events by engaging cognitive, behavioural and arousal systems specialised for survival. Part of responding in survival mode includes a loss of self-monitoring, an increased propensity to detect threat, increased irritability, and for some a tendency to dissociate. We have found that people intuitively recognize this aspect of their response to life-threatening events. Describing survival mode has been an important part of the psychoeducational component that we use following the affective processing component of our debriefing groups.

There are a number of survival-mode-specific cognitive distortions. These include the following, colloquially named for the purposes of educating affected people. (a) The 'in your face effect', that is the tendency to be overly preoccupied by the disaster to the extent of relatively neglecting to extend proportionate attention to predisaster events. Many people report that disaster-related preoccupations seem to crowd out other parts of one's experience. (b) The 'neon effect', which refers to an exacerbation of pre-existing issues at the individual, group and community levels. For example, a leader with a prior reputation for micro managing a group is likely to be seen as even more likely to engage in such a management style. Indeed, the leader may in fact do so, independently of the increased tendency to perceive him or her as doing so. An example of such exacerbation at the community level was seen on Kauai where there had been predisaster ambivalence about the election of a female mayor. During and following the hurricane, the mayor's performance was roundly criticized by some who attributed all difficulties in the response to the disaster to her gender. In reality, the mayor's performance was so good that she was given a special award by the Federal Emergency Management Agency, which is the primary agency for responding to national-scale disasters in the USA. Anecdotally, we have found that education about survival mode appears to help debriefing group participants better to integrate their group experience and helps them to restore self-monitoring.

Some examples of delayed uses of debriefing

In this section, several examples of delayed uses of psychological debriefing principles are presented to illustrate that the application of the concepts incorporated into this approach are not limited to the immediate aftermath of a stressful event. Indeed, implicit in the present argument is that trauma prevention requires time-extended attention and the creative design of trauma-preventive interventions fitted to each phase of recovery.

The examples that are presented are all drawn from our work following Hurricane Iniki, which struck Kauai in the Hawaiian Islands, on 11 September 1992. Hurricane Iniki carried sustained winds of 230 kilometres per hour with gusts up to 320 kilometres per hour, for over eight hours. Seventy-one per cent of homes on the island were damaged or destroyed. Damage affecting this community of only 50 000 people was estimated to be close to (US)$2 bn. Ranked as one of the most destructive disasters in US history, the impact of Iniki is nevertheless often underestimated. Living on an island, people were constantly re-exposed to destroyed homes and businesses, as well as to the ravaged natural environment. On an island, unlike with major disasters in mainland communities, affected people could not easily drive away to get respite. Moreover, the damage to the extraordinary beauty of the island, and to its hotels, caused a secondary economic disaster compounding the natural disaster's impact. This secondary economic damage clearly qualified Hurricane Iniki as a catastrophic disaster. There is an increasing recognition that traumatic events, natural disasters in particular, have longer-term psychological consequences. We had occasion to use a number of modified psychological debriefing procedures in the aftermath of Hurricane Iniki.

Using psychological debriefing methods some months after the index event

Because the state of Hawaii has a relatively sophisticated trauma community, there had been quite systematic efforts to provide psychological debriefing for large numbers of people on Kauai. It is estimated that several thousand people participated in some form of debriefing activity. As is usual in the post-disaster context, within two to three months most of the psychological helpers who had come to assist in the island's recovery went home or stopped coming over from the other islands to help. In the USA, the Federal Emergency Management Agency (FEMA) funds subsequent psychological outreach and counselling through an agreement with the Center for Mental Health Services. Three to four months after the hurricane, the author was asked to provide trauma and counselling training for the FEMA outreach peer counsellors and for the professionals working with them. It was known that quite extensive debriefing efforts had already occurred. Therefore, at a preliminary meeting with some of the staff that would be trained, it was assumed that much of their psychological recovery had already occurred. However, as the staff began to describe what they perceived as their training needs, it quickly became evident that they were still suffering substantial disaster-related symptoms. Given the staff's continuing distress, it became evident that training could not effectively proceed until support to resolve the persistent effects of their experience had been provided. As I continued to work on the island, it quickly became clear to me that this state of affairs was not limited to the staff of the psychological recovery project but certainly extended to many other members of the community.

In that instance, psychological debriefing procedures associated with critical incident stress debriefing were directly applicable. The major modification of technique was holding the debriefing groups several months after the event rather than in closer proximity to the event. The only other modification in technique that was undertaken was the addition of a period of direct didactic education (including describing survival mode) following the psychological debriefing. This didactic period, usually lasting two to three hours, seemed (1) to permit the participants a period of psychological integration of the emotional material that they had expressed and listened to, and (2) to provide a cognitive framework for disaster-related reactions that permitted the person to develop a self-regulatory set of reference points.

Because capacity limitations restricted the number of people who could be debriefed at one time, we had an opportunity to construct a quasi-experimental study (for details, please see Chemtob et al., 1997). Consequently, we treated two groups of people using a lagged-groups design such that one group served as a partial control for the passage of time. Our design clearly had limitations. Nevertheless, the results indicated that we could achieve 40% reductions in trauma-related symptoms as indexed by the Impact of Event Scale (Horowitz et al., 1979). This result was repeated when the comparison group was treated. While this was not a randomized controlled trial, and therefore required some caution in interpretation, the study suggested that substantial symptom reduction could be achieved and documented using a quasi-experimental design.

In other instances, where the debriefing was also presented in a delayed framework, but trauma-related feelings and thoughts were not as readily accessible, we have found it useful to use variations in technique which serve to restore the immediacy of the events that are being addressed. We have used two such variations successfully. One variation involved reviewing a videotape of Hurricane Iniki. Viewing the videotape seemed to serve to revive memories for participants and thus renewed the sense of immediacy of the event. The content of the group was then very similar to that experienced in more temporally proximate debriefing groups. Once activated, each person's story was told with vivid imagery and feeling. Another approach to revivifying memories involved asking the participants to imagine themselves back in the initial context. The process of imaginal re-exposure seems to refresh the sense of immediacy of the memory of the event(s) involved. As a result of this reactivation process, we found that groups have been able easily to access and work through experiences that they had felt compelled to avoid.

In conducting delayed debriefing groups, resistance to reactivating painful feelings must be dealt with. It is important to address these feelings thoughtfully and respectfully. They are reflective of the need that people feel to put aside feelings so that they do not interfere with their ongoing functioning. This should be explained and respected. However, it should also be addressed with information that the purpose of reactivating feelings that have been set aside is to assist with their resolution; to alleviate the continued distress that can result if they are not worked through.

In this regard, it is important to help people to make the link between the traumatogenic event and the current distress. The work of addressing these resistances should be seen as an adaptation to the task of providing education as part of psychological debriefing. The educational focus is on a later phase of trauma response. However, this aspect of stress response is increasingly well understood. I would argue that these specialized techniques to access distressing symptoms that have not yet constelled into a clinical disorder could be thought as supporting a later phase of the trauma recovery cycle.

Longer-term psychological recovery of children

The next case example also illustrates a delayed use of trauma prevention. It involves a public health inspired community-wide post-disaster psychosocial intervention that was undertaken by the author's group to reduce disaster-related psychological distress in elementary school children. Intervention with children in post-disaster environments is difficult because of the tendency of disaster-affected people, with the passage of time, to deny the existence or importance of the disaster-related symptoms that they and others are experiencing. Even when symptoms are acknowledged, people generally no longer attribute their distress symptoms to the disaster.

As a result, children's disaster-related symptomatology often fails to be identified by relevant adults even a few weeks after a disaster. Further contributing to this problem is the fact that children's disaster-related distress often manifests as internalizing symptoms (such as anxiety) rather than as externalizing problem behaviours (usually conduct problems) that more readily attract adult attention. For example, a child who was experiencing high levels of distress two years after the hurricane (including hiding under her bed when there were high winds) and difficulty concentrating at school was asked whether she had told her mother about her symptoms. She replied: 'No, my mother has too much to worry about with the hurricane already.'

It is clear that children experience substantial levels of persistent post-traumatic distress following exposure to a hurricane. Although for most children this distress diminishes with time, effective psychological intervention is needed to help children recover from hurricane-related distress and to prevent the development of chronic psychopathology. Two years after Hurricane Iniki, we used a school-based screening protocol community-wide ($n = 4259$) to identify children with continuing hurricane-related distress (Chemtob et al., 1996). Children with the highest levels of distress were provided with a manual-guided short-term psychosocial intervention by specially trained school counsellors. This method incorporated principles of psychological debriefing into a brief resource-friendly intervention with children during the mid-disaster phase of recovery (i.e. in the period of one to two years following the event). Children were randomly assigned to either group or individual counselling. The children were guided through a four-session process that involved working through feelings of helplessness, loss, anger and finally a memorialization process that put the focus on positive coping with the aftermath of the disaster. The intervention goal was defined as restoring and supporting the normal processes of recovery, rather than treating morbidity and pathology. The intervention was conceptualized as supporting normal processes of psychological recovery that were either slower for these children or had been interrupted by some cognitive distortion. Thus the intervention was aimed at facilitating the normative resolution of an abnormal event rather than focussed on treating specific symptoms. Intervention effectiveness was assessed using the children's self-report inventory and teacher ratings of the children's classroom behaviours. Children were followed up one year later to ensure that they had recovered. As a result of the intervention, children reported significant reductions in trauma-related distress. Teachers reported significant improvements in the children's ability to concentrate and significant reductions in their disruptiveness. Gains were maintained at one-year follow-up. Importantly, this intervention was designed as part of a process that included treatment follow-up one year later. At that time, children who were nonresponders to the secondary prevention intervention were identified and triaged to a more resource-intensive tertiary prevention level of care that clearly qualifies as traditional psychotherapy (Chemtob et al., 2000).

Renewing post-disaster school culture as a longer-term psychological debriefing intervention

This case example describes an approach to supporting the recovery of school faculty and staff in the middle phase of disaster recovery. Two years after Hurricane Iniki, it became clear that the schools with which we were working were suffering a great deal of internal friction among staff. Staff stress appeared to be manifested in reduced tolerance for student misbehaviours, as reflected in greatly increased suspension rates. The faculty and staff seemed to be experiencing a sense of exhaustion, depression and continued feelings of being overwhelmed. While the disaster appeared to have a great deal of continued after effects, resistance to further direct psychological work about its impact had emerged among some adults within the community. Yet restoring the vitality of these educators' commitment to educating the children in their care and assisting them in learning to identify children who were continuing to experience disaster-related distress was a crucial goal. The original requests for assistance from schools were quite diverse in form. For example, one high school asked for assistance with discipline problems, which had dramatically increased; another school asked for help with developing the relationship component of the teacher–student interaction. We therefore defined our intervention focus more broadly than disaster. We collaboratively evolved the notion of addressing reinforcing the 'teaching alliance', which we defined as

the joining of teacher, staff and parents in a common purpose of caring for and teaching children. As we began to implement our workshops, word of mouth led to invitations to give them in yet other schools.

Our assessment indicated that we should target our adaptation of psychological debriefing to address (1) education about longer-term effects of disaster; (2) revitalizing a sense of shared commitment and collaboration for a common purpose, in effect renewing a commitment to shared cultural values, in this case related to caring about children; (3) addressing through education, normalization and support the continued after effects of having served as de facto emergency workers during the hurricane and the impact of the hurricane on them as affected people. An important aim for us was to provide support to participants through acknowledging their caring and the extraordinary sacrifices they undertook to care for both their own families and the children they had had to teach during a catastrophic time.

The general level of resistance in the community required a relatively indirect approach. Consequently, we initiated one-day workshops with approximately 20 staff and faculty meeting with us at a time. Our project funding permitted us to free the teachers to participate by providing for substitute teachers. When we convened the groups, we began each group by giving flower leis (garlands) to each participant. In Hawaii, such flower leis are given to people to celebrate a variety of life transitions ranging from birthdays to graduations. They mark a change in status and celebrate it. We acknowledged each participant as we gave him or her a lei for their contribution to the children and for their efforts in the recovery of their community.

The next phase of the session involved participants recounting their experiences of the secondary impact of the hurricane on the school children, the staff and their community. This was focussed on more recent events but many chose to recount their actual experiences in surviving the hurricane. This phase was somewhat briefer than a more standard debriefing process. It led into an educational presentation linking what the participants had said about themselves and about the children they worked with to what is known about recovery from disaster, the emphasis being on long-term recovery issues. The presentation empha-sized the 'normal people in abnormal circumstances' theme, which is a key part of applying the principle of normalization in psychological debriefing.

A key goal of the intervention was to revitalize the commitment of the faculty and staff to the educational enterprise. A second goal was to revitalize a sense of community within schools that had become character-ized by factionalism. We accomplished these aims by inviting the participants to reassert the values that they believed characterized their school. We termed this process the creation of intentional culture. As the par-ticipants described what they believed their school stood for, they became re-energized by the assertion of a common purpose, specifically of a community of values. This process was particularly important be-cause, as a result of the hurricane, factionalism around ethnic lines had emerged. Asserting common values permitted the participants to commit to an intentional culture defined by shared commitments. Moreover, the hurricane's impact had interfered with the normal pro-cess by which new staff became acculturated. It brought them on board and made them known more intimately to other participants. This process was fol-lowed by an opportunity for each participant to let go anonymously of a hurt they had experienced from an-other participant during the post-hurricane recovery process. Participants were asked to describe anonymously very briefly such a hurt on a piece of paper. The papers were placed in a sand bucket and circulated. Each participant then drew a piece of paper and read the description of the slight. This was followed by a brief meditation focussed on letting go of the pain involved.

Finally, we asked the group to define shared goals they might have for their school. This was done by having people write ideas on poster paper. Participants then 'voted with their feet' by lining up with the ideas or projects that interested them. Participants were free to change groups at any time. This process led to the formation of common interest work groups that then presented their plans to the whole group. Groups agreed to present progress reports at faculty meetings. The follow-through on these projects was reported to be excellent by the school principals and by other par-

ticipants. Regrettably, despite our general commitment to putting in place evaluation measures as a standard practice when deploying debriefing-type procedures this was not done in this aspect of out intervention. Therefore, we are limited to anecdotal reports of sig-nificant positive impact.

Prescription for future research

The thesis of this chapter is that psychological debrief-ing has come to represent for many a description of a broad approach to trauma prevention. This is highly problematic for research on the efficacy of psychologi-cal debriefing, since efficacy research must depend on clear specification of the procedural steps involved in a given intervention. Without such procedural clarity it is not possible to implement treatment integrity and fi-delity controls. Failure to implement such controls means only that 'someone did something to someone somewhere'. This is hardly an appropriate standard on which to base scientific judgements about the value of specific approaches to trauma prevention. In this chap-ter, it has been proposed that one must distinguish between psychological debriefing as a general ap-proach to trauma prevention and specific procedural implementations of this approach. One can conceive of many procedures that are specific implementations of broad emerging principles of trauma prevention. It is these clearly specified procedures that must be studied for their efficacy.

Research on psychological debriefing procedures is often difficult to implement because of the intense and compelling level of need when one is responding to catastrophic situations. It is proposed that a potential strategy to surmount this problem is to convene groups of clinical researchers to consider many varieties of possible research design scenarios, together with re-quired assessment instruments. These designs and the associated measurement instruments could then be 'pre-positioned' so that they are ready for use. In order to succeed, this strategy will require practitioners of trauma prevention to make a commitment to changing the standard of practice so that evaluation of debriefing interventions always includes, as an essential part of their procedures assessment, post-debriefing assessment and follow-up. Including such routine assessment is necessary to fulfil the screening and monitoring requirement of responsibly designed psychological debriefing procedures. Such follow-up must be defined as a necessary part of responsible clinical practice in trauma prevention. It is therefore essential for the field to commit to undertaking clear descriptions of specific procedures, to evaluate the efficacy of these procedures, and to begin to enhance effective interventions. Failing to do so will ultimately prove profoundly divisive and undermine the credibility of psychological practices aimed at preventing the deleterious effects of traumatic events.

Acknowledgements

Much of the work described in this chapter was undertaken as part of the Maile Project, a hurricane recovery effort directed by Joanne Nakashima, of the Hawaii Department of Education, Kauai District. The Maile Project was funded by a special State of Hawaii appropriation to provide a 'systematic assessment and intervention program for disaster-affected children in Kauai public schools'. The author gratefully acknowledges Representative Bertha Kawakami for her assistance in making the Maile Project possible. The author is deeply appreciative of the cooperation of Kauai's school teachers, staff, and administrators, and of District Superintendent Shirley Akita's leadership, and salutes their steadfast caring about the children in the midst of the effects of the disaster on their own lives and families.

REFERENCES

Bisson, J. I., Jenkins, P. L., Alexander, J. & Bannister, C. (1997). Randomised controlled trial of psychological debriefing for victims of acute burn trauma. *British Journal of Psychiatry*, **171**, 78–81.

Butcher, J. N. & Hatcher, C. (1988). The neglected entity in air disaster planning: psychological services. *American Psychologist*. **43**, 724–9.

Chemtob, C. M., Roitblat, H. L., Hamada, R. S., Carlson, J. G. & Twentyman, C. T. (1988). A cognitive action theory of post-traumatic stress disorder. *Journal of Anxiety Disorders*. **2**, 253–75.

Chemtob, C. M., Nakashima, J. & Hamada, R. (1996). The Maile Project: A community-wide psychosocial intervention for elementary school children with disaster-related psychological distress. Unpublished paper presented at Symposium on Psychological Treatment for Disaster Affected Children, American Psychological Association, Toronto.

Chemtob, C. M., Tomas, S., Law, W. & Cremniter, D. (1997). Post-disaster psychosocial intervention: a field study of the impact of debriefing on psychological distress. *American Journal of Psychiatry*, **154**, 415–17.

Chemtob, C. M., Nakashima, J., Hamada, R. & Carlson, J. (2000). Brief treatment for Elementary School children with disaster-related PTSD: a field study. *Journal of Clinical Psychology*, in press.

Dunning, C. (1988). Intervention strategies for emergency workers. In M. Lystad (Ed.). *Mental Health Response to Mass Emergencies: Theory and Practice* (pp. 284–307). New York: Brunner/Mazel.

Flannery, R. B. (1990). Social support and psychological trauma: a methodological review. *Journal of Traumatic Stress*, **3**, 593–611.

Flannery, R. B., Penk, W. E., Hanson, M. A. & Flannery, G. J. (1996). The Assaulted Staff Action Program: guidelines for fielding a team. In G. R. VandenBos & E. Q. Bulatao (Eds.) *Violence on the Job: Identifying Risks and Developing Solutions* (pp. 327–41). Washington, DC: American Psychological Association.

Foa, E. B., Hearst-Ikeda, D. E. & Perry, K. J. (1995). Evaluation of a brief cognitive- behavioural program for the prevention of chronic PTSD in recent assault victims. *Journal of Consulting and Clinical Psychology* 63, 948–55.

Gist, R., Lubin, B. & Redburn, B. G. (1998). Psychosocial, ecological, and community perspectives on disaster response. *Journal of Personal and Interpersonal Loss*, **3**, 25–51.

Grainger, C. (1995). Occupational violence: armed hold-up – a risk management approach. *International Journal of Stress Management*, **2**, 197–205.

Green, B. L. (1995). Long-term consequences of disasters. In S. E. Hobfoll & M. W. De Vries (Eds.). *Extreme Stress and Communities: Impact and Intervention* (pp. 307–24). Dordrecht: Klüwer Academic.

Hobbs, M., Mayou, R. A., Harrison, B. & Worlock, P. (1996). A randomised controlled trial of psychological debriefing for victims of road traffic accidents. *British Medical Journal*, **313**, 1438–9.

Horowitz, M. J. (1976). *Stress Response Syndromes*. New York: Jason Aaronson.

Horowitz, M. J., Wilner, N. & Alvarez, W. (1979). Impact of Event Scale: a measure of subjective distress. *Psychosomatic Medicine*, **41**, 209–18.

Mitchell, J. T. (1983). When disaster strikes . . . The critical incident stress debriefing process. *Journal of Emergency Medical Services*, **8**, 36–9.

Mitchell, J. T. & Everly, G. S. (1996). *Critical Incident Stress Debriefing (CISD): An Operations Manual for the Prevention of Traumatic Stress among Emergency Service and Disaster Workers*, 2nd edn. Ellicott City, MD: Chevron Publishing.

Pennebaker, J. W. (1993). Putting stress into words: health, linguistic, and therapeutic implications. *Behaviour Research and Therapy*, **31**, 539–48.

Raphael, B. (1986). *When Disaster Strikes: How Individuals and Communities Cope with Catastrophe*. New York: Basic Books.

Raphael, B., Meldrum, L. & McFarlane, A. C. (1995). Does debriefing after psychological trauma work? *British Medical Journal*, **310**, 1479–80.

Young, M. A. (1988). Support services for victims. In F. M. Ochberg (Ed.) *Post-traumatic Therapy and Victims of Violence* (pp. 330–51). New York: Brunner/Mazel.

17

Debriefing in different cultural frameworks: responding to acute trauma in Australian Aboriginal contexts

Coralie Ober, Lorraine Peeters, Ron Archer and Kerrie Kelly

EDITORIAL COMMENTS

This chapter presents, clearly and intensely, a description of chronic traumatization and its effects, over many generations, and in many different forms, for Australian Aboriginal peoples. The past chronic and repetitive nature of such traumatization, and the fact that Aboriginal peoples are currently still not secure and safe for recovery highlights the complexity of any healing processes. As Ober et al. powerfully attest it is simplistic to suggest that acute trauma, when superimposed on this situation, is readily soluble by a short-term intervention according to a Western Model such as debriefing.

While this chapter reflects one indigenous culture, the themes therein are reflected in many others, particularly those 'First Nations' where there have been discrimination, attempts at assimilation and chronic traumatization and disadvantage. High rates of child abuse, drug and alcohol problems, premature mortality, suicide and mental health problems have all been reported in studies of Native American Indian and Alaska Native communities (Manson et al., 1982). They continue to be an important focus for prevention, and for treatment approaches.

An environment supporting indigenous populations so that they can take the necessary steps for recovery is the first essential. This must recognize and acknowledge the extent and contexts of traumatization and their contribution to the very adverse state of Aboriginal physical and emotional health and well-being. In addition, communities must be supported to build culturally appropriate models for healing, including those that may apply in acute situations of trauma superimposed on chronic.

Ober et al. acknowledge that such culturally based models fit more with crisis intervention in the acute sense and healing processes such as narrative therapy, developed and delineated in ways that meet indigenous needs. They point out that self-determination and culturally valid approaches are central to this.

This chapter serves to highlight an issue critical for the whole field of debriefing, that of prolonged traumatization and the impacts of disadvantage and other socially determined pervasive trauma and loss. Social action rather than mental health intervention, the authors challenge, may be the most appropriate model. These understandings are critical to all working in the field of trauma, and particularly so when one considers the needs of indigenous populations, many of which are similar across the world. This chapter, however, speaks for Australian Aboriginal peoples and is a powerful challenge to any simplistic view of interventions aimed at preventing adverse outcomes following acute traumatic experiences. It is a strong message to be considered not only in this context, but in many other fields of trauma (see also Silove, Chapter 25).

A supplication

Coralie Obers, Lorraine Peeters and Ron Archer, the Aboriginal authors, offer this chapter in the hope that our voice will not only be heard but listened to when professionals are responding to trauma in Australian Aboriginal communities and potentially in other indigenous settings. We are concerned about the increasing use of debriefing-type interventions world-wide and the potential risks these may pose for our people, a group exposed to state-sanctioned traumatization since the time of colonization. We are continuously aware of the traumas of the past and the suffering of the present. For many years we, the victims, have been blamed for our plight because it has not been in the best interests of wider society to recognize the source of our traumatization. Now that mainstream attention is turning to the effects of trauma we fear that we, perpetual survivors, will become the focus of another round of colonization and exploitation, this time by well-meaning but ill-equipped mental health practitioners and researchers with little awareness of the possible consequences of their actions on our lives. Our problems will never be overcome with person-centred or small-scale interventions, and ill-conceived and inappropriate responses are likely to amplify our distress and further destabilize our communities.

Healing from past and present trauma cannot be prescribed for us using dominant culture paradigms. Much of our trauma has its source in the oppressive attitudes and actions of the dominant culture. Since colonization, responsibility for deciding what constitutes our welfare has been effectively removed from us and placed in the hands of representatives of the dominant culture. We know what we need to do to respond to past and present traumatization. Our biggest barriers have been structural in the lack of access to resources – often the barriers have been influential non-Aboriginal mental health professionals who have failed to consult with us, have appropriated and misused our stories and knowledge, and responded with interventions which have been neither desired nor appropriate. We ask mental health practitioners to rethink their responsibilities towards Australian Aboriginal people. We recognize that positions of power and privilege are not willingly given up, but in this task we need the assistance of those who are willing to be taught by us how to help our people, and who wish to engage in a dialogue in which we can learn from each other. We are joined, in authoring this chapter, by a non-Aboriginal psychologist, Kerrie Kelly, who has shown herself willing not only to listen, but to hear what we say.

Introduction

A sound understanding of the colonization process is a prerequisite for understanding and responding to acute trauma in Australian Aboriginal settings today. In this chapter an overview of the Aboriginal experience of trauma is presented – the seeds of understanding and of responding to current trauma are contained within the past. Aboriginal attempts to define the scope and severity of their traumatization have been consistently frustrated by the denial of successive governments and their agencies. A disremembering of state-sanctioned traumatization has led mainstream responses to its social and emotional aftermath becoming further traumatic stressors in themselves, have subverted Aboriginal understandings of their situation, and have undermined attempts to heal from past and current traumatization. We argue for the need to situate any understandings and responses to acute trauma in Aboriginal settings today within a framework of collective and cumulative traumatization over several generations. While contemporary trauma issues cannot be explained only in terms of colonization, as with so much else in Aboriginal life, it cannot be properly understood outside this.

Few Australians are aware of the history of widespread and collective traumatization of Aboriginal Australians. The landfall of Europeans began momentous events that changed the course of Aboriginal history forever. Exposure to systematic and pervasive traumatization over several generations has led Australian Aboriginal people to become perpetual survivors – at considerable social cost. Morbidity, mortality, longevity, injury, suicide, violence, substance abuse... The social and health indicators are uniformly dismal and reflect the public health consequences of chronic and collective traumatization, but Aboriginal attempts to relate past and ongoing experience of traumatization to abysmal health and social indicators have yet to be accepted by successive governments. While there are obvious parallels with patterns of ill health among colonized indigenous peoples elsewhere, Aboriginal Australians are distinguished by having, relatively, the worst health status. Kunitz (1994) has sought explanations in terms of 'Anglo settler colonialism' (Canada, the USA and Australia). A number of correlates emerged in Kunitz's analysis, including health status being worse in those nations where no formal treaty had been concluded between the colonizing and indigenous populations. No treaties have ever been signed to regulate relations between Australian Aboriginal groups and successive governments. We suggest the presence or absence of a formal treaty influences the health status of indigenous peoples, including Australian Aborigines, by indicating: the quality of experience and relationship between colonizer and colonized; the ability of the indigenous population to gain some closure of their traumatization; and the potential for regaining some certainty and autonomy from which post-trauma recovery adaptation can take place.

Background to collective traumatization of Aboriginal Australians

The nation is now attempting to address the legacy of a history about which most Australians have only recently become aware. Rather than the peaceful process of settlement advanced by early historians, in recent decades an accumulating mass of historical evidence has emerged of the heartless extermination, exploitation and enduring social rejection of Aboriginal Australians since landfall. While traumatization was universal, Aboriginal experience of colonization varied greatly among individuals, families and communities. Australian Aboriginal people have never been, nor are now, a homogeneous cultural group. Great diversity existed at the time of settlement, there being some 500 autonomous tribal groups, each with their own land, language, law and culture. In turn, the colonizing experience was greatly influenced by factors such as geography and economic potential of land occupied by clan groups. For example, on the pastoral frontier, appropriation of both land and labour resulted in a pattern of small discrete settlements serving cattle and sheep stations. In areas of agriculture or mining, in contrast, Aboriginal peoples constituted an obstacle to appropriation of land and were dealt with by 'dispersal', euphemism for forced removal and killing. On the other hand, those groups occupying arid or inaccessible lands were left comparatively undisturbed for

decades. Some groups managed to retain association with traditional lands; some did not. In addition, each state varied somewhat in its approach to the management and control of its Aboriginal peoples. For example, Victoria and New South Wales placed less emphasis than other states on isolation and segregation.

None the less, wherever they were, Aboriginal Australians came under special legislations that treated them as different and inferior, and while the timing and impact may have varied, the colonization process followed broadly similar phases in each state as the frontier expanded from its original penal foothold along the eastern seaboard.

Collective and cumulative traumatization

The traumatization of Aboriginal Australians began within a short period after the arrival of the Europeans in 1788, the first wave a result of introduced diseases, particularly smallpox which decimated whole tribal groups, sometimes in advance of actual contact. This was soon followed by periods of uncontrolled conflict as the pastoral and mining frontier expanded into the continent. As Broome (1982, p. 36) observed 'each confrontation was a dramatic clash between Aboriginal people who saw the land religiously, as an intimate part of themselves and all life, and the Europeans who saw it economically, as a commodity to be taken, exploited, bought and sold'. Aboriginal resistance, when it occurred, was swiftly and violently suppressed, often invoked as a pretext for further rounds of indiscriminate killings, rapes and displacement. Survivors were forced from homelands into yet more inhospitable lands that were home to other, often hostile, tribes, where competition for scarce resources compounded what disease and massacre had started.

Their autonomy destroyed, the surviving remnants of tribes, dispossessed and no longer perceived to be a threat to colonists, were allowed to drift in to live on the outskirts of frontier towns (Reynolds, 1987). No longer able to feed themselves from traditional lands, they were forced to beg or to exchange menial work for food. Here, widespread exploitation of survivors occurred, particularly of women and girls. A combination of moral outrage at the progeny from this exploitation, a fear of diseases, and concern in Britain over the declining Aboriginal populations stimulated a further wave of traumatization through the drafting and implementation of policies to isolate and segregate mainland Aborigines from Europeans (Loos, 1982). While these policies were drafted with the aim of protecting Aboriginal Australians from the exploitation of unscrupulous Europeans, they were subsequently implemented in a way that contradicted the original intents. This was due largely to the influential views of Charles Darwin, then recently published in *The Origin of Species* (1859). The social application of Darwin's explanatory framework supported the economic agendas of colonial administrators and allowed a reinterpretation of the depopulation that had occurred since contact. Theories of evolution and 'survival or the fittest' were seized upon and used both to justify and to obscure past violence and brutality, and to place the blame for their 'extinction' with Aboriginal people themselves. Until this time, the role of colonists in the depopulation of Australian Aborigines was well acknowledged by both the colonial and British administrations. As historian Reynolds (1987, p. 104) has stated 'Racism was as functional to the squatter as the colt revolver. One cleared the land, the other cleared the conscience'. The aim of isolation and segregation became one of providing palliative care, a 'smoothing of the pillow' while waiting for what was considered to be a 'child race', to succumb to their own genetic weaknesses and to 'die out'.

From the end of the nineteenth century these policies, euphemistically labelled 'protection', resulted in the forced relocation of Aboriginal people to reserves or missions located some distance from frontier towns. This process of centralization and concentration brought Aboriginal Australians under the control and regulation of European administrators, and Aboriginal people effectively became exiles in their own country. As members of what was believed to be a 'child race', Aboriginal people were to be managed like children (Broome, 1982). In each colony and, subsequently, in each state, Aboriginal people were classified as wards of the state and had the legal status of minors. Supported by legislation, mission and station administrators controlled all major and most minor decisions at personal, family and community levels. In many states, activities such as travel, employment, medical treatment, access to alcohol and firearms, child rearing, management of wages, bank accounts, wills, ownership of land, marriage, and sexual activity of women were variously regulated, with infringements punishable by law.

Government control firmly established, it was assumed that the 'dying out' would proceed unhindered. However, by the early twentieth century it was clear that, far from disappearing, Aboriginal populations were increasing. While this might have suggested that the need for discriminatory protective legislations could have been revoked, this did not occur. In concert with eugenic theories gaining credence in Europe and the USA through the first half of this century, government policy shifted to embrace assimilation, which assumed that the future of Aboriginal Australians lay in absorption into the dominant Australian culture.

Reserves and missions, later relabelled 'communities', became training institutions where vigorous and sustained attempts were made to 'assimilate' Aboriginal peoples by prohibiting expression of their own cultures and replacing Aboriginal values, beliefs, lifestyles, languages, behaviours and spirituality with those of the dominant culture. Despite being defined as genocide in the United Nations Convention on the Prevention of the Crime of Genocide, which Australia ratified in 1948, assimilation policies allowed for the abduction of Aboriginal children from their families of origin and placement with Europeans. Tens of thousands of children were abducted and raised in institutions or dormitories where they were deprived of Aboriginal cultural points of reference. Ostensibly preparing Aboriginal boys and girls for entry into the Australian mainstream, such institutions were, instead, preparation for poorly paid service in European's homes and, not infrequently, their beds.

For some decades Aboriginal Australians remained isolated, segregated and powerless unless and until they embraced assimilation. Exemption from discriminatory legislations was possible, but conditional on the elimination of any vestiges of Aboriginal culture, a demonstrated capacity to live according to dominant cultural mores, and, in most states, a commitment to avoid all Aborigines other than their immediate family. Those whose application for exemption was successful were permitted to move into mainstream towns and suburbs and supposedly to assume the same human rights enjoyed by other Australians. Assimilationist policies were thus not only an assault on individual identity and psychological sense of self, but also on the links and connections between Aboriginal people and the patterns of relationships through which they defined themselves and gave meaning to their lives. Discriminatory legislations persisted in some form in most states until 30 years ago, at which time the Commonwealth government assumed control of Aboriginal affairs from state governments. One state, Queensland, continued isolation, segregation and assimilation policies until the early 1980s.

The last 30 years have seen a move towards self-determination and major social changes as Australian Aboriginal activists successfully placed their concerns on the national agenda. Central among these was the appalling state of Australian Aboriginal health. A demand, ultimately repeated mantra-like by Australian Aboriginal people and organizations, was the need for health services to take into account not only the physical well-being of individuals, but the social, emotional and cultural well-being of the whole community (National Aboriginal Health Strategy Working Party, 1989). However, mainstream health systems remained unresponsive and narrowly focussed on biomedical treatment services. Their manifest failure in the face of obvious Australian Aboriginal ill health and needs led to the setting up of Australian Aboriginal community controlled health services from the early 1970s, but these are few and remain dependent on government benevolence.

Recovery environment

Long-term outcomes after trauma are clearly influenced by the nature of the post-trauma environment. Repeated traumatization and enduring traumatic stress responses are thought to potentiate the impact of subsequent traumatic events and also prolong recovery from the initial trauma (Raphael & Wilson, 1993). Repeated traumatization can therefore take on a cyclical nature where the ability to cope becomes more and more compromised. The immediate impact of colonization on Aboriginal people was compounded by policies that suppressed or prohibited culturally informed coping mechanisms to deal with extreme stress such as ceremonies and ritual. In many instances, the cohesive structures of clan groups, and health, social, family, spiritual and other structures integral to the functioning and support of individuals, families and communities were destroyed or compromised, leaving many Aboriginal people powerless to summon the resources to adequately protect themselves or their families. Those who resisted the destruction of culture or openly expressed their distress ran the risk of being branded a deviant or 'uncontrollable', and became vulnerable to a variety of state-sanctioned punishments, including jail without trial and/or forced removal from their families and communities. Successive generations of Aboriginal Australians have existed in an environment of sustained assault on identity and culture, continued traumatization, and enduring grief, powerlessness, uncertainty and fear, with little opportunity to resolve or dissipate the emotional aftermath common to survivors of trauma (i.e. emotional numbness, shame, distrust, anxiety, anger, fear, guilt, grief, and a sense of powerlessness and meaninglessness).

Furthermore, dispossession and continued alienation from traditional lands has been an enduring predicament for many Australian Aboriginal people. This is not a matter of space or residence: the land formed the basis of cultural practices that served to maintain, enrich and restore the social, emotional and spiritual well-being of Aboriginal Australians. Dispossession of land has meant alienation from the very source of spiritual and community healing and restoration. For those who did remain or return, the social significance and healing power of traditional land has been compromised by degradation of land and sacred sites carried out in the name of 'improvement' or 'development'. Across this spectrum of experience, the cultural and spiritual basis of both traumatization and recovery of Aboriginal Australians has yet to be fully acknowledged or explored.

Despite years of rhetoric regarding self-determination, successive governments have consistently frustrated requests for increasing autonomy over Aboriginal affairs. Instead, control over Aboriginal lives has persisted through marginalization and welfare dependence, and provision of government services such as housing, health, policing and education, which remain essentially and blindly ethnocentric and within which strong traces of paternalism, social darwinism and assimilationist approaches can still be found. This not only has served to inhibit recovery from traumatization (past and present) but has contributed to a sustained assault on identity and culture, the effects of which have been amplified by enduring prejudice and discrimination by the wider community. Continued disadvantage, ill health and alienation from land have ensured that Aboriginal Australians have been largely preoccupied with the ongoing struggle for survival, recognition of land rights, social justice, and some form of autonomy. Healing and recovery from trauma has therefore taken second place for many Aboriginal groups, and in many ways could be seen as contingent on achieving the former. Thus, Aboriginal people have yet to achieve a sense of closure to their traumatization or a safe environment from which to appraise their experience and address recovery issues.

The lack of social acceptance, recognition or validation of Aboriginal experience or distress has ensured that when symptoms of distress emerged they were not recognized or accepted as being related to the aftermath of traumatization and have become subject to responses that have served to further disintegrate communities and intensify feelings of powerlessness, uncertainty and injustice.

Contemporary issues

Outcomes of those exposed to overwhelming trauma will vary depending, among other things, on how the wider society defines the event, develops a response and facilitates recovery (Raphael & Wilson, 1993). Whether or not a society regards the suffering of those exposed to trauma as 'legitimate' will influence how a society responds to their suffering.

While the casualties of the sustained social and emotional turmoil endured by Aboriginal Australians have been many, their mental health needs have yet to be systematically assessed or addressed. Rather than being inscribed in mental health databases, continued denial of Aboriginal experience of collective traumatization has meant that the consequences are more likely to be found in the records of social welfare, health and criminal justice systems. Alarmingly high rates of preventable morbidity and mortality, injury, suicide, violence, adult and juvenile arrest, incarceration, substitute care, substance abuse and low rates of fetal and infant growth, school retention, education and longevity tell a tale of ongoing distress and disadvantage. Such figures not only represent the social and emotional aftermath of chronic and collective traumatization, but in themselves constitute sources of acute trauma in Aboriginal communities today. Many Aboriginal people face reduced life circumstances in communities that exist in continuing states of crises, and in which trauma has become an endemic and accepted part of life.

A recent national survey revealed that one in five indigenous Australians over the age of 25 years reported being removed from his or her family by a church mission, the government or a welfare organization (Australian Bureau of Statistics, 1996). While the effect on those removed may be obvious, to this must be added the effects of removal on parents, siblings, extended families and communities. Not surprisingly, many Aboriginal people, and in some cases entire communities have exhausted their coping resources. Some have lost the vitality or motivation to repair the damage wrought by successive governments. Internalization of responsibility and self-blame is common and horizontal violence is widespread. Many elders have repressed or learnt to deny, and avoid talking about, their own or others' experiences, leaving subsequent generations with little ground from which to understand themselves or their parents.

Some suggest that if post-traumatic stress disorder (PTSD) is left unacknowledged and untreated, it can develop into depression, substance abuse, phobia, generalized anxiety disorder or other mental health problems (Matsakis, 1994). Raphael & Wilson (1993) reported that PTSD among survivors of disasters commonly coexists with depressive disorders, anxiety and substance abuse. Green (1993) has noted that, while little work has been done to examine or compare the outcomes of prolonged as opposed to acute traumatization, it is highly likely that the effects of multiple traumatic events would be more complicated, severe and long lasting.

The frequent coexistence of PTSD and substance abuse is thought to reflect an attempt by survivors to self-medicate in order to deal with the primary symptoms of PTSD. Substance abuse is a major concern among some Aboriginal Australians, historically dealt with by the criminal justice system and more recently through illness-oriented health services.

The Royal Commission into Aboriginal Deaths in Custody (1991), instigated after a series of Aboriginal suicides in police custody, found Aboriginal people to be massively overrepresented in the criminal justice system, largely for alcohol-related offences against good order. Some have suggested a strong subculture has emerged in some Aboriginal communities as a result of the lengthy periods of time that many young and adult men spend in jail (Human Rights and Equal Opportunity Commission, 1993). As the Royal Commission emphasized in framing their recommendations, their main thrust is 'directed toward the prime objectives – historically linked – of the elimination of disadvantage and the growth of empowerment and self-determination in Aboriginal society' (Royal Commission into Aboriginal Deaths in Custody, 1991, p. 27). Of the 99 deaths investigated, 30 were by suicide, only one person being over 30 years of age. Indeed, the increasing incidence of suicide and self-harming behaviours among young men has emerged as a major concern among Aboriginal populations in the last three decades. While uncommon prior to that time, suicide among young indigenous males is now not so, the rate for those aged 15–29 years in Queensland being 3.8 times that of their nonindigenous peers (Baume, 1997).

Many Australian Aboriginal people clearly see the sources of acute trauma that occur in Aboriginal communities today as transgenerational traces of the past in the present. Internalization of blame by Aboriginal people, reinforced by stereotyping and victimizing on the part of sections of the wider community, serves to locate responsibility for these tragedies with Aboriginal people themselves – blaming the victims. There is a certain chilling similarity in the social and emotional consequences of colonization of other indigenous peoples, as the following extract from the Canadian Royal Commission on Aboriginal People's (1995, p. 2) report on Aboriginal suicide illustrates.

We concluded that suicide is one of a group of symptoms, ranging from truancy and law-breaking to alcohol and drug abuse and family violence, that are in large part interchangeable as expression of the burden of loss, grief and anger experienced by Aboriginal people in Canadian society. On both grounds, we are convinced that an adequate response to the crisis of suicide among Aboriginal people cannot be limited – whether to crisis services in the absence of long-term family and community supports, or to narrowly focused suicide prevention programmes without reference to the web of related social problems in which community problems may be caught. An adequate response to suicide must entail an overall health strategy. It must speak to the many forms of self-destructive behaviour in Aboriginal communities and to its underlying causes. It is not enough to treat desperate individuals and the immediate sources of their despair – although such strategies must be the starting point of a comprehensive suicide prevention strategy. As well, Aboriginal people must gain the means to address long-standing needs of families and communities and redress the imbalance of power between themselves and other Canadians from which so much distress flows.

Mental health responses to Australian Aboriginal trauma issues

As with other health issues, Australian Aboriginal people have clearly expressed to mainstream mental health services their wish for contemporary mental health issues such as depression and anxiety, alcohol and substance abuse, family instability and violence and high levels of self-harming and suicidal behaviour to be understood and addressed within a holistic framework that takes account of the aftermath of colonization and enduring disadvantage. This has been repeatedly expressed in recommendations from the First National Aboriginal Mental Health Conference held in 1993, in the National Aboriginal Community Controlled Health Organization definition of mental health, in the Royal Commission into Aboriginal

Deaths in Custody (1991), in a national consultancy on Aboriginal and Torres Strait Islander mental health (Swan & Raphael, 1995), and in state Aboriginal and Torres Strait Islander mental health policy statements. While the stories and manifestations of trauma have been clearly and often painfully spelt out by Aboriginal people individually and collectively to mainstream mental health professionals there has been an unwillingness or inability to understand Aboriginal suffering from the framework provided by psychological traumatization. Yet the field of traumatology was more likely than any other to have offered Australian Aboriginal people a framework within which to understand their experience as normal adaptive processes to extreme and destructive events – that not only were these types of problem to be expected within a context of prolonged and repeated traumatization, but that it was possible to transcend such experiences. Several factors may have contributed to the inaction of state-controlled mental health services in the face of high levels of psychological and social distress. These include the genuine ignorance of many mainstream mental health professionals of the real history and its profound impact on Aboriginal people (who had been segregated out of sight and out of mind), the infancy of the field of traumatology, and the limitations of contemporary nosological frameworks. However, we would suggest that a major factor has been a reluctance on the part of non-Aboriginal Australians, including mental health practitioners, to recognize Aboriginal suffering and explore its causes.

This situation has been compounded by governmental reluctance to officially acknowledge responsibility for past policies, which it is argued, may carry implications in terms of restitution and compensation. The latest national enquiry, the Human Rights and Equal Opportunity Commission's (1997) *Inquiry into the Separation of Aboriginal and Torres Strait Islander Children from their Families* detailed practices carried out until the late 1960s. The report called for a national apology as well as compensation for the victims, probably the most massively traumatized group of all. Both of these recommendations were rejected by the existing national government. The national debate that followed included justifications for the widespread practice of abduction and detainment of Aboriginal children as being 'for their own good'. The national government response is a mental health package, which totals approximately one-eighth of the amount cut from the budget of the Aboriginal and Torres Strait Islander Commission when the current government came to power. Without an apology, expressions of remorse, and recognition of harm caused, indigenous Australians have little reason to expect the traumatization and continued removal of children through welfare systems to cease.

The quality of care offered by state mental health services has been crucial for Aboriginal Australians, since accessibility to other services has been restrained by financial and, for rural and remote dwellers, geographical considerations. State services have traditionally adopted a clinical approach that focusses on the diagnosis and cure of disorders. Apart from leaving Aboriginal people vulnerable to misdiagnosis, this has had the effect of individualizing and pathologizing what are complex social and historical issues. The continued discrepancy between the stated needs of Aboriginal Australians and service provision by state mental health services and the frustration of Aboriginal people was captured by Swan (1988, p. 12) when she stated, 'Today there is no framework by which Aboriginal mental health problems can be usefully understood. Without this framework, services that are accessible and acceptable will never become available, and the mental distress of our people will remain as it is today – largely unrecognised and untreated'. The apparent inability of state-funded mental health systems to respond to the mental health needs of Aboriginal Australians has led to the recent federal funding of a range of community-based initiatives to address Aboriginal mental health needs. This has seen the emergence of parallel systems of Commonwealth-funded Aboriginal controlled social and emotional health (mental health) initiatives using a holistic approach to mental health, leaving state mental health services to continue to rely on treatment services for mental disorders.

None the less, this approach may bring some clarity to the confusion and frustration about roles and responsibilities in relation to Australian Aboriginal mental health issues. While traumatization can exact a toll on emotional and social well-being it should be considered not simply in pathological terms. Appropriate referral points for treatment services will always be necessary for those disabled by their experience, but in most cases human suffering and survival is not a disease or disorder that requires treatment by mental health professionals and the urge to pathologize Aboriginal experience and suffering should be resisted. Nor is knowledge about mental health and ways of achieving social and emotional well-being the sole province of mental health practitioners, particularly since such understandings are multifaceted and tend to reflect cultural views of what it means to be a person of well-being.

Theoretical framework for chronic and acute traumatization

The collective traumatization endured by Aboriginal Australians and its social and emotional sequelae is immensely complex. Clearly, it is not possible to locate traumatization to a discrete place or time. Within Aboriginal experiences of colonization it is possible to identify many of the dimensions proposed by Green (1990) to be generic to a variety of personal traumatic experiences. While such approaches to assessing the nature and impact of trauma move somewhat towards an acknowledgement of the multidimensional nature of acute trauma and recognize that within a collective experience of trauma the experience of individuals will vary widely, they none the less still fail to capture the Aboriginal experience of layered, cumulative and collective traumatization of several generations. In such situations common to indigenous peoples, the traumatization as well as the processes of coping and adaptation have spread out over time so that one cannot see a simple cause and effect, but rather prolonged and repeated waves of traumatization with several feedback loops likely to have impacted on several generations (Marsella et al., 1996). A similar view is proposed by Australian Aboriginal authors who see linear causal models as trivializing their experience. As Robin et al. (1996), drawing widely on traumatology research have noted in discussing cumulative trauma among

native Americans, appropriate assessment must give close scrutiny to several factors.

First, the nature and extent of prolonged and repeated trauma in American Indian populations needs to be more extensively documented, so that non-Indian clinicians and researchers can better understand the history of trauma in American Indian populations... Second, the impact of a single, acute, traumatic incident within the context of cumulative, multi-generational trauma needs to be examined... Finally, the concept of community trauma, or trauma as experienced by entire communities, needs to be developed (Robin et al., 1996, p. 246).

In an attempt to address the earlier perceived limitations of the concept of PTSD, consideration was given to the inclusion of disorder of extreme stress not otherwise specific (DESNOS) in *The Diagnostic and Statistical Manual for Mental Disorders* (DSM-IV; American Psychiatric Association, 1994) to cover reactions to prolonged interpersonal violence, childhood incest, repeated domestic violence, prolonged captivity, or protracted torture. Herman (1992) argued that such experiences can lead to symptoms of somatization, dissociation, changes in affect, impact on relationships and identity, self-injury, suicidal behaviour and revictimization as a result of ongoing trauma. If ultimately incorporated, this diagnostic formulation may assist mental health professionals towards a more comprehensive understanding of the distress of victims of chronic traumatization but it still does not adequately describe the impact of collective and chronic traumatization on an entire social group across several generations.

Furthermore, in an indigenous context of severe and ongoing socioeconomic disadvantage, all such constructions are at risk of what Klienmann (1987) has termed a 'category fallacy'. Klienmann used this term to refer to the nosological reification of what may be termed 'normal' reactions to adversity, such as the unremitting poverty, illness, violence, incarceration and unemployment that characterize the lives of many in Aboriginal communities. Indeed, to focus on individual distress rather than the social and political context may only deflect energy and attention away from social, political and community solutions.

This raises questions about the utility of healing and recovery work in an environment of continued traumatization. Those who have recovered after incest, torture, captivity and/or interpersonal violence have either escaped or been released from the source of their traumatization. Indigenous people have not, as a group, had the benefit of regaining some form of autonomy which would allow cultural intrusions to be limited or controlled, and few have escaped the cycle of poverty, enduring discrimination and ongoing trauma and distress. In Australia, Aboriginal people have yet to have their rights as a first nation recognized and have remained dependent and enmeshed within a system of 'welfare colonialism' or 'paternal welfarism' (Bernardi, 1997). Recovery cannot reasonably be expected to gain momentum until there is, as Dudgeon (1993) suggested in evidence to the Human Rights and Equal Opportunity Commission (1993, p. 718): 'real progress on the fundamental cause, which is to ensure access to Aboriginal mental health through Aboriginal self-determination in all aspects of life – to make possible a dignified Aboriginal life which is viable and meaningful as seen and experienced and constructed by Aboriginal people themselves'.

Responses to acute trauma in Aboriginal settings

Chronic and acute trauma in Australian communities exist in a volatile and dynamic relationship. In considering appropriate responses to acute trauma it is unlikely that conventional debriefing interventions will be sufficient or meaningful. However, the principles of crisis intervention in acute trauma situations may still be applied with some effectiveness in Aboriginal contexts of collective and cumulative traumatization. The disruption caused by discrete traumatic event(s) is likely to precipitate acute personal, family and community distress, may evoke meanings and reactions similar to those of previous trauma(s), and trigger a resurgence of post-traumatic symptoms. However, the crisis precipitated by the current trauma may be used as an opportunity to allow individuals, families and communities to make connections between the past and present situation and to begin the recovery process from both

present and past traumatization. The nature and approach to such issues is none the less exquisitely sensitive and potentially volatile. If handled poorly or insensitively the process can be fraught with dangers such as the precipitation of overwhelming reactions and exacerbation of associated syndromes such as substance abuse, self-harming behaviours, family violence and suicide. In Aboriginal contexts of interconnectedness, the secondary effects of individual distress are likely to have, via the extended family, a community-wide reach. Distress can reverberate and multiply in this way in communities for extended periods. One would therefore be ill advised to raise or address issues related to acute and/or chronic traumatization without a range of culturally appropriate resources, supports and interventions already in place to contain or deal with any such eventuality. Rather than a conventional medical paradigm, support is required for a paradigm that focusses not only on the healing and restoration of equilibrium of individuals or high-risk groups, but also on community healing and the restoration of a sense of hope, dignity and empowerment.

The imposition of interventions that rely on the language and symbols of the dominant culture, and discount the rich sources of meaning and symbolism available in Australian Aboriginal cultures, would merely continue the process of colonization. Clearly, those best placed for this sensitive work are Aboriginal people themselves, using cultural frames of reference. Indeed, in the face of state denial and lack of interest, Aboriginal individuals and communities have, of necessity, been providing for healing and recovery needs for generations. As the Central Australian Aboriginal Congress told the Human Rights and Equal Opportunity Commission (1993, p. 717) 'Our strength is that we have survived. We are strong, or we would not have survived. Our culture is alive, and it is central to our strength. The colonization process of dispossession made us strong. We depend on each other, we understand and support each other'. Indeed, many Aboriginal people have undertaken the painful journey from victim to survivor and some have devoted lives to assisting others to do the same. Programmes have recently been developed specifically for this task. One such initiative, We Al-Li in Queensland, seeks to 'transform the present and the future by reawakening the powerful past' through processes that 'decolonize' individuals, families and communities (Atkinson & Ober, 1995, p. 205). For several decades the particular needs of the 'stolen generation' have occupied a New South Wales Aboriginal organization called Link Up. Considerable expertise has been developed in responding to episodes of acute trauma not uncommonly precipitated during the process of reconnecting chronically traumatized individuals, families and communities.

A recent Federal Government initiative has funded several Indigenous Social and Emotional Regional Centres across the nation. These centres will draw on the considerable indigenous expertise in healing from trauma and give it a voice, one largely rendered silent until now. Other strategies have included: the working through of the effect of local, state and national histories on personal and family lives (e.g. Stewart et al., 1997); reclaiming parts of, or returning to, family, culture, country and community; and participation in healing ceremonies where participants grow stronger by overcoming pain and suffering together. Particularly promising has been the use of narrative therapy to address collective experiences of loss and grief, originally funded in the early 1990s following the Royal Commission into Aboriginal Deaths in Custody and subsequently expanded to broadly address recovery from traumatization (Aboriginal Health Council of South Australia, 1995).

There has been active debate regarding the appropriateness of the therapeutic aims of Western models of debriefing interventions that emphasize self-efficacy, interpersonal independence and control through externally oriented instrumental behaviour in non-Western cultures (Marsella et al., 1996). Indeed Aboriginal Australian concepts of positive mental health are more likely to include interdependence, reciprocal relationships and systems of social exchange and obligation, and spiritual reference points to provide meaning and facilitate recovery. There are few concepts of mental health that are entirely free from particular cultural points of view (Shotter, 1990) and the unthinking application of Western approaches to trauma recovery may unwittingly serve to further undermine the basis of Australian Aboriginal social and emotional health and

well-being. It is therefore particularly inappropriate for Western blueprints for mental health to be imposed on Aboriginal Australians during the process of healing and reintegration of self, family and community.

Conclusion

Australian Aboriginal people are well aware that recovery from acute, chronic and collective traumatization defies a wholesale remedy and cannot be adequately addressed by any short-term methods. Given the salience of disempowerment and loss of control to the experience of trauma for Aboriginal people, it is crucial that they now be in control of the pace, rate and extent of any initiatives to address trauma-related issues. To be meaningful, interventions must be long range and aim to establish or restore an integrated sense of self, family and community. The means of achieving this are likely to be as diverse as the Aboriginal peoples, cultures and groups that exist in Australia today. Each community is unique in its history, culture(s) and aspirations and may preclude the development of a standard approach. Initiatives should be responsive to this diversity and to the changing needs of individuals, families and communities over time, and should mobilize and build on resources and strengths that already exist in Aboriginal communities. To this end, it is important that Aboriginal people are resourced and supported to do such work themselves, using cultural frameworks that contain the accumulated knowledge of some 40 000 years of successful adaptation to a unique and complex environment. The contribution and participation of mental health practitioners willing to work for Aboriginal ends, by Aboriginal direction, would be welcomed.

Acknowledgements

The authors wish to acknowledge the feedback, direction and endorsement provided by the following members of an Aboriginal Advisory group: Val Stanley, Townsville, Queensland; Lyn Johnson, Mossman, Queensland; Mary Graham, Brisbane, Queensland; Priscilla Iles, Rockhampton, Queensland; Cindy Shannon, Rockhampton, Queensland; Bronwyn Fredericks,

Rockhampton, Queensland; Dr Noel Hayman, Brisbane, Queensland; Tom Brideson, Sydney, New South Wales. This chapter has been endorsed by the New South Wales Link Up Organization. Kerrie Kelly wishes to acknowledge the influence of her cross-cultural mentors, Lorraine Peeters, Ron Archer, Val Stanley and Lyn Johnson, who, during the process of development of Social and Emotional Health and Healing curricula, took the time to ensure that her understanding of Aboriginal trauma issues reflected theirs.

REFERENCES

Aboriginal Health Council of South Australia (1995). Reclaiming our stories, reclaiming our lives. An initiative of the Aboriginal Health Council of South Australia. *Dulwich Centre Newsletter*, **1**, 1–40.

American Psychiatric Association (1994). *Diagnostic and Statistical Manual of Mental Disorders*, 4th edn. Washington, DC: American Psychiatric Association.

Atkinson, J. & Ober, C. (1995). We Al-Li 'Fire and water'. A process of healing. In Hazelhurst, K. (Ed.) *Populate Justice and Community Regeneration. Pathways of Indigenous Reform.* Westport, CT: Praeger Publishers.

Australian Bureau of Statistics (1996). *National Aboriginal and Torres Strait Islander Survey.* Canberra: Australian Government Publishing Service.

Baume, P. (1997). Suicide in the family context. Suicide and families towards better research and practice. Paper presented at a conference at the Gold Coast, Queensland, 26 November.

Bernardi, G. (1997). The C.D.E.P. scheme, a case of welfare colonialism. Australian Aboriginal Studies, **2**, 36–46.

Broome, R. (1982). *Aboriginal Australians. Black Response to White Dominance 1788–1980.* George Allen & Unwin: Sydney.

Dudgeon, P. (1993). Head, Centre for Aboriginal Studies, Curtin University. Evidence to Human Rights and Equal Opportunity Commission. In *Report of the National Inquiry into the Human Rights of People with Mental Illness* (p. 218). Canberra: Australian Government Publishing Service.

Green, B. (1990). Defining trauma terminology and generic stressor dimensions. *Journal of Applied Psychology*, **20**, 1632–41.

Green, B. (1993). Identifying survivors at risk for trauma and stressors across events. In J. Wilson & B. Raphael (Eds.) *International Handbook of Traumatic Stress Syndromes* (pp. 135–44). New York: Plenum Press.

Herman, J. L. (1992). *Trauma and Recovery.* New York: Basic Books.

Human Rights and Equal Opportunity Commission (1993). *Report of the National Inquiry into the Human Rights of People with Mental Illness.* Canberra Australian Government Publishing Service.

Human Rights and Equal Opportunity Commission (1997). *Bringing Them Home Report of the National Inquiry into the Separation of Aboriginal and Torres Strait Islander Children from their Families.* Canberra: Australian Government Publishing Service.

Klienmann, A. (1987). Anthropology and psychiatry. The role of culture in cross-cultural research on illness. *British Journal of Psychiatry*, **151**, 447–54.

Kunitz, S. J. (1994). *Disease and Social Diversity. The European Impact on the Health of non-Europeans.* New York: Oxford University Press.

Loos, N. (1982). *Invasion and Resistance. Aboriginal–European Relations on the North Queensland Frontier 1861 to 1897.* Canberra: Australian National University Press.

Manson, S. M., Taturn, E. & Dinges, N. G. (1982). Prevention research among American Indian and Alaska native communities: charting future causes for theory and practice in mental health. In Manson, S. M. (Ed.), *New Directions in Prevention among American Indian and Native Alaskan Communities* (pp. 11–90). Oregan: NIMH.

Marsella, A. J., Friedman, J., Gerrity, E. T. & Scurfield, R. M. (1996). Ethnocultural aspects of PTSD. Some closing thoughts. In A. J. Marsella, M. J. Friedman, E. T. Gerrity & R. M. Scurfield (Eds.) *Ethnocultural Aspects of Post-traumatic Stress Disorder* (pp. 529–38). Washington, DC: American Psychiatric Association Press.

National Aboriginal Health Strategy Working Party (1989). *A National Aboriginal Health Strategy.* Canberra: Department of Aboriginal Affairs.

Raphael, B. & Wilson, J. (1993). Theoretical and intervention considerations in working with victims of disaster. In J. Wilson & B. Raphael (Eds) *International Handbook of Traumatic Stress Syndromes* (pp. 105–17). New York: Plenum Press.

Reynolds, H. (1987). *Frontier. Aborigines, Settlers and Land.* Sydney: Allen & Unwin.

Robin, R. W., Chester, B. & Goldman, D. (1996). Cumulative trauma and PTSD in American Indian Communities. In A. J. Marsella, M. J. Friedman, E. T. Gerrity & R. M Scurfield (Eds.) *Ethnocultural Aspects of Post-traumatic Stress Disorder* (pp. 239–54). Washington, DC: American Psychiatric Association Press.

Royal Commission into Aboriginal Deaths in Custody (1991). *Final Report*. Canberra: Australian Government Publishing Service.

Royal Commission on Aboriginal Peoples (1995). *Choosing Life. Special report on Suicide among Aboriginal People*. Ottawa: Communication Group.

Shotter, J. (1990). Social individuality versus possessive individualism. The sounds of silence. In I. Parker & J. Shotter (Eds.) *Deconstructing Social Psychology*. London: Routledge.

Stewart, P., Gray, R. & Millard, M. (1997). Reclaiming futures; making lives a story about stories, mental and healing. Paper presented at an Australian Psychological Society National Conference, Cairns, Australia.

Swan, P. (1988). 200 years of unfinished business. *Newsletter*, September, pp. 12–17. Redfern: Aboriginal Medical Service.

Swan, P. & Raphael, B. (1995). *'Ways Forward' National Consultancy Report on Aboriginal and Torres Strait Islander Mental Health*. Canberra: Australian Government Publishing Service.

18

The concept of debriefing and its application to staff dealing with life-threatening illnesses such as cancer, AIDS and other conditions

Jane Turner and Brian Kelly

EDITORIAL COMMENTS

The ubiquity of the conceptualization of debriefing as an appropriate intervention to deal with 'stress' has meant that it is now frequently applied in health care settings to deal with emergency health workers' experience and also that of other workers perceived to work in stressful settings such as with terminally ill patients as well as more widely.

This detailed review examines the types of stressor experienced by health care workers, and their relationship to burnout and other work-related stress is considered. Critical incident stress debriefing as a model in such contexts is critically reviewed, although Turner and Kelly note that there is no empirical research validating its use for health care staff in these settings.

Of particular value, and applicable to many other worker and stress situations is the detailed review of factors that need to be considered as sources of stress. These include factors relating to the situation of the patient and the illness, for example type of illness, stage of lifecycle, suffering and other clinical problems, and patient characteristics. Factors relating to the individual worker include maturity and past experience, personality style, interpersonal relationships, expectations, requirement for emotional support, education and training experiences of staff, pre-existing psychological vulnerability and morbidity, and protective factors. External factors include administrative issues, team membership, and volunteer status. Sociocultural factors include personal and social attitudes to death and dying and cultural requirements for these. Such factors serve as a model for the many contributions to

stress affecting workers in any setting, not simply health care. And they highlight the fallacy of any simplistic conceptualization of critical incident stresses that may be superimposed on, or even arise from, these underlying problems.

In addition, this review highlights the chronicity of the stressor background for workers and thus challenges the validity of a model more focussed on specific acute stressors. It highlights other administrative, organizational and training interventions and more specifically the significance of supervision and support and what they may contribute to the prevention and managements of the stressor effects for workers.

Like debriefing models, other possible models to be applied in such settings, including clinical supervision, also lack empirical research testing their effectiveness in preventing negative outcomes. In addition the linking of acute models such as debriefing to models for prevention and management of chronic stressors needs to be explored. This is relevant in many workplace settings, as well as in sociocultural contexts such as that experienced by indigenous and disadvantaged populations who may face chronic and severe stressors as well as acute ones (see Ober et al., Chapter 17; Silove, Chapter 25).

Introduction

Concepts of trauma and trauma response have become widely applied to a broad range of human experiences. This has extended to occupational experiences and formed the basis for the development of interventions to lessen traumatic stress reactions in groups of personnel such as emergency workers (Mitchell & Everley, 1995). Similarly, the experiences of those working in health care, particularly in areas involving the care of the dying, in oncology and human immunodeficiency virus (HIV) treatment units, paediatric services, in emergency departments or in other potentially distressing medical settings, have also received attention. Concepts such as 'burnout' (Maslach & Jackson, 1981) have been used to describe the adverse emotional effects of such experiences, particularly among health professionals, and a considerable body of mostly descriptive reports has examined the role of interventions in assisting such staff in their work, and to prevent the development of psychological morbidity. Debriefing is one such model of intervention.

Implicit in the concept of burnout is that the symptoms arise as a direct result of, and are referable to, the workplace experiences. The symptoms are thus manifest in terms that relate to response to work demands (e.g. feelings of distance, noninvolvement or dissatisfaction). Evaluation of the role of workplace stress, in addition to a range of other factors that may impinge on an individual's emotional well-being, therefore needs to be incorporated in any model of intervention in this setting.

This chapter reviews concepts of stress as applied to health care professionals, the perceived extent of the problem, the factors that have been identified as contributing to the psychological symptoms and distress of health care professionals, and the models of interventions that have been used in some settings, as part of a critical evaluation of the role of Critical Incident Stress Debriefing (CISD) in these settings. Training and professional needs and the role of institutional factors are examined alongside critical examination of the application of a traumatic stress paradigm to the experience of nurses, doctors and other health professionals in their work.

The nature of trauma

Debate continues regarding the severity of the events that can typically precipitate a post-traumatic stress disorder (PTSD) or contribute to other morbidity (American Psychiatric Association, 1994, pp. 424–9).

It has been argued that the threat to life represents the common feature of trauma events (Lifton, 1993) and that it is the encounter and confrontation with death that represent the traumatic component of an event, differentiating trauma events from other forms of adverse life events. This is an important issue in assessing the role of experiences arising in the care of individuals with cancer, acquired immune deficiency syndrome (AIDS), or other life-threatening illness, and the psychological impact on health professionals.

Comorbidity of traumatic stress syndromes with other psychiatric syndromes remains an important issue in assessing psychological responses to trauma and risks to both those directly affected and to health care professionals working in these fields (Breslau et al., 1991; Davidson et al., 1991; Helzer et al., 1987; McFarlane, 1993; Yehuda & McFarlane, 1995). This has not generally been incorporated in the evaluation of occupational trauma or in interventions to deal with it.

McFarlane (1993) has proposed that the comorbidity of major depression or anxiety disorder may be important determinants of the exacerbation of traumatic stress symptoms, for example intrusive memories of trauma during an episode of major depression. These findings from PTSD research have direct relevance to the methods by which preventive interventions such as CISD are applied. The very real issue is that there is a need to examine aetiology, taking such factors into account in order to support any potential role of stress debriefing or CISD in health care systems.

Green et al. (1985) and Green (1993) summarized a range of theoretical issues in PTSD research that need to be considered in this context: the nature of the stressor criterion, including the role of individual vulnerability and the development of PTSD, whether to 'emphasize the trauma or the person'; and the need to consider the specific characteristics of the individual and the characteristics of the recovery environment. Such issues need to be included in any consideration of trauma occurring in a health care setting.

Models of 'stress'

'Stress' is a concept that has been broadly applied to a range of physiological and psychological responses to physical or emotional demands on the individual. Its common usage to describe a broad range of psychological responses and events has contributed to confusion in this field. Stress may have adaptive outcomes – it may not be freedom from adversity that promotes psychological health, but how the individual responds to adversity (Vaillant, 1995). The potential for growth and development in response to adversity needs to be acknowledged, along with our limited understanding of the developmental linkages between adversity and a range of outcomes (Rutter, 1994).

Stress can be construed as an experience that provokes a range of emotional and physiological responses. The early work of Selye (1976) outlined the autonomic response to psychological stress. Similarly, recent traumatic stress research has indicated important variations in physiological responses to distress among individuals with PTSD, indicating the role of trauma experiences in altering physiological responsiveness (van der Kolk, 1994).

Individual response may be adaptive or maladaptive, according to the consequences, distress experiences, and degree to which the reality of the events is able to be acknowledged and understood (Vaillant, 1995). Literature concerning the consequences of life events has attempted to deal with the issues of individual variation in response to any life events, particularly the contextual threat and meaning that may be critical factors in determining outcome. These may also reflect cultural differences and meanings, social context and past experiences. These concepts have a direct bearing on how the experiences of health care providers are understood and addressed – the contextual threat, the meaning of experiences, and the individual response style may be critical factors that contribute to outcome, along with the social environment of the institution (e.g. hospital ward).

Social support has also been recognized as a critical variable affecting psychological outcome to adversity. Nevertheless, some argue that the perception of social support is more closely linked to aspects of personality, and represents an individual characteristic that may affect outcome (Henderson et al., 1981). Bereavement research has also highlighted the potential negative aspects of social interaction that may inhibit open expression of distress, promote maladaptive responses or not provide the 'fit' to the individual's needs (Stylianos & Vachon, 1993). Aspects of social support have frequently been addressed in regard to the needs of caregivers, reflected in the development of interventions to enhance the support available for health professionals caring for cancer patients. It is important to note that the perception of such support may be affected by institutional factors (e.g. confidence in leaders, degree of trust in co-workers), and may not be automatically developed in the workplace.

Application in health care settings

The applicability of traumatic stress models to experience in health care fields is evidenced by the nature of stressors themselves. These may involve confrontation with death and disfigurement, sometimes in the setting of complex ethical concerns. The health professional must also deal with the beneficial as well as adverse effects of treatments, potential helplessness and frustration in the face of chronic and terminal illness, and concerns about the emotions of patients and families. This occurs alongside the health professional's own life experiences. Loss is a universal experience, and loss experiences in the workplace may resonate with personal vulnerabilities or experiences to accentuate the risk of escalating distress in the caregivers. Loss and death may become an embedded component of their work, so that no single event can be readily identified among a cumulative set of losses, particularly deaths of patients in general and of children in particular. Psychological reactions may then become chronic, reflecting defences to this long-term distress, and shape reactions to new experiences as they arise.

A model is required that gives adequate recognition to the role of individual attributes, the social context (in this instance institutional practices that may exacerbate or mitigate the experiences of caregivers), alongside recognition of the distressing human experiences to which many health professionals are exposed in their workplace.

Chronic exposure to trauma needs to be considered also for many health professionals. Where an event is shared in a community, acute in onset and extraordinary for a group (e.g. a community disaster), this is likely to have sequelae different from those encountered in the experience of a health professional for whom events may be repeated and covert, often not fully acknowledged by others. This may contribute to a private level of trauma that is often not acknowledged or for which there may be few avenues for expression, and which are seen as the expected consequences of one's career choice. This latter feature of the workplace experiences of health professionals has contributed to the development of interventions that have at their basis the provision of sharing experiences, gaining validation and support (Burr, 1996; Sowney, 1996), and these have been recognized by health staff as the more beneficial aspects of CISD in this setting.

It is important therefore to delineate the trauma component of experiences of health professionals in such settings. If confrontation with death and threat to bodily integrity to others are considered to be potential traumatic events, then the workplace for those caring for the dying and those with life-threatening medical illness provides a range of potential triggers. Difficulties in conducting research on CISD and supporting its role may be due to generalization from acute trauma to other settings without consideration of the differing nature of experiences, and other forms of adaptation and responses that might result from other events and experiences that individuals face.

Any consideration of traumatic stress syndromes in the health care setting needs to acknowledge the role of the climate of interpersonal relationships and institutional factors in the workplace. For instance, workplace conflict may precipitate and accentuate psychological distress and maladaptive responses through dysfunctional group interactions where the source of anxiety is not addressed, leadership role is unclear, and interdisciplinary tensions develop. In such a setting the capacity to address the psychological demands on the team is likely to require external intervention and some degree of recognition by the team of their own ongoing emotional needs, as distinct from those precipitated in relation to traumatic experiences.

A dilemma can evolve in such considerations: how to sensitively and effectively acknowledge the role of the individual and individual vulnerability in the workplace, while not ignoring the general experiences, workplace practices and institutional environment that may have a bearing on caregivers' well-being. Individual needs can be addressed in a framework of continuous individual supervision alongside interventions for groups of staff and clinical teams. Education, in-service development and efforts to maintain competency, as well as support of staff, are important. These will assist in the ability of staff to gauge their own psychological responses, become more familiar with the impact on patient care and the potentially intense and disorienting effects for themselves of close contact with the suffering, distress and at times death of their patients (Miller, 1995).

Levels of stress experienced by staff

As described, the concept of workplace stress and burnout has gained widespread popularity, and there is considerable literature about the levels of stress experienced by staff who care for those with HIV and cancer. Most studies have relied on measures such as the General Health Questionnaire (GHQ), the Maslach Burnout Inventory (MBI), with some also employing the Impact of Event Scale (IES), and AIDS Impact Scale. As described above, many studies uncritically accept that any documented levels of stress or dysfunction can be attributed to work, without elucidating the particular facets of professional and personal life that may have contributed to the difficulties, and the effects or otherwise of particular 'events'.

Oncology settings

As early as 1978, Vachon explored stress experienced by staff in a newly opened palliative care facility in Canada (Vachon et al., 1978). Nurses in this facility had twice the score levels of other staff in an active treatment Cancer Centre on the GHQ. In contrast, one study of 29 hospice nurses and 28 hospital oncology nurses found hospice nurses to have significantly lower stress scores (Bram & Katz, 1989). Two other studies of oncology nurses assessed respectively 185 and 152 oncology nurses (Yasko, 1983; Jenkins & Ostchega, 1986). Both studies reported higher levels of stress in those staff who were younger and who had less support in the ward.

More recently, there have been studies of larger numbers of consultant medical staff. Whippen & Canellos (1991) assessed 598 oncologists by means of a postal self-report questionnaire. Fifty-six per cent of respondents described some degree of burnout in their professional life. A UK study assessed 882 consultants, comprising gastroenterologists, surgeons, clinical radiologists, and oncologists (Ramirez et al., 1996). Twenty-seven per cent of consultants had a GHQ score of 4 or more, indicating likely psychiatric morbidity, with no significant differences across the four specialist groups. Of these specialists, 27% to 35% scored high emotional exhaustion scores. In an earlier study of 392 oncologists (Ramirez et al., 1995), 31% reported high levels of emotional exhaustion. The estimated prevalence of psychiatric disorder using the GHQ was 28%.

In a review of the literature dealing with staff stress in hospice and palliative care, Vachon (1995) discussed the finding that stress and burnout in palliative care are not universal. She noted that alcohol and drug use, anxiety and depression and suicidal ideation may be experienced by staff working in this area, as well as difficulties in dealing with the issues of death and dying. The factors underpinning staff difficulty in coping are discussed further in the next section.

HIV settings

Several studies have described the extent of concerns experienced by staff working in the area of HIV, documenting varying levels of stress. The AIDS Impact Scale and MBI were administered to 410 nurses working with patients with HIV (Visintini et al., 1996). Although a small proportion had a high level of burnout, overall the level of burnout was considered by the authors to be low.

In contrast, of 108 health professionals working with patients with AIDS (including doctors, social workers and nurses), 22% reported 'a lot' of stress (Ross & Seeger, 1988). More recent studies have also reported high levels of stress for staff working in that area. Bennett et al. (1994b) assessed 84 staff by means of the MBI, GHQ, and the AIDS Impact Scale. Thirty-four per

cent experienced high levels of burnout, and 34% experienced medium levels of burnout. A similar picture was obtained by Miller & Gillies (1996), who assessed 103 staff working with HIV patients, 36% experiencing high levels of emotional exhaustion on the MBI. This study also found 41% of staff qualified as cases on the GHQ. This compared with caseness on the GHQ amongst 42% of 100 oncology staff assessed, of whom 25% also had high emotional exhaustion scores. Thus there are a range of reports indicating stress or its effects, although their relation to other variables, including the individual's personal life, organizational matters and so forth are not clear.

Staff in other settings

High levels of stress have been reported in studies assessing burnout in other areas of health care. For example, Catalan et al. (1996) assessed 41 doctors and nurses caring for patients with serious illness. More than one-third of staff had substantial levels of psychological morbidity as measured by the GHQ and approximately one-fifth had significant levels of work-related stress. In an assessment of physician burnout, of 342 physicians assessed, 58% reported high emotional exhaustion, scores being higher in those who were younger (Deckard et al., 1994). This is consistent with the finding of lower stress in older intensive care unit nurses (Keane et al., 1985).

Comparisons of staff stress across differing settings

Several studies have compared stress in nursing staff working across a variety of treatment settings. Most have compared staff working in intensive care units, operating theatres and oncology units. The majority of studies reported no significant differences in the level of stress between nurses working across these different treatment settings (Cronin-Stubbs & Rooks, 1985; Foxall et al., 1990; van Servellen & Leake, 1993; Papadatou et al., 1994; Tyler & Ellison, 1994). One earlier small study (Stewart et al., 1982) reported that levels of stress were comparable for 40 female nurses working in the areas of cancer, cardiology, operating theatre and intensive care, although the nurses working with cancer patients reported more enduring stress.

Factors which may contribute to stress in staff

Any effort to offer preventive interventions or treatment for staff working in oncology, AIDS and other health care settings must, of necessity, incorporate a comprehensive understanding of the issues for individuals, in terms of both personal and external factors, including the nature of the patient's illness and the environment in which the person works. A further dimension of complexity is added by the chronicity of exposure to suffering, distress and death, with the relative absence of clearly defined events that may be followed by respite.

Factors relating to the patient and the illness

Type of illness

Since the earliest descriptions of HIV and AIDS, there has been strong sentiment and stigma surrounding the illness. A number of authors have alluded to the fear of contagion for staff working in the area (Dworkin et al., 1991; Cooke, 1992; Maj, 1991), this fear sometimes being expressed as anger or revulsion towards such patients (Silverman, 1993). The stigma about HIV and AIDS may also extend to those staff who work in the area (Bennett, 1992). Outsiders may question the sexuality and values of staff working in the area (Bennett & Kelaher, 1993). Some staff working with HIV patients may receive less support from their families than, for example, those staff working in oncology (Miller & Gillies, 1996).

Other conditions, such as cancer, may involve highly mutilating and deforming treatment. In addition to the personal grief and distress experienced by such patients, staff must also deal with secretions, smells and patients' loss of bodily control, for which their training may have offered them inadequate preparation. Junior nursing staff involved, for example, in dressing changes on a woman who has had a radical vulvectomy may feel not only threatened about their own personal vulnerability in this context, but be the recipient of envious attacks from patients who perceive their carer as 'whole and undamaged'. Many patients and their families have had past experience directly or indirectly with cancer, and there remain social connotations of cancer as being a 'death sentence'. A major source of stress for staff is having to inform patients of the diagnosis of cancer (Herschbach, 1992).

The cognitive changes consequent upon some conditions, for example dementia in AIDS, may be associated with major behavioural difficulty with which staff feel ill trained to cope. Furthermore, in some areas such as neurooncology, many patients not only require assistance with activities of daily living, but are unable to communicate, necessitating staff involvement with family members who are acting as the patient's surrogate (Horowitz et al., 1994).

Although diseases such as cancer and AIDS may be fatal in the longer term, in many instances, the patient endures deteriorating health for many years before succumbing, which may prove a painful and ongoing reminder to staff of their perceived professional impotence.

Stage of the lifecycle

Dealing with younger patients for whom the illness seems particularly incongruous has been described as stressful for staff (Catalan et al., 1996). Dealing with the deaths of children has also been described as particularly difficult for staff (Burns & Harm, 1993), and this is consistent with trauma research (Robinson & Mitchell, 1993). Staff perceptions of positive attributes of patients and their families may, in fact, represent a way of coping with a highly emotionally charged situation in paediatric oncology (Grootenhuis et al., 1996) and a defence to mitigate the suffering and deaths of children.

Those patients who have dependent children may also represent a source of emotional distress to staff who may closely identify with the person, perhaps because of similarities of age of their own family members. This may cause anxiety and further erode the person's sense of professional competence.

Suffering of patients and clinical problems

Technological advances mean that patients can now be offered a greater array of treatments, but many of these may be particularly adversive. A measure of concern about the perceived toxicity of treatments is gleaned by use of terms such as 'poison peddler' to denote oncologists in some settings (Wise, 1977). The toxicity of treatment, and the potential for errors to occur, have also more recently been described as sources of stress for oncologists (Ramirez et al., 1995).

Particularly in the areas of HIV and cancer, pain relief is a major concern for patients and their families. Unrelieved pain, due for instance to peripheral neuropathy (Glare & Cooney, 1996), may engender a sense of professional impotence, but also arouses distress and anger in families and patients, these in turn, contributing to staff stress.

Treating patients who are dying and, in particular, being unable to relieve their suffering as fully as one would wish, have been described as being associated with a sense of powerlessness and impotence in staff (Spikes & Holland, 1975; Keane et al., 1985; Kent et al., 1994). It may also lead to negative coping strategies, for example higher alcohol consumption (Cooper et al., 1989).

Characteristics of patients

Major medical illness does not occur in a vacuum, and many patients facing terminal illness have grappled with complex psychosocial problems before the onset of illness. For instance angry, demanding, or resentful patients may engender powerful feelings of rage in staff (Spikes & Holland, 1975). Such feelings may, of course, engender shame and guilt as 'good nurses don't have bad feelings' (Vachon et al., 1978).

Even for those who have habitually employed mature ego defences, regression and the use of immature defences such as spitting, rejection, or acting out, are commonly seen in the context of pain, disability and the disempowerment imposed by illness (Blacher, 1991).

The development of mental illness is common in the cancer population, up to 20% to 25% of patients attracting a diagnosis of major depression (Massie et al., 1994). In an Australian study of HIV-positive men, 49% were considered likely to be classified as psychiatric cases, using a cut-off of 4 on the GHQ (Kelly & Raphael, 1993). Recognition of, and dealing with, mental illness may pose a major burden on staff, who feel anxious or react angrily when confronted by patients whose behaviour deviates from the norm. Of especial concern is the stress posed for staff when patients commit suicide. Cancer patients are recognized as being at increased risk of suicide (Breitbart, 1995), as are patients with HIV/AIDS. Although the issue of patient suicide has received some attention in the general psychiatric literature (Little, 1992), development of measures to help staff deal with patients' suicide do not appear to have been applied in either oncology or HIV settings.

Factors relating to the individual

Motivation and past experience

Motivation to work in a particular area may be complex, and it is important to draw the distinction between those who elect to work in a particular area, and those who work there by chance, or because of particular delegation (Barbour, 1994).

Certainly, past experience of loss will shape response to new trauma and challenges (Raphael, 1986), and some studies at least have reported a higher proportion of those working with AIDS as having a history of chronic or life-threatening illness in close family members (Miller & Gillies, 1996).

The relative contribution of age has not been studied extensively, although younger staff members are described as experiencing more stress (Yasko, 1983; Deckard et al., 1994). Other personal dynamics such as caring for others to meet one's own deprived needs for care should be taken into account.

Personality style

It is simplistic to assume that all staff will adjust to particular difficulties at work in the same way. In a review of burnout in staff working in the area of AIDS, Miller (1995) considered that the individual's perception of work stress is a critical factor affecting adjustment. Similarly, Vachon (1995) highlights the fact that it is the balance between personal strengths and weaknesses, and the demands and benefits related to the work environment, that will determine adjustment.

Several studies have considered adjustment in terms of internal versus external locus of control, finding that an external locus of control is associated with higher levels of burnout (McElroy, 1982; Bennett & Kelaher, 1993; Bennett et al., 1994a). The capacity to engage empathically with patients has also been considered by some workers in the trauma area as leading to compassion fatigue (Figley, 1995). However, in contrast with work in the trauma field, the care of patients with terminal illness is not a time-limited, discrete event. Such staff are often immersed in suffering, from which there is little respite from the need to demonstrate warmth and empathy (Abeloff, 1991).

Interpersonal relationships

Stable, supportive interpersonal relationships are proposed as providing some protection against burnout (Cronin-Stubbs & Brophy, 1985). One study of stress experienced by physicians and nurses in a cancer ward found that, for nurses, interpersonal stress was the main link with physical complaints (Ullrich & Fitz-Gerald, 1990).

The obligation to work shiftwork may pose significant relationship and family problems for nursing staff. Shiftwork may erode social contacts, many staff finding themselves unable to participate in family and other activities (Waterhouse et al., 1992).

The quality and complexity of marital relationships of doctors have been considered in some detail in the literature (Gabbard et al., 1987). The medical practitioner may face expectations of their spouse regarding earning potential, and in turn exert pressure on themselves to fulfil these expectations and may well experience a range of stresses in relation to their work and roles. Furthermore, there may be difficulties with the practitioner who is used to delegation and a position of authority at work, who finds the transition to family life awkward. There may also be expectations that a medical partner will 'fix' minor medical maladies in their own family and extended family, despite the fact that to do so may involve a transgression of boundaries, and the conditions may be outside the area of the doctor's clinical expertise. Feeling overloaded at work and its effect on home life has been cited as a source of stress for oncologists (Ramirez et al., 1995).

Expectations of caregivers

Many health professionals come into their field of practice with unrealistic expectations. Many medical practitioners, for instance, view themselves as powerful healers, attempting to defend against their own anxiety about death (Spikes & Holland, 1975). Furthermore, junior medical staff in particular may have a strong feeling of the need to be in control in clinical situations, often unfavourably comparing their own performance against an idealized perception of peer performance (Ziegler et al., 1984). For staff exposed to repeated and often untimely death, unrealistic expectations of how they should cope may be compounded by the concern that discussion of their concerns with their peers will diminish their professional standing.

Emotional support of others

Recognition of, and dealing with the emotional problems of patients and their families have been cited in the literature as sources of stress for staff in the area of HIV and oncology (Barbour, 1995; Catalan et al., 1996). Ross & Seeger (1988) in a study of 108 health professionals working with patients with AIDS, reported that a frequently cited source of stress for staff was needing more information about the patient's emotional needs.

Traditional expectations about the role of caregivers in providing emotional support or caring for patients and their families may have important implications in particular for female staff members. Women are socialized from an early age to be nurturing and caring (Notman & Nadelson, 1973), and may experience expectations in their work environment that they will automatically address the emotional concerns of patients and their families, or even other staff. These factors, operating against a background of the role conflicts experienced by women as they juggle competing family and work needs, may contribute greatly to personal stress (McBride, 1990).

Despite the expectations of patients and families that staff will provide emotional support, there is evidence that the ability of staff to detect distress in their patients varies considerably, one study reporting that oncologists tend to underrecognize distress in their patients (Ford et al., 1994). This provides clear implications for intervention, particularly in view of research that reveals that burnout is more prevalent among clinicians who feel less well-trained in communication skills (Ramirez et al., 1996).

Education and training experiences

The above clinical and emotional demands occur against a background of medical education and training that continues to focus heavily on cure of patients as the only acceptable outcome, and in which death is seen as a failure (Hanson, 1994).

Particularly in the training of medical students, there is powerful socialization for students beginning early in their course to learn to deny their feelings, and to seek the active approval of their peers, who, in turn, minimize their own feelings (Coombs & Fawzy, 1986). Medical training has often been conducted in a rigid hierarchy, in which more junior staff may be denigrated or even abused. The banter 'Don't do that, you'll kill the patient' may seriously erode the sense of professional competence of junior staff, particularly as their training has often led to a narrowing of the social repertoires (Coombs & Fawzy, 1986) that might otherwise have helped them to cope.

Research also suggests that training provides little preparation for entry into the workforce, as opposed to the acquisition of theoretical knowledge. One study of 65 oncology nurses found newly qualified nurses to be consistently more anxious than those more experienced (Wilkinson, 1994). For medical students also, the transition to physician seems to be a difficult one (Reuben et al., 1984). Junior staff do seem to be more vulnerable to experiencing higher stress (Jenkins & Ostchega, 1986). Many students emerge from training with little grasp of the multifaceted and chronic health problems encountered in clinical practice, and even

less awareness of the grief and distress such problems may engender and how to deal with these.

Psychological morbidity in staff

Although staff from a variety of professional backgrounds clearly play significant roles in caring for patients with cancer, AIDS, and other serious illness, there is scant literature examining their mental health. In contrast, there is considerable published evidence attesting to the extent of psychological problems experienced by medical practitioners.

The previous section alluded to high levels of stress experienced by staff working with patients with cancer and AIDS. However, it is simplistic to attribute these difficulties to work alone. The experience of distress clearly is the result of an interplay between a doctor's personality (or that of other health workers), factors within relationship and work demands, and the sociocultural context in which the person works (Kelly & Varghese, 1997). There is a very real risk that those staff who are suffering from depression, for example, are inappropriately considered to be suffering from stress or burnout, thus undermining opportunities for effective treatment.

Although there is a paucity of reliable and valid data concerning the rates of serious illness in doctors, rates of suicide are higher (Steppacher & Mausner, 1974), implying that depression is a significant problem for medical practitioners, as there is evidence that the majority of cases of suicide are suffering from mental illness (Barraclough et al., 1974). Additionally, possibly up to 7% to 8% of doctors have a problem of significant alcohol abuse (Lawrence, 1992).

Protective factors

There is, as yet, little research on what may protect staff against the development of stress while they are working in settings in which they are treating patients with HIV and cancer, and other serious illnesses.

Some studies report that stress may be lower in those with children (Tyler & Ellison, 1994), and that the risk may be higher in those with fewer children (Yasko, 1983). The reported finding that stress is less prevalent in those workers who are older (Ullrich & FitzGerald, 1990) may be an artefact, in that staff who are more highly stressed may leave the field. Alternatively, it may be that, with increasing age, staff members gain further experience and expertise in dealing with problems. The importance of supportive relationships outside work has been suggested as having a role of protecting against burnout (Cronin-Stubbs & Brophy, 1985).

The concepts of hardiness and resilience have not been explored in detail in the context of occupational functioning. In general terms, it appears that more hardy individuals appraise stressors as less threatening than those of low hardiness (Funk, 1992), and that competence and empowerment are factors that underpin a sense of personal well-being (Cowen, 1991). The notion that stress is inevitably damaging is not supported in the developmental literature, which, instead, highlights that encountering stress in such a way that confidence and competence are increased through mastery and appropriate responsibility may promote resilience (Rutter, 1985). High self-esteem is a strong predictor of subjective well-being (Diener, 1984), with job satisfaction also appearing to be linked.

It is crucial that any interventions developed for staff working in the areas of HIV, cancer or other life-threatening illness must incorporate notions of self-esteem, personal empowerment, and the promotion of job satisfaction.

External factors

Administrative issues

Fiscal restraint and the shrinking of the health budget may mean that staff really are expected to perform more tasks with fewer resources, posing a significant burden. Indeed, the enthusiastic acceptance by some administrators of a concept of burnout may represent displacement of imperatives for intervention away from administration onto staff themselves. An increased emphasis on quality assurance measures to improve patient care and clinical practice may also mean that for staff there is a sense of escalation of paperwork that they may perceive to be of little clinical utility. This may pose a source of stress for staff, and

this is reinforced by research that highlights the burden posed by organizational responsibilities (Ramirez et al., 1995).

Increasing litigation may engender a sense of a need to practise defensive medicine, this of itself posing a further burden.

Team membership

Conflict amongst team members has been described by several authors as contributing to staff stress (Price & Bergen, 1977; Heim, 1991; Riordan & Saltzer, 1992). Professional communication and boundaries and clarity of role definition are key factors underpinning cohesive team functioning (Jamieson, 1994; Plante & Bouchard, 1995–6; Vachon, 1995), and, as described above, the capacity of the team members to recognize their own emotional needs may influence what resources are employed to assist in coping.

Volunteers

Particularly in the AIDS field, volunteers play a prominent role in the care of patients. Although many intuitively regard the role of volunteers as very valuable, in some respects their contribution may pose difficulties for patients and staff. There are major ethical issues surrounding the training of volunteers, their accountability, and their motivation to become involved in this area of work. Certainly, some studies have suggested that there are significant levels of distress in AIDS volunteers. Raphael et al. (1990) assessed 157 volunteers, finding 37% to score above a cut-off mark of 4–5 on the GHQ, with 14% scoring above the 10–11 cut-off (conventionally thought to reflect serious psychiatric morbidity). More recently, Bennett et al. (1996) studied 174 AIDS helper volunteers, concluding that lack of training and an absence of personal effectiveness (presence of stress and absence of reward) were both independently associated with burnout frequency. Maslanka (1996) has also highlighted the need to intervene early when volunteers are being trained in order to diminish problems before they arise.

Sociocultural issues

Personal attitudes to death

Staff caring for patients with HIV, cancer and other serious illnesses bring with them into their professional setting values that are determined, in part at least, by their own life experiences. However, a major influence is exerted by sociocultural factors, and nowhere is this more true than in attitudes towards death and dying.

In the health care setting where death is frequently seen as equating with professional failure (Schulz & Aderman, 1976), it is easy to understand how staff may feel overwhelmed, particularly when they are faced with the death of large numbers of patients which may lead to 'accumulative loss' phenomena (Killeen, 1993). Exposure to seriously ill people may be a sharp reminder of one's own mortality ('It could have been me'), perhaps leading to a sense of being overburdened, particularly in the context of having to support the patient's family also (Schaerer, 1993). Being confronted with insoluble clinical problems poses a challenge to the indestructible self-image of the clinician (Spikes & Holland, 1975), the specific response relating to experiences of training and previous life experiences (Delvaux et al., 1988).

Social attitudes to death and dying

Aries (1974) has described the history of Western attitudes towards death from the Middle Ages into the late twentieth century. He proposed that, in the past, before medical advances, death was accepted as an inevitable consequence of serious illness, thus profoundly influencing people's acceptance of it, both personally and within their cultural setting. Technological advances, particularly from the 1930s to the 1950s saw the development of hospitals as places where technological treatment and care could be delivered, effectively removing the patient from treatment that may previously have been given at home. With this shift, the initiative in coping with illness and control of illness effectively passed from the patient, who had previously been surrounded by family, ultimately to hospital staff. Illness had moved from the personal and family do-

main into the public arena, where there were sanctions against active expression of feelings. In addition, the requirements of different cultures about the networks and practice surrounding death and dying may impose extra demands on workers in such settings.

Against this background, it is interesting that the pioneering work of Kübler-Ross (1969) has been so enthusiastically embraced. However, the richness of her clinical observations has been reduced to a 'formula' by many health professionals who conceptualize patients as conforming to rigidly defined stages, without recognition of the person's unique personality attributes and social concerns.

Models of Critical Incident Stress Debriefing

CISD has been outlined in other chapters in this volume (see e.g. Mitchell and Everly, Chapter 5) and has been summarized in other publications by Robinson & Mitchell (1993) and Mitchell & Everly (1995). The role of CISD for health care workers has developed as an extension from its application in emergency personnel and other groups (Wilson, 1995). The trauma components of the work of health care personnel and the complex background of, and interaction with, personal, social, workplace, illness and other factors have been outlined above. The use of CISD has been described for emergency medical services personnel (Lane, 1994), and among emergency nurses (Burns & Harm, 1993). Similar interventions have also been described for research teams (Pickett et al., 1994), paediatric oncology nurses (Waters, 1985; Harding, 1996) and those working with patients with AIDS (Grossman & Silverstein, 1993). The majority of these do not appear to have encompassed the complexity of the issues involved.

With regard to the needs of health care staff in areas such as oncology, emergency care and HIV services, a wide range of interventions has been described, but in few instances evaluated. Common elements to these interventions have included the provision of peer support, education, opportunities to share difficult workplace experiences in a supportive group framework, identification of key stressor experiences, and discussion of the demands of care (Bolle, 1988; Cooke,

1992; Deahl et al., 1994; Horowitz et al., 1994; Lane, 1994; Burr, 1996). Debriefing has become a term applied to a range of interventions in the health care setting, often containing these common elements.

Little attention has been given to evaluating the specific components of such interventions that may be most helpful, and the framework under which they need to be conducted (e.g. the frequency, timing and structure of such interventions). A survey of experiences of debriefing among emergency nurses identified the most helpful component as the opportunity to talk about the incident, and sharing their experiences with others (Burns & Harm, 1993). Less helpful aspects were group leaders not having had the relevant experience, difficulties in sharing the experience with other members of the group, and the timing of the intervention being too long after the incident. Other reviews (Vachon, 1995) have emphasized the importance of individual staff recognizing their own responsibility to care for themselves physically and emotionally, and to monitor their reactions. This highlights the need to integrate group-based interventions, which recognize the value of interpersonal support in a health care team, with an improved understanding and recognition of individual psychological responses, and appropriate interventions for these vulnerabilities.

Much work conducted among health workers has recognized the important role of formal and informal mutual support (Wade & Simon, 1993) as well as the function of these supportive interventions in providing an outlet for discussion of distressing experiences in a structured framework, where ventilation along with containment can be concurrent (Talbot et al., 1992; Robinson & Mitchell, 1993; Jamieson, 1994). Other interventions have incorporated strategies to assist staff to recognize and deal with difficulties in the team, and concerns about patients' families (Gray-Toft, 1980). It is important to consider to what extent these interventions provide specific benefits for staff, or whether they represent common elements of a range of therapeutic or supportive interventions that may be useful in this setting.

Evaluation of CISD as an intervention in such populations needs to consider the beneficial aspects, as well as those that are perceived by staff as unhelpful, or

counterproductive. Many of the publications in this area are descriptive, with lack of empirical data and evaluation (Kahill, 1988). In cases where evaluation has been described, the absence of a control group makes interpretation of results problematic (Bisson & Deahl, 1994). The theoretical framework underpinning interventions has not always been clearly delineated, or, conversely, there has been an uncritical application of traumatic stress models to a range of adverse experiences in widely divergent groups. Furthermore, implicit in many interventions is the notion that the workplace experiences are inevitably psychologically damaging, a finding not supported in a long-term follow-up of police body handlers (Alexander, 1993). A deficiency of any application of the CISD model in health care settings is its failure to incorporate attention to the pervasive background stress experienced by such staff. Critical incidents as such may be relatively few, with the risk that the cumulative effect of exposure to repeated death and loss is not fully acknowledged. In addition, grotesque and horrifying exposure for emergency workers in disasters is clearly outside the range of normal human experience, and implies the normality of subjective distress, compared with the area of health care where exposure to suffering and distressing or disgusting experiences is more likely to be conceptualized as an inevitable part of the job, and less worthy of acknowledgement. Even in areas where a specific traumatic event has occurred, CISD does not appear to reduce psychological stress or prevent the onset of PTSD (Wessely et al., 1998).

Methodological problems underpinning the evaluation of interventions for staff are extensive. Not least of these are the expectations of staff that debriefing be available (Sowney, 1996), and the high rate of turnover in some clinical settings (Lansdown et al., 1990). Particularly noteworthy is the enthusiasm of staff for support groups and perception of their helpfulness, although formal evaluation fails to demonstrate any significant benefit (Amaral et al., 1981).

Of especial concern is the risk that interventions may aggravate staff distress. In the HIV setting, some workers have been critical of debriefing that has been perceived as breaching confidentiality, or pressured staff into conceptualizing their work as problematic

(Barbour, 1995). A randomized controlled trial of psychological debriefing for victims of road traffic accidents showed no evidence that debriefing has been helpful, with indications that it may have been disadvantageous (Hobbs et al., 1996). Such research highlights the need to clarify the role of specific interventions and their relationship to models of identified needs in health care staff.

It is important to note the limited research on the development in clinical fields such as medical/surgical units, oncology or HIV care, of individual clinical supervision as a means of providing training, support, mentorship, and monitoring of clinical functioning. A long tradition of the important role of supervision exists in mental health and other disciplines, but there is little empirical research that evaluates such supervision and its functions. The research that exists indicates the importance of the supervisor's competence and clinical role, capacity to be empathic and supportive, as well as being able to take responsibility when needed (Kozlowska et al., 1997). Promoting a model for professional and ethical standards, for appropriate attitudes in their professional role, and for enhancing the understanding of therapeutic relationships and a realistic monitoring of the psychological impact of one's work experience are important functions (Clarke, 1993).

Structured clinical supervision provides opportunities for health professionals to concentrate on their clinical skills and experiences in the workplace, with a clear focus on the feelings, difficulties and impact of their work with patients. This should be clearly delineated from therapy of the health professional, which may in some instances be needed to address personal vulnerabilities and assist the health professional to gain understanding of the personal origin of their reactions. A priority given to supervision, clear lines of responsibility and clinical duties can represent an acknowledgement of, and respect for, the health professional's general training and experience. This model may provide the necessary support and intervention to lessen the risk of burnout and other psychosocial morbidity related to this type of workplace stress, rather than identify distress in these settings as being highly pathogenic.

Recommendations

Perhaps one of the most important issues emerging from the burgeoning literature on emotional well-being of health care staff has been the recognition of the emotional and interpersonal consequences of some aspects of work for many doctors, nurses and other health care workers and the implications this may have for the effective functioning of health care teams and individuals within those teams, and the potential impact on patient care. There needs to be a recognition, also, of the interaction of individual factors, such as strengths and vulnerabilities that individuals may bring to their experience in the workplace, along with other tasks and current events that may affect emotional well-being. One's capacity to adapt to the clinical demands posed in acute medical settings can also be affected by emotional well-being. Burnout has become a widely accepted term, the literature often failing to clarify the nature of emotional issues that are present in the workplace, attributing these to workplace stress. There is a real risk that symptoms, and at times disorders such as depression and anxiety requiring specific assistance and intervention, are attributed to burnout phenomena rather than addressing the needs of the individual for clinical care.

A range of approaches have been described and less frequently evaluated in a systematic fashion. Of particular concern is the failure of many researchers to acknowledge that some interventions may make things worse (Raphael et al., 1995). Common elements to most interventions include the provision of interpersonal support, and explicit recognition of the shared experience of many difficulties in units such as oncology wards or emergency care, or in the care of patients with illnesses such as HIV infection and AIDS. The provision of a respected and trusted leader of a group who can facilitate discussion in a directive manner has been recognized as valuable. The boundaries between the provision of assistance in the workplace, and other forms of intervention such as debriefing or indeed therapy, need to remain clear.

Given the data that support of patients and their families' emotional needs may pose a burden for staff, coupled with evidence of the poor communication skills of many staff, communication skills training must emerge as a key area for further intervention. It is crucial that staff at an early stage of their training recognize that there are few, if any, medical problems in which psychological, social and emotional issues neither contribute to the presentation of a patient's complaints, nor powerfully affect the acceptance of reassurance, advice and treatment decisions (Fallowfield, 1992). There is increasing evidence that particular techniques are useful for discussing diagnosis and prognosis with cancer patients (Bennett & Alison, 1996; Maguire et al., 1996b), and that interviewing and communication skills can be effectively taught (Maguire et al., 1996a).

Institutional administrative practices can provide considerable opportunities for prevention and enhancement of competence. The formal provision of individual and group supervision can provide an ongoing and long-term opportunity for the development of skills, identification of key problem areas, and establishment of an environment in which these issues are given status alongside the development of clinical skills in staff caring for physically ill patients. It may be that in many instances, the provision of formal supervision and support in educational programmes provides important recognition to staff that their educational, training and other needs in the workplace are understood by the institution in which they work. Implementation of such programmes must incorporate adequate time and explicit encouragement to attend, and planning to ensure that clinical duties do not preclude attendance.

Identification of factors in the work experience such as training, rostering for duty, levels of staffing, and duration of time on a particular clinical rotation, may provide opportunities to develop a working environment that is supportive of staff needs, and acknowledges their concerns.

It is also important to take into account the impact of workplace trauma on patient care. In services that experience recurrent and multiple deaths, such as in oncology or HIV units, staff are often confronted with conflicting ethical demands. Facing the real limitations of a curative model of medicine may engender emotional reactions that, if unaddressed, may affect the capacity of staff to support and care for patients. At an institutional level, depersonalization of care and the avoidance of the psychosocial demands of good medical treatment can be concerning consequences that further adversely affect patients and their families. All these factors may constitute a background onto which further traumatic experiences may be implanted.

Individuals must also accept some responsibility for their own professional development and training, recognizing the need to care for themselves physically, emotionally and spiritually (Vachon, 1995). Further research that attempts to understand the factors that contribute to resilience, particularly the experiences of those working in areas such as oncology or HIV medicine for many years, may enhance our understanding of those strategies and adaptations that are effective in enhancing the well-being of the staff member without jeopardizing the quality of patient care.

Finally, systematic research is required to evaluate a range of interventions, particularly comparison of different styles of group and individual intervention and administrative system-based interventions, while appropriately recognizing individual, workplace and social factors. While the model of traumatic stress and CISD has been increasingly applied in this setting, and has bearing on some of the experiences faced by health care professionals in their work, there is further scope for research that explores the nature of the experiences that generate distress for staff, and appropriately enhances their competency and well-being. Training needs to provide appropriate recognition of the emotional vulnerability of health care professionals and appropriate mechanisms of support and intervention that are readily available and nonstigmatizing.

REFERENCES

Abeloff, M. D. (1991). Burnout in oncology – physician heal thyself. *Journal of Clinical Oncology*, **9**, 1721–2.

Alexander, D. A. (1993). Stress among police body handlers – a long-term follow-up. *British Journal of Psychiatry*, **163**, 806–8.

Amaral, P., Nehemkis, A. M. & Fox, L. (1981). Staff support group on a cancer ward: a pilot project. *Death Education*, **5**,

267–74.

American Psychiatric Association ((1994). *Diagnostic and Statistical Manual of Mental Disorders*, 4th edn. Washington, DC: APA Press.

Aries, P. (1974). *Western Attitudes towards Death: From the Middle Ages to the Present*. Baltimore, MD: Johns Hopkins University Press.

Barbour, R. S. (1994). The impact of working with people with HIV/AIDS: a review of the literature. *Social Science Medicine*, **39**, 221–32.

Barbour, R. S. (1995). The implications of HIV/AIDS for a range of workers in the Scottish context. *Aids Care*, **7**, 521–35.

Barraclough, B., Bunch, J., Nelson, B. & Sainsbury, P. (1974). A hundred cases of suicide: clinical aspects. *British Journal of Psychiatry*, **125**, 355–73.

Bennett, L. (1992). The experience of nurses working with hospitalised AIDS patients. *Australian Journal of Social Issues*, **27**, 125–43.

Bennett, L. & Kelaher, M. (1993). Variables contributing to experiences of grief in HIV/AIDS health care professionals. *Journal of Community Psychology*, **21**, 210–17.

Bennett, L., Kelaher, M. & Ross, M. W. (1994a). The impact of working with HIV/AIDS on health care professionals: development of the AIDS Impact Scale. *Psychology and Health*, **9**, 221–32.

Bennett, L., Kelaher, M. & Ross, M. (1994b). Quality of life in health care professionals: burnout and its associated factors in HIV/AIDS related care. *Psychology and Health*, **9**, 273–83.

Bennett, L., Ross, M. W. & Sunderland, R. (1996). The relationship between recognition, rewards and burnout in AIDS caring. *AIDS Care*, **8**, 145–53.

Bennett, M. & Alison, D. (1996). Discussing the diagnosis and prognosis with cancer patients. *Postgraduate Medical Journal*, **72**, 25–9.

Bisson, J. I. & Deahl, M. P. (1994). Psychological debriefing and prevention of post-traumatic stress. *British Journal of Psychiatry*, **165**, 717–20.

Blacher, R. S. (1991). Brief psychotherapy for medical and surgical patients. In F. Judd & G. Burrows (Eds.) *Handbook of Studies in General Psychiatry* (pp. 143–52). Amsterdam: Elsevier.

Bolle, J. L. (1988). Supporting the deliverers of care: strategies to support nurses and prevent burnout. *Nursing Clinics of North America*, **23**, 843–50.

Bram, P. J. & Katz, L. F. (1989). A study of burnout in nurses working in hospice and hospital oncology settings. *Oncology Nursing Forum*, **16**, 555–60.

Breitbart, W. (1995). Identifying patients at risk for, and treatment of major psychiatric complications of cancer. *Support Care Cancer*, **3**, 45–60.

Breslau, N., Davis, G. C., Andreski, P. & Peterson, E. (1991). Traumatic events and posttraumatic stress disorder in an urban population of young adults. *Archives of General Psychiatry*, **48**, 216–22.

Burns, C. & Harm, N. J. (1993). Emergency nurses' perceptions of critical incidents and stress debriefing. *Journal of Emergency Nursing*, **19**, 431–6.

Burr, C. K. (1996). Supporting the helpers. *Nursing Clinics of North America*, **31**, 243–50.

Catalan, J., Burgess, A., Pergami, A., Hulme, N., Gazzard, B. & Phillips, R. (1996). The psychological impact on staff of caring for people with serious diseases: the case of HIV infection and oncology. *Journal of Psychosomatic Research*, **40**, 425–35.

Clarke, D. M. (1993). Supervision in the training of a psychiatrist. *Australian and New Zealand Journal of Psychiatry*, **27**, 306–10.

Cooke, M. (1992). Supporting health care workers in the treatment of HIV-infected patients. *Primary Care*, **19**, 245–56.

Coombs, R. H. & Fawzy, F. I. (1986). The impaired-physician syndrome: a developmental perspective. In C. D. Scott & J. Hawk (Eds.) *Heal Thyself: The Health of Health Care Professionals* (pp. 44–55). New York: Brunner/Mazel.

Cooper, C. L., Rout, U. & Faragher, B. (1989). Mental health, job satisfaction, and job stress among general practitioners. *British Medical Journal*, **298**, 366–70.

Cowen, E. L. (1991). In pursuit of wellness. *American Psychologist*, **46**, 404–8.

Cronin-Stubbs, D. & Brophy, E. B. (1985). Burnout: can social support save the psych nurse? *Journal of Psychosocial Nursing*, **23**, 8–13.

Cronin-Stubbs, D. & Rooks, C. A. (1985). The stress, social support, and burnout of critical care nurses: the results of research. *Heart and Lung*, **14**, 31–9.

Davidson, J. R., Hughes, D., Blazer, D. G. & George, L. K. (1991). Post-traumatic stress disorder in the community: an epidemiologic study. *Psychological Medicine*, **21**, 713–21.

Deahl, M. P., Gillham, A. B., Thomas, J., Searle, M. M. & Srinivasan, M. (1994). Psychological sequelae following the Gulf War: factors associated with subsequent morbidity and the effectiveness of psychological debriefing. *British Journal of Psychiatry*, **165**, 60–5.

Deckard, G., Meterko, M. & Field, D. (1994). Physician burnout: an examination of personal, professional, and organisational relationships. *Medical Care*, **32**, 745–54.

Delvaux, N., Razavi, D. & Farvacques, C. (1988). Cancer care – a stress for health professionals. *Social Science Medicine*, **27**, 159–66.

Diener, E. (1984). Subjective wellbeing. *Psychological Bulletin*, **95**, 542–75.

Dworkin, J., Albrecht, G. & Cooksey, J. (1991). Concern about AIDS among hospital physicians, nurses and social workers. *Social Science Medicine*, **33**, 239–48.

Fallowfield, L. (1992). The ideal consultation. *British Journal of Hospital Medicine*, **47**, 364–7.

Figley, C. R. (1995). Compassion fatigue: toward a new understanding of the costs of caring. In B. H. Stamm (Ed.) *Secondary Traumatic Stress* (pp. 3–28). Lutherville, MD: Sidran Press.

Ford, S., Fallowfield, L. & Lewis, S. (1994). Can oncologists detect distress in their out-patients and how satisfied are they with their performance during bad news consultations? *British Journal of Cancer*, **70**, 767–70.

Foxall, M. J., Zimmerman, L., Standley, R. & Captain, B. B. (1990). A comparison of frequency and sources of nursing job stress perceived by intensive care, hospice and medical-surgical nurses. *Journal of Advanced Nursing*, **15**, 577–84.

Funk, S. C. (1992). Hardiness: a review of theory and research. *Health Psychology*, **11**, 335–45.

Gabbard, G. O., Menninger, R. W. & Coyne, L. (1987). Sources of conflict in the medical marriage. *American Journal of Psychiatry*, **144**, 567–72.

Glare, P. A. & Cooney, N. J. (1996). HIV and palliative care. *Medical Journal of Australia*, **164**, 612–15.

Gray-Toft, P. (1980). Effectiveness of a counselling support program for hospice nurses. *Journal of Counselling Psychology*, **27**, 346–54.

Green, B. L. (1993). Identifying survivors at risk: trauma stressors across events. In J. P. Wilson & B. Raphael (Eds.) *International Handbook of Traumatic Stress Syndromes* (pp. 135–44). New York: Plenum Press.

Green, B. L., Lindy, J. D. & Grace, M. C. (1985). Posttraumatic stress disorder ' toward DSM-IV. *Journal of Nervous and Mental Disease*, **173**, 406–11.

Grootenhuis, M. A., van der Wel, M., de Graaf-Nijkerk, J. & Last, B. F. (1996). Exploration of a self-protective strategy in paediatric oncology staff. *Medical and Paediatric Oncology*, **27**, 40–7.

Grossman, A. H. & Silverstein, C. (1993). Facilitating support groups for professionals working with people with AIDS. *Social Work*, **38**, 144–51.

Hanson, E. J. (1994). An exploration of the taken-for-granted world of the cancer nurse in relation to stress and the person with cancer. *Journal of Advanced Nursing*, **19**, 12–20.

Harding, R. (1996). Children with cancer: managing stress in staff. *Paediatric Nursing*, **8**, 28–31.

Heim, E. (1991). Job stressors and coping in health professions.

Psychotherapeutic Psychosomatics, **55**, 90–9.

Helzer, J. E., Robins, L. N. & McEvoy, L. (1987). Post-traumatic stress disorder in the general population. Findings of the epidemiologic catchment area survey. *New England Journal of Medicine*, **317**, 1630–4.

Henderson, A. S., Byrne, D. G. & Duncan-Jones, P. (1981). *Neurosis and the Social Environment*. Orlando, FL: Academic Press.

Herschbach, P. (1992). Work-related stress specific to physicians and nurses working with cancer patients. *Journal of Psychosocial Oncology*, **10**, 79–99.

Hobbs, M., Mayou, R., Harrison, B. & Worlock, P. (1996). A randomised controlled trial of psychological debriefing for victims of road traffic accidents. *British Medical Journal*, **313**, 1438–9.

Horowitz, S. A., Passiki, S. D., Brish, M. & Breitbart, W. S. (1994). A group intervention for staff on a neuro-oncology service. *Psycho-Oncology*, **3**, 329–32.

Jamieson, S. (1994). Developing staff support. *Nursing Standard*, **8**, 44–6.

Jenkins, J. F. & Ostchega, Y. (1986). Evaluation of burnout in oncology nurses. *Cancer Nursing*, **9**, 108–16.

Kahill, S. (1988). Interventions for burnout in the helping professions: a review of the empirical evidence. *Canadian Journal of Counselling*, **22**, 162–9.

Keane, A., Ducette, J. & Adler, D. C. (1985). Stress in ICU and non-ICU nurses. *Nursing Research*, **34**, 231–6.

Kelly, B. & Raphael, B. (1993). AIDS: coping with ongoing terminal illness. In J. P. Wilson & B. Raphael (Eds.) *International Handbook of Traumatic Stress Syndromes* (pp. 517–25). New York: Plenum Press.

Kelly, B. & Varghese, F. (1997). The emotional hazards of medical practice. In M. R. Sanders, C. Mitchell & G. J. A. Byrne (Eds.) *Medical Consultation Skills* (pp. 472–88). Melbourne: Addison-Wesley.

Kent, G., Wills, G., Faulkner, A., Parry, G., Whipp, M. & Coleman, R. (1994). The professional and personal needs of oncology staff: the effects of perceived success and failure in helping patients on levels of personal stress and distress. *Journal of Cancer Care*, **3**, 153–8.

Killeen, M. E. (1993). Getting through our grief. *American Journal of Hospice and Palliative Care*, September/October, 18–24.

Kozlowska, K., Nunn, K. & Cousens, P. (1997). Training in psychiatry: an examination of trainee perceptions. Part 1. *Australian and New Zealand Journal of Psychiatry*, **31**, 628–40.

Kübler-Ross, E. (1969). *On Death and Dying*, London: Tavistock.

Lane, P. S. (1994). Critical incident stress debriefing for health care workers. *Omega*, **28**, 301–15.

Lansdown, R., Pike, S. & Smith, J. (1990). Reducing stress in the cancer ward. *Nursing Times*, **86**, 34–8.

Lawrence, J. M. (1992). The impaired doctor. *Medical Journal of Australia*, **157**, 4–6.

Lifton, R. J. (1993). From Hiroshima to the Nazi doctors: the evolution of psychoformative approaches to understanding traumatic stress syndromes. In J. P. Wilson & B. Raphael (Eds.) *International Handbook of Traumatic Stress Syndromes* (pp. 11–23). New York: Plenum Press.

Little, J. D. (1992). Staff response to inpatient and outpatient suicide: what happened and what do we do? *Australian and New Zealand Journal of Psychiatry*, **26**, 162–7.

Maguire, P., Booth, K., Elliott, C. & Jones, B. (1996a). Helping health professionals involved in cancer care acquire key interviewing skills – the impact of workshops. *European Journal of Cancer*, **32A**, 1486–9.

Maguire, P., Faulkner, A., Booth, K., Elliott, C. & Hillier, V. (1996b). Helping cancer patients disclose their concerns. *European Journal of Cancer*, **32A**, 78–81.

Maj, M. (1991). Psychological problems of families and health workers dealing with people infected with human immunodeficiency virus 1. *Acta Psychiatrica Scandinavica*, **83**, 161–8.

Maslach, C. & Jackson, S. E. (1981). The measurement of experienced burnout. *Journal of Occupational Behaviour*, **2**, 99–113.

Maslanka, H. (1996). Burnout, social support and AIDS volunteers. *Aids Care*, **8**, 195–206.

Massie, M. J., Gagnon, P. & Holland, J. C. (1994). Depression and suicide in patients with cancer. *Journal of Pain and Symptom Management*, **9**, 325–40.

McBride, A. B. (1990). Mental health effects of women's multiple roles. *American Psychologist*, **45**, 381–4.

McElroy, A. M. (1982). Burnout – a review of the literature with application to cancer nursing. *Cancer Nursing*, **5**, 211–17.

McFarlane, A. C. (1993). PTSD: synthesis of research and clinical studies: the Australia bushfire disaster. In J. P. Wilson & B. Raphael (Eds.) *International Handbook of Traumatic Stress Syndromes* (pp. 421–30). New York: Plenum Press.

Miller, D. (1995). Stress and burnout among health-care staff working with people affected by HIV. *British Journal of Guidance and Counselling*, **23**, 19–31.

Miller, D. & Gillies, P. (1996). Is there life after work? Experiences of HIV and oncology health staff. *Aids Care*, **8**, 167–82.

Mitchell J. T. & Everly, G. S. (1995). Critical incident stress debriefing (CISD) and the prevention of work-related traumatic stress among high risk occupational groups. In G. S.

Everly, Jr & J. M. Lating (Eds.) *Psychotraumatology* (pp. 267–80). New York: Plenum Press.

Notman, M. T. & Nadelson, C. C. (1973). Medicine: a career conflict for women. *American Journal of Psychiatry*, **130**, 1123–6.

Papadatou, D., Anagnostopoulos, F. & Monos, D. (1994). Factors contributing to the development of burnout in oncology nursing. *British Journal of Medical Psychology*, **67**, 187–99.

Pickett, M., Brennan, A. M. W., Greenberg, H. S., Licht, L. & Worrell, J. D. (1994). Use of debriefing techniques to prevent compassion fatigue in research teams. *Nursing Research*, **43**, 250–2.

Plante, A. & Bouchard, L. (1995–96). Occupational stress, burnout, and professional support in nurses working with dying patients. *Omega*, **32**, 93–109.

Price, T. R. & Bergen, B. J. (1977). The relationship to death as a source of stress for nurses on a coronary care unit. *Omega*, **8**, 229–38.

Ramirez, A. J., Graham, J., Richards, M. A., Cull, A., Gregory, W. M., Leaning, M. S., Snashall, D. C. & Timothy, A. R. (1995). Burnout and psychiatric disorder among cancer clinicians. *British Journal of Cancer*, **71**, 1263–9.

Ramirez, A. J., Graham, J., Richards, M. A., Cull, A. & Gregory, W. M. (1996). Mental health of hospital consultants: the effects of stress and satisfaction at work. *Lancet*, **347**, 724–8.

Raphael, B. (1986). The problems of mental health and adjustment. In *When Disaster Strikes: How Individuals and Communities Cope with Catastrophe* (pp. 179–221). New York: Basic Books.

Raphael, B., Kelly, B., Dunne, M. & Greig, R. (1990). Psychological distress among volunteer AIDS counsellors. [Letters to the Editor]. *Medical Journal of Australia*, **152**, 275.

Raphael, B., Meldrum, L. & McFarlane, A. C. (1995). Does debriefing after psychological trauma work? *British Medical Journal*, **310**, 1479–80.

Reuben, D. B., Novack, D. H., Wachtel, T. J. & Wartman, S. A. (1984). A comprehensive support system for reducing house staff distress. *Psychosomatics*, **25**, 815–20.

Riordan, R. J. & Saltzer, S. K. (1992). Burnout prevention among health care providers working with the terminally ill: a literature review. *Omega*, **25**, 17–24.

Robinson, R. C. & Mitchell, J. T. (1993). Evaluation of psychological debriefings. *Journal of Traumatic Stress*, **6**, 367–82.

Ross, M. W. & Seeger, V. (1988). Short communication: determinants of reported burnout in health professionals associated with the care of patients with AIDS. *AIDS*, **2**, 395–7.

Rutter, M. (1985). Resilience in the face of adversity: protective factors and resistance to psychiatric disorder. *British Journal of Psychiatry*, **147**, 598–611.

Rutter, M. (1994). Beyond longitudinal data: causes, consequences, changes, and continuity. *Journal of Consulting and Clinical Psychology*, **62**, 928–40.

Schaerer, R. (1993). Suffering of the doctor linked with the death of patients. *Palliative Medicine*, **7** Suppl. 1, 27–37.

Schulz, R. & Aderman, D. (1976). How the medical staff copes with dying patients: a critical review. *Omega*, **7**, 11–21.

Selye, H. (1976). *Stress in Health and Disease*. Boston, MA: Butterworths.

Silverman, D. C. (1993). Psychosocial impact of HIV-related caregiving on health providers: a review and recommendations for the role of psychiatry. *American Journal of Psychiatry*, **150**, 705–12.

Sowney, R. (1996). Stress debriefing: reality or myth? *Accident and Emergency Nursing*, **4**, 38–9.

Spikes, J. & Holland, J. (1975). The physician's response to the dying patient. In J. J. Strain & S. Grossman (Eds.) *Psychological Care of the Medically Ill* (pp. 138–48). New York: Appleton-Century-Crofts.

Steppacher, R. C. & Mausner, J. S. (1974). Suicide in male and female physicians. *Journal of the American Medical Association*, **228**, 323–8.

Stewart, B. E., Meyerowitz, B. E., Jackson, L. E., Yarkin, K. L. & Harvey, J. H. (1982). Psychological stress associated with outpatient oncology nursing. *Cancer Nursing*, October, 383–7.

Stylianos, S. K. & Vachon, M. L. S. (1993). The role of social support in bereavement. In M. S. Stroebe, W. Stroebe & R. O. Hansson (Eds.), *Handbook of Bereavement* (pp. 397–410). New York: Cambridge University Press.

Talbot, A., Manton, M. & Dunn, P. J. (1992). Debriefing the debriefers: an intervention strategy to assist psychologists after a crisis. *Journal of Traumatic Stress*, **5**, 45–62.

Tyler, P. A. & Ellison, R. N. (1994). Sources of stress and psychological well-being in high-dependency nursing. *Journal of Advanced Nursing*, **19**, 469–76.

Ullrich, A. & FitzGerald, P. (1990). Stress experienced by physicians and nurses in the cancer ward. *Social Science of Medicine*, **31**, 1013–22.

Vachon, M. L. S. (1995). Staff stress in hospice/palliative care: a review. *Palliative Medicine*, **9**, 91–122.

Vachon, M. L. S., Lyall, W. A. L. & Freeman, S. J. J. (1978). Measurement and management of stress in health professionals working with advanced cancer patients. *Death Education*, **1**, 365–75.

Vaillant, G. E. (1995). *Adaptation to Life*. London: Harvard University Press.

Van der Kolk, B. A. (1994). The body keeps the score: memory and the evolving psychobiology of posttraumatic stress. *Harvard Reviews of Psychiatry*, **1**, 253–65.

Van Servellen, G. & Leake, B. (1993). Burn-out in hospital nurses: a comparison of acquired immunodeficiency syndrome, oncology, general medical, and intensive care unit nurse samples. *Journal of Professional Nursing*, **9**, 169–77.

Visintini, R., Campanini, E., Fossati, A., Bagnato, M., Novella, L. & Maffei, C. (1996). Psychological stress in nurses' relationships with HIV-infected patients: the risk of burnout syndrome. *Aids Care*, **8**, 183–94.

Wade, K. & Simon, E. P. (1993). Survival bonding: a response to stress and work with AIDS. *Social Work in Health Care*, **19**, 77–89.

Waterhouse, J. M., Folkard, S. & Minors, D. S. (1992). Shiftwork health and safety, an overview of the scientific literature 1978–1990. *HSE Contract Research Report*, no. 31/1992 (pp. 1–30). London: Health & Safety Executive.

Waters, A. L. (1985). Support for staff in a paediatric oncology unit. *Nursing*, **43**, 1275–7.

Wessely, S., Rose, S. & Bisson, J. (1998). A systematic review of brief psychological interventions ('debriefing') for the treatment of immediate trauma related symptoms and the prevention of post traumatic stress disorder (Cochrane Review). *The Cochrane Library*, **3**. Oxford: Update Software.

Whippen, D. A. & Canellos, G. P. (1991). Burnout syndrome in the practice of oncology: results of a random survey of 1,000 oncologists. *Journal of Clinical Oncology*, **9**, 1916–20.

Wilkinson, S. M. (1994). Stress in cancer nursing: does it really exist? *Journal of Advanced Nursing*, **20**, 1079–84.

Wilson, J. P. (1995). Traumatic events and post traumatic stress disorder and prevention. In B. Raphael & G. Burrows (Eds.) *Handbook of Studies on Preventive Psychiatry* (pp. 281–99). Amsterdam: Elsevier.

Wise, T. N. (1977). Training oncology fellows in psychological aspects of their specialty. *Cancer*, **39**, 2584–7.

Yasko, J. M. (1983). Variables which predict burnout experienced by oncology clinical nurse specialists. *Cancer Nursing*, April, 109–16.

Yehuda, R. & Mcfarlane, A. C. (1995). Conflict between current knowledge about posttraumatic stress disorder and its original conceptual basis. *American Journal of Psychiatry*, **152**, 1705–13.

Ziegler, J. L., Kanas, N., Strull, W. M. & Bennet, N. E. (1984). A stress discussion group for medical interns. *Journal of Medical Education*, **59**, 205–7.

19

Traumatic childbirth and the role of debriefing

Philip Boyce and John Condon

EDITORIAL COMMENTS

This chapter considers the potential application of the debriefing model of intervention to women adversely affected by the experience of childbirth, particularly an occasion that might be traumatic. Boyce and Condon provide evidence suggesting that, although postnatal depression has been readily recognized, post-traumatic stress disorder (PTSD) can also occur, and may rarely be detected. They hypothesize that it may also significantly interfere with the mother's attachment to her new infant.

It is suggested that antenatal education could contribute to stress inoculation and have a preventive benefit, as does such training in other trauma situations. However, to date there is no evidence that, in its present form, it does. This may, however, also relate to the relevance of childbirth education, for its aim usually is to be reassuring and not to prepare the woman for potential but rare catastrophies. It may, therefore, be inappropriate in the specific sense, but it could prepare a woman to deal with the general rather than specific stressors, and provide coping strategies for these.

On the other hand, the work presented suggests that where the childbirth is traumatic, the opportunity for the woman to talk through her experience may be helpful, both perceived as such and potentially lessening her vulnerability. This reflects, the authors believe, good clinical care, and is probably best provided by the midwife or obstetrician, rather than trained debriefers who may not be able to answer the woman's questions about her experience and may provide a more patho-logical orientation to this experience. Boyce and Condon conclude that women, particularly those who may have had a traumatic birth, should be offered the opportunity to talk through their experience and feelings associated with it; this is good clinical care. It should not, however, be forced on women, or be made compulsory.

This chapter thus considers the use of a debriefing context for women potentially traumatized by childbirth. This highlights the types of controversy associated with debriefing. Here it is recognized as part of the support associated with good clinical care. But the very use of the term debriefing and its powerful connotations presume an activity with a formalized structure derived from a militaristic model of intervention. The authors strongly recommend against the provision of formal debriefing in the obstetric setting. This issue of the now widespread use of the term to cover all potential psychological interventions in association with life experience must be a cause for concern, as is any suggestion of the universal or widespread use of this type of intervention for what is, in the majority of instances, a normal and joyful experience. Furthermore, it is particularly in this context that normal forgetting of childbirth distress may provide understandings relevant to normal recovery from other major life experiences, a recovery that should be understood and facilitated, not interfered with and pathologized. This is not to deny that in some circumstances of childbirth, including infant loss as well as psychological trauma, specific and appropriate psychosocial intervention may be required.

Introduction

It is now generally accepted that there can be adverse mental health outcomes after traumatic events. While the focus has been principally on post-traumatic stress disorder (PTSD), other mental health problems also arise, such as depression and anxiety disorders. Psychological debriefing has been proposed as a primary preventative measure aimed at reducing the incidence of such disorders. Debriefing has become common-place after traumatic events and disasters, not only for the victims but also for emergency workers using the model developed by Mitchell (Robinson & Mitchell, 1993). But disasters are not the only traumatic events that can lead to the onset of PTSD. Illness and medical interventions can also be categorized as traumatic (Fisch & Tadmor, 1989; Fones, 1996) and may similarly have adverse mental health outcomes.

Stress and childbirth

Childbirth is a major and generally positive life event in a woman's life. For the majority of women, their recollection of the childbirth experience is a joyous one, albeit intermingled with memories of anxiety, fear and physical pain. However, for a minority, the latter experiences predominate and their overall recollection is of a highly stressful and traumatic event. While childbirth is now considered to be a relatively safe and even commonplace event, it has not always been so. Prior to the introduction of modern obstetrics, women were at risk of dying during childbirth. If they survived, significant morbidity could follow. The infant was also at risk of dying during childbirth or of being disabled. In Australia in the triennium 1964–1966, 30 women per 100 000 confinements died during childbirth, whereas in the triennium 1988–1990 this fell to 5 women per 100 000 (NH&MRC, 1993). While the rates of morbidity and mortality have fallen, the potential for danger still remains, a fact which is commonly brought home to women in the popular literature, television and films.

A number of issues are relevant when one considers childbirth as an event or stressor. First, there are the profound psychosocial stresses associated with becoming a mother. There can be few events that have as much an impact as childbirth on all facets of a woman's life (Oakley, 1980; Cox, 1988a,b), affecting her self-concept, social role and interpersonal relationships.

Secondly, there are the profound physiological and hormonal changes during the course of childbirth and in the subsequent days. Such physiological changes can also be stressful and impact on a woman's coping style, as illustrated by the onset of the 'blues' on the third to fifth day post partum (Kendell et al., 1984; Kennerley & Gath, 1989; Harris, 1994).

Thirdly, childbirth is a physically demanding and painful process. The pain of childbirth was one of the driving forces in developing anaesthesia; it is noteworthy that Queen Victoria was one of the first to give birth using an anaesthetic. While some women will be amnesic for the pain during childbirth, it is for many an extremely painful process and one that may be remembered for many years (Simpkin, 1991). This pain may have an impact on how a woman bonds with her infant, and women who have experienced excessive pain may have difficulty in early attachment.

Fourthly, there is the possibility that women may have to undergo an obstetric intervention such as a forceps delivery, caesarean section or episiotomy – procedures that can be very stressful. Such interventions are becoming more common (Boyce & Todd, 1992; King, 1993; Treffers & Pel, 1993; Editorial, 1997) and may contribute to increased psychological morbidity for the woman (DiMatteo et al., 1996; Waldenström et al., 1996; Fisher et al., 1997).

Finally, some women will have pre-existing psychopathology, complicating their pregnancy, which may be exacerbated by the childbirth experience. Such psychopathology can range from the psychotic illnesses through to anxiety and depression. Women, in addition to this may also experience ongoing major stressors such as domestic violence during pregnancy and post partum, which can increase the impact of childbirth especially if it is traumatic. If domestic violence is prevalent during the pregnancy (Gelles, 1975), the level of violence may decrease for some during pregnancy (Adams-Hillard, 1985) but may well increase as shown in a study by Webster et al. (1994), who reported that 5.8% of women reported being abused during early pregnancy, and 8.9% being abused by 36 weeks' gestation. Among women who have experienced physical abuse during the pregnancy, the pain associated with childbirth may bring to the fore the cumulative stress of the previous assaults on her.

In addition to these stressors associated with childbirth, there are a number of characteristics of the birth experience of some women that may specifically predispose to the development of PTSD. First, the *Diagnostic and Statistical Manual of Mental Disorders* (DSM-IV; American Psychiatric Association, 1994, p. 427) highlights 'threatened death or serious injury, or a threat to the physical integrity of self or others' as important attributes of events leading to PTSD. In our clinical experience, if intense pain accompanies childbirth, many women subsequently report that they believed their bodies were being permanently damaged, or even that they might not survive. Some women equate this experience to being 'torn in two' or 'split open'. For many women suffering traumatic deliveries, fears that the baby will be damaged, born deformed or stillborn, transcend those relating to their own welfare. Anxieties relating to the well-being of the baby during labour have been shown to outweigh those relating to all other aspects, including pain (Arizmendi & Affonso, 1987). Fetal monitoring results in women being very aware of any dangers that may arise for the unborn baby. In a controlled study using hormonal measures of psychological stress, Shalev et al. (1985) demonstrated significantly higher stress levels in women who had fetal monitoring during labour compared with those who did not. In addition, the use of the term 'fetal distress' can provoke considerable fear and anxiety, since it is usually equated, in the lay mind, with 'suffering'. Moreover, if there are major obstetric complications resulting in death or damage to the infant, the woman may be exposed to 'actual death or serious injury'. This is the central characteristic of events, as highlighted in the DSM-IV, which can lead to PTSD.

Secondly, the DSM-IV highlights the importance of the experience of 'helplessness' in situations leading to the development of PTSD. In the usual labour ward delivery setting, women often feel they have little or no control over what is occurring. Some feel that their communications are ignored, and this in turn can result in helplessness giving way to panic and a sense of being out of control. Simultaneously, there are strong social pressures to not display these very powerful emotions, and a sense of guilt that they are letting down both their partner and their baby. This constellation of helplessness, panic, loss of control, guilt and shame are common reactions in veterans stressed in combat who may develop PTSD as a consequence.

Thirdly, as described by Rhodes & Hutchinson (1994), women who have been victims of childhood sexual abuse (or sexual assault in adulthood) may find the experience of delivery particularly traumatic, recapitulating the same kind of pain they experienced in the past and causing memories of the assault to intrude into awareness. Some women also reported that they felt trapped or 'tied down' by the intravenous line or monitoring equipment, recapitulating the restraint experienced during assault. These women may also have a pre-existing anxiety, depression or PTSD, as a consequence of having been a victim of sexual abuse (Mullen et al., 1996). This will compound their risk of having an adverse outcome.

The male partner is generally present at delivery, and powerful social pressures operate to ensure this. Unlike in past times, he will often be permitted to remain, even if complications develop. We believe the latter stance is usually appropriate. However, with the exception of physical pain, all of the above elements of a traumatic delivery may also impact upon the male partner. He may experience a profound sense of helplessness as a bystander witnessing the pain and injury being suffered by his partner and child. Berry (1988) has identified that a major source of stress for fathers at delivery is a perceived need to hide the feelings they experience. The male is now also frequently present at Caesarean deliveries. Mutryn (1993, p. 1276) made the point that this is the 'only circumstance in modern medicine where a lay person is witness to a major surgical procedure performed on a family member'. Even if the outcome is good, the male may be traumatized by exposure to such an event.

Stress inoculation and psychoprophylaxis

In the terminology used for PTSD, antenatal classes are essentially seeking to provide stress inoculation (SI, see

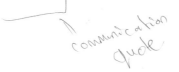

Chapter 1, this volume). The core ingredients of SI include instilling realistic expectations of both the event and the emotions that may be experienced during it. Such emotions are portrayed as normal under the circumstances in order to diminish incapacitating anxiety, guilt and shame that might otherwise accompany them. In addition, SI provides a battery of coping strategies aimed at dealing with the event itself, as well as the accompanying emotions.

Childbirth education hopefully provides women and their partners with realistic expectations of the delivery experience and a range of coping strategies (e.g. controlled breathing). If it provides unrealistic expectations, for example the expectation that most women should be able to experience natural childbirth as painless (Brownridge, 1995), it could, at least in theory, increase rather than decrease the likelihood of PTSD. Stewart (1982) has described the development of diverse psychiatric symptoms in women following traumatic attempts at natural childbirth, and also in women who had attended childbirth education classes that fostered unrealistic expectations (Stewart, 1985).

There is a consensus in the military literature that individuals who have undergone SI, or have been trained and briefed 'function better in action'. Evaluation studies of childbirth psychoprophylaxis would be largely consistent with this view, although some studies have failed to find any significant impact (Astbury, 1980). Beck & Siegel (1980) have critically reviewed the literature on psychoprophylaxis at that time. However, there is no consensus that SI or equivalent preparatory techniques reduce the incidence of PTSD or other psychological morbidity in those exposed to the trauma of combat. Neither has there been any assessment of whether this model, applied as antenatal education, protects against the development of psychological morbidity should there have been a traumatic childbirth.

Childbirth as a routine

Childbirth has now become relatively safe, and this has resulted in de-emphasizing the impact of childbirth as an event of special significance. There has also been the demystification of childbirth; women are now better informed than ever before about the process, through self-help books, information provided by the media and antenatal classes. This has also encouraged the perception of childbirth as a commonplace, unremarkable event. This loss of importance of the *rite de passage* has meant that women are denied the opportunity to talk about and work through their labour experiences. Failure to work through this important life experience may be associated with adverse psychological outcomes, especially for psychologically vulnerable women who have had a relatively straightforward labour and delivery.

Psychological outcomes following childbirth

Over the past 20 years there has been a considerable amount of research examining the psychological outcomes following childbirth. Most of this research has focussed on the development of postnatal depression; however, anxiety (panic disorder, obsessive–compulsive disorder) and functional psychoses can also be precipitated by childbirth.

A series of epidemiological studies conducted over the last five years all report a prevalence rate close to 10% for postnatal depression (Kumar, 1994; O'Hara & Swain, 1996). There are, in addition, a further 20% to 30% of women who, while not reaching criteria for major depression, will have some symptoms of depression and/or anxiety causing distress and dysfunction. While the prevalence of postnatal depression appears high, it is in fact no higher than the prevalence rate of depression among women at other times of the life cycle (Cox et al., 1993; Boyce & Stubbs, 1994). The proximity of the onset of the depression to childbirth suggests that the stress associated with childbirth, particularly for vulnerable women, precipitates the depression.

PTSD is now recognized as one possible outcome of childbirth. The literature is small and largely anecdotal and is described briefly below.

One of the earliest accounts of PTSD following an obstetric procedure is that of Fisch & Tadmor (1989). The patient suffered classic symptoms of PTSD continually for $2\frac{1}{2}$ years after the therapeutic abortion of a hydatidiform mole.

Reynolds (1997) has recently reviewed the sparse literature on PTSD following childbirth. He summarized one of the few epidemiological studies of PTSD following delivery, which has only appeared in the French literature. In a sample of 4400 women, the authors estimated a prevalence rate of post-delivery PTSD to be 0.2%. Goldbeck-Wood (1996) reported a prevalence of 1.5% in 500 consecutive women following gynaecological or obstetric procedures, and Ballard et al. (1995), on the basis of 163 consecutive deliveries, found a prevalence of obstetric-related PTSD of 1%.

Reynolds (1997) also pointed out that population prevalence rates for PTSD in the USA are more than twice as high in women as compared with men. In the recent survey of health and well-being carried out in Australia, the rate of PTSD for women was 4.2% compared with 2.3% for men (McLennan, 1998). Sexual assault (and child abuse) could largely account for this difference. However, McLennan makes the point that obstetric trauma may also contribute.

Reynolds (1997) cited two Swedish studies of caesarean section performed at the woman's request in the absence of any obstetric indications. Most of these women had had previous traumatic deliveries, including giving birth to a severely compromised baby. Reynolds suggested that this behaviour might reflect the avoidance dimension of PTSD. The possibility is raised that some terminations of pregnancy may be similarly motivated.

Moleman et al. (1992) presented three cases of women who experienced symptomatology consistent with PTSD following childbirth. All three had a dissociative reaction during delivery and had histories of infertility, the latter possibly exacerbating their fear of losing their babies. All three had difficulties attaching to their infants. In two of these cases, symptoms persisted beyond one-year post partum. Reynolds also provided a brief description of one of his own cases in which the patient clearly dissociated during delivery and developed PTSD.

Ballard et al. (1995) described four cases of PTSD following traumatic delivery. In one case the baby suffered cardiac arrest and in the other three the women experienced severe pain (including failure of epidural anaesthesia during caesarean). The authors noted that depression was also a feature of these presentations. Onset of symptoms was within the first two days and three of the four had marked attachment difficulties.

Condon (1987) has also published an account of PTSD symptomatology in a woman giving birth to an infant with major deformity.

Debriefing following obstetric trauma

Brant (1972) has highlighted some of the difficulties that may arise with a process such as postnatal debriefing. These include the reluctance of some women to mention negative aspects of their birth experience because they equate this with criticism of the midwife or obstetrician. Brant also pointed out that other women may be so relieved that they have a healthy baby that they understate the trauma experienced in obtaining that baby. Goldbeck-Wood (1996) noted that the patient's view of what constitutes trauma during delivery (e.g. helplessness) may be quite different from that of the obstetrician or midwife, constituting another obstacle to debriefing. Beech & Robinson (1985) described other potential obstacles to debriefing, including excessive defensiveness or antagonism in obstetric staff who may feel unfairly criticized.

Ralph & Alexander (1994), on the other hand, viewed debriefing as part of the midwife's role and advocated that it should be offered to all women.

Arizmendi & Affonso (1987) believed that women may experience the full psychological impact of the stresses of labour and delivery several weeks *after* childbirth. Women may continue 'to review the process of actual labour and delivery perhaps as a way of attempting to understand and integrate it ... to help gain control of it in anticipation of the next childbirth ... as a way of evaluating their behaviour during delivery ... as a method of diffusing the enormous anxiety related to such a traumatic event' (ibid., p. 753).

Nepean study

Some evidence for this proposition comes from a prospective study of women examining the psychological outcome, especially postnatal depression, following childbirth (Boyce et al., 1996; Hickey et al., 1997). Five hundred and twenty-two women delivering consecutively at the Nepean Hospital were recruited shortly after delivery. They were followed up at six-weekly intervals using the Edinburgh Postnatal Depression Scale (EPDS) (Cox et al., 1987) until 24 weeks post partum. The majority of women had a spontaneous vaginal delivery (76.8%), 6.3% had an elective caesarean section, 10% an emergency caesarean section and 5.9% an instrumental delivery.

The rates of postnatal depression between the groups differed significantly: at three months post partum 10% of women who had a spontaneous vaginal delivery suffered from postnatal depression; 8.7% of women who had had an elective caesarean section and 12.5% of women who had had a forceps delivery were depressed, whereas none of the women who had an emergency caesarean section suffered from postnatal depression. This was a counterintuitive result. It seemed improbable that emergency caesarean section was protective. One explanation for this finding was that the midwives in the postnatal ward, having become aware of our project and the potential increased risk for postnatal depression after an emergency caesarean section (Boyce & Todd, 1992), were providing additional clinical care to women who had had an emergency caesarean section. The women were encouraged to talk about their birth experience with the midwives, who were willing to listen to the women's stories in a nonjudgemental manner. The women were given permission to talk about their feelings, disappointment at needing to have a caesarean section, or about other aspects of becoming a mother. They could also talk about the positive aspects of the delivery and their new baby. The midwives spent time with the women discussing strategies for coping with physical discomfort as well as providing them with information about caring for their newborn infant and coping with motherhood. It appeared that the increased clinical care provided for this group of women (and not the other women) may have had a prophylactic effect and reduced the likelihood of these women developing postnatal depression. It may also be that the positive outcome of the emergency and possibly even life-threatening situation also contributed.

A brief intervention programme has now been developed, allowing women the opportunity to work through their labour and birth experiences. As with stress inoculation programmes, this intervention also aims to provide women with information about the role of being a mother, the stresses that may accompany it, a series of coping strategies to deal with them, as well as information about postnatal depression and how it can be dealt with. This brief intervention is currently being evaluated. While it is described as a brief intervention, it is in reality no more than good clinical care.

Debriefing after miscarriage

Fifteen per cent of pregnancies are miscarried and there is abundant evidence that spontaneous miscarriage is a highly traumatic event for many women who experience it. Moreover the severity of this trauma continues to be underestimated by health professionals. Surprisingly, the relatively large literature on the psychological sequelae of miscarriage focuses almost exclusively on depression and anxiety (Lilford & Braunholtz, 1996), with PTSD rarely mentioned.

In a study of 27 women, Jackman et al. (1991) demonstrated significantly lower scores on the General Health Questionnaire in women who had had an opportunity to discuss their miscarriage at a follow-up visit.

Only one controlled study of structured debriefing after miscarriage has been published to date. Lee et al. (1996) randomly allocated 39 women to either a debriefing or a control group. They used the Hospital Anxiety and Depression Scale and the Impact of Event Scale at one week and four months post miscarriage, with subjects receiving the intervention at two weeks. Intrusion and avoidance scores at one week were as high as those in post-trauma victims, but declined at four months. In contrast, anxiety scores remained significantly elevated relative to community norms. Although subjects perceived debriefing as helpful, there were no significant differences in outcome between the two groups.

An important finding of the above study is that the debriefing was conducted by a psychologist who had no knowledge of the relevant medical aspects of miscarriage. Women commented that they needed to be debriefed by someone who could answer their questions, as well as provide emotional support. Lee et al. cited similar findings by others. This may be one explanation for the lack of efficacy of the intervention. Extrapolating to the childbirth setting, it would seem that debriefing should be conducted by the midwife actually present at the birth rather than a 'trained debriefer'.

Discussion

There can be little doubt that the characteristics of traumatic childbirth (and other traumatic obstetric events) are of a kind that could be expected to result in PTSD in a subgroup of women (and men) exposed to them. A sparse and largely anecdotal literature supports this view. Perceived danger to the baby, feelings of being helpless and/or out of control, perceived danger to self and excessive pain appear to be factors of major importance (probably in the order listed). A dissociative experience during delivery may also be a significant risk factor for subsequent PTSD.

Aside from the distressing nature of the core PTSD symptomatology itself, avoidance of reminders of the event is likely to cause major problems in the maternal–infant relationship, the baby obviously being an ever-present reminder for both parents. The attachment difficulties that have been reported after traumatic delivery may also stem from the feelings of detachment that commonly accompany PTSD. Additional problems that may arise in women with obstetric-related PTSD include sexual dysfunction, avoidance of cervical smear tests and termination of a wanted pregnancy (Goldbeck-Wood, 1996).

Women may also be fearful of having a further child, and if they become pregnant again may experience high levels of anxiety during the pregnancy and fearful anticipation of the delivery.

There is almost a complete absence of research addressing the question of whether some form of debriefing can diminish adverse psychological outcomes following childbirth. Our own opinion could be summarized as follows:

1. An opportunity to discuss their delivery experience should ideally be offered to all women after childbirth. Preferably this should be with the midwife involved. The resource implications probably render this unfeasible in many settings. This really represents basic good quality clinical care.

2. If a woman's delivery has been characterized by the risk factors listed above, every effort should be made to offer her an opportunity to discuss the delivery with the midwife, and ideally also with the obstetrician. Aside from the question of whether or not this might reduce adverse psychological sequelae, it may help to markedly reduce subsequent litigation (Condon, 1992).

3. We would oppose the view that formal Critical Incident Stress Debriefing, as carried out by 'trained debriefers' should be used in obstetric settings. There is the possibility that, by encouraging women to describe the negative aspects of their childbirth experience, they may do so at the expense of positive aspects thereby distorting their recollection. Critical Incident Stress Debriefing is usually used after negative and atypical events such as disasters, whereas childbirth will have positive components, unless the outcome is a stillbirth. Focussing on the negative aspects in this way will pathologize their experience, which may, in turn, interfere with normal adaptation to childbirth.

4. We would also oppose the notion that any form of debriefing or counselling should be imposed upon women (regardless of their delivery experience). We believe women should be offered the opportunity to discuss their experiences and if this is handled sensitively and empathically, the risks of this type of intervention being damaging are low.

5. In the case of women at risk (as in (2) above), we would recommend a follow-up appointment with the midwife at eight weeks post partum. If clinical depression, anxiety or PTSD are present, appropriate psychiatric referral should be made.

6. When women present with postnatal depression, or other adverse sequelae of childbirth, there should be some exploration of the childbirth experience as it may have been traumatic for her and the stress unresolved.

7. Although empirical data are lacking, the possibility

that the male partner may be adversely affected by the delivery experience should not be overlooked.

REFERENCES

Adams-Hillard, P. J. (1985). Physical abuse in pregnancy. *Obstetrics and Gynaecology*, **16**, 185–90.

American Psychiatric Association (1994). *Diagnostic and Statistical Manual of Mental Disorders*, 4th edn. Washington, DC: American Psychiatric Press.

Arizmendi, T. & Affonso, D. (1987). Stressful events related to pregnancy and post-partum. *Journal of Psychosomatic Research*, **31**, 743–56.

Astbury, J. (1980). The crisis of childbirth: can information and childbirth education help? *Journal of Psychosomatic Research*, **24**, 9–13.

Ballard, C. G., Stanley, A. K. & Brockington, I. F. (1995). Post traumatic stress disorder (PTSD) after childbirth. *British Journal of Psychiatry*, **166**, 525–8.

Beck, N. & Siegel, L. (1980). Preparation for childbirth and contemporary research on pain, anxiety, and stress reduction: a review and critique. *Psychosomatic Medicine*, **42**, 429–47.

Beech, A. B. & Robinson, J. (1985). Nightmares following childbirth. *British Journal of Psychiatry*, **147**, 586.

Berry, L. (1988). Realistic expectations of the labour coach. *Journal of Obstetrics, Gynaecology and Neonatal Nursing*, **17**, 354–5.

Boyce, P. M. & Stubbs, J. M. (1994). The importance of postnatal depression. *Medical Journal of Australia*, **161**, 471–2.

Boyce, P. & Todd, A. (1992). Increased risk to postnatal depression following caesarian section. *Medical Journal of Australia*, **157**, 172–4.

Boyce, P. M., Starick, D., Hickey, A. & Price, J. (1996). A brief intervention to lower the risk for postnatal depression: a step forward or turning the clock back? *Marce Bulletin*, December, 14–19.

Brant, M. (1972). The post-delivery interview. In *Psychosomatic Medicine in Obstetrics and Gynaecology: Third International Congress, London*. Basel: Karger.

Brownridge, P. (1995). The nature and consequences of childbirth pain. *European Journal of Obstetrics and Gynaecology and Reproductive Biology*, **59**, Suppl. S9–S15.

Condon, J. T. (1987). Prevention of emotional disability following stillbirth – the role of the obstetric team. *Australian and New Zealand Journal of Obstetrics and Gynaecology*, **27**, 323–9.

Condon, J. T. (1992). Medical litigation. The aetiological role of psychological and interpersonal factors. *Medical Journal of Australia*, **157**, 768–70.

Cox, J. L. (1988a). Childbirth as a life event: socio-cultural aspects of postnatal depression. *Acta Psychiatrica Scandinavica*, Suppl. 344, 75–83.

Cox, J. L. (1988b). The life event of childbirth: socio-cultural aspects of postnatal depression. In R. Kumar & I. F. Brockington (Eds.) *Motherhood and Mental Illness, 2: Causes and Consequences* (pp. 64–77). London: Wright.

Cox, J. L., Holden, J. M. & Sagovsky, R. (1987). Detection of postnatal depression: development of the 10-item Edinburgh Postnatal Depression Scale. *British Journal of Psychiatry*, **150**, 782–6.

Cox, J. L., Murray, D. & Chapman, G. (1993). A controlled study of the onset, duration and prevalence of postnatal depression. British Journal of Psychiatry, **163**, 27–31.

DiMatteo, M. R., Morton, S. C., Lepper, H. S., Damush, T. M., Carney, M. F., Pearson, M. & Kahn, K. L. (1996). Cesarean childbirth and psychosocial outcomes: a meta-analysis. *Health Psychology*, **15**, 303–14.

Editorial (1997). What is the right number of caesarean sections? *Lancet*, **349**, 815.

Fisch, R. Z. & Tadmor, O. (1989). Iatrogenic post-traumatic stress disorder [letter]. *Lancet*, **2**, 1397.

Fisher, J., Astbury, J. & Smith, A. (1997). Adverse psychological impact of operative obstetric interventions: a prospective longitudinal study. *Australian and New Zealand Journal of Psychiatry*, **31**, 728–38.

Fones, C. (1996). Posttraumatic stress disorder occurring after painful childbirth. *Journal of Nervous and Mental Disease*, **184**, 195–6.

Gelles, R. (1975). Violence and pregnancy: a note on the extent of the problem and needed services. *Family Coordinator*, **24**, 81–6.

Goldbeck-Wood, S. (1996). Post-traumatic stress disorder may follow childbirth [news]. *British Medical Journal*, **313**, 774.

Harris, B. (1994). Biological and hormonal aspects of postpartum depressed mood. Working towards strategies for prophylaxis and treatment. *British Journal of Psychiatry*, **164**, 288–92.

Hickey, A., Boyce, P., Ellwood, D. & Morris-Yates, A. (1997). Early discharge and risk for postnatal depression. *Medical Journal of Australia*, **167**, 244–7.

Jackman, C., McGee, H. M. & Turner, M. (1991). The experience and psychological impact of early miscarriage. *Irish Journal of Psychology*, **12**, 108–20.

Kendell, R. E., Mackenzie, W. E., West, C., McGuire, R. J. & Cox,

J. L. (1984). Day-to-day mood changes after childbirth: further data. *British Journal of Psychiatry*, **145**, 620–5.

Kennerley, H. & Gath, D. (1989). Maternity blues. III. Associations with obstetric, psychological, and psychiatric factors. *British Journal of Psychiatry*, **155**, 367–73.

King, J. (1993). Obstetric intervention and the economic imperative. *British Journal of Obstetrics and Gynaecology*, **100**, 303–6.

Kumar, R. (1994). Postnatal mental illness: a transcultural perspective. *Social Psychiatry and Psychiatric Epidemiology*, **29**, 250–64.

Lee, C., Slade, P. & Lygo, V. (1996). The influence of psychological debriefing on emotional adaptation in women following early miscarriage: a preliminary study. *British Journal of Medical Psychology*, **69**, 47–58.

Lilford, R. J. & Braunholtz, D. (1996). The statistical basis of public policy: a paradigm shift is overdue [see comments]. *British Medical Journal*, **313**, 603–7.

McLennan, W. (1998). *Mental Health and Wellbeing: Profile of Adults, Australia*. Canberra: Australian Bureau of Statistics.

Moleman, N., van der Hart, O. & van der Kolk, B. (1992). The partus stress reaction: a neglected etiological factor in postpartum psychiatry disorders. *Journal of Nervous and Mental Disease*, **180**, 271–2.

Mullen, P. E., Martin, J. L., Anderson, J. C., Romans, S. E. & Herbison, G. P. (1996). The long-term impact of the physical, emotional, and sexual abuse of children: a community study. *Child Abuse and Neglect*, **20**, 7–21.

Mutryn, C. S. (1993). Psychosocial impact of caesarean section on the family: a literature review. *Social Science Medicine*, **37**, 1271–81.

NH&MRC (1993). *Report on Maternal Deaths in Australia (1988–1990)*. Canberra: Australian Government Printing Service.

Oakley, A. (1980). *Women Confined. Towards a Sociology of Childbirth*. Oxford: Martin Robertson.

O'Hara, M. W. & Swain, A. M. (1996). Rates and risk of postpartum depression – a meta-analysis. *International Review of Psychiatry*, **8**, 37–54.

Ralph, K. & Alexander, J. (1994). Borne under stress. *Nursing Times*, **90**, 28–30.

Reynolds, J. L. (1997). Post traumatic stress disorder after childbirth: the phenomenon of traumatic birth. *Canadian Medical Association Journal*, **156**, 831–5.

Rhodes, N. & Hutchinson, S. (1994). Labour experiences of childhood sexual abuse survivors. *Birth*, **21**, 213–20.

Robinson, R. & Mitchell, J. (1993). Evaluation of psychological debriefings. *Journal of Traumatic Stress*, **6**, 367–82.

Shalev, E., Eran, A., Harpaz-Kerpel, S. & Zuckerman, H. (1985). Psychogenic stress in women during foetal monitoring (hormonal profile). *Acta Obstetrica et Gynaecologica Scandinavica*, **64**, 417–20.

Simpkin, P. (1991). Just another day in a woman's life? Women's long-term perceptions of their first birth experience. Part 1. *Birth*, **18**, 203–10.

Stewart, D. E. (1982). Psychiatric symptoms following attempted natural childbirth. *Canadian Medical Association Journal*, **127**, 713–16.

Stewart, D. E. (1985). Possible relationship of post-partum psychiatric symptoms to childbirth education programs. *Journal of Psychosomatic Obstetrics and Gynaecology*, **4**, 295–301.

Treffers, P. & Pel, M. (1993). The rising trend for caesarean birth. *British Medical Journal*, **307**, 1017–18.

Waldenström, U., Borg, I. M., Olsson, B., Skold, M. & Wall, S. (1996). The childbirth experience: a study of 295 new mothers. *Birth*, **23**, 144–53.

Webster, J., Sweett, S. & Stolz, T. A. (1994). Domestic violence in pregnancy. A prevalence study. *Medical Journal of Australia*, **161**, 466–70.

20

Debriefing health care staff after assaults by patients

Raymond B. Flannery Jr

EDITORIAL COMMENTS

This chapter reports an interesting and reportedly effective programme used to lessen the stressor impact of assaults by patients on staff in psychiatric inpatient settings. The programme is structured in an organizational health and safety approach and is associated with a positive framework of peer support, i.e. it emphasizes positive coping and outcomes, including reinforcing attachments. The peer support team members who respond immediately are backed by supervisors and a team leader.

The model provides for direct support to the assaulted staff member in this way, while at the same time, if the event is very severe or involves others, critical incident stress debriefing is provided. Follow-up occurs to check whether the individual needs referral for more specialized care. This model has been widely tested and found to be effective in returning staff to functioning, lessening staff loss and decreasing assaults in the hospitals where it has been implemented. Flannery also reports significant cost savings.

Although this is not reported as a controlled trial, the replication of this intervention appears to support its effectiveness. As an intervention, it fits in the broader context of stress management, particularly Critical Incident Stress Management. The incidents, while disturbing, have a relatively low prevalence of post-traumatic stress disorder (PTSD) associated with them. It appears that the intervention is helpful in the ways claimed, and does not claim to prevent PTSD in this population, although it appears to be associated with lessening distress.

This model of a primary response, with peer support and fitting within the organizational framework, appears to reflect some of the emphasis in other chapters. Furthermore, the focus on stressors at this level may fit better with a stress management model.

Again, these are very interesting and potentially useful findings. Where they sit with the context of theoretical understanding of trauma and prevention needs to be further analysed and, ideally, a controlled study undertaken to investigate further the opportunities that the framework presents.

Introduction

In many nations throughout the world, violence and crime are frequent and unwelcome visitors at home, in the community and in the workplace. These acts of aggression vary, but usually include the major violent acts of homicide, rape, robbery and assault. In many countries the extent of this violence has increased significantly during the past 35 years. In the USA, for example, homicides have doubled, robberies and rapes have tripled, and aggravated assaults have increased six-fold (Dobrin et al., 1996).

Work violence

Settings and assailants

Violence at work refers here specifically to the increased risk of being a victim of workplace violence because of the nature of the work itself (e.g. policing, health care, emergency services) or the nature of the work site (e.g. hotels/motels, convenience stores, liquor stores). Violence is encountered in corporate/industrial settings, police/corrections, schools/colleges, health care, and in most other settings where individuals are employed (Flannery, 1995). In these settings, assault is the most frequently encountered violent act (National Research Council, 1993). For example, in the USA, of every 1000 episodes of violence 800 are assaults (National Research Council, 1993).

These acts may result in death, permanent disability, major medical injury, psychological suffering, lost productivity, and medical and legal expense. If left untreated, this psychological suffering may result in untreated post-traumatic stress disorder (PTSD) (Flannery, 1994a).

Contrary to common opinion, employees are not most highly at risk from fellow disgruntled employees. These events are relatively rare (Flannery, 1995), but often involve multiple murders that garner extensive media coverage. Such coverage alters the perception of the risk for violence in the workplace. More common are murders of taxi drivers, and robberies of stores and petrol stations. These acts usually occur singly, are reported singly, and the collective impact of such events is lost. Much of this mayhem is perpetuated by five other types of assailants.

First is the angry customer. Herein are included average citizens who become violently angry over price, quality and/or service, and strike out at the workforce. Examples include assaulting lawyers, bus drivers and parking meter maids or traffic wardens. The second group of possible assailants is the medically ill. Some medical conditions such as serious mental illness (e.g. psychosis), organic personality syndrome and substance abuse are associated with increased frequencies of assault.

Domestic batterers form a third class of aggressors. Batterers are frequently angry, fear rejection and behave in entitled ways. Often, they are also intoxicated. Treating spouses and children as property, batterers begin the violence at home and continue it in the workplace, for example after an assailant has stalked his wife to her work site.

Juvenile delinquents and adult career criminals comprise the next two groupings. Here, poverty, inadequate schooling, substance abuse and easily available weapons have exacted a human toll that results in cruelty towards persons and property.

Lastly, there is the disgruntled employee of which we have already spoken. Usually older, possibly with an interest in guns and social contacts, the disgruntled employee is often depressed and abusing substances. The job has become the sole meaning in his or her life so that its loss or threat of its loss may lead to violence.

Causes

The biological, sociological, and cultural theories of violence in the workplace are similar to those of the culture at large (Flannery, 1997). In the biological sphere, there appears to be no consistent evidence to support genetic theories of aggression, although there may be some genetic basis for impulsivity. Similarly, there are a few medical conditions, when not properly treated, that cause subsequent, uncontrollable violence. Organic personality syndrome, some forms of mental retardation, some dementias, and impulsive personality disorder are rare exceptions. Substance abuse, which alters brain chemistry and cognitive controls, is frequently associated with violence, but is not a medical condition beyond the individual's control.

Common sociological factors that contribute to violence are poverty, inadequate schooling, discrimination, domestic violence, substance abuse, easily available weapons, and violence in the media. As a general rule of thumb, the greater the number of sociological risk factors present, the greater the likelihood of aggression.

The recent sharp upswings in crime may be accounted for in part by the cultural theory of Durkheim, known as *anomie* (Durkheim, 1897/1951). Culture may be defined as the customary beliefs, social forms and material traits of a people. Cultural mores are learned from society's basic societal institutions, including business, government, family, school and religion. These institutions show individuals how they are to behave and interact with others in socially adaptive ways. These social norms create a sense of attachment amongst its members and maintain a sense of community.

During periods of great social upheaval, this sense of integrated community becomes disrupted and the societal institutions may lose their force to regulate social behaviour. Durkheim (1897/1951) referred to this situation as *anomie*. He documented sharp increases in suicides, mental illness, general distress and violent crime during these periods.

Our own age is considered by many to be one of these periods of disruption as we move from the industrial state with its manufactured goods to the post-industrial knowledge-based state with its emphasis on information, advanced technology and research. This change has been accompanied by the emergence of the global marketplace, in which most countries of the world are exploring new economic options for growth. During such a period, the major societal institutions themselves undergo a major transformation, and the earlier rules for family, business, government and the like are no longer as helpful in providing guidance for constructive social behaviour. Social disorganization often follows, and an increase in violence and crime may be one of the outcomes. This may be especially true when the cultural factors for violence interact with known biological and sociological causes.

Psychological aftermath

Workplace violence may end in death, serious injury, lost productivity and human suffering, as we have seen. While the medical needs of employee victims are attended to, less attention is usually addressed to the psychological impact of these events in the victims' lives. Violence often results in acute stress, psychological trauma, and, if left untreated, PTSD; (Flannery, 1994a).

Psychological trauma refers to the person's physical and psychological response to a sudden, unexpected, potentially life-threatening event over which the victim has no control, no matter how hard the victim tries. These events are accompanied by intense anxiety, and the victim's response is usually one of being numbed in a state of shock, then intense fear, followed by anger.

The cardinal domains of good mental health, reasonable mastery of one's environment, caring attachments to others, and a sense of meaningful purpose to life, are all disrupted. The victim also often has the symptoms of distress associated with psychological trauma and PTSD. The most common include hypervigilance, sleep disturbance, intrusive memories and an avoidance of the site of the violence.

For many, the acute, angry, protesting phase passes within a few weeks or months, and normal life continues. But not all, for many others the painful memories are etched into vivid consciousness and this psychological awareness becomes a state of chronic numbed feelings, and continuous depressive affect. Untreated PTSD, with the full weight of its human misery, may last until death.

Psychiatric assaults

I conclude this general overview of violence in the workplace by specifically examining the primary nature of health care violence: assaults by psychiatric patients against staff.

These assaults are usually grouped into four categories (Flannery et al., 1995a). Physical assaults refer to any unwanted touching with intent to harm, and include biting, kicking, punching, slapping, etc. Sexual assaults refer to any unwanted sexual behaviour, and may include rape, attempted rape, fondling, exposure or other unwanted sexual contact. Nonverbal intimidation refers to situations in which patients use material objects to threaten and frighten staff. Examples of nonverbal intimidation might include kicking the door at the nurses' station or hurling an ashtray across the ward. Finally, verbal threats are verbal statements meant to frighten staff. These may include death threats, threats of retaliation, racial epithets, or threats against property or loved ones.

Twenty-five years of empirical research (for reviews, see Carmel & Hunter, 1989; Blair, 1991; Davis, 1991; Flannery et al., 1994) have documented consistent findings concerning the nature of psychiatric patients who are likely to become assaultive and the characteristics of the employee victims most at risk.

The most violent patients tend to be younger male patients with a diagnosis of psychosis with impaired thinking or other neurological abnormality, and histories of violence towards others and of substance abuse (Flannery et al., 1994).

The employees most at risk are younger male employees who are less senior mental health workers with less formal psychiatric training and education. These assaults may be precipitated by denials of services or benefits, are apt to occur during meal time periods, and may be sustained in restraint and seclusion procedures (Flannery et al., 1994).

When health care employees are victims of assaults by patients or any of the other forms of violence in the workplace that we have noted, how do they cope with the psychological aftermath?

One common response is to blame one self for having been attacked and to withdraw in shame. Another is to use denial and to believe that the event had no impact at all. A third strategy may be to talk to peers or supervisors about what has happened. A fourth is to believe that 'violence comes with the turf,' and employees should live with this possibility.

The problem with these solutions is that, for many, they are not helpful, and often contribute to the development of PTSD (Caldwell, 1992). To prevent this needless human suffering, Flannery and colleagues (Flannery et al., 1991, 1995b, 1996; Flanner, 1998) designed and fielded a post-incident response debriefing unit to provide needed support to employee victims. Known as the Assaulted Staff Action Programme (ASAP), this voluntary, peer-help approach provides an array of crisis intervention procedures to the individual employee victim and to the greater hospital community in time of need.

The Assaulted Staff Action Program

Philosophy

The ASAP (Flannery et al., 1991, 1995a,b, 1996; Flannery, 1998) is a voluntary, systems-wide, peer-help, crisis intervention approach for dealing with the psychological aftermath of patient assaults on staff.

Several basic assumptions inform the programme.

First is that aggression does not 'come with the turf'. While aggressive outbursts may occur, employees are not expected to place themselves at undue risk (Occupational Safety and Health Administration, 1996). Secondly, acts of patient assault may precipitate acute distress in the life of the staff member (Caldwell, 1992). Thirdly, ASAP believes that employee victims are worthy of the compassionate care extended to any injured human being. ASAP also believes that episodes of violence are not the employee's deliberate fault. Employees may make mistakes in service delivery that contribute to assaults, but most employees do not deliberately inflict harm. (Criminal acts by employees are dealt with according to law.) Finally, ASAP assumes that discussing the event early on will result in immediate relief and minimize the development of PTSD in the longer term.

ASAP is based on the characteristics of stress-resistant persons (Flannery, 1994b). In a 12-year study, Flannery followed 1200 persons to study who coped adaptively with life stress and what skills they employed in this process. Six characteristics were observed. These included: (1) reasonable mastery of the environment; (2) personal commitment to an important life task; (3) wise lifestyle choices that included few dietary stimulants, aerobic exercise, and periods of relaxation; (4) active social support; (5) a sense of humour; and (6) concern for the welfare of others.

All ASAP crisis interventions are directed towards reducing any symptomatology associated with psychological trauma and PTSD and towards strengthening the employee victim in the domains of mastery, attachment and meaning by means of fostering or restoring the skills of stress-resistant persons.

Structure

ASAP is highly modular and flexible and has been adapted for a variety of health care settings. The basic model for state hospitals is used here for illustrative purposes.

ASAP hospital teams comprise 15 volunteer members from all clinical disciplines as well as mental health workers and administrators. Eleven of the volunteers are first responders who provide individual crisis intervention debriefings for each incident of patient-to-staff assault. When an incident occurs, the charge nurse is required to notify the hospital switchboard so that the ASAP member on-call may be beeped. The ASAP member arrives on-site within 15 minutes, and offers the ASAP service. If it is accepted, the team member debriefs the employee victim; strengthens the basic domains of mastery, attachment and meaning; and contacts that employee victim three and ten days later to see whether further ASAP services are needed.

First responders rotate coverage on a daily basis, attend weekly ASAP team meetings during those weeks that they are on-call, and participate in monthly ASAP inservice trainings.

Three ASAP supervisors support the first responders. On-call by page beeper, supervisors provide second opinions, if needed, conduct individual crisis interventions in cases of multiple assaults, and co-lead Critical Incident Stress Debriefings (CISD; Mitchell & Everly, 1993). Supervisors attend each weekly ASAP team meeting as well as in-service training sessions.

The ASAP team leader administers the programme and monitors the quality of all ASAP services rendered. The leader co-leads CISD interventions (Mitchell & Everly, 1993), conducts a weekly support group for staff victims, provides in-service training, leads the weekly clinical team meeting, and is responsible for all data collection. The team leader also monitors ASAP team members for possible vicarious traumatization (McCann & Pearlman, 1990), and debriefs any ASAP team member who is assaulted in the line of duty during their regular duties.

Services

Consistent with a Critical Incident Stress Management approach (CISM; Everly & Mitchell, 1997), ASAP offers a wide range of crisis intervention services to support the needs of the employee victim and others in the hospital community. ASAP services include individual crisis intervention, CISD (Mitchell & Everly, 1993) for entire ward units, a staff victims' support group, employee victim family counselling and professional referrals, when indicated.

1. *Individual crisis counselling.* As noted earlier, when an assault occurs, the ASAP first responder is summoned and offers ASAP services. If the employee victim accepts the service, the facts of the assault are reviewed, the presence of any symptoms associated with psychological trauma are noted, and the employee is encouraged to discuss his or her thoughts and feelings about what has happened. Emphasis is on accepting the fact of the event, ventilating feelings, and developing an action plan that includes restoring mastery and caring attachments, and making some meaningful sense of what has happened.

2. *Critical Incident Stress Debriefing.* Some episodes of assault are so frightening that the entire ward unit is negatively impacted. In these cases, CISD (Mitchell & Everly, 1993) is employed. The basic CISD approach is used and includes a review of the facts of the event and of the thoughts, feelings and symptoms that it may have generated. It closes with a discussion for adaptive strategies for coping in the coming days. It is co-led by the ASAP team leader and one or more ASAP supervisors.

3. *Staff victims' support group.* Some assaults are more difficult to cope with than others, and employee victims may need additional support. ASAP accomplishes this by means of a weekly support group to discuss these particular incidents in greater detail. The group is co-led by the team leader and an ASAP supervisor. It is held in mid afternoon to maximize the attendance of employees from all shifts. Employees are paid their hourly wage for attendance, if they attend the group during off-shift periods.

4. *Employee victim family interventions.* On occasion, the families of employees become distressed when the employee family member is assaulted at work. This is especially true in single-parent families. The children may be fearful of the employee's return to work. In these cases, ASAP family outreach may prove helpful in permitting family members to receive support and discuss their fears.

5. *Professional referrals.* Sometimes an assault by a patient reminds the employee victim of past episodes of personal victimization unrelated to work. For example, the patient assault may serve as a reminder of childhood abuse at the hands of a step-parent. In cases such as these, the ASAP team leader meets

with the employee victim and, in due time, refers the employee victim to a specialist in psychological trauma counselling.

Unless the employee victim reports a crime, all ASAP services are confidential, and do not become part of the employee's personnel record or medical record. Except for any needed private counselling, all ASAP services are free employee benefits, and have the full support of management and the union.

Findings

The first ASAP was begun in a US state mental hospital in April 1990. By June 1997, ASAP procedures were fielded in ten sites. These settings included hospitals, community residences and shelter programmes. There are currently 150 ASAP team members who provide services to 2000 employees who are providing care for 3000 patients. ASAP teams have volunteered over 170,000 hours of service to the facilities in which they work.

The preliminary findings of the ASAP (Flannery, 1998) are presented here in three categories: clinical care, declines in assaults, and US dollar cost savings. The data reported are from four state hospital settings, and include the original team from 1990 to 1992 and three additional facilities from 1994 to 1995.

Clinical care

The original ASAP team responded to 327 episodes of patient assault on staff before the facility was closed due to a severe state fiscal crisis. The team completed 278 calls for assistance and was declined in 49 incidents.

Assaults were usually unprovoked (62%), occurred during meal times, and were perpetrated by a male (56%), psychotic (95%) patient. The assault ratio for male and female staff victims was 60:40, and most frequently involved less-senior mental health workers (63%) and registered nurses (16%). Bruises with swelling (34%) were the most common type of injury.

Several staff victims reported feelings of fright and anger, and symptoms of hypervigilance, sleep disturbance, and intrusive memories. For most staff, these

passed within ten days, but fully 9% of the employee victims continued to experience significant impairment in symptomatology and in the domains of mastery, attachment and meaning.

The next three ASAP hospital teams responded to 125 calls for assistance during their first year of operation. ASAP was accepted in 109 cases and declined in 16 episodes. Again, assaults were usually unprovoked and occurred during meal times. The assailant was a female (60%) or male (40%) patient with a diagnosis of psychosis (57%) or personality disorder (17%). The assault ratio for male and female staff victims was 62:38 with bruises (33%) the most common injury. Less-senior mental health workers were again at greatest risk (90%).

Employee victims reported symptoms of hypervigilance, sleep disturbance and intrusive memories. Again, these disruptions passed within ten days for most of the employees, but 15% of these victims continued to experience distress.

Declines in assaults

An unexpected finding in the first hospital with an ASAP team was a sharp decline (63%) in the frequency of assault after the ASAP team was fielded. Assaults declined from a base rate of 30 assaults per month prior to ASAP to a base rate of 11 per month two years later when the hospital was closed (Student's $t(8) = 16.47$; $p < 0.005$).

A similar reduction in the assault rate (over 40%) was found in each of the three facilities after ASAP procedures were fielded in each of these facilities. The assault rate declined from an average base rate of 32 assaults per month for all three facilities to an average base rate of 7 per month within one year (F [4/40] $= 80.85$; $p < 0.0001$).

Hospital costs

Each ASAP team costs an estimated (US)$40 000 per year in ASAP staff salaried hours. Since ASAP team members continue to do all of their regular duties as well as ASAP services, these costs are actually less.

In the original hospital where ASAP was fielded, 15 employees on average left the facility each year for reasons related to patient assaults. After ASAP was fielded, only one employee left the facility for this reason. With an estimated cost of $12 000 to replace an employee, and allowing for the cost of the ASAP team, this one outcome measure saved the facility $268 000 over a two-year period (Flannery et al., 1994).

Additional savings were realized in all four hospitals due to declines in assaults, which resulted in less medical injury, less sick leave, sustained productivity and less human suffering.

Discussion

The preliminary findings from these four ASAPs suggest at least three important findings for further study. The first is the apparent utility of the ASAP approach in addressing employee victim needs. Second is its flexibility for various workplace settings, and third is the demonstration that empirical studies of CISM programmes (Everly & Mitchell, 1997) can be successfully undertaken.

Clinical care

The reported findings from these four ASAPs document that employee victims of patient assaults do suffer from the symptoms associated with psychological trauma, and this is consistent with previously reported findings (Caldwell, 1992). Untreated acute distress from psychological trauma associated with assaults may result in impaired employee victim functioning. The weight of the empirical evidence suggests that the ASAP appears to be efficacious and cost-effective in providing support for these employee victims of patient assault. ASAP appears: to reduce symptomatology; to restore and strengthen mastery, attachments, and meaning; and to mitigate the development of long-term PTSD. ASAP also appears to strengthen the sense of community that is subject to disruption in this age of *anomie* (Durkheim, 1897/1951).

The demonstration of declines in violence in four different hospitals was a serendipitous finding that warrants further enquiry. The mechanisms for this outcome remain unclear at present. These findings may reflect non-ASAP factors such as the halo effect, advances in psychopharmacology, or experienced staffing. However, it may also be that ASAP itself is a contributing factor to the observed outcome. ASAP may support staff who become less anxious when they feel supported. As the staff become less anxious, the patients may become less anxious, and the threshold for violent outbursts is raised. ASAP may also be teaching staff to pay more attention to the early warning signs of impending loss of patient control, and to deploy alternatives to restraint and seclusion early on. ASAP may also be modifying the hospital's culture of toughness (Morrison, 1990), which relies on physical force by staff to maintain order among the patient community. The nonverbal presence of an ASAP team member on-site after each episode of violence is a strong message of the need for prevention (Occupational Safety and Health Administration, 1996).

ASAP flexibility

As noted earlier, many different types of work site continuously experience assaults and other types of crimes committed against employees. ASAP is modular and flexible in design, and can easily be adapted to these various types of setting. Corrections facilities, schools and industrial settings could field ASAP teams adapted to their agency needs. In addition, if assaults are infrequent in one agency, but that agency would like to field an ASAP team, one solution is to group similar agencies together. In health care settings, community residences and homeless shelters have each grouped themselves with similar programmes. For example, whereas one residence might have two assaults per month on average, 18 residences would have 36 assaults per month on average. A mobile ASAP team could be fielded to serve all 18 sites. Further flexibility may be obtained by not offering all types of ASAP services initially and by responding to only the most pressing form of violence in a facility first.

Research

The present findings from the ASAPs demonstrate that CISM approaches (Everly & Mitchell, 1997) can be subject to rigorous experimental enquiry. While research on the impact of natural or human-engendered disasters is more difficult, health care, corrections and school settings offer the opportunity for more effective experimental control. Operational definitions could be developed, procedures could be standardized across studies and pre- and post-measures could be adequately obtained (Flannery & Penk, 1996).

A recent review of perceived CISD shortcomings (Kenardy et al., 1996) demonstrated the need for such experimental precision. Kenardy and his colleagues (1996) reviewed the literature on CISD procedures (Mitchell & Everly, 1993) and found the approach to be inadequate in some settings. While this, in fact, may be true, it is difficult to arrive at this conclusion on the basis of the studies that were cited. In these studies, the CISD procedure used and the training of those who conducted these procedures are not presented in sufficient detail to assess whether the CISD model was correctly fielded. Our knowledge of the strengths and limitations of CISM approaches (Everly & Mitchell, 1997) will be strengthened as needed methodological refinements increase.

With violence a daily companion in many work places, including those of health care, the ASAP procedure, with its dual role of treatment and prevention, is one approach that may provide some of the tools needed to reduce human suffering.

REFERENCES

Blair, D. T. (1991). Assaultive behaviour: does provocation begin in the front office? *Journal of Psychosocial Nursing*, **29**, 21–6.

Caldwell, M. E. (1992). The incidence of PTSD among staff victims of patient violence. *Hospital and Community Psychiatry*, **43**, 838–9.

Carmel, H. & Hunter, M. (1989). Staff injuries from inpatient violence. *Hospital and Community Psychiatry*, **40**, 41–6.

Davis, S. (1991). Violence in psychiatric inpatients: a review. *Hospital and Community Psychiatry*, **42**, 585–90.

Dobrin, A., Wiersema, B., Loftin, C. & McDowell, D. (1996). *Statistical Handbook of Violence in America*. Phoenix, AZ: Ornyx Press.

Durkheim, E. (1951). *Suicide: A Study in Sociology*, G. Spaulding & G. Simpson (Transl.) New York: Free Press. (Originally published in French, 1897.)

Everly, G. S. Jr & Mitchell, J. T. (1997). *Critical Incident Stress Management (CISM): A New Era and Standard of Care in Crisis Intervention*. Ellicott City, MD: Chevron Publishing.

Flannery, R. B. Jr (1994a). *Post-traumatic Stress Disorder: The Victim's Guide to Healing and Recovery*. New York: Crossroad Press.

Flannery, R. B. Jr (1994b). *Becoming Stress-resistant Through the Project SMART Program*. New York: Crossroad Press.

Flannery, R. B. Jr (1995). *Violence in the Workplace*. New York: Crossroad Press.

Flannery, R. B. Jr (1997). *Violence in America: Coping with Drugs, Distressed Families, Inadequate Schooling, and Acts of Hate*. New York: Continuum.

Flannery, R. B. Jr (1998). *The Assaulted Staff Action Program (ASAP): Coping With the Psychological Aftermath of Violence*. Ellicott City, MD: Chevron Publishing.

Flannery, R. B. Jr, & Penk, W. E. (1996). Program evaluation of an intervention approach for staff assaulted by patients: preliminary inquiry. *Journal of Traumatic Stress*, **9**, 317–24.

Flannery, R. B. Jr, Fulton, P., Tausch, J. & DeLoffi, A. Y. (1991). A program to help staff cope with psychological sequelae by patients. *Hospital and Community Psychiatry*, **42**, 935–8.

Flannery, R. B., Jr., Hanson, M. A. & Penk, W. E. (1994). Risk factors for psychiatric inpatient assaults on staff. *Journal of Mental Health Administration*, **21**, 24–31.

Flannery, R. B. Jr, Hanson, M. A. & Penk, W. E. (1995a). Patients' threats: expanded definition of assault. *General Hospital Psychiatry*, **17**, 451–3.

Flannery, R. B. Jr, Hanson, M. A., Penk, W. E., Flannery, G. J. & Gallagher, C. (1995b). The Assaulted Staff Action Program (ASAP): an approach to coping with the aftermath of violence in the workplace. In L. R. Murphy, J. J. Hurrell, Jr, S. L. Sauter & G. P. Keita (Eds.) *Job Stress Intervention: Current Practices and Future Directions*, vol. III (pp. 199–212). Washington, DC: American Psychological Association.

Flannery, R. B. Jr, Hanson, M. A., Penk, W. E. & Flannery, G. J. (1996). The Assaulted Staff Action Program (ASAP): guidelines for fielding a team. In G. R. Vandenbos & E. Q. Bulatao (Eds.) *Violence on the Job: Identifying Risks and Developing Solutions* (pp. 327–41). Washington, DC: American Psychological Association.

Kenardy, J. A., Webster, R. A., Levin, T. J., Carr, V. J., Hazell, P. L. & Carter, G. L. (1996). Stress debriefing and patterns of recovery following a natural disaster. *Journal of Traumatic Stress*, **9**, 37–49.

McCann, L. & Pearlman, L. A. (1990). *Psychological Trauma and the Adult Survivor: Theory, Therapy, and Transformation*. New York: Brunner/Mazel.

Mitchell, J. T. & Everly, G. S. Jr (1993). *Critical Incident Stress Debriefing (CISD): An Operation Manual for the Prevention of Traumatic Stress among Emergency Services and Disaster Workers*. Ellicott City, MD: Chevron Publishing.

Morrison, E. F. (1990). The tradition of toughness: psychiatric nursing care by non-professional staff in institutional settings. *Image*, **20**, 222–34.

National Research Council (1993). *Understanding and Preventing Violence*. Washington, DC: National Academy Press.

Occupational Safety and Health Administration (1996). *Guidelines for Preventing Workplace Violence for Health Care and Social Service Workers*. Publication no. 3148. Washington, DC: OSHA Publications Office.

21

Multiple stressor debriefing as a model for intervention

Keith Armstrong

EDITORIAL COMMENTS

Multiple stressor debriefing has evolved as an adaptation of debriefing processes to a framework for dealing with the multiple and often prolonged stresses involved in disaster relief work, for instance in the weeks and months following an earthquake in a devastated community. As Armstrong points out the stresses in these circumstances are multiple and not so clearly identifiable as those in the acute rescue phase. Workers may come from multiple settings, may not have been trained to work together, and may not have been adequately briefed or prepared for their contribution.

The author describes the model he and his group have evolved and provides examples of its implementation. The model is reported to be flexible and able to be used in individual, family or group situations according to specific need. It is of interest to see the potential of family-based interventions in this context and their possible normalizing roles. The intervention or debriefing model proposed is more positive and involves four phases: disclosure of events; feelings and reactions to these; coping strategies; and a termination phase that focusses on learning and integration. This more positive model may in and of itself have benefits as it appears not to pathologize the experience. Furthermore, as described, the model appears to provide for implementation in frameworks linked to need and also for opportunities for a screening approach to identify those in need of more ongoing clinical services. Armstrong also demonstrates significant sensitivity to the complex group process and dynamic issues that are relevant to group debriefing but are rarely addressed.

The model described has a clinical and positive orientation, and is generally supportive. How it relates to other debriefing formats highlights the confusion in this field about which interventions can be classified as debriefing, and, if they are, what this means. The group appears to have commenced some research on their model. Here, as elsewhere, however, it is critical that systematic research establishes the benefits or otherwise of these processes and what can be learned that is useful. There is a powerful belief that such interventions are inherently good and inherently needed, that they represent a good and humanitarian response. Evaluation does not have to stop this response, but rather to identify its achievements, its dangers, and how it may be developed better in the future. In this context a focus on aims, processes to achieve these and monitoring of outcomes are critical to development of the field.

Introduction

The purpose of this chapter is to provide a comprehensive discussion of the concept and practice of multiple stressor debriefing (MSD). Various types of MSD are outlined, strategies for improving debriefing, including coordinating the intervention with management, are proposed, research regarding the model is reviewed, and finally concerns and limitations of the model are discussed.

MSD was originally developed to debrief American Red Cross (ARC) personnel following a lengthy disaster relief operation in connection with the 1989 San Francisco earthquake (Armstrong et al., 1991). ARC personnel who responded to this relief effort were faced with a combination of stressors not previously encountered in a large urban community in North America. These stressors include multiple contracts with trauma survivors, long working hours, a dangerous work environment, shifting in Red Cross policy, fear of aftershocks, inexperience of some ARC personnel, recent exposure to a previous disaster relief effort (Hurricane Hugo), working with a population of victims who had been homeless prior to the disaster, being away from home, a hostile political environment, and negative press coverage.

While under 'ordinary' disaster relief circumstances, emergency service response to a traumatic incident is brief; ARC personnel were involved in this relief effort for an extended period lasting up to three months. These unique circumstances provided an opportunity to develop effective debriefing interventions for workers engaged in responding to extended disaster relief operations (Armstrong et al., 1991). Our research team realized that group debriefing of personnel after large-scale, long-term disasters must allow for a variety of issues to be addressed. What is traumatic or painful for one person may be experienced differently by another. In order for an intervention to be useful it must address both the variety of individual concerns raised by participants and the common themes and similarities among these individual experiences.

MSD addresses the thoughts and feelings about the stressors that personnel encounter while participating in a disaster operation. The model provides education about stress responses, coping strategies, and the transition back to the home environment. MSD is a one-session individual, family or group intervention consisting of four stages. The goals of MSD are as follows:

1. Encouraging disclosure of troubling events experienced by participants during the disaster relief effort.
2. Facilitating discussion of associated thoughts and feelings about the troubling events.
3. Encouraging discussion about, and use of, effective coping strategies. An important assumption underlying this model is that people are aware of some internal coping strategies on which they are able to

draw. These strategies are discussed explicitly and encouraged. Participants are also specifically educated about typical stress reactions and are provided with written materials describing adaptive and maladaptive coping strategies to such reactions.
4. Facilitating discussion of positive accomplishments during the disaster relief effort while preparing participants for the transition back to the home environment. Assessing participants' need for future services is also a goal of this stage.

An underlying theoretical assumption in this model is that talking about traumatic events to an accepting audience is helpful to most participants. In addition, providing participants with the experience of successfully talking about their experience may allow for a continuation of this process in other settings, whether it be with friends, family or co-workers. The participant's telling of the story also provides an opportunity for others to aid in reworking the meaning that the participant has the experience.

The model of debriefing is applicable to many other trauma-response groups such as medical, police and fire personnel, Federal Emergency Management Agency (FEMA) workers, as well as direct victims. Specific modifications in this model may be warranted to serve adequately a particular population.

Group, individual and family debriefing

The debriefing literature is divided on the question of whether a single individual can be successfully debriefed and often describes debriefing as a group-only format. Mitchell (1996) contended that debriefing cannot occur in an individual format. He used the term 'one to ones' to refer to the individual meetings that take place during, rather than at the conclusion of, the disaster relief operation, and argued that the characteristics of group interactions are critical to the concept of debriefing.

However, I believe that MSD, like psychotherapy, can take place in an individual, family or group context and that in some instances an individual debriefing is the intervention of choice. The social context in which the response to the traumatic event and relief effort occurs will influence intervention strategies. The skills of the providers, the organizations involved, the access to family, and the specifics of the event can all affect which type of intervention(s) will be preferable. Similar to a psychotherapist, MSD facilitators need to have specific skills to conduct a useful intervention. Although some of those skills are universal to any intervention (e.g. forming an alliance or joining with the participant(s)), other skills are more specific and vary according to the type of intervention used. If the facilitators are competent, each format of debriefing can be successful.

Group debriefing advantages

A group debriefing may be advantageous in that it provides an opportunity for members to support each other and share information within the group, creates a format for members to discuss the common themes of their experiences, and provides a less costly and more time efficient intervention. In addition, group debriefing offers participants a context in which to re-examine their misperceptions about their roles in the event, and to develop a more realistic understanding of their own actions and/or inactions.

Individual debriefing advantages

The primary advantage of an individual debriefing is that it provides an opportunity to aid persons who might not otherwise receive an appropriate level of individual attention. An individual debriefing may be a superior intervention for people who are not comfortable talking about their experiences in a group, for those who have been relieved of their duties because of behavioural problems on the job, for those who may be disruptive in or to the group, and for those who, due to psychological make-up or the specifics of the disaster relief operation, are at risk for decompensation within a group. In addition, an individual debriefing would be warranted for those persons who experienced unique events within a large-scale, long-term disaster. For example, an ARC worker who was mugged while working in a disaster relief effort benefited from an individual rather than a group intervention. A group facilitator

would not have been able to provide her with enough individual attention to discuss her concerns nor would the group facilitator have been likely to obtain enough information to determine whether a referral for additional services would be appropriate.

Family debriefing advantages

An important goal of debriefing is to provide support for participants and to encourage them to ask for support from the larger social system in which they participate. A primary advantage of a family debriefing is that families can be quickly and effectively mobilized to provide support for the affected person. Because little is written on family debriefings, this section outlines some of the rationale for the intervention.

Although exposure to a traumatic event does not necessarily lead to psychiatric problems such as posttraumatic stress disorder (PTSD) (American Psychiatric Association, 1994), it frequently leads to problems in family functioning. In the extreme case of war, the manner in which the veteran has been affected may significantly impact on his or her partner when he or she returns home. In Solomon et al's (1992) study of couples who were together prior to the male partner's participation in the 1973 Arab–Israeli conflict, families in which the veteran was diagnosed with either warzone-related PTSD or a stress reaction were found to include partners who reported more psychiatric problems than those in families of veterans without stress-related symptoms. These couples had not had significant problems prior to the veteran's war experience, strongly suggesting that traumatic events can negatively impact on the entire family, even those members who have not directly witnessed the trauma.

Involving the family as a source of support through an individual family debriefing intervention may provide a useful advantage over a typical intervention where the focus is only on the individual in the context of the work/disaster environment. In the last stage of any debriefing, facilitators typically encourage participants to utilize their social supports effectively. Rather than just encouraging participants to use their families to help them to talk about their feelings and reactions, a family debriefing helps directly to facilitate the support. In addition, a family debriefing engages family members in an active discussion of the ways in which the event that was traumatic to their loved one has affected them as well.

The facilitator's adept assessment of pretrauma family roles and negotiation with the family about how to include the directly affected member in the day-to-day functioning may help in the readjustment process. In addition, this intervention can help to prevent the member of the family who had direct exposure to the event from becoming the identified patient within the family, or retaining a prolonged focus on the disaster experience rather than reintegrating in family life. The debriefer's role is to help the family to mobilize useful responses for all participant(s) without placing the responsibility for change on the survivor. Families can be encouraged to give the member who was most directly involved in the disaster relief some time to make sense of the experience without making the individual completely extraneous to family functioning.

Education about typical responses to stressful situations may aid the family in understanding the affected member's current state. Knowing that after a disaster a family member is likely to be irritable, more quiet and withdrawn, or more emotional than usual can be helpful to the family. Handouts describing typical responses that people go through after traumatic events, the typical course of response, and adaptive coping strategies can provide the family with a framework in which to understand the behaviour and also can assist them in retaining this information after the session is over.

Another method of structuring a family/group debriefing may involve several simultaneous group meetings: one for those persons exposed to the traumatic event and another for their spouses or significant others (R. J. Green, personal communication). Spouses or significant others are encouraged to express the reactions to their partners' reactions to the traumatic event. The two groups may then meet together, with leaders educating the larger group about family difficulties that typically occur when one member goes through a traumatic event, as well as leading a discussion of coping strategies. For example, the irritable behaviour of a survivor of a traumatic incident may initially result in the partner's withdrawal. After both members attend the group, the traumatized member may be better prepared to discuss his or her disappointment and feelings of guilt regarding the incident, rather than push the partner away. In turn, the partner may be less likely to withdraw and more inclined to ask helpful questions or provide the their opposite number with time to talk.

Debriefing may be particularly useful for families who have experienced a traumatic loss. A debriefing can normalize the grieving process and help to mobilize support within and outside the gamily. For example, an adult family of five (including parents, adult son and wife, and unmarried daughter) met with a therapist to discuss the death of another son, who was killed in a drive-by shooting. During this meeting, they worried about their father, who had lost weight, feared going outside, and was extremely depressed. The therapist educated the family about traumatic stress, referred the family on for further treatment, including a medication evaluation for the father, and linked the family to support groups with specialized services for families of murder victims.

Group debriefing case example

Although family and individual debriefings are intervention options, debriefing most commonly takes place in a group format. The following case example illustrates an MSD group debriefing during a disaster relief effort after the 1994 Los Angeles earthquake. To protect the confidentiality of the participants, composite case examples rather than specific cases are used.

After four workers signed up at the mental health services table, the two facilitators walked with them to the debriefing site. During this walk, the facilitators engaged in getting to know the members informally prior to the start of the debriefing. All four members in this debriefing had been at the disaster site for approximately three weeks and were in the process of exiting the relief effort. At the start of the debriefing the group was informed of the purpose and rules of the meeting, as well as the limits of confidentiality according to state law.

Bob and Priscilla were Caucasian, had been married

to each other for 29 years, and resided in a suburb of Akron, Ohio. Priscilla had been volunteering for the last three years on national assignments; Bob had been involved for 20 years and had volunteered on numerous national assignments. Priscilla was a homemaker and began volunteering after their second child left home to get married. Bob worked as a supervisor at a steel plant. They had been assigned during this relief effort to work together on an emergency response vehicle (ERV) distributing food in damaged areas of the San Fernando Valley.

Sarah was a 34-year-old single African-American woman from Buffalo, New York, employed as a private practice psychologist and was attending her first national disaster relief effort. Her role on this assignment was to provide mental health services to ARC workers, including those experiencing difficulties with job performance.

Mark was a 46-year-old divorced Caucasian from Edmonton, Alberta, employed as an administrative assistant. He was involved in his first large-scale disaster relief effort and was assigned to Staffing, which involved providing administrative support to ARC personnel.

In the Disclosure of Events phase, a facilitator asked each member to describe what had been most troubling or stressful to them during the disaster relief effort. Priscilla described seeing the destruction the earthquake had caused and how it affected the families to whom she served food. Sarah spoke of having to recommend removal of a supervisor who was not handling his responsibilities effectively. Bob recounted his concerns with the inefficiency of the food distribution mechanism. Mark stated that he had not been assigned to the job he had anticipated. All group members identified stress from the long working hours with little chance to sleep and eat. One of the facilitators framed these experiences as 'challenges' faced by workers during this disaster and asked group members to comment about the feelings or reactions they had to these experiences.

In the Feelings and Reactions phase, Priscilla described her feelings of sorrow about the plight of the victims. Bob expressed his anger at the bureaucratic delays with the delivery of food. Upon further questioning by one facilitator, Bob also expressed disappointment that he could not do more for the victims. Sarah expressed feelings of guilt about having to confront someone who was not doing his assigned job well, an aspect of her work which she always found difficult. Mark disclosed disappointment and frustration at having to perform an administrative 'paper pushing' job after coming all the way from Canada with the expectation of working directly with victims.

Both facilitators then led a discussion of the common themes that had emerged from the group, beginning with the wish that the workers could do more to help, and characterized the emotional reactions expressed as normal.

In the Coping Strategies phase, members discussed what they found useful in helping them through these stressful experiences. Bob and Priscilla stated that they relied on talking to each other about these experiences. Priscilla, who had develop friendships with other volunteers on this and past disasters, said she also found it helpful to discuss her reactions about the devastation with friends who were working on the disaster relief effort. Bob stated that all he needed was to talk to Priscilla about his experiences in order to feel better. Sarah described receiving support from her supervisor and co-workers. Priscilla remarked that having to confront people was difficult but important if it helped the operation run more smoothly. Bob commented that workers had a hard time realizing that the jobs to which they were assigned might be too much for them. Mark was asked by a facilitator how he coped with not doing what he expected to be doing on the disaster. Mark responded that he had come to realize that each person's job served an important function for the success of the mission as a whole. Priscilla quickly remarked that if his job wasn't done they would have a difficult time leaving, since everyone needed to go through Staffing prior to leaving the disaster relief effort. Sarah talked about going to the beach with co-workers to take a break from the long days at work. Group members commented on the fact that making phone calls to family and friends at home and laughing with co-workers had been useful in helping them to cope with the current stresses of their work.

Facilitators provided information on stress and coping and gathered information on how group members had been sleeping and eating. Members discussed their difficulties in sleeping and problems with remembering to eat, and keeping track of what day it was. These experiences were described by one co-facilitator as typical reactions to the stressors of disaster relief work.

In the Termination phase, the facilitators encouraged members to discuss their most positive experiences during the disaster relief effort. Each member described a particular situation in which they believed they had helped others or provided a valuable service to the ARC. Group members discussed important relationships that they had developed during the operation, and how they planned to say goodbye to their colleagues.

The facilitators then shifted the discussion to going home. Priscilla discussed how supportive and interested her children were in hearing about what she and Bob had done. Bob told the group about the feelings of disorientation upon returning home after his first disaster and how he was planning a day or two of rest before he returned to his regular work responsibilities. Members were encouraged to identify people in their support system who could listen to them talk about their experiences in the disaster relief operation. Sarah and Mark planned to present their experiences to a local psychological association and a local Red Cross chapter.

Group members were cautioned to remember that even though they had been working at the disaster, their loved ones would need time to tell them about what happened during their absence from home. No one in the group appeared to be in need of follow-up mental health intervention.

Guidelines for fine tuning debriefing

Prescreening individuals for one-session interventions to assess level of functioning and to explain goals is useful in preparing for group psychotherapy (Block, 1985). However, prior to debriefing at disaster sites there is usually little or no chance to prescreen members (Wollman, 1993). Facilitators are responsible for managing participants' anxiety levels during the intervention while working to accomplish the goals of de-

briefing. By structuring the debriefing, creating an alliance with the participant(s), and carefully observing interactions, facilitators can determine how often and in what ways to intervene (Armstrong et al., 1995).

The purpose, rules, and phases of the intervention need to be outlined at the beginning of the meeting. Members value knowing the norms or fundamental rules of the group (Schopler & Galinsky, 1981). A lack of structure, confusion about norms, and low task orientation can lead to problems in any group, especially a single-session group (Galinsky & Schopler, 1977). It is advisable when possible to meet briefly, provide potential members with information about the group, and make a contract with them prior to starting the group (Block, 1985). Rules of confidentiality should be explained, an emphasis being put on the need for group members to refrain from discussing other members' experiences outside the group. It should be stated explicitly that the intervention is not a critique of the event nor is it psychotherapy.

Similar to conducting inpatient psychotherapy groups, leaders of a group debriefing must be prepared to be verbally active throughout the entire session (Yalom, 1983; Armstrong, 1990). Facilitators must be careful in managing the high level of anxiety associated with debriefing. The leader encourages the exploration of troubling events while creating a safe environment. Leaders must carefully assess the ability of members to tolerate anxiety-laden material. Depending on the composition and size of the group, the leaders may emphasize educational components of the debriefing or the detailed discussion of troubling events. In addition, debriefings should be provided in a fashion that is convenient, private, and accessible for participants.

The advantages of using two leaders in a one-session debriefing group include an increased ability to solve problems, to manage group issues, to provide structure, and to reinforce leader interventions, as well as to minimize potential countertransference issues that can arise when discussing anxiety-laden material (Galinsky & Schopler, 1980; Armstrong et al., 1995). A co-leadership model tends to reduce the potential for countertherapeutic behaviours in the group. Peer co-leaders are often used in debriefing with emergency services personnel and can be especially effective in groups with high levels of suspicion and scepticism towards mental health professionals. Group members may feel that they receive more attention with two leaders.

The debriefing should incorporate a discussion of positive aspects or moments in which the participants feel proud of their contributions (Raphael, 1986). Such discussion is helpful to persons in integrating their experience into their lives. Facilitators must remain aware, however, that the members may emphasize positive themes in order to avoid discussing the difficult events and feelings; the discussion should be balanced between focussing on troubling and on positive aspects of the experience.

An important aspect of running an effective debriefing is establishing the group as a safe place for members to discuss what was troubling to them without criticizing other group members. Leaders must be adept in creating an atmosphere that allows members to discuss events without other members feeling criticized about what they did or did not do.

Debriefing should be encouraged but not be made mandatory. The multitude of effective ways that people care for themselves should be respected and encouraged. In addition, it is important to recognize that individuals who use avoidance, denial, and repression as primary coping mechanisms may not benefit from, and may in fact be made more anxious by, a group debriefing intervention focussed on reworking the traumatic event (Shalev, 1994). By the conclusion of a debriefing, facilitators should be able to identify members who would benefit from further mental health services and should refer these individuals appropriately.

Issues of difference – gender, race, culture, ethnicity, or even a lack of familiarity with the requirements of someone's job – are important variables to account for when providing an intervention. If the facilitators are 'too different' or not knowledgeable about the participants, the intervention may fail to be effective because of participants' concerns about not being understood. Allowing time to acknowledge differences between facilitators and participants may help to improve the alliance and allow for a more productive intervention.

Leaders should obtain as much information as possible regarding the event and the participants prior to debriefing. In debriefing emergency relief workers, it is important to obtain information in advance about specific task assignments in order to avoid extended discussions about logistics. Unlike traditional outpatient therapy groups, in which there is ordinarily little overlap between members outside the group, debriefings are often conducted with persons who have worked closely together before, during and after a highly stressful time. This overlap can present a challenge to the group leaders as there may be unspoken issues that can mitigate the group's effectiveness.

Emergency services personnel may be comfortable in identifying others who need help but may have difficulty asking for assistance for themselves. It can be productive for the facilitators to reframe 'obtaining help for oneself' as a way to become a 'more effective worker', or to suggest that, although certain individuals may not themselves need services at this time, they can be of help to their colleagues by participating in the group debriefing. Once group members begin to disclose troubling personal experiences, the facilitators encourage all members to empathize and to discuss their own difficult experiences.

In providing debriefing services for disaster relief workers, a continuum of mental health services should be provided. These should include:

1. *Pre-disaster briefings*: these are to help relief workers recognize problematic acute stress reactions in themselves and others, and to prepare relief workers for disaster work. These briefings are often effectively presented in a large group, psychoeducational format.

2. *Informal individual or group meetings*: these should take place during extended rescue operations. These meetings have been referred to as individual or group defusings (Mitchell, 1983), and are a valuable resource for workers who are experiencing stress reactions or who simply need to talk with someone outside a particular work environment about how things are going.

3. *Exit debriefings*: these are for workers who are finished with the disaster relief effort and who are preparing to leave the disaster site. Workers identified as interested in follow-up should be referred at this time for short- or long-term therapy.

Coordinating with management

For traumatic events that impact on a workplace, careful coordination with management is an important step in providing comprehensive care. Gathering an organization's history can reveal useful information to help to determine an appropriate intervention within the company. If there is considerable tension between management and line workers, an intervention initially separating both groups may be warranted. If no such tension exists, a debriefing that involves the entire staff may be preferable. Working carefully with management to keep them informed of what will take place during the intervention without violating confidentiality and teaching them how to provide services to affected employees is critical. The stance that management takes after a traumatic event may have a significant effect on the health of the staff. Providing limited time off for affected employees may send the message that the organization is interested in their well-being.

Management should be informed that a decline in staff productivity may occur after exposure to a work-related traumatic event. Appropriate services will vary depending on the traumatic event and the perceived needs of management and employees. If, for example, the traumatic event is caused by a significant error made by a worker, it may be useful to provide education about normal stress responses and to provide easy access to individual debriefing meetings to aid in the resolution of the situation. When members of the institution have been assaulted or harmed by an outside assailant, a group or family debriefing may be quite useful in helping employees to return to their previous level of functioning.

Debriefing post intervention

Evaluating the effectiveness of debriefings through anonymous questionnaires or by asking participants for their feedback at the conclusion of the debriefing is an important step in creating a useful intervention. Questionnaires provide participants with a method of communicating their responses with less concern about how the facilitators will experience their comments, while asking participants for feedback can engender more brainstorming on how the intervention could be more helpful to participants.

Finally, it is suggested that facilitators should be offered a debriefing by a nonfacilitator mental health professional to prevent secondary traumatization or compassion fatigue among group leaders (Talbot et al., 1992).

MSD research

Numerous authors assert that debriefing prevents or minimizes stress reactions and is considered useful by participants (Mitchell, 1983; Dyregrov, 1989; Armstrong et al., 1991, 1995). However, there are few empirical studies to substantiate these claims (Robinson & Mitchell, 1993; Stallard & Law, 1993) and a few studies have indicated that debriefing has little or no measurable effect on symptom reduction (Deahl et al., 1994; Kenardy et al., 1996).

Although few hard data currently exist that indicate that debriefing decreases symptoms, there is evidence that talking or writing about troubling past experiences may improve physical health, and that not talking about troubling experiences can be harmful (Pennebaker, 1989).

In one research study (Armstrong et al., 1998), the MSD model was used to debrief 112 American Red Cross workers individually or in groups after their participation in the 1994 Los Angeles earthquake relief effort. A questionnaire that examined workers' experience of debriefing was completed by 95 workers.

No significant differences were found when comparing individual with group debriefings, years of experience, or gender. Any correlation between participant to facilitator ratio and each of the questionnaire items was examined for participants in-group debriefing. Size of the groups varied from 2 to 12 persons. Only the correlation between participant to facilitator ratio and the question ('I expressed my feelings and reactions') reached significance ($r = -0.35$, $p = 0.002$). Participants were more likely to feel that they had expressed their opinions and feelings when there were fewer participants per facilitator.

Participants in this study appeared to express a

desire for an intimate or smaller-size meeting in which to talk and listen to other participants and leaders, suggesting that the opportunity for receiving individual attention may be more important than receiving large-group support. During a large scale disaster in which it is not possible to provide small-group interventions for most people, such interventions should be targeted specifically at those determined to be at high risk for developing psychiatric problems after the disaster relief effort.

General debriefing concerns

Although debriefing appears to be helpful for many individuals exposed to traumatic events, numerous concerns remain about this type of intervention. A static model of intervening is not useful, yet the chaos that ordinarily surrounds a traumatic event makes it difficult to customize an intervention. Debriefers must be prepared to assess the specific situation quickly and be ready to offer an array of appropriate services. For example, if an individual has been implicated in causing a particular problem, it may be important to refrain from having him or her attend any group debriefing and instead to provide an individual or family intervention. Another general concern about debriefing is that participants may be less likely to use their natural supports because they attended a debriefing and discussed the event. Participants may attempt to keep their work experience from family life as a way to protect families. Unfortunately, not sharing with the family a brief explanation of the work difficulties generally produces more problems for the family.

Training for debriefers

Debriefers who are poorly trained or unskilled as facilitators pose a serious potential liability to the success of an intervention. Creating a peer and participant evaluation system as well as a method for continued training of the debriefers is essential. Since debriefing provides little or no prescreening, a facilitator can misjudge what might be most helpful to his or her audience. It is critically important that facilitators have access to participant feedback in order to learn from participant

experiences. Care should be taken to match facilitators with participants who are similar, or to match those facilitators who have experience in working with individuals of a particular gender, culture, race, ethnicity, or work environment in order to provide the most useful and applicable intervention.

Debriefing: mandatory or optional?

The organizational setting and culture will often determine whether a debriefing is mandatory or optional. Both approaches have limitations. Mandatory debriefing is not universally useful for all participants and in fact may be contraindicated for those persons who rely heavily on an avoidant-coping style. If debriefing is optional, the intervention may fail to attract large numbers of participants in an environment where mental health interventions are suspect. Participants who are required to attend against their own inclinations may create a problematic environment that can impact on the effectiveness of the intervention. Paying close attention to the perceived needs of the organization and the prospective participants will be helpful in designing a useful intervention. Working within the organizational structure can help to create an atmosphere of acceptance of a debriefing intervention rather than one of hostility and suspiciousness. Care providers must also be aware that those who have responded to a traumatic event may not immediately be in a position to determine what is best for them. Facilitators must, in a respectful manner, suggest that attending an intervention may be helpful to them or to their colleagues.

Single-session versus multi-session debriefing

A single meeting may not be the ideal format for intervening. It may send a message that traumatic events are easy to overcome. Conversely, an extended session or sessions may send a message that traumatic events are always difficult to resolve. Two or three meetings over several days or weeks may provide a more useful service than a one-off intervention, although there is a risk that participants will not attend all of the meetings

A full service intervention comprising mental health professionals who follow up people over a period of time after the event may aid in the identification of those who need more help, and may provide a more complete service. An Employee Assistance Programme within the organization may be well situated for a longer term follow up with participants.

Misuse of debriefing

Despite its potential benefits, debriefing may be subject to misuse or misapplication. It is possible that debriefing may give the impression that management is providing help to workers in distress when in fact, the workers need a much more fundamental change in their occupation or its organization. In the most extreme example, debriefing may help soldiers to return to the front to continue fighting, but it begs the question of whether fighting is ever in itself healthy for the individual. Organizations can use debriefing as a superficial attempt to cover over problems that are much more serious than a one-off intervention can meaningfully address. For example, some organizations that are downsizing have used debriefing to help take the 'sting' out of impending job losses, while failing to make any meaningful attempt to help workers relocate, find new jobs or obtain new skills.

Group debriefing concerns

Group debriefing with co-workers

Participants attending a debriefing with co-workers may not feel comfortable revealing their thoughts and feelings with people with whom they need to have a long-term relationship. Debriefing with co-workers may be so uncomfortable that some participants would not be able to use the intervention in a meaningful way. Although the information in a debriefing is confidential, the session inevitably changes the relationships among co-workers. This change may improve the relationship among co-workers or could in some cases lead to greater difficulties. Thus, facilitators need to be sensitive to participants and explain the possible ramifications of the intervention.

Size and composition of group debriefings

The size and composition most appropriate for group debriefings is difficult to assess. Recent research suggests that a large participant-to-facilitator ratio may negatively impact on group debriefing (Armstrong et al., 1998). Group debriefings can become so big that the intervention loses its effectiveness. Dividing groups into smaller units may give members more individual attention at the expense of important information that other group members could provide. A group lecture with a focus on stress, coping and answering questions from the audience might be an appropriate intervention after members have had the opportunity to relate briefly accounts of their experience in an informal way. Some participants may feel as though they have not received enough individual attention in a group debriefing. Debriefers should remain aware of these possibilities and be flexible enough to respond to the needs of the participants.

Individual debriefing concerns

Although individual debriefing may at times be the ideal intervention, it may not be cost-effective. Because the views of other participants are nonexistent in an individual intervention, individual debriefing does not provide a chance for group or family members to challenge the distorted thinking and the sense of overresponsibility that are common sequelae after a traumatic event. Consequently, the facilitator's work in challenging any potential distortions can be made more difficult without the input of other supportive group or family members.

Family debriefing concerns

Although a family intervention may be desirable in theory, it may be difficult to determine how and when to involve a family in debriefing. Families, like co-workers, are not always supportive and may be driven by hidden and complex agendas. Unsupportive comments can lead to problems in facilitating a smooth intervention and consequently may prolong maladaptive coping on the part of the individual. However, the family system may be the most important variable to which the trauma-exposed individual will return. By working with the family, the facilitator can more accurately assess with participants whether or not they would benefit from future interventions in couples, family, individual or group settings. A family debriefing may be impractical in situations where family members are not readily available. In large-scale disasters, for example, many ARC personnel are flown into a disaster site from all over the country, leaving family members at home.

Essential aspects of debriefing

Talking about troubling events whether it be in an individual, family or group context, can be a healing experience. The telling and retelling of the story provides participants with a chance to develop a coherent narrative of what happened and also to experience the process of desensitization to the traumatic aspects of the experience. Although telling the story usually occurs only once in a debriefing, facilitators encourage participants to continue their work with supportive individuals who can help them process their experiences more fully. The facilitators also have a responsibility to aid the participants in remembering the positive and negative aspects of the event (Raphael, 1986). The power of an individual, group or family intervention can aid participants in more deeply examining their role in a traumatic event. Facilitators, family or group members may provide alternative perspectives that may allow a more realistic appraisal of participants' roles in the traumatic event. These perspectives can be essential for participants who feel guilt or shame for what they did or did not do during or after a traumatic event. However, there is here as elsewhere the need for significant further research to evaluate the effects of debriefing and its outcomes, be they positive or negative.

Individual, family or group debriefing provides an opportunity to review the disaster experience with others, share coping styles and learn about typical reactions to stress. This process helps participants to engage in a cathartic experience, provide and receive information, and gain hope for the future. All forms of debriefing may also communicate a caring message to workers that the sponsoring institution is interested in employee well-being. Debriefing may, over the long-term, help to decrease job burnout, aid in workers' ability to perform their jobs, decrease family problems and/or highlight the need for additional intervention.

Acknowledgement

The author thanks Barbara Ustanko and Mia Laurence for their comments on this chapter.

REFERENCES

American Psychiatric Association (1994). *Diagnostic and Statistical Manual of Mental Disorders*, 4th edn. Washington, DC: American Psychiatric Press.

Armstrong, K. (1990). The discharge issues group: a model for acute psychiatric inpatient units. *Social Work with Groups*, 13(1), 93–101.

Armstrong, K., O'Callahan, W. & Marmar, C. (1991). Debriefing Red Cross disaster personnel: the multiple stressor debriefing model. *Journal of Traumatic Stress*, 4, 581–93.

Armstrong, K., Lund, P., Townsend-McWright, L. & Tichenor, V. (1995). Multiple stressor debriefing and the American red cross: the East Bay hills fire experience. *Social Work*, 40(1), 83–90.

Armstrong, K., Zatzick, D., Metzler, T., Weiss, D., Marmar, C., Garma, S., Ronfeldt, H. & Roepke, L. (1998). Debriefing of American Red Cross personnel: pilot study in participants' evaluations and case examples from the 1994 Los Angeles earthquake relief operation. *Social Work in Health Care*, 27(1), 33–50.

Block, L. (1985). On the potentiality and limits of time: the single session group and the cancer patient. *Social Work with Groups*, 8(2), 81–99.

Deahl, M. P., Gillham, A. B., Thomas, J., Searle, M. M. & Srinivasan, M. (1994). Psychological sequelae following the Gulf War: factors associated with subsequent morbidity and the effectiveness of psychological debriefing. *British Journal of Psychiatry*, 165, 60–5.

Dyregrov, A. (1989). Caring for helpers in disaster situations: psychological debriefing. *Disaster Management*, 2(1), 25–30.

Galinsky, M. & Schopler, J. (1977). Warning: groups may be dangerous. *Social Work*, March, 89–94.

Galinsky, M. & Schopler, J. (1980). Structuring co-leadership in social work training. *Social Work with Groups*, **3**(4), 51–63.

Kenardy, J. A., Webster, R. A., Lewin, T. J., Carr, V. J. & Hazell, P. L. (1996). Stress debriefing and patterns of recovery following a natural disaster. *Journal of Traumatic Stress*, **9**(1), 37–49.

Mitchell, J. (1983). When disaster strikes . . . the critical incident stress debriefing process. *Journal of Emergency Medical Services*, **8**, 36–9.

Mitchell, J. (1996). Panel presentation on debriefing. International Society of Traumatic Stress Studies, San Francisco.

Pennebaker, J. (1989). Confession, inhibition and disease. *Advances in Experimental Social Psychology*, **22**, 211–44.

Raphael, B. (1986). *When Disaster Strikes: How Individuals and Communities Cope with Catastrophe*. New York: Basic Books.

Robinson, R. C. & Mitchell. J. T. (1993). Evaluation of psychological debriefings. *Journal of Traumatic Stress*, **6**, 367–82.

Schopler, J. & Galinsky, M. (1981). When groups go wrong. *Social Work*, September, 424–9.

Shalev. A. Y. (1994). Debriefing following traumatic exposure in individual and community responses to trauma and disaster: the structure of human chaos. In R. J. Ursano, B. G. McCaughey & C. S. Fullerton (Eds.) *Individual and Community Responses to Trauma and Disaster: The Structure of Human Chaos* (pp. 201–19). New York: Cambridge University Press.

Solomon, Z., Waysman, M., Levy, G., Fried, B., Mikulincer, M., Benbenishty, R., Florian, V. & Bleich, A. (1992). From front line to home front: a study of secondary traumatisation. *Family Process*, 31 September, 289–302.

Stallard, P. & Law, F. D. (1993). Screening and psychological debriefing of adolescent survivors of life-threatening events. *British Journal of Psychiatry*, **163**, 660–5.

Talbot, A., Manton, M. & Dunn, P. (1992). Debriefing the debriefers: an intervention strategy to assist psychologists after a crisis. *Journal of Traumatic Stress*, **5**, 45–62.

Wollman, D. (1993). Critical incident stress debriefing and crisis groups: a review of the literature. *Group*, **17**(2), 70–83.

Yalom, I. (1983). *Inpatient Group Psychotherapy*. New York: Basic Books.

PART IV

Debriefing overview
and future directions

22

Concerns about debriefing: challenging the mainstream

Cynthia Stuhlmiller and Christine Dunning

EDITORIAL COMMENTS

Stuhlmiller and Dunning challenge some of the basic concepts and beliefs surrounding debriefing. They describe its evolution from military to civilian settings (emergency workers), and then its rapid expansion as a panacea for all trauma experiences. They hypothesize that debriefing has evolved in a medical or pathologizing model and that its processes may encourage pathology outcomes in a process of medicalization of normal life experience. Debriefing has evolved in a technological age, as a technological solution. They go on to discuss the impetus of its popularization.

The authors also contest the universal application of debriefing, suggesting that this is inappropriate, as all events, even the most traumatic, do not universally lead to morbidity or post-traumatic stress disorder. They see as problematic the failure to substantiate debriefing as effective, the differences in what is defined as a critical incident, the assumption of adverse effects, and the failure to separate stress and trauma responses psychologically and in terms of their inherent biochemical phenomena.

The appropriateness of self-reflection is also explored, particularly when it is associated with the potential for negative rumination, and in circumstance of ongoing stress or the need to remain active in response to it. Stuhlmiller and Dunning question what should be disclosed and also the capacity of this to be helpful to those who are traumatized and may be suffering significant cognitive distortion or dissociation. There may be the capacity to retraumatize. Furthermore, assumptions of positive group process may be inappropriate.

The potential for positive processes, resilience and growth are explored and the possibility of a salutogenic approach to intervention suggested. This would build on theories of resilience, and the theories of salutogenics and sense of coherence. This framework also requires research, but the authors consider that it would be a valuable and hopeful paradigm shift. It is seen as lessening the likelihood of doing harm and would contribute to the building of human resilience.

Introduction

Psychological debriefing after disastrous events has become a widespread and popular trend over the past 15 years. Conceptualization and interventions, as generated by, and promoted from, the framework of psychology, have been generally accepted with little debate or critique. Despite a few early challenges and more recent evidence questioning its efficacy, psychological debriefing currently stands as the panacea organizational response for stressful conditions. It is argued here that approaches derived from a pathogenic framework overshadow positive outcomes, undermine individual and collective restorative capabilities and responsibility, and can have iatrogenic effects.

Underpinning the discussion is the effect of the diagnostic culture in creating and maintaining the deficit view of experience and the role of professionals in treating clients. A critical rethink is called for to incorporate a more balanced perspective that includes discovery and promotion of self-reliance, resilience, efficacy and support for positive utilization of everyday occupational and personal connections for recovery.

After commentary regarding the medical context from which current debriefing practices have evolved, research data are used to illustrate several concerns. An alternative conceptualization based on the salutogenic paradigm is outlined.

Medicalization of life

For millennia, people have been exposed to and withstood life-threatening and traumatic events. Why then have these basic facts of human existence become a medical condition demanding psychological intervention? Part of the answer can be traced back from the mid-nineteenth century, when madness – formerly considered deviant behaviour – became transformed into mental illness and the responsibility of 'mad doctors'. Because of the value placed on scientific understandings in academic training, doctors became knowers of what constitutes sickness, what shall be done about it, and who is at risk. With the industrialized society and its emphasis on producing social order, there is a progression of the medicalization of life, enabling a whole litany of disorders to evolve and a corresponding rise of the professional disciplines to serve the needs they created (Illich, 1977).

Today more than ever society is defined by the culture that defines risk, symptoms and outcomes. In fact, living itself has become an object of risk.

By definition, the person exposed to a life-threatening or extremely stressful event (abnormal situation) is at risk of developing negative psychological symptoms (a normal reaction). Therefore a normal reaction, i.e. having a pathological response, is one expected outcome.

Post-traumatic stress disorder (PTSD) has become a household term and, based on a collective professional wisdom, a need for psychological intervention has developed. Traumatologists are now dispatched to treat this pathological norm in all kinds of emergencies, disasters and situations defined as having the potential to create stress reactions.

In addition, new conditions known as compassion fatigue, vicarious traumatization, and secondary traumatization, are emerging to accommodate those who absorb trauma second-hand, because of their work with traumatized persons.

Debriefing: a technological solution

The modern solution for dealing with the psychological aftermath of traumatic situations is to get help from an expert. Help once rendered by family, friends or other members of the community has now fallen into the domain of a new breed of professionals known as traumatologists, who intervene with strategies of response known as demobilization, defusing and debriefing.

If one looks at the history of debriefing, it is important to note that the modality had its genesis in attempting to address stress, not trauma (Wagner, 1979; Dunning & Silva, 1980; Dunning, 1995, 2000). First used in combat to address battle fatigue, the modality was transplanted by military combat veterans in the early 1970s to the profession of law enforcement as well as other emergency services (Blakemore, 1975; Kroes & Hurrell, 1975). Served by the rising field of police psychology, former military psychologists used the rubric of debriefing to introduce mental health counselling in emergency and critical incident situations. Their ministrations were embraced as the profession accepted that the duties performed by those in the protective emergency services produced a high incidence of stress in personnel.

Stress management training and reduction programmes flourished in the 1970s in response to the need to mitigate stress to improve officer performance and health. The physiological reaction called stress or 'fight or flight' was well understood and its presence easily identified and monitored by both officers and administration. The dramatic increase in the number of stress claims for workers' compensation substantially drove the trend to develop formal organizational responses to stress, to contain both the financial drain and the productivity problems that were of concern to administration. Programmes that offered claims of great success and did not burden the organization with cost or disruption were highly valued.

Debriefing to mitigate stress had been supported by Roberts (1975) and Davidson (1979) in relation to the professional response to post-shooting, aeroplane and train crash, and civilian massacre incidents. Initially developed as a military tactic to keep soldiers at the battle front, an adapted form of debriefing was used by

Roberts in his work with the San Jose, California, Police Department upon his return from military service as a psychologist in Vietnam. Roberts used the psychological debriefing as a mechanism to reduce stress and anxiety levels and facilitate return to service for police officers involved in a variety of incidents, predominantly shootings and riots. The military debrief technique was further extended by Dunning and colleagues to address the emotional stress associated with police work in rescue, recovery and disaster mitigation incidents.

Where once conducted as an individual intervention modality, the debrief as a group process gained popularity in response to the need to cover, with a minimum of intrusion and cost, a large group of responders to stressful assignments. Mantell (1986) compared the effects of group debriefing for stress in his study comparing interventions in 1978 after a Pacific Southwest Airlines aeroplane crash and in 1982 in the San Ysidro McDonald's massacre, noting the drop in claims for disability rehabilitation and retirement. By early 1981, Roberts serving San Jose, California, Police Department, and Wagner, serving the Chicago Police Department, had travelled the country giving in-service training to police administrators and psychologists about the benefits of group intervention following significant operations as a mechanism to reduce stress (Wagner, 1981a,b). The sessions were touted to have two benefits. It was purported that: (1) the opportunity to talk about disaster recovery experience helped some police officers who responded to the 25 May 1979 American Airlines Flight 191 crash at O'Hare airfield in Chicago to avoid stress symptoms and to lessen the intensity of the symptoms that did occur, and (2) that a discussion of critical incidents and individual reactions of rescue personnel could be used to educate the participants about the nature of stress reactions and provide stress inoculation to prevent future stress. By 1984, debriefing had become the accepted modality to reduce stress in the police services, as evidenced by Federal Bureau of Investigation Training Keys, police magazine articles, and training presentations on the subject by the Consortium of Police Psychologists (COPS). No claims were made that the protocol had any effect on trauma, which by then had been codified by the American Psychiatric Association (APA) (1980) the *Diagnostic and Statistical*

Manual of Mental Disorders (DSM-IV) as PTSD.

Despite several problems and shortcomings later identified by Dunning (1988), the approach was taken up by Mitchell (1983), who purported that debriefing had the ability to reduce trauma among emergency workers. The generic use of the word trauma led many to believe that what was being offered was a technological fix for the more serious and long-lasting effects of PTSD.

Legal liability issues in the USA have caused concern for work-related trauma to ebb and flow over the last two decades. When debriefing resulted in large numbers of workers' compensation, payments and insurance or civil claims, the modality was rejected by the police administrators who perceived it as instigating malingering and secondary gain (Dunning, 1990a). Some administrators perceived control of debriefing as a mechanism for controlling later access to treatment. Concurrently, unions picked up the protocol as a safety programme for mental injuries and made its formalization as part of the organizational response mandatory as an employee benefit (Dunning, 1985a,b).

Critical Incident Stress Debriefing (CISD), presented by Mitchell (1983, 1988) and Mitchell and colleagues (Mitchell & Bray, 1990; Mitchell & Everly, 1993) caught on as the programme of choice, and has become the standard of care in human resource response to traumatic organizational experience. A technological solution had been found to address a human resource or personnel problem, not one of mental health.

The impetus for the popularization of debriefing

The field of protective and emergency medical service personnel management has essentially been acculturated to believe that being exposed to, or witnessing, an event that most people would consider as traumatic has a great potential to cause emotional harm in virtually anyone. This assumption emanates from a marketing strategy rather than empirical fact. Repeated studies involving such personnel responding to traumatic incidents in an occupational capacity to perform rescue or mitigation have found a low incidence of PTSD symptomatology (Paton & Violanti, 1996; Violanti, 1996). Even then, spontaneous remission and informal coping strategies generally result in a reduction of symptomatology within six months.

Why has the phenomenon of debriefing occurred? To a large extent it was driven by those gratified that such a job-related injury was being validated, and in fact normalized, thus removing the stigma that had previously been attached. It is important to note that over the years the sentiment once expressed by the medical director of American Airlines following the Flight 191 crash in 1979 still imbued the profession:

These are professionals ... from the sheriff, police, ambulance crew, and so forth. They've seen it all before, this is what they are trained to do. If any of them needs help dealing with a situation such as this, perhaps the worker really is not suited for this type of job (Staver, 1979).

Clearly, the movement has been driven by product development and marketing strategies rather than from data analysis and hypothesis testing. What has evolved has been characterized as a repetitive catechism of presumption and postulates delivered in what has been called testimonials proffered by adherents to the debriefing movement. One might construe embracing the debriefing movement as a result of its validation of risk experienced by exposed workers rather than any documentation of effectiveness. Proselytizing and identification appear to have replaced sound empirical and professional judgement, as previous relevant experience and research in mental health, cognitive psychology and rehabilitation medicine were ignored.

Over the years, adaptations and variations of the model have emerged and gained widespread appeal as a mainstream intervention across a range of events and populations outside of group and work applications. Mitchell adjusted his approach to accommodate varying populations and cultures, thereby broadening the application to include critical incident stress management. Soon debriefing was seen as the acute intervention of choice for any work group, ad hoc group and even for individuals. Additional momentum for debriefing has also been achieved as a result of revisions made in the DSM-IV. The new diagnosis of acute stress disorder as lasting from two days to one month and the new criteria for PTSD beyond one month added to the urgency felt in intervention.

What's really going on after traumatic incidents?

Evidence that exposure does not lead inevitably to PTSD or trauma is well documented (Sledge et al., 1980; Silver et al., 1983; Veronen & Kilpatrick, 1983; Thompson, 1985; Burt & Katz, 1987; Kahane, 1992). Also well documented, but infrequently cited, is the possibility of positive impact of negative events and the potential and possible prophylaxis of resilient factors that can lead to post-traumatic growth (Raphael, 1986; Tedeschi & Calhoun, 1996; Tedeschi et al., 1998).

As the protocols involved in helping victims of disasters or other traumatic events increased so too did the need to examine ethical aspects of research and of clinical interventions in this field. Respected members of the field of mental health have pointed out that it is important to question whether acute post-trauma interventions are truly in the best interest of those expected to benefit. They argue that the ethical implications of trauma work when dealing with people in extreme situations make professionals much more obliged to give special thought to ethical issues related to their role and function. It has been argued that individuals experiencing trauma are in particularly vulnerable situations, and therefore at risk of exploitation or further abuse. Survivors are easily suggestible to the idea that some intervention is necessary after specific types of incident. The old adage that 'thousands can't be wrong' has done much to add to the credibility of acute trauma intervention protocols lacking substantive validation.

Some problematic aspects of debriefing

Aside from adjustments made by Mitchell, several fundamental aspects of debriefing approaches remain problematic. To make the point, the model synthesis of Tehrani & Westlake (1994), and an inclusion of the US military model as described by Samter et al. (1993) illustrate the line of enquiry taken.

What each model shares is a common pathogenic framework. The basic assumption is that individuals who have experienced or witnessed events that could commonly be construed as traumatic need to be treated. The treatment choice is talk therapy. The therapeutic vehicle of choice is group, selected for its basic economy and its facilitation of disclosure and social sharing. The focus is on obtaining a directed chronicle of an incident from what happened (the facts) to how the person was affected (emotionally). Each model, however, varies in its emphasis on eliciting the negative aspects of the encounter. Positive experiences are minimized in the military, Mitchell & Everly (1993) and Dyregrov (1989) models, while Raphael (1986) is mindful of the potential of good feelings.

As with all theoretical understandings that lead to formulated models and guidelines for interventions, the information solicited by the facilitator or debriefer is that which experts have identified as important. By using standardized context-free formats, the debriefer is actually helping to co-construct experience by directing the narrative according to a predetermined set of concerns. In a group format, the pressure to conform and fulfil expectations such as following the line of enquiry of the group leader will undoubtedly have a major impact on understandings and interpretations of the experience. Because each of these models has its roots in the theoretical orientations of learned helplessness, with an assumption of potential post-incident difficulty, individuals become sensitized towards vulnerability while significantly less attention is paid to strengths, resilience and positive outcomes.

Given the fact that the efficacy of psychological debriefing after trauma remains uncertain and unsupported by research (Dunning, 1988, 1990b; Bisson & Deahl, 1994; Raphael et al., 1995; Kenardy et al., 1996) it is indeed puzzling that it continues to be a mainstream intervention.

Between 1989 and 1995, research focussing on the psychological impact of several major Californian disasters was conducted with a variety of occupational groups (see Stuhlmiller, 1992, 1994a,b, 1995, 1996a,b). The method of obtaining data was based on both on-site participant observation at disaster scenes and an interpretative phenomenological approach: asking people to describe their experiences in detail at different points after the event. Psychological debriefing was one aspect of experience discussed in their narratives.

Among their concerns about debriefing were questions regarding what is a critical incident, who should receive it voluntarily or involuntarily, who should facilitate it and when should it be done?

What is a critical incident?

A standard definition developed for occupational groups is, 'any unplanned, unexpected, or unpleasant situation faced by emergency services personnel that causes them to experience unusually strong emotional reactions and which have the potential to interfere with their ability to function either at the scene or later' (Mitchell, 1983, p. 36).

Strong emotional reactions may not be shared by all people exposed to the same event. What is traumatic to one may not be to another. For example, on a medical call several responders may find the incident to be rather routine, while one responder may be shocked and upset by the sight of a victim who happens to be wearing the same pyjamas as his own child, thus triggering specific significance. Even the most obvious stress events may be similarly experienced as threatening and disruptive but personal meanings and interpretations will vary from person to person and from culture to culture.

As an example, the 1989 Loma Prieta earthquake in northern California was considered by most traumatologists to be a highly stressful event, meeting the definitional criteria of a critical incident. Despite only 60 deaths out of a population of five million in the affected area, debriefing services were deemed necessary and organized throughout the locale. While a member of a psychological team responding to a freeway collapse that resulted in 43 deaths, the first author (C.S.) heard a much different interpretation of the event than that expected. The quake had indeed been sudden, life-threatening, and challenged assumptions of life, death and personal invulnerability. For some, usual coping skills were rendered ineffective. However, those who helped in the highly dangerous rescue effort, by and large found their experience to be rewarding because of the opportunity created by helping to 'undo the tragedy'. So, while the event, by definition, met the criteria of a critical incident, the risk to develop difficulties was, in part, mitigated by the fact that, for many, it was an opportunity to do what they had practised doing and found important and sustaining in their work. The following interview excerpts (Stuhlmiller, 1992) illustrate the ubiquitous nature of trauma:

The big events – more exciting, more memorable. You know, more of a challenge to do what you practice to do. I can understand somebody having problems because it was ferocious, the earthquake itself. But like myself, it's harder to understand what would bother somebody. I don't see it any different than what we do all along. So something bothered them that day. They've probably been prone to something disturbing them all along, whether it be an automobile accident or . . .

It was three days of my life that I wouldn't trade for anything because of the excitement and being there. How many people in this country, or in this world, did what we did. The opportunity to do what we did – it was exciting, interesting, and rewarding.

Further evidence to support the above claims was found by Marmar et al. (1996), who conducted a quantitative investigation of the freeway rescuers' response. Their data failed to show symptoms and social functioning disturbances. This underscores the need for research designs to incorporate a better contextual understanding of specific events into research questions. Additionally, it highlights the conceptual flaws of traumatic stress studies that suggest that experiences can be defined, operationalized, generalized and measured with consistency.

Is critical incident stress trauma?

First, it should be noted that stress and traumatic stress are two different phenomena, representing different physiological, neurobiological and psychological responses. It is unfortunate that the word 'stress' even exists in the diagnosis of post-traumatic stress disorder. It is not uncommon to find individuals, especially clinicians, who see stress and traumatic stress as existing on a continuum, traumatic stress being the most intense, severe form of stress – the ultimate 'flight or fight' response. This is a misconception. While stress relates to anxiety and the adrenaline response of fight or flight,

traumatic stress involves the way in which the brain in its physical structures and chemistry takes in information, encodes it, stores it and is able to retrieve it as memory. It is important for any clinician involved in the intervention of trauma subsequent to crisis to have a basic understanding of the neurobiological differences between stress and traumatic stress (Yehuda & McFarlane, 1997; Yehuda, 1998). This is especially true as the confusion as to whether critical incident stress comprises stress or traumatic stress causes an overstatement in support of the efficacy of debriefing. A police officer involved in a community riot asked:

Do you think I'm traumatized? I thought I was just stressed. I feel like this a lot after something heavy goes down? Does that mean I'll get PTSD, I've never had it before? I thought I was immune, after all I've done this for years . . .

Traumatic stress appears to result in a reduction of HPA function as the cortisol, which in fact is released in great amount, is consumed at a significantly higher rate by glucocorticoid receptors. Traumatic stress is then characterized as increased cortisol production and consumption, thus resulting in low cortisol levels. It is this physiological response that can be found in short-term traumatic reaction called acute stress disorder (lasting from immediately after to one month subsequent to the traumatic event) and in PTSD (occurring from one month to years or decades after the trauma), which can be exacerbated by events occurring subsequently.

You get a kind of 'runner's high' out there . . . and its hard to come down. Sometimes your knees don't start shaking until after, when you realize you could have been killed out there . . .

It has been suggested that debriefing accentuates the stress response causing prolongation of the hypothalamus–pituitary–adrenal gland (HPA) reaction, thus fostering depression (sustained high cortisol) or PTSD (engagement of increased glucocorticoid reception (Yehuda & McFarlane, 1997). It is also possible that debriefing exacerbates the traumatic stress response, further activating the physiological structures that result in acute stress and ultimately PTSD (Herman, 1992; Dunning, 1995; Paton & Stephens, 1996). The traumatized person in a group debriefing may be triggered into the same neurobiological response as the traumatic event when confronted by the disclosure of others.

> You know, I didn't start feeling bad till we went over it in the group . . . I though we had done a good job . . . should be proud. Now I guess I was wrong, and that bothers me a lot . . . I wish I hadn't gone . . . (Koval, 1987)

In affective overload, the cognitions involving imagery, sensory-motor memory, and interpretative sense of meaning held by persons who experienced the event, the traumatized person may confabulate and bring such material into their trauma set. What would appear problematic, then, is when group debriefing exacerbates or intensifies the physiological process that causes stress or traumatic stress.

One criticism of contemporary research in post-traumatic sequelae has been the reactionary bias in favour of identifying pathology resulting from traumatization in the move to validate negative consequences to victims. Hence, all research on debriefing has centred on its efficacy in preventing or ameliorating the 'golden wound' of PTSD.

> We told those docs what they wanted to hear, how we couldn't sleep and were drinking and all . . . Then we could get some mental health days off free on the taxpayers' tab . . . they owe us big . . .

It would appear that research has rarely looked at the effect of debriefing on anything other than PTSD, for instance anxiety and depression. Nor has the research explored the positive growth that might accompany traumatic experience.

Should participation involve self-reflection?

The offer, at least of a formal nature, to seek assistance within the framework of a group exercise may be the only support offered. On the assumption that ventilation is healthy, and that social sharing is cathartic, debriefing has institutionalized myths and assumptions that may not be valid. The intrusive nature of debriefing requires a reconsideration of the research on the effectiveness of disclosure, especially in identifying its underlying mechanisms. While disclosure is most often thought of as verbalization, traumatized individuals might use other expressive methods such as writing, art, kinaesthetic movement, role-playing, stress inoculation rehearsal or other experiential therapies. An insistence on verbalization is to ignore and devalue other effective coping modalities.

> You know, I really didn't like being put on the spot like that . . . it was like show and tell, show me your trauma and I'll get the chief to lay off . . . Either they accuse you of not being tough enough or being a cry baby. Am I supposed to get these symptoms or what? If I do, is that good or bad? The old-timers say they had it worse and they never had problems. But it seems you're supposed to . . .

Furthermore, several studies have shown that self-focussed attention or rumination is associated with more severe and long-lasting periods of distressed mood and subsequent depression (Lyubomirsky & Nolen-Hoeksema, 1993). People induced to self-focus ruminatively on their feelings and personal characteristics endorse more negative, biased interpretations, are more pessimistic about positive events in their future, and generate less-effective solutions (Lyubomirsky & Nolen-Hoeksema, 1995). Why, then, would one consider debriefing with its parallel focussing, to be restorative.

We know that ruminative thought characterized by a focus on personal problems combined with a negative tone, self-criticism and self-blame for problems, as well as reduced self-confidence, optimism and general perceived control are found to be counterproductive to trauma recovery. Ruminators, as compared with those who use distraction, rated their problems as severe and unsolvable, but did not reduce their confidence in the effectiveness of their solutions. However, ruminators reported a low likelihood of actually implementing their solutions. This finding suggests that rumination in the presence of a depressed mood may deplete motivation to solve one's problems. Lyubomirsky & Nolen-Hoeksema (1995) found that activities of active distraction that interfere with rumination have been found to be strongly positive in terms of avoiding or reducing the psychological impact of trauma on cognitive dysfunction. It would appear that activities to distract would prove just as useful as disclosure and social sharing in preventing or ameliorating the deleterious effects of trauma.

One might consider the self-reflective group approach that is required by debriefing to be antithetical to occupational groups whose work depends on lack of reflection and confidence in team strength. Rehashing can create anxiety about future situations, questioning of others' ability to respond, can inhibit performance and can undermine occupational values. US military pararescuers are one such group who are specifically selected and socialized into practice to be omnipotent and hold positive illusions of invincibility in order to transcend the dangers that they will face. Firefighters also describe their work as requiring action over reflection. Therefore the approach to debriefing that increases selfconsciousness and vulnerability may render a firefighter ineffective. In addition, if team strength depends on not publicly admitting weakness, the group forum may not be appropriate. As firefighters say:

People don't want to muck around in that because they have to go right back out there again … I think you can overdo it. You can over-dwell. If you're having trouble coping with it, I'd say it is great to have it available but I don't think it should be mandatory.

You're not going to spill your guts in front of the guys you work with that you feel emotional, that you felt drained. Shit no. 'Man, I'm ready to go.' You want that feeling.

Emergency personnel are often involved in different aspects of a rescue operation. Thus not all are exposed to the same things at the scene. Some may be involved in live rescues, while others are performing extrication of dead bodies. The thrill of saving a life can thus be reduced when one is forced to listen to others not involved in successful rescue efforts. As firefighters indicate:

Some guys weren't even in an incident and they were debriefed. There was an engineer at the hydrant, three blocks away and at 3.00 a.m. in the morning they're debriefing. 'Well, I want to go to bed.' No, you have to be debriefed. What the fuck are we doing here. You know, debriefing has lost its point. So the whole crew had to stay up and they had to debrief.

What should be disclosed, if anything?

The protocols that developed simultaneously and subsequent to the interest in debriefing in the 1980s all had an orientation to disclosing the worst fear, sight, experience or meaning. In addition, the educational component dwelt on pathology, the emergence of symptomatology associated with being touched by traumatic events. Participants are encouraged to disclose symptoms. It is natural to assume that there would be considerable stress and anxiety. Finding no trauma subsequently could then be construed as effectiveness. Finding trauma brings a response that, without treatment, the rate would have been much higher. It is a win–win situation, the lack of documentation that the problem ever existed or to what extent it existed allows the purveyors of the protocol to claim success.

It is known from numerous studies that there is a high spontaneous remission rate among trauma survivors who receive no treatment and that a placebo effect surely accounts for some of the success reported by many participants.

Can traumatized individuals effectively participate in a debrief?

Lacking an understanding of the most basic tenets of the psychobiology of trauma, the debrief protocol ignores the need for a higher level of abstraction and cognitive reasoning that is not generally found in the dissociative and concrete mental processing of the traumatized person. The debrief process fails to recognize that the reflective approach it requires only adds to the fears and frustration of traumatically impaired individuals, who may become anxious, confused, or 'shut down' in the debriefing process.

There is a need for evidence of the value of cathartic recounting of one's trauma story, and the psychological relief or comfort it is seen to bring. One wonders why individuals using concrete reasoning, emotional numbing and techniques of dissociation would benefit by the forced ventilation. In fact, the traumatized individual with acute stress disorder may dissociate during the debriefing, or the use of dissociative coping to avoid loss of control may be reinforced. An individual required to attend and participate may have their sense of identity as a 'mentally injured' individual reinforced.

Debriefings have in many instances become mandatory mental health treatment programmes. Employing agencies want to cover themselves to be sure that they meet the 'standard of reasonable care', which means they compel this treatment modality so that the courts cannot find them negligent in consideration of employee safety. In fact, we use the argument that traumatized individuals would resist or forego treatment if not otherwise compelled. It is 'in their best interest' to have an external support system 'look out for their injury and recovery' by compelling attendance as a function of work assignment or fitness for employment assessment. Thus what an agency accomplishes is the creation of a second group of coerced clients to be treated in a mental health system. Mandatory, inescapable mental health treatment is generally associated only with those found criminally insane or in need of protection of self or society. To refuse to participate, even when it is voluntary, creates problems associated with the recovery of civil or workers' compensation. It is inconceivable that the traumatized person be placed in a position of being compelled to receive a therapeutic modality that the provider cannot guarantee has benign, at best, or positive results.

Should the group be the treatment vehicle of choice for acute intervention?

Debriefing modalities appear to have often ignored long held tenets of group dynamics. Since debriefing protocols were developed in an environment where the groups under consideration were of long standing, being members of an employment organization, it was assumed that the stages of 'forming, storming, norming and performing' were already accomplished. Issues of safety in a group, the existence of trust and expectation of helpful assistance and of group norms about the value of the individual and the group were assumed to be positively established.

Simply because a work group has existed over a period of time, the mental health professional cannot assume that all members feel safe, trust other group members, or believe that membership in the group will have positive results. A work group cannot be construed as a therapeutic group. Nor can most work groups be transformed into functioning task groups in one session. Group process formation is not accom-

plished simply because the group shares a common employer, organization or experience.

Rather than engaging in optimizing and prioritizing steps to be taken to effect change of whatever is bothersome to the individual, the debriefing group members are focussed on a narrow set of expectations and responses associated with the trauma – all of which are negative. Changing practice to include a wider range of diagnostic and intervention goals and strategies rarely occurs in the formal debriefing model.

Resistance to incorporating other brief intervention protocols, especially those with a salutogenic focus, in the practice of debriefing can be seen in the current battle being played out between the International Critical Incident Stress Foundation and other organizations, associations and agencies dealing with traumatized persons.

Is acute intervention even necessary?

In incorporating definitions of events construed to be traumatic or critical incidents, and in using the threshold of the occurrence of the event as the impetus for treatment, the mental health field has failed to follow steps to even consider whether their services are necessary. Using the occasion of the event as the instigating decision point for initiating intervention, the debriefing is relieved of the need to conduct an assessment of whether any mental injury has occurred. Rather than following parsimony or least intrusive approach when none is needed, the field of acute intervention has rushed in and enveloped a population who might not ever need their services. What has ensued has been the 'carving out of turf'. Having established themselves as a necessary and integral component to the critical incident event experience, debriefers seem reluctant to give up participation. By hiding behind the 'disease' model, trauma is considered a progressive disorder and the course of the 'illness' is expected to worsen unless 'treated by debriefers'. Starting where the client is at and what they want to accomplish in the debriefing does not seem to be a consideration.

Practitioners have failed to keep pace with the changing research on the psychobiology of trauma, on changing paradigms for treating trauma problems. The increasing attention to individuals with varying responses to trauma, emphasizing wellness over illness, parallels the attention given to health promotion and early intervention strategies in the health care system in general. To attend to the diversity of clients seen for trauma exposure, greater emphasis needs to be placed on a variety of intervention approaches reflecting the continuum of symptoms, behaviours, coping capacities and needs of the diverse client group. Rather than reinforcing notions of illness, dependency and the need for immediate and possible long-term treatment, wellness suggests another paradigm. Brief interventions, if needed at all, should convey the optimistic message that with the support of spouses or significant others, the individual has the inherent coping resources to deal with what 'trauma has wrought in their perception, what it means to them personally'.

An approach that involves brief nontherapeutic intervention is based on the expectation that potential for growth and recovery is possible for those exposed to traumatic events, without the interventions of a mental health therapist. This approach is aimed at enhancing self-directed efforts to resolve the traumatic event as a self-efficacy experience rather than reinforcing the notion that the ultimate outcome will be illness and the need for treatment. By conveying the optimistic message that, with the support of others, the individual has the inherent coping resources to find meaning in the event and recovery from the mental injuries it inflicts, the focus changes to the positive aspects of trauma experience. This brief intervention approach is grounded in the principle of natural recovery.

Who should do it, if it is done?

As pointed out by Deahl et al. (1994), mental health professionals in many settings suffer from a lack of status and recognition, for example peer counsellors who have not yet achieved sufficient respect by their peers (Stuhlmiller, 1992). It is a common belief that the debriefer should be a mental health professional; someone who is able to facilitate disclosure and discussion of sensitive issues is warranted. Lazovik (1995), however, provided a strong argument that a person who is trusted and respected in terms of professional integrity and competence is sufficient. A major criticism of group debriefing is that, when it occurs in an environment in which the participant does not feel safe, varying levels of acceptance and support can result in secondary wounds. This creates additional pressure for a facilitator, often a stranger to the group, to ensure safety and support. The debriefing frequently occurs without the necessary development of a therapeutic alliance between the facilitator and group members.

Acknowledgement and timing

It is not uncommon to find debriefers at disaster scenes, advising that intervention be provided between 24 to 48 hours after an incident. As Everstine & Everstine (1993) posited, it is not conducive to recovery to encourage a traumatized person to 'let go' of or 'vent' feelings at a time when the person is struggling to regain composure and to make sense of chaos, horror or loss. They pointed out that emotions may be the only thing that the traumatized person feels they can control.

Disasters and traumatic events can continue for days, and sometimes longer. Body recovery after the Pan Am Lockerbie crash continued for seven months. Persons conducting acute intervention need to be sensitive to the unfolding nature of rescue and mitigation operations. Common sense should overrule procedural dogma regarding timing. The reality is that workers often have to return repeatedly to the same site or situation, not only to continue with recovery efforts but also to conduct normal work operation.

Help or hindrance?

Debriefing has become a politically 'sexy' trend for good reason. As our world becomes increasingly global and crises are part of our everyday reality where trauma and tragedy surround us, efforts to control and cope with situations that fall outside human command will undoubtedly increase. Creating specific technologies for widespread application is also part of progress.

Striving to conquer the unconquerable may be a way to defend against a shared vulnerability that tragedy brings out and that binds us to one another. People are compelled to want to do something, to want something in place, to feel that all bases have been covered to deal with mental, as well as physical, injuries.

Because these are in times where social contact and interpersonal connections have been replaced by coaxial cable, it is perhaps good news that people will show up to help each other in emotionally difficult times. 'And counsellors were called' seems to be the tag ending of every media story dealing with mass catastrophe. Depending upon the event, there can even be a surplus of willing helpers. It seems to have been forgotten, though, that on an everyday basis individual personal traumas occur that go unnoticed and unaided.

It is important to recognize that debriefing is a growth industry in affluent societies and has largely ignored the more insidious, yet every bit as tragic, individual events that befall people. This is probably fortuitous because it is highly unlikely that this model is at all appropriate for such circumstances.

Whether debriefing is thought of as helpful or not, open debate is a crucial professional responsibility because organizational response systems are guided by social and scientific constructions of psychological risk and illness. As a result, the ideologies of professional 'experts' affect the lives and activities of hundreds of thousands of human beings who have come to be identified as being 'at risk'. These representations, when applied to other populations and societies, can seriously undermine restorative capabilities, especially in situations where they do not relate to local understandings. In order to broaden post-trauma understanding, reduce iatrogenic concerns and create the everyday caring culture, a paradigmatic shift is called for and, certainly, our professional ethics should further compel us in that direction.

Ethics of debriefing: *primum non nocere*

Primum non nocere. First, do no harm. The ancient medical motto does not seem to have permeated the mental health profession as clients are inundated with modalities and protocols that stand no rigour of testing to determine whether the benefits of treatment outweigh hidden risks. Unlike the stringent scrutiny of the US Food and Drug Administration in relation to psy-

chopharmacological treatment, our profession has gone blithely ahead and subjected thousands of suffering, and nonsuffering, clients, presumed to have psychological wounds, with all manner of intrusive treatment protocols. As a discipline, we have never heard, or seem to have forgotten, the most basic tenets of the helping profession. That is, in an age where the urge to do something, anything, often overpowers prudence, we seemed to have forgotten that often it is better to do nothing. Hippocrates (400 BCE) exhorted us to embrace the ethic that 'I will follow that system of regimen which, according to my ability and judgement, I consider for the benefit of my patients, and abstain from whatever is deleterious and mischievous'.

It is difficult to achieve a sense of virtue in defending a modality that does not address the first needs of the traumatized – for safety, for restoration, for acknowledgement of strength. Instead, we point out the nobility of our provision of validation and normalization to support our role in the recovery process. Who are we to think we are the only source to provide that?

Shifting the paradigm from pathogenesis to salutogenesis

The issues identified by emergency workers underscore a need for a modification of current strategies and even a rethink of the tenets of debriefing. There is no question that some people find value in talking, sharing and expressing emotions. There is disagreement that it is necessary for all people and that guided group format focussing on emotional content is helpful.

Integration of experience occurs according to a combination of individual, group and societal meanings that cannot always be readily identified or teased out. To achieve greater understanding, the framework must enable identification of sources of hope, courage and recovery, which would require a shift away from the disease orientation to a health-oriented conceptualization.

The framework for such investigation has long been developed by Antonovsky (1980, 1988, 1990a,b, 1991) in his salutogenic model. The central concern in salutogenesis is on how people manage to stay healthy after stressful encounters in contrast to why people become sick (i.e. pathogenesis). It is believed that the differences between health breakdown and wellness may depend more upon one's outlook on life than upon the avoidance of stress. According to Antonovsky, stress is omnipresent. A person's coping ability and sense of health or well-being is connected to the degree of that person's 'sense of coherence' (SOC) or to what extent stress is experienced as coherent, manageable and meaningful. This is similar to the treatise of Janoff-Bulman (1992) in *Shattered Assumptions* and the meaning discussed by Herman (1992) in *Trauma and Recovery*. Antonovsky has demonstrated that the stronger the person's SOC, the more likely the person will be able successfully to deal with life stressors. These notions, not to be discussed here, are not unlike Rotter's (1966) locus of control, Bandura's (1977, 1982) notion of self-efficacy and Kobasa's (1979, 1982; Kobasa et al., 1985) concept of hardiness and Taylor's (1983, 1989) concept of positive illusions.

By adopting the salutogenic model, many of the issues outlined by emergency workers become eliminated. Instead of the assumption that stress, traumatic stress and critical incidents cause people to develop, or put them at risk of developing negative outcomes, a salutogenic perspective acknowledges the ubiquitous nature of stress and that consequences are not necessarily pathological but possibly salutary. This idea affirms what is already known – that even people who experience extreme stress survive and do well.

By opening up the view, debriefing strategies would include not only illness-susceptibility factors (sources of stress) but resistance factors such as SOC. By enhancing or strengthening the resources of the person, one is maximizing resistance. A strengthened sense of coherence during periods of crisis may result in improved ability to withstand future stress as well as modifying the deleterious effects of the immediate crisis.

By shifting the paradigm, mental health professionals are asked to consider the wealth of research that documents the positive aspects of trauma incident experience. In changing the perception of experience from being injurious to facilitating growth, the potential protocols for acute intervention that do not exacerbate traumatization widen considerably. Research is needed here also to substantiate the effectiveness or otherwise of this model.

Positive aspects of trauma experience

It seems to have been forgotten that research conducted on community or group-experienced disaster also consistently documents that a honeymoon period generally exists in which survivors support and enhance a collective sense of strength. That strength can be found not only in what was just experienced but also in a future ability to control and respond to the demands occasioned by the event (Dynes, 1970). Sociologists that studied disaster in the 1960s and 1970s talked about the importance of interventions that would support the group in its strengths and acknowledge survivorship in facing and recovering from 'what God or man has wrought'. Higgins (1994) suggested that resilience, like the term 'survivor', best captures the active process of self-righting and growth. By viewing resilience as a process in which the person experiences learned resourcefulness, a worker contributes internal strengths, which are validated by the natural honeymoon process of the group. Lyons (1991) supported this orientation in suggesting that it is imperative not to err in the opposite direction of attempting to identify pathology resulting from traumatization.

While individuals may have differing core resilient dynamic capacities, all people possess to some degree the ability to learn and grow from the traumatic experience. Lyons suggested that there are natural holding environments that promote the growth of these capacities. In order to facilitate the maximization of these capabilities, the holding environment must attend to the culture and climate that surrounds the event. Just as individual characteristics influence outcome, so too do group norms, values, interpretations and meanings that are communicated to its members. Yalom (1975) and others have long noted the impact of the group as a source of healing and recovery or of exacerbation and decline. What is done in the group has not been as widely examined, although benefits of the group for protective service personnel have been suggested

(Paton & Stephens, 1996). There is a need for research on positive holding environments after traumatic incidents, that pays attention to organizational culture and behaviour rather than turning attention to the individual as the patient.

It is important that any formal response subsequent to a traumatic event builds upon the strengths and capabilities of those affected. Most individuals who experience traumatic events are normal people, who are generally capable of functioning in an effective manner, both physically and emotionally. They have been subjected to severe stress and it is not unusual that they may show signs of emotional strain. This transitory disturbance is to be expected and does not necessarily imply mental illness or post-traumatic reaction. Few studies have sought to determine how marginally impaired and successful individuals cope with the aftermath of trauma. In fact, while the literature gives brief mention to hardiness and resilience little attention has been paid to the assessment of positive outcome from traumatic experience. One author (C.M.D.) has repeatedly heard from police officers that:

The [shooting, disaster, tornado], ... was the greatest thing that happened to me. I proved to myself that I could do it, that my training worked. I feel more confident now about my ability to respond to emergency situations. I know what I'm made of ... I've got the right stuff.

Raphael (1986) described positive findings in disaster workers after a major disaster when workers reported a feeling of greater value in life and relationships. Tedeschi & Calhoun (1995, 1996) suggested the possibility of positive impact of negative events and the potential, and possible prophylaxis, of resilient factors that can lead to posttraumatic growth (Sledge et al., 1980; Silver et al., 1983; Veronen & Kilpatrick, 1983; Thompson, 1985; Burt & Katz, 1987; Kahane, 1992). Some of the positive effects of trauma are the enhancement or reinforcement of the responder's ability to cope with adversity, development of self-discipline, and the realization of an appreciation of the value of life. Individuals experience a sense of accomplishment, competence and resilience that come as a result of the traumatic experience. Tedeschi & Calhoun (1996)

found at least three broad categories of perceived benefit that individuals have identified in connection with their traumatic experience: changes in self-perception, changes in interpersonal relationship and a changed philosophy of life.

People who have experienced exposure to horrific traumatic events have extolled the importance of consequent positive growth benefits, identification of meaning and of connection with others as salutary consequences of their sorrow (Frankl, 1959; Eitinger, 1964; Krystal, 1968; Bettleheim, 1979). It would appear that the identification of benefits and measurement of growth add significantly to the perception of meaning that survivors derive from their traumatic experience. What is significant, according to Higgins (1994), is that resilience can be cultivated, that the group can influence the individual, and that 'good company' can change the course of individual reaction from traumatic decline to traumatic growth. Ursano et al. (1986) and Sledge et al. (1980) also suggested that coping style and social cohesion can act to integrate cognitively the traumatic experience. The salutogenic effects of resilience and social perception inform us that the group can facilitate the active process of self-righting and growth. Interestingly, the Raphael (1986) Australian debriefing protocol contained many of the same positive-directed questions to be asked by the debriefer. Yet, subsequent iterations of debriefing have focussed on negative, worst case, worst outcome orientation.

Conclusions

What needs a re-examination is that which we have always known. There is a saying that there is nothing new to be learned, only the need to return to past lessons. We need to go back to the wealth of research that exists outside of that specific to trauma populations such as combat veterans, firefighters or sexual assault survivors. We need to revisit the building block of human cognition, disastrous experience, and recovery in an ecological environment. It is here that the research of A. Antonovsky and others has much to inform us and much to contribute in a hopeful appreciation of human resilience.

REFERENCES

American Psychiatric Association. (1980). *Diagnostic and Statistical Manual of Mental Disorders*, 3rd edn. Washington, DC: American Psychiatric Press.

Antonovsky, A.(1980). *Health, Stress, and Coping*. San Francisco: Jossey-Bass.

Antonovsky, A. (1988). *Unravelling the Mystery of Health: How People Manage Stress and Stay Well*. San Francisco: Jossey-Bass.

Antonovsky, A. (1990a). Pathways leading to successful coping and health. In M. Rosenbaum (Ed.) *Learned Resourcefulness: On Coping Skills, Self- Control, and Adaptive Behaviour* (pp. 31–63). New York: Springer-Verlag.

Antonovsky, A. (1990b). The salutogenic model of health. In R. Ornstein & C. Swencionis (Eds.) *The Healing Brain: A Scientific Reader* (pp. 231–43). New York: Guilford Press.

Antonovsky, A. (1991). The structural sources of salutogenic strengths, In C. Cooper & R. Payne (Eds.) *Personality and Stress: Individual Differences in the Stress Process* (pp. 67–104). London: England: John Wiley and Sons.

Bandura, A. (1977). Self-efficacy: Toward a unifying theory of behavioural change. *Psychological Review*, **84**, 191–215.

Bandura, A. (1982). Self-efficacy mechanism in human agency. *American Psychologist*, **37**, 122–47.

Bettelheim, B. (1979). *Surviving and Other Essays*. New York: Knopf.

Bisson, J. I. & Deahl, M. P. (1994). Psychological debriefing and prevention of post-traumatic stress: more research is needed. *British Journal of Psychiatry*, **165**, 717–20.

Blakemore, J. (1975). Are police allowed to have problems of their own? *Police Magazine*, March, 47–55.

Burt, M. R. & Katz, B. K. (1987). Dimensions of recovery from rape: focus on growth outcomes. *Journal of Interpersonal Violence*, **2**, 51–81.

Davidson, A. D. (1979). Air Disaster: coping with stress. *Police Stress*, 1(2), 20–2.

Deahl, M. P., Ernshaw, N. M. & Jones, N. (1994). Psychiatry and war: learning lessons from the former Yugoslavia. *British Journal of Psychiatry*, **164**, 441–2.

Dunning, C. M. (1985a). Prevention of stress in disaster workers. In American Psychological Association (Ed.) *Role Conflict and Support for Emergency Workers, National Institute for Mental Health* (pp. 126–39). Washington, DC: U.S. Government Printing Office.

Dunning, C. M. (1985b). The burden of duty and psychosocial trauma resulting from life threatening and extinguishing events. In A. D. Mangelsdorff, J. M. King & D. E. O'Brien (Eds.) *Proceedings of the Fifth Users' Workshop on Combat Stress* (pp. 32–8). Fort Sam Houston, TX: US Army Health Services Command.

Dunning, C. M. (1988). Intervention strategies for emergency workers. In M. Lystad (Ed.) *Mental Health Response to Mass Emergencies: Theory and Practice* (pp. 384–407). New York: Brunner/Mazel.

Dunning, C. M. (1990a). Mitigating the impact of work trauma: administrative issues concerning intervention in J. Reese, J. Horn & C. M. Dunning (Eds.) *Critical Incidents in Policing* (pp. 73–82). Washington, DC: US Government Printing Office.

Dunning, C. M. (1990b). Mental health sequelae in disaster workers: prevention and intervention. *International Journal of Mental Health*, **19**, 91–103.

Dunning, C. M. (1995). Fostering resiliency in rescue workers. In A. A. Kalayjian (Ed.) *Disaster and Mass Trauma: Global Perspectives on Post Disaster Mental Health Management* (pp. 174–84). Long Branch, NJ: Vista Press.

Dunning, C. M. (2000) Strategies to support performance of police officers responding to traumatic incidents. In J. Violanti, D. Paton & C. Dunning (Eds.) *Traumatic Stress Intervention: Changing Perspectives on Debriefing*. Springfield, IL: Charles C. Thomas, in press.

Dunning, C. M. & Silva, M. (1980). Disaster-induced stress in rescue workers. *Victimology: An International Journal*, **5**, 287–97.

Dynes, R. (1970). *Organised Behaviour in Disasters*. Lexington, KY: Health-Lexington.

Dyregrov, A. (1989). Caring for helpers in disaster situations: psychological debriefing. *Disaster Management*, **2**, 25–30.

Eitinger, L. (1964). *Concentration Camp Survivors in Norway and Israel*. Oslo: Universttetsfordaget.

Everstine, D. S. & Everstine, L. (1993). *The Trauma Response: Treatment for Emotional Injury*. New York: WW Norton & Co.

Frankl, V. (1959). *Man's Search for Meaning*. Boston, MA: Beacon Press.

Herman, J. (1992). *Trauma and Recovery: Aftermath of Violence from Domestic Abuse to Political Terror*. New York: Basic Books.

Higgins, G. O. (1994). *Resilient Adults: Overcoming a Cruel Past*. San Francisco: Jossey-Bass.

Hipocrates (400 BCE). 'The Oath'. Transl. F. Adams. See: http://classics.mit.edu/Hippocrates/hippooath.sum.html

Illich, I. (1977). *Disabling Professions*. London: Salem & Boyars.

Janoff-Bulman, R. (1992). *Shattered Assumptions: Toward a New Psychology of Trauma*. New York: Free Press.

Kahane, B. (1992). Late life adaptation in the aftermath of extreme stress. In M. Wykel, E. Kahane & J. Koval (Eds.) *Stress and Health among the Elderly* (pp. 151–71). New York: Springer- Verlag.

Kenardy, J. A., Webster, R. A., Lewin, J. J., Carr, V. J., Hazell, P. L. & Carter, G. L. (1996). Stress debriefing and patterns of recovery following a natural disaster. *Journal of Traumatic Stress*, **9**, 37–49.

Kobasa, S. C. (1979). Stressful life events, personality, and health: an inquiry into hardiness. *Journal of Personality and Social Psychology*, **37**, 1–11.

Kobasa, S. C. (1982). Commitment and coping in stress resistance among lawyers. *Journal of Personality and Social Psychology*, **37**, 1–11.

Kobasa, S. C., Maddi, S. R., Puccetti, M. C. & Zola, M. A. (1985). Effectiveness of hardiness, exercise and social support as resources against illness. *Journal of Psychosomatic Research*, **29**, 525–53.

Koval, S. (1987). Midwest Flight 151: trauma and rescuers. MA thesis, Cardinal Stritch University.

Kroes, W. & Hurrell, J. Jr (1975). *Job Stress and the Police Officer – Identifying Stress Reduction Techniques*. Washington, DC: US Government Printing Office.

Krystal, H. (1968). *Psychic Traumatizations*. New York: International Universities Press.

Lazovik, J. (1995). Remembering how to stay well: a regenerative tool for counselling centre staff. *Journal of College Student Psychotherapy*, **9**(4), 57–77.

Lyons, J. A. (1991). Strategies for assessing the potential for positive readjustment following trauma. *Journal of Traumatic Stress*, **4**, 93–112.

Lyubomirsky, S. & Nolen-Hoeksema, S. (1993). Self-perpetuating properties of dysphoric rumination. *Journal of Personality and Social Psychology*, **65**, 339–49.

Lyubomirsky, S. & Nolen-Hoeksema, S. (1995). Effects of self-focused rumination on negative thinking and interpersonal problem solving. *Journal of Personality and Social Psychology*, **69**, 176–89.

Mantell, M. (1986). When the badge turns blue: the San Ysidro massacre. In H. Goldstein, J. Reese & J. Horn (Eds.) *Psychological Services for Law Enforcement* (pp. 357–60). Washington, DC: US Government Press.

Marmar, C. R., Weiss, D. S., Metzler, T. J., Ronfeldt, H. M. & Foreman, C. (1996). Stress responses of emergency services personnel to the Loma Prieta earthquake Interstate 880 freeway collapse and control of traumatic incidents. *Journal of Traumatic Stress*, **9**, 63–85.

Mitchell, J. T. (1983). When disaster strikes: the critical incident stress debriefing process. *Journal of Emergency Medical Services*, **8**, 35–9.

Mitchell, J. T. (1988). The history, status and future of critical incident stress debriefings. *Journal of Emergency Medical Services*, **13**, 49–52.

Mitchell, J. T. & Bray, G. (1990). *Emergency Services Stress*. Upper Saddle River, NJ: Prentice-Hall.

Mitchell, J. T. & Everly, G. S. (1993). *Critical Incident Stress Debriefing: An Operations Manual for the Prevention of Traumatic Stress Among Emergency Service Workers*. Ellicott City, MD: Chevron Publishing.

Paton, D. & Stephens, C. (1996). Training and support for emergency responders. In D. Paton & J. Violanti (Eds.) *Traumatic Stress in Critical Occupations: Recognition, Consequences and Treatment* (pp. 173–205). Springfield, IL: Charles C. Thomas.

Paton, D. & Violanti, J. M. (Eds.) (1996). *Traumatic Stress in Critical Occupations: Recognition, Consequences and Treatment*. Springfield, IL: Charles C. Thomas.

Raphael, B. (1986). *When Disaster Strikes: How Individuals and Communities Cope with Catastrophe*. New York: Basic Books.

Raphael, B., Meldrum, L. & McFarlane, A. C. (1995). Does debriefing after psychological trauma work? *British Medical Journal*, **310**, 1479–80.

Roberts, M. (1975). *Debriefing and Peer Counselling of Police Officers Subsequent to Shootings and Crises*, FBI Training Key. Washington, DC: FBI.

Rotter, J. B. (1966). Generalised expectancies for internal versus external locus of control of reinforcement. *Psychological Monographs*, **80**, 1–28.

Samter, J., Fitzgerald, M., Braudaway, C., Leeks, D., Padgett, C., Swartz, A., Gary-Stephens, M. & Dellinger, N. (1993). Debriefing: from military origin to therapeutic application. *Journal of Psychosocial Nursing*, **31**, 23–7.

Silver, R. L., Boon, C. & Stoves, M. (1983). Searching for meaning in misfortune: making sense of incest. *Journal of Social Issues*, **39**, 81–102.

Sledge, W. H., Boydstun, J. A. & Rahe, A. J. (1980). Self-concept changes related to war captivity. *Archives of General Psychiatry*, **37**, 430–43.

Staver, S. (1979). Victim's relatives ignored M.D. claims. *American Medical News*, **15**, 7–8.

Stuhlmiller, C. M. (1992). An interpretive study of appraisal and coping of rescue workers in an earthquake disaster: the Cypress collapse. Ph.D. thesis. University of California, San Francisco.

Stuhlmiller, C. M. (1994a). Rescuers of Cypress: work meanings and practices that guided appraisal and coping. *Western Journal of Nursing Research*, **16**, 268–87.

Stuhlmiller, C. M. (1994b). Narrative methodology in disaster studies: rescuers of Cypress. In P. Benner (Ed.) *Interpretive Phenomenology: Embodiment, Caring and Ethics in Health and Illness* (pp. 323–49). Thousand Oaks, CA: Sage Publications.

Stuhlmiller, C. M. (1995). The construction of disorders: exploring the growth of PTSD and SAD. *Journal of Psychosocial Nursing and Mental Health Services*, **33**, 20–3.

Stuhlmiller, C. M. (1996a). *Rescuers of Cypress: Learning from Disaster*. Book no. 2 of the International Health Care Ethics Series. New York: Peter Lang Publishing.

Stuhlmiller, C. M. (1996b). Studying the rescuers. *Sigma Theta Tau International Reflections*, **22**(6), 18–19.

Taylor, S. E. (1983). Adjustment to threatening life events: a theory of cognitive adaptation. *American Psychologist*, **38**, 1161–73.

Taylor, S. E. (1989). *Positive Illusions: Creative Deception and the Healthy Mind*. New York: Basic Books.

Tedeschi, R. G. & Calhoun, L. G. (1995). *Trauma and Transformation: Growing in the Aftermath of Suffering*. Thousand Oaks, CA, Sage.

Tedeschi, R. & Calhoun, L. (1996). Posttraumatic growth inventory: measuring the positive legacy of trauma. *Journal of Traumatic Stress*, **9**, 455–71.

Tedeschi, R., Park, C. & Calhoun, L. (Eds.) (1998). *Posttraumatic Growth: Positive Change in the Aftermath of Crisis*. New York: Lawrence Erlbaum.

Tehrani, N. & Westlake, R. (1994). Debriefing individuals affected by violence. *Counselling Psychology Quarterly*, **7**, 251–9.

Thompson, S. C. (1985). Finding positive meaning in a stressful event and coping. *Basic Applied Social Psychology*, **6**, 279–95.

Ursano, R. J., Wheatley, R., Sledge, W., Rahe, A. & Carlsen, E. (1986). Coping and recovery styles in the Vietnam era prisoner of war. *Journal of Nervous and Mental Disease*, **174**, 707–14.

Veronen, L. J. & Kilpatrick, D. G. (1983). Rape: a precursor to change. In E. Callahan & K. McCluskey (Eds.) *Lifespan Development Psychology: Non-normative Life Events* (pp. 167–91). New York: Academic Press.

Violanti, J. M. (1996). Trauma stress and police work. In D. Paton & J. M. Violanti (Eds.) *Traumatic Stress in Critical Occupations: Recognition, Consequences, and Treatment* (pp. 88–96). Springfield, IL: Charles C. Thomas.

Wagner, M. (1979). Stress debriefing: Flight 191. *Chicago Police Star*, August, 4–7.

Wagner, M. (1981a). Airline disaster: aA stress debrief program for police. *Police Stress Magazine*, **2**, 16–19.

Wagner, M. (1981b). Trauma counselling and law enforcement. In R. Thomlinson (Ed.) *Perspectives on Industrial Social Work Practice* (pp. 133–9). Ottawa, Canada: Family Service Canada.

Yalom, I. (1975). *The Theory and Practice of Group Psychotherapy*, 2nd edn. New York: Basic Books.

Yehuda, R. (1998). *Psychological Trauma*. Washington, DC: American Psychiatric Press.

Yehuda, R. & McFarlane, A. (1997). *Psychobiology of Posttraumatic Stress Disorder. Annals of the New York Academy of Sciences*, **821**.

23

Is consensus about debriefing possible?

Philip L. P. Morris

EDITORIAL COMMENTS

This chapter is a brief presentation of an attempt to attain consensus on some key questions in the field of debriefing, derived from a consensus conference held in 1996 in Australia. What becomes very clear is that even with those supportive of debriefing and those critical of it working together personally, there was extreme difficulty in gaining agreement on common issues. The result might be suggested to be a general and perhaps polite recognition of the other points of view, but nevertheless a strong commitment to the original respective beliefs.

While this specific consensus meeting was held some years ago the themes of difficulty in reaching agreement are reflected in more recent debates and in this book. The same proponents are profoundly committed, despite a growing body of scientific evidence questioning benefits. The International Society for Traumatic Stress Studies has also recently addressed the need for a stronger evidence base and is developing Evidence Based Guidelines. Nevertheless, the belief that something must be done and the need to give this a structure make it difficult to challenge the commitment to debriefing. Thus moving to a consensus continues to be difficult.

This book shows that there has been some movement, particularly in the fields of establishing a stronger scientific base for both points of view. Nevertheless, the widespread and often uncritical usage of debriefing models by those who may have little training and experience with respect to the situations in which they apply their techniques must call for major concern – first, do no harm.

In the absence of demonstrated effectiveness for wide population use it is perhaps safest to consider the application of debriefing only in the contexts for which it was originally developed: for stress (not psychological trauma) in emergency service workers. There appears little scientific justification of its use more widely, but some cause for concern. Because it represents a humane and caring response in situations of acute distress, most workers are keen to retain it. Perhaps its utility as a supportive measure can be justified, but even with emergency workforces there is a need, as identified by all workers in this field, for further research, and indeed a growing body of negative findings.

Introduction

On 22 October 1996, the Australian National Centre for War-related Post Traumatic Stress Disorder held a conference at its Melbourne offices entitled 'Debriefing Consensus Forum'. The Debriefing Consensus Forum brought together senior Australasian academics, practitioners and researchers to discuss traumatic stress debriefing. A wide range of views were sought and the forum included participants who were strong advocates of debriefing as well as those who were critical of the intervention.

The National Centre for War-related Post Traumatic Stress Disorder is a collaborative project of the Department of Veterans' Affairs, the University of Melbourne and the Austin and Repatriation Medical Centre. One of the National Centre's roles is to advance knowledge about prevention of post-traumatic stress disorder (PTSD) and to inform the professional and veteran communities about new interventions for the treatment of traumatic stress disorders. With these objectives in mind, the National Centre sought to use the Debriefing Consensus Forum as a method of focussing expert opinion on the role of debriefing as an intervention for traumatic stress. The timing of the Consensus Forum was topical for two reasons. First, the then recent publication of articles critical of debriefing by Raphael et al. (1995) and Bisson & Deahl (1994) had provoked much discussion among interested professionals about this technique. Secondly, the presence in Australia of Professor Arieh Shalev as the first visiting professor at the National Centre provided an opportunity for the National Centre to use an external overseas consultant as a participant in the forum.

Providing debriefing to those who have experienced or witnessed a traumatic incident remains a controversial issue for mental health professionals. However, in the general community (and in legal circles), debriefing appears to have become an expected response to traumatic exposure and is frequently perceived as the responsibility of the employer when traumatic incidents occur in the workplace. The extent to which debriefing has become a routine response to traumatic incidents is a testament to the effectiveness of the protagonists of debriefing in Australasia. But this situation ignores the problem of scientific credibility of the technique, particularly its effectiveness. The very nature of what are the core elements of debriefing is questioned, the appropriateness of its use as a response to traumatic stress is debated, and evidence of its effectiveness in either improving adjustment of individuals to traumatic incidents or preventing psychiatric sequelae is seriously doubted.

In order to provide some discussion of the controversies surrounding debriefing, the National Centre conducted the Debriefing Consensus Forum. The Forum had two main objectives. The first was to discuss a number of key questions about debriefing:

1. What are the key elements that characterize debriefing?

2. For what types of traumatic incident is debriefing appropriate?
3. What individuals or populations should be offered debriefing?
4. What training and accreditation should those who carry out debriefing have?
5. What outcomes can be expected from debriefing?
6. Is there evidence to support the use of debriefing?
7. In what way can knowledge about debriefing be advanced?

The second objective was to identify whether any common ground could be established about these questions. In other words, could consensus be reached about answers to these issues and, if not, could an agreed approach be recommended to resolve outstanding problems. Although a consensus view was an objective of the Forum, it was appreciated that full agreement about all these questions was unlikely. However, establishing some agreed positions and identifying unresolved issues was considered an important task.

Each of the invited participants made a brief, formal presentation to the forum. Each presentation was followed by questions and later in the day the forum moved into a plenary discussion of the main questions. While much fruitful dialogue resulted from this debate and many issues were clarified, it was clear that the Forum could not reach a final consensus view about debriefing. The issues dividing the protagonists of debriefing from those who were more critical remained, but the distance between these two viewpoints narrowed substantially. Perhaps the best way to illustrate this movement of views is to discuss each of the Forum questions in terms of what was agreed by most participants and what remained contentious or unresolved.

1. What are the key elements that characterize debriefing?

Most participants considered that the Mitchell (1983) model of debriefing, later termed 'psychological debriefing' by Dyregrov (1989), was the one that had the widest currency and was the prototype debriefing intervention. The agreed key elements of debriefing were that it is usually a group intervention, it is confidential, it occurs soon after a traumatic event, it is led by one or more trained counsellors, and it involves the sharing of emotions, the teaching of coping skills and the validation of individual experiences among those who share a similar exposure. It also provides an opportunity for identification of subjects at risk, it allows for the evaluation of stress reactions and it provides information about traumatic stress responses. Key elements of debriefing that were thought to be important but had not been given much emphasis so far were the qualities of the debriefer such as his or her acceptance by the group, empathy, genuineness and the ability to facilitate group cohesiveness. It was agreed that the seven-stage Mitchell model is a confrontational technique in that it encourages participants to process the traumatic experience through an emotional review. The necessity of having a confrontational element as a core component of the technique was challenged by some participants. A nonconfrontational approach to debriefing (termed 'supportive debriefing') was proposed that included many of the other elements of the Mitchell model. This alternative model of debriefing might be appropriate for most situations to which debriefing is applied currently and could be extended to populations of traumatized individuals or survivors. This proposal was discussed briefly but a consensus position was not reached. Participants agreed that the literature was notable for an absence of empirical studies relevant to identifying the key components of debriefing and determining what elements of debriefing are responsible for positive (or negative) outcomes. These issues need to be addressed in further work.

2. For what types of traumatic incident is debriefing appropriate?

There was general agreement that the traumatic stressors for which debriefing might be appropriate would be those that fall within the description of the *Diagnostic and Statistical Manual of Mental Disorders* (DSM-IV; American Psychiatric Association, 1994) definition of trauma (criterion A) for PTSD. While there was consensus about the appropriateness of debriefing for the more severe stressors, the role of debriefing for less

distressing traumatic incidents that might be expected in everyday life (such as bereavement or miscarriage) remained unresolved. One of the participants drew the distinction between critical incident stress (experienced as part of the job by emergency service workers) and traumatic stress (unexpected, disaster-type events). It was proposed that debriefing would be best limited to critical incident stress rather than traumatic stress situations. However, consensus was not reached on this issue. It was agreed that the types of critical incident that might be most appropriate for debriefing have not been well canvassed in the literature.

3. What individuals or populations should be offered debriefing?

On this question there was a consensus that debriefing is most applicable for emergency service workers, police and defence force personnel who have experienced critical incident stress in the line of duty. There was some agreement that debriefing might be appropriate for medical teams, welfare workers and other groups assisting the primary victims (or survivors) of disasters. Agreement was not reached as to whether debriefing had a role in the management of primary or secondary victims of traumatic incidents. The role of debriefing in children is controversial. Many participants felt that unmodified use of the Mitchell model for children is inappropriate. There seem to be virtually no data from which to judge the effectiveness of debriefing for children.

4. What training and accreditation should those who carry out debriefing have?

There was a consensus view that those conducting debriefing should be knowledgeable and skilled mental health professionals. Participants agreed that outside of the emergency service organizations, police and defence forces, the training and experience of debriefers was often inconsistent and inadequate. Many Forum participants called for a uniform training programme for debriefers. There was agreement that debriefers need not only to be well trained but also to have experience in the application of this technique in the field.

The need for uniform standards of training, supervision and experience highlighted the need for some form of accreditation. This issue was not discussed in detail but the question of whether there should be one national body for accreditation or whether accreditation should be the responsibility of professional associations remained unresolved.

5. What outcomes can be expected from debriefing?

One of the more obvious disagreements between participants was the question of what can be expected of debriefing. Debriefing was originally intended as a preventive measure for individuals exposed to critical incidents. A reduction in short- and long-term adverse outcomes (e.g. days off work or the incidence of PTSD) might then be expected. However, over time the expected outcomes of debriefing have changed; now many practitioners of the technique see it as a brief therapeutic tool designed to help to validate feelings, confront inappropriate responsibility/guilt, normalize stress reactions and integrate the traumatic event, rather than to prevent complications. This dual view of outcome was reflected among forum participants. Those supportive of debriefing expected it to help to facilitate general adjustment to traumatic incidents rather than prevent psychiatric or other adverse outcomes, whereas participants more critical of debriefing expected it to have some preventive effects.

There was general agreement that the brief nature of debriefing and its timing so soon after the traumatic incident was unlikely to produce a substantial effect on the long-term consequences of traumatic exposure. The prevention of PTSD and other trauma-related psychiatric disorders was thought unlikely as a result of debriefing. This viewpoint has implications for current medico-legal practice.

Although debriefing may have little effect on long-term psychological consequences of traumatic exposure, it may have an effect on short-term outcomes. These outcomes could include improved morale in the workforce, reduced levels of subjective distress, improved workplace and team cohesion, the mobilization of social supports, decreased days off work, improved productivity and less use of medical services. The protagonists of debriefing claimed that there was evidence for these short-term benefits but other forum participants were not as convinced. This issue remained unresolved.

6. Is there evidence to support the use of debriefing?

The absence of evidence supporting the effectiveness of debriefing from randomized controlled studies was acknowledged by all participants. This was regarded as a major weakness in the literature on debriefing and needs to be corrected. The protagonists of debriefing thought that anecdotal evidence and uncontrolled studies provided substantial evidence of a positive role for debriefing, particularly on short-term outcomes. These participants criticized studies showing no effects or possibly deleterious effects of debriefing, as being methodologically flawed on a number of counts. These flaws included inadequate description of the debriefing technique, inappropriate use of debriefing in situations that it was not designed for, debriefers who lacked appropriate training and experience, and uncontrolled study designs.

Those participants critical of debriefing were less impressed by the anecdotal and uncontrolled study data and raised the point that some studies suggest that debriefing might be harmful. Participants critical of debriefing proposed that this intervention should be abandoned, particularly for primary and secondary victims of traumatic incidents, until clear evidence of effectiveness is available from randomized controlled studies.

Other participants held opinions that were somewhere between these two viewpoints. Clearly consensus was not reached on the question of whether there was enough evidence to support the practice of debriefing.

As a postscript it is worth noting that three randomized controlled studies of debriefing have been published since the Debriefing Consensus Forum. In these three studies (Hobbs et al., 1996; Lee et al., 1996; Bisson et al., 1997) the Mitchell model was used for individual or couple debriefing but not in a group setting. In none of these studies did debriefing have a beneficial effect on short-term (three to four months) or long-term outcome. In two studies (Hobbs et al., 1996; Bisson et al. 1997) the intervention group fared worse. A recent systematic review of published randomized controlled studies of brief early psychological interventions following trauma (Rose & Bisson, 1998) identified only six studies, of which two showed positive effects, two were neutral and two showed negative outcomes. The two positive studies were early ones in Australia (Bordow & Porritt, 1979; Bunn & Clarke, 1979) before the Mitchell model of debriefing was published. This review concluded that there was little evidence for the utility of debriefing and further trials of group debriefing are needed.

7. In what way can knowledge about debriefing be advanced?

Participants agreed that the promise of debriefing as a potential preventive intervention in mental health should not be abandoned, despite the limitations and inconsistency of the evidence supporting its effectiveness. The consensus view was that further work should be undertaken to explore the role of debriefing in more specific ways. Studies directed at examining the most appropriate populations that need to be debriefed, the parts of the debriefing technique that are most effective, the types of traumatic incident that are most appropriate for debriefing, the immediate, early and late effects of debriefing, the personal qualities and skill of the debriefer, and the effect of training and experience of debriefers on outcome should be commissioned as a matter of urgency. The application of debriefing techniques at different times following trauma exposure should be studied in order to determine whether there are critical periods where interventions may be most effective. Controlled and randomized studies must have a high priority. One view (not a consensus) put forward at the Forum was that, until we are better informed, debriefing should be confined to use within emergency services organizations, police and defence forces. It is imperative that these organizations place an emphasis on quality control of the technique and the assessment of short-term effects of the intervention.

The role of debriefing for other trauma-exposed populations was not resolved at the Forum.

Summary

The Debriefing Consensus Forum was conducted by the National Centre to provide an opportunity to discuss controversies surrounding debriefing and to see whether consensus could be reached on some of the key questions concerning this intervention. The meeting canvassed many viewpoints and provided a setting for a robust discussion of the role of debriefing. A number of issues were clarified and agreement was reached on some basic understandings of the key elements of debriefing, situations and populations where it could be applied, and the need for training of debriefers. Unfortunately, a number of areas remained where consensus was not achieved. These issues included accreditation of debriefers, what outcomes can be expected from debriefing and evidence for its effectiveness. It is disappointing that, after 13 years since the introduction of critical incident stress debriefing, so much remains unknown about this intervention. More positively, the Forum highlighted the need for further research and suggested how future studies could make useful contributions to knowledge about debriefing.

Acknowledgements

I would like to acknowledge the valuable assistance of Professor Beverly Raphael, co-chair of the Consensus Forum, and the staff of the National Centre who were responsible for organizing the meeting.

REFERENCES

American Psychiatric Association (1994). *Diagnostic and Statistical Manual of Mental Disorders*, 4th edn. Washington, DC: American Psychiatric Press.

Bisson, J. & Deahl, M. (1994). Psychological debriefing and prevention of post-traumatic stress. More research is needed. *British Journal of Psychiatry*, **165**, 717–20.

Bisson, J. I., Jenkins, P. L., Alexander, J. & Bamister, C. (1997). Randomised controlled trial of psychological debriefing for victims of acute burn trauma. *British Journal of Psychiatry*, **171**, 78–81.

Bordow, S. & Porritt, D. (1979). An experimental evaluation of crisis intervention. *Social Science and Medicine*, **13a**, 251–6.

Bunn, T. & Clarke, A. (1979). Crisis intervention: an experimental study of the effects of a brief period of counselling on the anxiety of relatives of seriously injured or ill hospital patients. *British Journal of Medical Psychology*, **52**, 191–5.

Dyregrov, A. (1989). Caring for helpers in disaster situations: psychological debriefing. *Disaster Management*, **2**, 25–9.

Hobbs, M., Mayou, R., Harrison, B. & Worlock, P. (1996). A randomised controlled trial of psychological debriefing for victims of road traffic accidents. *British Medical Journal*, **313**, 1438–9.

Lee, C., Slade, P. & Lygo, V. (1996). The influence of psychological debriefing on emotional adaptation in females following early miscarriage. *British Journal of Medical Psychology*, **69**, 47–58.

Mitchell, J. T. (1983). When disaster strikes . . . the critical incident debriefing process. *Journal of the Emergency Medical Services*, **8**, 36–9.

Raphael B., Meldrum, L. & McFarlane, A.C. (1995). Does debriefing after psychological trauma work? Time for randomised controlled trials. *British Medical Journal*, **310**, 1479–80.

Rose, S. & Bisson, J. (1998) Brief early psychological interventions following trauma: a systematic review of the literature. *Journal of Traumatic Stress*, **11**, 697–710.

24

Can debriefing work? Critical appraisal of theories of interventions and outcomes, with directions for future research

Alexander McFarlane

EDITORIAL COMMENTS

This chapter draws together historical, social and psychotherapeutic strands as they contribute to the background of debriefing and its evolution. Its relation to military psychiatry, crisis intervention, narrative tradition, psychoeducation, grief counselling, group psychotherapy, behavioural and cognitive therapies, and psychopharmacology are touched upon and their implications for an 'eclectic model' considered.

McFarlane provides a framework for synthesis but one where the reader will be called upon to expand and explore underlying detail. Possible theoretical bases for the effects of debriefing, either positive or negative, are explored. Of particular interest is the view that the acute response period may be more amenable to pharmacological than to psychological interventions.

The lack of good outcome data on debriefing, both through the difficulties of researching this type of intervention or indeed ensuring its fidelity, lead to the important emphasis on the need for further research. As McFarlane suggests, this may require a previously developed set of instruments, an on-line funding source and an international consortium to answer the questions that must be addressed about the effects of this type of intervention. This is the more so with the recent *Cochrane Review*, as well as other studies that indicate few findings of benefit and some concern over potential for negative outcomes. Furthermore, financial, legal and occupational health and safety requirements may place demands for the provision of debriefing with the belief that it will lessen costs and workforce damage. The fact that debriefing may not be provided either with integrity or effectiveness, by suitably qualified and skilled persons, may mean that the potential to harm is greatly heightened. While clinical guidelines can be helpful, in the absence of evidence as to what is effective and best practice, there is potential for widespread use of interventions which may potentially adversely affect some of those for whom they are provided. At the same time, there is a profound socially driven expectation that everyone must be debriefed after any potentially traumatic experience. The importance of bringing quality control, research and evaluation into the debriefing movement is emphasized, as well as the need for caution – for 'first, do no harm' in the urgency of the wish to help others and assuage their suffering.

McFarlane concludes that there is a 'need to work cooperatively and tolerate uncertainty rather than seeking definitive answers in polemics'.

Introduction

The desire to rescue, protect and save those in danger must be one of the most powerful human motivations. This sense of group survival is critical to the motivation of health professionals. Perhaps one of the most alluring opportunities is the field of trauma where there is an imperative to prevent and minimize chronic post-traumatic reactions. In contrast to many areas of mental health, there appears to be an unusual opportunity to prevent the onset and relapsing course associated with many psychological disorders. This chapter discusses the theoretical basis and the origins of this work.

This is a challenging task because often clinical practice has been driven by the immediacy of the imperative to help, rather than the development of the sophisticated theory that is being carefully trialled for its widespread implementation.

In many ways, acute preventive interventions have been as much social movements as interventions driven out of progressive refinement in clinical practice.

The issue of moral and social attitudes to trauma survivors

Acute preventive interventions can be implemented only if there is a broad acceptance of a notion of collective responsibility and the value of group survival of caring for such individuals. Examination of the effects of trauma is not a neutral issue either at the individual or societal level. It reflects a core concern that drives many social and political ideals: to what extent should an individual be responsible for his or her own destiny?

Do we have the right to attribute our predicament to others or do we have to live with our suffering and not expect any particular dispensation from our pain? Societies that become too focussed on their trauma may fail to focus on the future. Thus, while the traumatized individual may benefit from recognition of his or her suffering, society as a whole may be depleted when it becomes centred on blame, rather than endurance and individual responsibility. This has led to often dichotomized views about the effects of trauma. On one side, there is the idea that traumatic events in themselves are not particularly toxic. Rather, it is that they lead to the manifestations of an individual's vulnerability.

The inner tensions associated with this dilemma are particularly important to emergency service organizations and the military. Acute preventive interventions become a realistic option only if the general culture of these organizations recognizes that there is a broad responsibility and benefit for addressing the nature of fear and horror and its capacity to disrupt the functioning of even the bravest individuals. The greatest military minds were generally accepting of these views. For example, according to Lady Frances Shelley, the Duke of Wellington said 'Next to a battle lost, the greatest misery is a battle gained'.

Acute preventive interventions are only realistic options when there is a genuine understanding of these issues in the broader social structures. Hence the effectiveness and theoretical underpinning of acute treatment and debriefing is critically dependent upon the general systems of leadership and the management of morale. It entails an essential series of beliefs about the dignity of the individual and his or her importance to the broader social group.

Organizations that escape high levels of psychological trauma frequently turn the issue of causation into one of predisposition.

Prolonged military struggles such as World Wars I and II have tended to slowly undo these prejudices. It is in these settings of recognizing the impact of prolonged combat that the culture emerges that allows the implementation of acute interventions.

This has a broader relevance because leadership structures that allow and encourage these concepts also permit a vocabulary of fear manifest in training and a variety of other organizational structures. For example, the two armies, namely the German and Russian armies, that continued to have high rates of conversion disorders in World War II are those that treated soldiers with acute combat stress disorders extremely harshly (R. Ball, personal communication). This included execution, as well as putting these soldiers in special troop battalions to lead assaults.

The theoretical origins of debriefing come from a variety of sources. The most pragmatic routes are from the management of acute combat stress disorders, a school of treatment that emerged in World War I and then was rediscovered in World War II. The proximity, immediacy and expectancy (PIE) model is based on three principles (Solomon & Bebenishty, 1986). The first is proximity, where any stress casualties should be treated in a familiar but safe environment that is not unduly medicalized. Thus the normal routines of the service organization in which the individual works are maintained albeit in a supportive environment.

The concept of immediacy is that the intervention should be applied in the immediate aftermath of the traumatic event. This prevented the pattern of maladaptation from becoming an established pattern. The benefits of this approach have been demonstrated in a number of settings but perhaps most objectively in the Israeli military services at the time of the Lebanon war. The outcome of these soldiers was compared with a group who were withdrawn from the front and treated more in a hospital-based setting. There was both a significantly better return to the fighting force as well as lower rates of chronic post-traumatic stress disorder (PTSD) in the group treated in the forward positions. However, it is important to state that over 50% in the longer-term developed a PTSD (Solomon & Bebenishty, 1986).

This emphasizes that while this method of intervention is highly effective at returning people to immediate functioning, it does not prevent the longer-term development of PTSDs. In many ways, the aim of the use of the PIE model for acute interventions is slightly different from that for which these interventions were developed. That is to say, the demonstrated value is in returning to immediate function rather than having a substantially more preventive effect.

The narrative tradition

One of the traditions of debriefing also grew out of the work of the American historian Brigadier General S. L. A. Marshall (Shalev & Ursano, 1990; Shalev, Chapter 1). His work represented a major shift in developing an understanding of how men behave in the face of fear. It was progressively realized that men did not fight in battles according to the rules of military tactics, but that behaviour in battle could be better understood by understanding human behaviour.

Marshall believed that obtaining personal accounts was critical to truly recording the events of what occurred in combat. Marshall was the leading historian of the European theatre of World War II (Keegan, 1991).

He employed a methodology where he would interview combat platoons for long periods of time, up to seven hours, to ascertain the events of a day in combat. He argued that the capacity of an Army to fight effectively depends upon it fostering quite close attachments amongst its soldiers. It would be then that they would be fighting as a group of friends. He states, 'When a soldier is ... known to the men around him, he ... has reason to fear losing the one thing he is likely to

value more than his life – his reputation as a man among other men'. The outcome of Marshall's work was to persuade the American army that its structure was inappropriate to the task. His work led to the creation of small groups of 'fire teams' centred on a natural fighter.

He noticed that the consequence of deciphering the events of battle appeared to have a beneficial effect on the well-being of the troops. In a sense, his exploration of the events of battle gave the troops an opportunity to develop a narrative, or internal verbal representation of the experience. Individual soldiers had little understanding of the pattern of events that had surrounded their platoon. It was only when this process occurred in the group that they began to have some realistic verbal representation of their combat. This is what appeared to provide them with the opportunity to organize their emotional reactions to the situation.

The aim of this process was not one of catharsis, but more that of documentation. This indirect origin of the idea that debriefing has much to do with the maintenance of group function is seldom recognized.

Group psychotherapy

Another paradigm employed in the critical incident debriefing model is that of group psychotherapy. The differences between the use of individual and group approaches for trauma victims have not been the focus of any extensive discussion. This is an issue of some interest because attachment behaviours are critical to the soothing of an individual's distress responses after traumatic events (van der Kolk & McFarlane, 1996). One only has to look at photographs or television footage of communities that have been devastated by a traumatic event to see the huddling together of the survivors, often in close physical contact. The need to be held, and to be close to friends and relatives is an instinctive reaction at times of threat and loss (Green & Solomon, 1995). The desire to be with one's family is a prime motivator of much disaster behaviour and not infrequently leads to death because people put themselves in needless danger simply to return to where family members are. Lindy et al. (1983) has spoken of the 'trauma membrane' that forms around the community involved in disaster. This speaks of an in-ward recognition of people who have suffered similarly. These principles are central to the use of group intervention, which uses the therapeutic forces within the group and constructive support and interaction to modify and heal people's reactions.

Group psychotherapy in England was introduced because of the pressure to treat large numbers of soldiers who were traumatized during World War II. One of the main advocates was W. R. Bion (1961, cited by Sadock, 1975), who interestingly had served in the tank corps in World War I (Main, 1989). He had a high degree of combat exposure and was decorated for his bravery. His autobiography is remarkable for its lack of introspection, considering that he became a psychotherapist. However, his life in the military seems to have been an important factor influencing his notion that the group had its own mental life. He spoke of there being two primary dynamics within a group: the work and maintenance functions. He suggested that the group should be worked with as a whole rather than that there should be a focus on the individual.

One can see the relevance of these ideas, particularly in the context of Marshall's ideas of attempting to support members of emergency services or groups who have been through similar traumatic experiences. The adaptive outcome of the group is the primary aim rather than the focus on individuals.

Crisis intervention

The legacies of military psychiatry are often forgotten. Social psychiatry as a discipline owes much to the training and experience gained by a generation of mental health professionals who served in the armed services in World War II. This led to a rapid growth of social psychiatry, with a particular focus on the role of life events as a cause of psychiatric illness. The accompanying arm of intervention was crisis intervention championed by G. Caplan (1964, cited by Zusman, 1975) and E. Lindemann (1944, cited by Zusman, 1975). The essence of crisis intervention is that a clear precipitant exists and that the individual's distress is clear. It attempts to remove such distress from the

domain of illness and presumes that the patient has experienced an offence that has caused this disequilibrium because of its suddenness; it has not allowed the individual time to master his or her emotional response. The essence of the intervention is that the temporary support of the mental health professional will bring about mastery. It is a model of intervention based on the premise that the event is over and the symptoms exhibited by the patient are no longer appropriate. The therapist provides a reorganizing influence that assists the individual who is feeling overwhelmed. The critical dimension is to assist the person in re-establishing rational problem solving. It should be recognized that this is the same approach as is used in other psychiatric emergencies (Fauman, 1995).

There are two particular perspectives that a therapist must bring. First, the patient probably will not have had an opportunity to discuss the breadth of response and sense of distress about the experience and particularly the less acceptable reactions that may have provoked feelings of guilt. Secondly, discussion of these events frequently arouses anger associated with a sense of abandonment. The therapist can become the object of these feelings which more appropriately have their origin in the event. This can be used as in other forms of brief psychotherapy to assist the working through of this conflict.

Grief counselling

The concepts of crisis intervention rapidly extended into the management of the bereaved. Bereavement was used as a model for depression. Lindemann's (1944) work after the Coconut Nightclub fire in Boston, Massachusetts, led to an investigation both of the stages of grief and the interventions that could be successful. Progressively, grief counselling grew away from crisis intervention as a separate discipline. Raphael's (1977) work with widows at high risk of negative outcomes from bereavement highlighted the value of interventions in this context. These therapies included: an educational component aimed at normalizing the feelings and behaviours associated with grief; and the importance of expression of the range of complex emotions associated with loss, often assisted by visiting memorials and possessions of the dead person. The relationship with the deceased had to be focussed on to allow the development of the individual's new sense of identity and integrated self-image.

Singh & Raphael (1981) used this approach to assist the bereaved following the Granville train disaster in Australia. This led them to advocate the importance of acute interventions and support after disasters.

Behavioural/cognitive therapies

Although behaviour therapy is largely a clinical practice of the last half of the twentieth century, the principles were well understood in the first half of the century, but behaviour therapy has only become widely used in clinical practice since the 1960s. Two aspects have contributed to debriefing (Kaplan & Sadock, 1995). First, the idea of desensitization is an explicit rationale for minimizing avoidance, particularly in the immediate aftermath of traumatic experiences. The exploration of the cognitive schemas associated with traumatic memories is a further contribution that this field has made. The role of cognitive behaviour therapy in PTSD has emerged with roughly the same time frame as preventive interventions. This is not, therefore, an area of clinical practice that has had a major theoretical impact. However, the idea of manualized treatments is one that was brought to psychotherapy research by behaviour therapy. Manualized debriefings have become an important component of this field.

Psychoeducation

In many respects, debriefing is a form of psychoeducation. This is an important component of many cognitive-behavioural treatments. It raises the question of the extent to which treatments of psychological trauma owe their treatment effects to nonspecific factors. There is little doubt that giving traumatized individuals a psychological map from which to understand their reactions does much to contain their distress and to allow them to institute a series of self-regulatory processes.

Psychopharmacology

The use of alcohol is one of the oldest methods of self-regulation and its abuse by soldiers has a long historical record. Also, many disaster victims resort to a range of sedatives to assist in the modulation of their distress and sleep disturbance. There are no published studies of prescribed psychotropic drugs and their use to control acute distress. However, there is an established clinical practice for using medications based on clinicians conceptualization of the nature of the acute stress response. The healing qualities of sleep have a long tradition in medicine. There is also the experimentation with drugs in combat settings to assist soldiers to cope with fear. These drugs have been both of a prescribed and nonprescribed nature. For example, it is alleged that the Iraqi soldiers in the Gulf War were given amphetamines to assist in their fear control. The use of drugs in highly competitive sports is also indicative of the extent to which there are some theoretical and practical reasons to attempt to modify human physiology to optimize performance. Despite the relevance of this field, the knowledge base is, at the time of writing, entirely inadequate.

Catharsis

The expression of affect associated with the memory of an event is also a central component of debriefing. The notion of catharsis in relation to trauma was discussed in Breuer & Freud's (1893) first lecture 'Psychical mechanisms of hysterical phenomena; preliminary communications'. In this lecture, they argued that trauma does not simply act as a releasing agent for symptoms. Rather, they proposed that psychic trauma or 'more precisely the memory of the trauma acts like a foreign body which long after entry must continue to be regarded as the agent that still is at work' (ibid., pp. 56–7). They also discussed the process of treatment where the 'individual hysterical symptom immediately and permanently disappeared when we succeeded in bringing clearly to light the memory of the event by which it was provoked and in arousing the accompanying affect and when the patient has described the event in the greatest possible detail and put the affect into words' (ibid., p. 57).

An eclectic model

This brief review indicates that debriefing has its origins in a variety of sources. It has a clear intellectual and practical lineage with the original theories about traumatic neurosis from the 1890s, but it has been significantly modified by crisis theory and models of group intervention. The latter two owe their influence to the models of intervention provided in the services in World War II. Much of the interest in disaster research and subsequently PTSD came out of the social psychiatry movement. One of the intellectual struggles that emerged during this time, was the question of whether symptoms arising in relation to an event were simply a distress response or indicative of a more substantial psychiatric disorder. The psychoanalytical school very much argued the role of social and intrapsychic factors as being the critical determinants of psychological symptoms. Implicit in this idea is that modulation and direction of the individual's processing of the event would minimize or prevent any pathological or prolonged distress.

The theoretical difficulty with this argument emerges with the evidence that in PTSD it appears that there is an abnormal acute stress response of a biological nature (McFarlane et al., 1997). This is a provocative finding because it implies that a pathological outcome is not a direct extension of the normal response to an abnormal event (Yehuda & McFarlane, 1995). Furthermore, this challenging biological evidence suggests that the use of beta-blocker drug may decrease the probability that pathological memories will be indelibly imprinted (McGaugh et al., 1996). If individuals with a normal biological stress response do not develop PTSD, it raises questions of whether early and immediate interventions may modify the nature of the acute stress response in such a way as to increase the risk of PTSD. Given the dictum first, do no harm, the challenge is to demonstrate that, in individuals who have a predicted normal outcome, some form of acute intervention does not modify the adaptive restorative response.

In their separate domains, the contributing theories to debriefing appear sound. Hence, the issue arises of the appropriateness or otherwise of the way in which they have moulded the practice of debriefing.

Outcome research

Outcome research in the domain of debriefing is extremely difficult. The recruitment of people into treatment studies requires a careful process of planning and a collaboration with the populations and clinicians from whom subjects may be drawn. Given that disasters and traumatic incidents happen in situations of extreme emotion and unpredictability, it is very difficult to conduct systematic research. In particular, given the state of distress of the people when they are approached, it is difficult to explain the experimental process and get informed consent in these settings. Also, the idea of random allocation to 'treatment' and 'no treatment' groups goes against the immediate imperative of caring for people in these situations.

Conducting such trials also depends upon the adequate provision of funding to pay research staff who would conduct the assessments as well as doing the longitudinal follow-ups. Given the unpredictable nature of major disasters, it is difficult to establish a research fund that allows the implementation of such research projects.

For these reasons, much of the research has been done in situations that provide less than optimal design or have investigated somewhat atypical patient populations.

A further issue is that the available research tools for studying acute stress reactions and the nature of psychological distress in response to traumatic incidents are relatively poorly developed and still need ongoing testing of their reliability. Thus these instruments are trying to test fluid phenomena in a setting where there are often very considerable practical disruptions to people's lives.

It is also possible that the mere process of assessment may have a significant impact on psychological outcomes. The positive effects of short-term interventions of disclosure were shown in the Kings Cross disaster study where those who discussed their difficulties with others appear to have had better outcomes

(Turner et al., 1993). On the other hand, some studies have used similar approaches without there being any demonstrable benefits. For example, (Weisæth, 1989) conducted the study of a factory fire where very detailed discussions of the disaster experience were included, beginning two days after the disaster. PTSD emerged in a significant percentage of this population, suggesting that this process was by no means substantially effective in decreasing post-traumatic psychopathology.

While there is common sense in the idea that an acute intervention that decreases immediate distress would lead to a decreased prevalence of PTSD, this is not established. Shalev (1992) found that the intensity of acute memories are not necessarily a predictor of who develops long-term severe PTSD. Hence, the basic premise on which much intervention research is based does not necessarily hold up.

A further issue is that, in emergency service personnel, the role of repeated events also needs to be assessed. For example, while it may be possible to lessen the acute distress and the recurring memories of an event, this may encourage emotional numbing and social withdrawal. Such patterns can have very negative impacts on personal relationships. Monitoring alcohol usage should also be an important adjunctive measure.

Another issue that is important from a methodological point of view, both in terms of the validity of assessments and the ability of subjects to use interventions, is cognitive impairments which the individuals may experience at the time or in the immediate aftermath of the event. This creates a significant dilemma.

A further fundamental question is which type of coping style might be most adaptive in these circumstances. Particularly for highly trained individuals, their skill base may allow them to function using narrative memory. In other words, they do not primarily react to the affect and threat in the situation, but rather use specific skills that contain the circumstances. A surgeon or ambulance officer working in an emergency setting has technical procedures and practices that minimize any degree of personalization of the experience. If such an individual were to further examine the meaning context of what had occurred, this might in-

crease their degree of traumatization and inability to cope with very difficult experiences. In other words, for people who take functional or technical roles in disasters, unless specific circumstances call for it, the emotional retelling of an experience may undo effective coping mechanisms.

Background issues

The outcome of traumatic events and particularly the ability to demonstrate the value of debriefing needs to take account of other factors that might influence an individual's outcome. Many people involved in disaster work complain that it is the background organizational administrative and structural issues that are the predominant causes of stress. The traumatization of an individual may often be modified considerably by this context and debriefing may fail to recognize or have no mandate to deal with these matters.

For the majority of individuals it may be relevant to focus on the central role of a recent trauma in explaining people's distress. On the other hand, there will be a variety of intercurrent issues in people's lives, such as divorce, illness and financial problems. The context may be an important determinant of the nature and the severity of a person's response.

There is also a need to consider the occupational health and safety regulations and the possibility of litigation in determining outcomes. The issue of possible compensation claims can significantly modify the relationship between an individual and a provider who is seen to be part of the company who is wishing to minimize their long-term liability. Given the importance of compensation in this area, one could argue the importance of compensation insurers to fund the necessary research to answer a number of these questions.

A recent case in Australia, *Howell vs NSW State Rail* (1998), addressed the employer's obligation to provide debriefing. The absence of unequivocal evidence about the effectiveness of debriefing in the long term is problematic to the argument. At this stage, it seems that the most salient information is to recommend the importance of the early identification of people who may develop acute post-traumatic reactions and to provide them with optimal treatment.

A further matter that was addressed in the *Howell vs NSW State Rail* case was the importance of training as a method of minimizing long-term trauma. Another question that requires consideration is the capacity of training to minimize long-term post-traumatic reactions. The work of Ursano et al. (1994) has demonstrated that training can have an important impact on the distress of emergency service workers, by providing them with a variety of strategies for coping with difficult situations. Debriefing may well have a synergistic effect with these interventions.

Another issue is that one can never presume that outcomes demonstrated by highly trained providers will be transferred into situations that are less ideal and where the individuals have less knowledge and a smaller skill-base. Hence it is critical that there is ongoing quality assurance in settings providing debriefing. It is easy to argue against the negative outcomes that have been found in debriefing (Raphael et al., 1995) because the studies cited have certain deficiencies. Those in favour of debriefing could argue that in other situations, with different groups or different counsellors, better results could have been obtained. The obligation remains to demonstrate such beneficial effects.

This raises important questions about the level of clinical training and the range of skills required by practitioners working in this field. One of the difficulties that has emerged in recent years is that there are many people who descend on disaster sites claiming to have counselling skills that can be used for debriefing. This argues that some credentialling and vetting processes should be put in place. This is a complex political issue as there are a variety of vested interests who may wish to assert their role in providing credentials in this situation. Again, outcome research needs to be conducted to compare professionals with different levels of training. This is not a trivial issue because the treating of trauma is one of the few areas where the degree of clinician's experience has been shown to have an important impact on the outcomes of treatment (McFarlane, 1988). The distress of some therapists can interfere with the effectiveness of interventions offered, so it is important that practitioners do not work in isolation.

A further area that requires investigation is the possibility of negative effects. It would be interesting to compare those who stand to gain from debriefing with those who appear to be deriving little benefit or in fact seem to be becoming worse. It is important that any intervention does not undermine the natural resilience of the group who is likely to have a positive outcome anyway. In following traumatized populations it is obvious that some people develop depression or a range of other psychiatric disorders other than PTSD. In some regards, these disorders are more easily treatable than PTSD. Hence one does not wish to shift individuals from one outcome group to the other.

The outcomes research

The recent Cochrane Collaboration review (Wessely et al., 1998) summarizes the interventions that have been done and can be subjected to some critical analysis. Most of the studies have been done on individuals, independently of whether they had significant symptomatology. These studies have aimed to decrease the initial distress of the individual as well as preventing the onset of psychiatric disorders such as PTSD and depression. The available six randomized controlled trials have used an individual approach rather than group interventions. They have evaluated single treatments from a range of traumas. The available studies have had a series of short comings, including small sample sizes and lack of standardized treatments. The study of K. L. H. Stevens and G. Adshead (1993, cited by Hobbs & Adshead, 1997) also excluded subjects who appeared not to be able to tolerate intervention, thus creating a bias in the results.

Of these studies, two found some negative effects, two demonstrated no overall effect and the other two revealed some evidence for a positive outcome. The two positive ones are those of Bunn & Clark (1979) and Bordow & Porritt (1979).

The no effective outcome is that of Lee et al. (1996). Hobbs et al.'s (1996) and Bisson et al.'s (1997) studies showed negative outcomes.

These data are published in the *Cochrane Report* and further information will be provided in the treatment guidelines of the International Society for Traumatic Stress Studies.

There are a number of other studies that have investigated the question: Kenardy et al. (1996) and Watts (1994) pointed to far from positive findings in this arena. As hinted before, it is possible to raise a number of criticisms of such studies, such as lack of statistical power, difficulties with blind post-intervention assessments and inadequate long-term follow-ups. Other interventions have been conducted that are not in the strict outline criteria used. For example, Raphael (1977), Brom et al. (1993) and Chemtob et al. (1997) have conducted interventions one month after the traumatic event. Raphael's study was of high-risk widows and demonstrated the benefit of intervention. Chemtob et al.'s intervention looked at a group of helpers after a hurricane and demonstrated a significant reduction in Impact of Event Scale scores. These studies beg the interesting question of whether a more optimal time for intervention may occur some months after the disaster, rather than in the immediate post-disaster period.

Future directions for research

The methodological issues described point to the difficulty of conducting future research in this field. One could argue that there is a need to have a large international consortium attempting to answer these questions in a systematic way. Furthermore, there needs to be a stream of funding that can be moved according to the site of a disaster to facilitate the answering of these questions.

The role of these interventions should not be isolated from the broader culture in which they are provided. An understanding of psychological trauma has become an essential part of modern society. The media and other organizations frequently imply the importance of providing for victims in this way.

The openness to discuss some people's psychological reactions and an understanding about the longer-term effects of trauma in themselves have changed the social dynamic and the broader societal response to individuals. Debriefing can therefore be seen to be part of this broader social movement and the specific role of a one-hour intervention may miss the wider values and benefits that have been accrued from improving people's acceptance of the nature of the distress that arises from these experiences.

Conclusion

Unfortunately, the theoretical basis of debriefing, with its long tradition from the military and subsequently crisis intervention, has tended to be lost. As often happens with schools of psychotherapy, views become polarized and often misrepresented. Inevitably, to function in the face of chaos one needs belief. However, belief can at times interrupt critical scrutiny. An attempt to tease apart the different therapeutic ingredients from debriefing and to look at their different values is therefore as important a task as is the design of adequate outcome measures and ensuring the appropriate recruitment of subjects.

There is an important empiricism and questioning in these situations because this is a field that is only too readily subjected to polarization, which then has long-term negative effects. Hence those within the field need to work cooperatively and tolerate uncertainty, rather than seeking definitive answers in polemics.

Acknowledgement

I would like to thank Emily Collins for assistance in the preparation of the manuscript.

REFERENCES

Bisson, J., Jenkins, P., Alexander, J. & Bannister, C. (1997). A randomised controlled trial of psychological debriefing for victims of acute burn trauma. *British Journal of Psychiatry*, **171**, 78–81.

Bordow, S. & Porritt, D. (1979). An experimental evaluation of crisis intervention. *Social Science and Medicine*, **13a**, 251–6.

Breuer, J. & Freud, S. (1893). Psychical mechanisms of hysterical phenomena: preliminary communication. In J. Breuer & S. Freud, *Studies on Hysteria*, vol 3 (pp. 53–68). Harmondsworth, Middx: Penguin Books.

Brom, D., Kleber, R. J. & Hofman, M. (1993). Victims of traffic accidents: incidence and prevention of post-traumatic stress disorder. *Journal of Clinical Psychology*, **49**, 131–40.

Bunn, T. & Clark, A. (1979). Crisis intervention: an experimental study of the effects of a brief period of counselling on the anxiety of relatives of seriously injured or ill hospital patients. *British Journal of Medical Psychology*, **52**, 191–5.

Chemtob, C., Tomas, S., Law, W. & Cremniter, D. (1997). Post-disaster psychosocial interventions: a field study of the impact of debriefing on psychological distress. *American Journal of Psychiatry*, **154**, 415–17.

Fauman, B. J. (1995). Other psychiatric emergencies. In H. I. Kaplan & B. J. Sadock (Eds.) *Comprehensive Textbook of Psychiatry* VI, vol. 2 (pp. 1752–65). Baltimore, MD: Williams and Wilkins.

Green, B. L. & Solomon, S. D. (1995). The mental health impact of natural and technological disasters. In J. R. Freedy & S. E. Hobfoll (Eds.) *Traumatic Stress: From Theory to Practice* (pp. 163–80). New York: Plenum Press.

Hobbs, M. & Adshead, G. (1997). Preventative psychological intervention for road crash survivors. In M. Mitchell (Ed.) *The aftermath of road accidents* (pp. 159–71). London: Routledge.

Hobbs, M., Mayou R., Harrison, B. & Warlock, P. (1996). A randomised trial of psychological debriefing for victims of road traffic accidents. *British Medical Journal*, **313**, 1438–9.

Kaplan, H. I. & Sadock, B. J. (Eds.) (1995) *Comprehensive Textbook of Psychiatry* VI, vol. 2. Baltimore, MD: Williams and Wilkins.

Keegan, J. (1991). *The Face of Battle*. London: Pimlico.

Kenardy, J., Webster, R., Lewin, T., Carr, V., Hazell, P. & Carter, G. (1996). Stress debriefing and patterns of recovery following a natural disaster. *Journal of Traumatic Stress*, **9**, 37–49.

Lee, C., Slade, P. & Lygo, V. (1996). The influence of psychological debriefing on emotional adaptation in women following early miscarriage: a preliminary study. *British Journal of Medical Psychology*, **69**, 47–58.

Lindy, J. D., Green, B. L., Grace, M. C. & Titchener, J. (1983). Psychotherapy with survivors of the Beverley Hills supper club fire. *American Journal of Psychotherapy*, **37**, 593–610.

McFarlane, A. C. (1988). The longitudinal course of post-traumatic morbidity: the range of outcomes and their predictors. *Journal of Nervous and Mental Disease*, **176**, 30–9.

McFarlane, A. C., Atchison, A. & Yehuda, R. (1997). The acute stress response following motor vehicle accidents and its relation to PTSD. *Annals of the New York Academy of Sciences*, **821**, 437–41.

McGaugh, J. L., Cahill, L. & Roozendaal, B. (1996). Involvement of the amygdala in memory storage: interaction with other brain systems. *Proceedings of the National Academy of Sciences, USA*, **93**, 13508–14.

Main, T. (1989). *'The Ailment' and Other Psychoanalytic Essays*. London: Free Association Press.

Raphael, B. (1977). Preventative intervention with the recently bereaved. *Archives of General Psychiatry*, **34**, 1450–4.

Raphael, B., Meldrum, L. & McFarlane, A. C. (1995). Does debriefing after psychological trauma work? *British Medical Journal*, **310**, 1479–80.

Sadock, B. J. (1975). Group psychotherapy. In A. M. Freedman, H. I. Kaplan & B. J. Sadock (Eds.) *Comprehensive Textbook of Psychiatry*, II vol. 2 (pp. 1850–76) Baltimore, MD: Williams and Wilkins.

Shalev, A. (1992). Posttraumatic stress disorder among injured survivors of a terrorist attack: predictive value of early intrusion and avoidance symptoms. *Journal of Nervous and Mental Disease*, **180**, 505–9.

Shalev, A. & Ursano, R. J. (1990). Group debriefing following exposure to traumatic stress. In J. E. Lundeberg, U. Otto & B. Rybeck (Eds.) *War Medical Services* (pp. 192–207). Stockholm: Försvarets Forskningsanstalt.

Singh, B. & Raphael, B. (1981). Post-disaster morbidity of the bereaved. A possible role for preventative psychiatry? *Journal of Nervous and Mental Disease*, **169**, 203–12.

Solomon, Z. & Bebenishty, R. (1986). The role of proximity, immediacy and expectancy in frontline treatment of combat stress reaction among Israelis in the Lebanon War. *American Journal of Psychiatry*, **143**, 613–17.

Turner, S. W., Thompson, J. & Rosser, R. M. (1993). The King's Cross fire: early psychological reactions and implications for organizing a 'phase Two' response. In J. P. Wilson & B Raphael (Eds.) *International Handbook of Traumatic Stress Syndromes* (pp. 451–9). New York: Plenum Press.

Ursano, R. J., McCaughey, B. G. & Fullerton, C. S. (Eds.) (1994). *Individual and Community Responses to Trauma and Disaster*. Cambridge: Cambridge University Press.

van der Kolk, A. C. & McFarlane, B. A. (1996). Trauma and its challenge to society. In B. A. van der Kolk, A. C. McFarlane & L. Weisæth (Eds.) *Traumatic Stress: the Effects of Overwhelming Experience on Mind, Body and Society* (pp. 24–46). New York: Guilford Press.

Watts, R. (1994). The efficacy of critical incident stress debriefing for personnel. *Bulletin of the Australian Psychological Society*, **16**(3), 6–7.

Weisæth, L. (1989). The stressors and post-traumatic stress syndrome after an industrial disaster. *Acta Psychiatrica Scandinavica*, **80**, Suppl. 355, 25–37.

Wessely, S., Rose, S. & Bisson, J. (1998). A systematic review of brief psychological interventions ('debriefing') for the treatment of immediate trauma-related symptoms and the prevention of posttraumatic stress disorder (Cochrane Review). *The Cochrane Library*, **3**. Oxford: Update Software.

Yehuda, R. & McFarlane, A. C. (1995). Conflict between current knowledge about PTSD and its original conceptual basis. *American Journal of Psychiatry*, **152**, 1705–13.

Zusman, J. (1975). Primary production. In A. M. Freedman, H. I. Kaplan & B. J. Sadock (Eds.) *Comprehensive Textbook of Psychiatry* II, vol. 2 (pp. 2326–32). Baltimore, MD: Williams and Wilkins.

25

A conceptual framework for mass trauma: implications for adaptation, intervention and debriefing

Derrick Silove

EDITORIAL COMMENTS

Silove's contribution provides a comprehensive and integrative framework for drawing together the multiple issues that may affect traumatized populations. Its value lies in its holistic nature, and the encompassing of the multiple domains that may be relevant in situations of gross trauma. It is also, however, relevant to other human experience in the situation described in this book. It recognizes that the burden of traumatization in the world arises in developing countries and those with complex emergencies as a result of ethno-nationalist conflicts, human rights violation, torture, systematic violence, refugee status and displacement. The domains of threat and safety, loss and attachment, justice, meaning, identity and role, are all relevant in all these contexts, but also in many other disasters and contexts of psychological traumatization.

The model and its underpinning also recognize the different cultural interpretations and meanings of psychological traumatization. It provides a conceptual basis that is meaningful across cultures and settings and obviates arguments that these are simply western cultural interpretations. It also gives an appropriate framework for acute and longer-term interventions that is respectful of the human adaptations of so many of those affected. It cuts across the universalization of formal debriefing, which was never developed or intended for all settings, and sets up a system of meaning for human and compassionate response, as well as practical assistance. In this, it is also relevant for the smaller disasters of life.

Introduction

The burden of trauma world wide extends far beyond the events of accidents, critical incidents and even combat. Understanding the various components of stressors that may affect people takes on a new meaning when mass trauma and conflict, as they affect large segments of the world's population, are taken into account.

The communities and individuals at risk are diverse and heterogeneous both in their backgrounds and in the nature of the traumas they experience. They include populations who have experienced natural and technological disasters as well as those exposed to individual forms of civilian trauma such as assault, domestic violence, sexual abuse and accidents.

This chapter focuses primarily on persons exposed to intentional human violence occurring on a mass scale, although, with modification, the principles outlined may be applicable to other trauma-affected populations. Even within the group exposed to mass violence are complex and overlapping categories including political activists and dissidents, persecuted minorities and separatist groups, populations affected by genocide and other large-scale massacres, and those exposed to war and other forms of social, internecine and ethnic conflict.

The actual events subsumed under the term 'trauma' also are varied, not only in their objective details, but in the range of impacts and potential meanings of the experiences for individuals and their societies: at one end of the spectrum, individuals may be exposed to a distant or ill-defined threat such as living under an oppressive regime or in a society being threatened by outside invasion, while at the other, targeted groups may be subjected to the most egregious forms of human rights abuses such as torture, detention in political prisons and incarceration in concentration camps.

Unlike single-event traumas such as accidents, the traumas of mass human violence are not generally circumscribed in time, but usually trigger a concatenation of further traumas and stresses that may compound each other (Silove et al., 1991). Displacement and forced migration add a further layer of complexity to the stresses experienced by such populations. Thus statelessness itself has become a 'trauma', carrying with it many threats and stresses (Silove et al., 1997).

The sheer size of violence-affected populations also requires consideration. If those experiencing civilian forms of violence are counted with populations exposed to mass violence, then the problem can be considered to have reached epidemic proportions. In 1997, the United Nations High Commissioner for Refugees listed 23 million people as refugees, and an almost equal number who were 'of concern' to that agency (for example, the internally displaced). Many marginalized and persecuted communities are not accounted for by these estimates. In addition, the largest portion of these populations reside in developing countries, many of which face problems of widespread poverty, endemic communicable diseases, poorly developed infrastructures and limitations in expertise, particularly in fields such as mental health. The scale of the population numbers affected by mass violence, and the context in which such conflict often occurs, thus pose major challenges in relation to conceptualizing the problem and in offering realistic strategies to mitigate the adverse consequences.

In attempting to establish a sufficiently inclusive perspective on the problem, experts tend to draw on a pluralistic set of disciplines and paradigms. Aid agencies providing emergency assistance to populations exposed to mass conflict tend to mirror this eclecticism. At present, mental health professionals make a small contribution to such programmes, the leadership usually being given to administrators, planners, voluntary and religious organizations, peacekeepers, engineers and experts in logistics.

The personnel involved often are sceptical of mental health professionals, regarding their input variously as being unnecessary, ineffective, or based on obtuse principles not compatible with the practical mission of providing emergency aid and reconstruction. In order to engage the larger contributors to the aid process, and to ensure that they understand the strategies mental health professionals wish to implement, it is essential therefore that the concepts and language that are used make sense within the framework of social reconstruction and adaptation.

Tensions in the field of trauma conceptualization

Research in this field has tended to be dominated by a preoccupation with post-traumatic stress disorder (PTSD). Although the emphasis on PTSD has had positive consequences in that it has created a common basis for research across diverse areas of trauma (Mollica & Caspi-Yavin, 1992), the dominance of the Western trauma model has drawn criticism from various quarters in recent years (Summerfield, 1999). For convenience, such concerns can be subdivided into two major domains: those arising directly from the results of research on PTSD, and those of a more theoretical type. The latter set of concerns is considered first.

From a theoretical perspective, the anti-PTSD lobby has drawn its arguments from several wide-ranging contemporary sources that focus on fundamental issues relating to the theory of knowledge, the philosophy of scientific enquiry, the meaning of subjectivity and the influence of geopolitics on medical thinking and priorities. The converging endpoint of such deliberations, however, is a fundamental challenge to the appropriateness of applying the Western-based trauma model to culturally diverse societies that have experienced mass violence and social upheaval (Summerfield, 1997a, 1999). Western traditions of psychiatric research and nosology have been criticized for adhering to a reductionist framework based on an outmoded legacy of logical positivism (the epistemological argument). PTSD, it is argued, has been reified as a pathological entity when there is little empirical support for such an assumption. So-called PTSD is characterized by its opponents as an artefact created by Western traumatologists, a set of normative experiences to challenging events, or as a convenient banner that suits the designs of victim groups, politicians who are attempting to mitigate the suffering they have created, or lawyers and therapists who profit from the trauma industry. From a scientific perspective, critics raise concerns about what is seen as a simplistic linear model in which 'trauma' leads to 'PTSD'. Although such a paradigm is convenient for quantitative research and the statistical methods that support that endeavour, critics point out that such a formulation fails to capture the rich and diverse human experiences associated with extreme events. Thus, the modern trauma model stands accused of reverting to a 'black box' paradigm, in which the subjective experience of the person is lost.

Adherents of a social constructivist position, in particular, depict Western-trained traumatologists as being 'culture-blind'. They rightly state that an equivalent term for trauma does not exist in the lexicons of many cultures, even though other concepts such as suffering, grief and injustice invariably do (Silove, 1998). Western traumatologists, it is averred, adopt a naively universalistic belief in the salience of PTSD, thereby overlooking the extent that culture and context shape the subjective experience of adverse experiences. Culture is therefore posited as a powerful force that transduces the perception and meaning of trauma, and provides the belief system that largely governs the individual's response to such events.

Peace on the terms of the most powerful is best served by encouraging forgetting in those who are plagued by memories of the price that was paid (ethnic cleansing followed by memory cleansing). By pathologizing the problem, and placing it in the hands of mental health professionals, the more fundamental issues of human rights, power politics and economic underdevelopment can be obscured (Summerfield, 1999).

Traumatologists have been challenged on more practical levels. Prevention strategies such as debriefing, it is claimed, remain largely unproven (Solomon, 1999), and are costly in terms of expertise and time. Logistic and economic constraints also raise doubts about the appropriateness and effectiveness of

recommending debriefing or other interventions on a mass scale in post-conflict societies. Concerns are raised that careers and livelihoods have been built on the 'PTSD industry', and that the priority of trauma debriefing and counselling has been oversold to aid agencies and other donor organizations. These latter criticisms have had practical impacts – certain non-government organizations have withdrawn funding from traumatic stress programmes in post-war situations. An important debate has led therefore to some unforeseen consequences that threaten the very foundations of advances made in providing psychological assistance for survivors of trauma. Nevertheless, such events do compel us to recognize that a turning point has been reached that requires a closer analysis of the weaknesses and strengths of contemporary conceptualizations of trauma and its consequences.

Salient findings from recent research

Findings from recent investigations help to throw some light on the salience of PTSD in post-conflict situations. As indicated, strong claims have been made that the problem of PTSD has been exaggerated. Communities are often referred to as 'traumatized', the implication being drawn, often too readily, that most exposed persons are in need of intensive assistance such as debriefing, counselling or other forms of therapy. In fact, recent research has revealed relatively low rates of PTSD in post-war societies. A rigorous epidemiological study of Cambodian residents living in a refugee camp on the Thai border found that 15% suffered from PTSD (Mollica et al., 1993), even though the majority had experienced multiple forms of trauma. Displaced persons ($n = 1052$) who fled persecution in Bhutan and who were living in camps in Nepal showed relatively low rates of PTSD (14% for those who were tortured versus 4% who were not tortured) (Shrestha et al., 1998). The prevalence for PTSD in an unselected sample of Vietnamese refugees ($n = 145$) entering Norway was 9% (Hauff & Vaglum, 1993). Even lower rates (3.5%) were reported for Vietnamese refugees ($n = 209$) attending a compulsory health screening service in San Francisco (Hinton et al., 1993). Such rates should be contrasted with a lifetime prevalence for PTSD of 8% amongst the general USA population (Kessler et al., 1995).

Several factors may account for the relatively low rates of PTSD found in epidemiological studies focusing on refugees fleeing from persecution. These include the validity and reliability of measurement instruments, particularly when used across cultures (Mollica & Caspin-Yavin, 1992), and the period that elapsed since trauma exposure. There is evidence that, in the first few years, the natural recovery curve for PTSD leads to remission in the majority of cases (Kessler et al., 1995), and this may account in part for the lower rates of PTSD in refugee groups; torture survivors studied soon after exposure to trauma tended to show higher rates of PTSD. Nevertheless, existing data suggest that experts in the field should be cautious in their statements regarding the typical outcome of exposure to mass violence. Most importantly, it seems clear that, as in other areas of trauma, the majority of exposed persons do not develop chronic forms of PTSD. An additional issue that warrants further investigation is the extent to which PTSD is associated with overall psychosocial disability. For example, the study of Mollica and co-workers (1993) showed that Cambodians living in refugee camps were often capable of productive activity in spite of ongoing PTSD symptoms. A more recent study in a Bosnian refugee camp found that only a minority of people – those with PTSD and depression – suffered severe disability (Mollica et al., 1999).

An important associated finding of recent research is that there are diverse psychological outcomes associated with exposure to mass violence, and that a multiplicity of influences affect such outcomes (Silove, 1999). Depression may be at least as common as PTSD, and other psychiatric categories such as somatization, drug and alcohol abuse, panic disorder, separation anxiety and pathological forms of anger may occur. Comorbidity is commonly found; in particular, PTSD is often associated with depression, and there are several possible explanations for that finding, including definitional overlap between those categories. Nevertheless, there is also some evidence of specificity in the relationship of trauma categories and diagnostic outcomes. The extent of trauma exposure, and the type of

trauma experienced, does appear to influence risk of PTSD. For example, several investigators (Mollica et al., 1993, 1998; Silove et al., 1997) have shown a dose–response relationship between trauma events and severity of the PTSD symptoms (although memory disturbances associated with PTSD itself may account in part for this apparent relationship). In addition, the most egregious traumas, such as torture and detention in concentration camps, do appear to increase the prevalence, severity and chronicity of PTSD (Basoglu et al., 1994; Mollica et al., 1998; Shrestha et al., 1998; Steel et al., 1999).

In addition, a large range of stresses occurring in the post-traumatic period may influence the outcome of PTSD and other disorders. Some of these stresses appear to be specific in their impact on particular diagnostic categories, and others appear to have a generic effect on psychosocial disability as a whole. More general stresses include social and economic adversity, with unemployment, low family income, poverty and racial discrimination emerging as important factors associated with persisting psychosocial impairment (Beiser et al., 1993; Chung & Kagawa-Singer, 1993; Lavik et al., 1996; Silove et al., 1997; Gorst-Unsworth & Goldenberg, 1998). Loss of social networks and separation from family members are important factors that appear to perpetuate psychiatric symptoms, particularly of depression (Gorst-Unsworth & Goldenberg, 1998). In an 18-month follow-up of Vietnamese refugees resettled in the USA, Ladson Hinton and coworkers (1997) found that premigration trauma variables were less powerful predictors of persisting depression than were demographic variables such as age, marital status and English language proficiency – factors that, in turn, may be associated with level of integration into the new environment.

Important to the planning of intervention strategies is the growing recognition that protective factors may act as a buffer against the psychosocial impact of mass violence and persecution. Political activism, preparedness for abuse and an expectation that a regime will act malevolently, all appear to confer some protection against PTSD in those exposed to torture (Basoglu et al., 1996, 1997). Religious belief, particularly adherence to Buddhism, has been found to cushion the effects of trauma in Asian communities (Allden et al., 1996; Shrestha et al., 1998). Evidence is accruing therefore, that social, political and cultural mechanisms may be important in determining whether the individual and, the community as a whole, are able to adapt to the challenges of exposure to mass violence.

In summary, it is important for practitioners in the field to recognize that only a minority of people exposed to mass violence or other forms of disaster are at risk of developing debilitating PTSD in the long run. Other outcomes, especially depression, may be at least as common. Apart from pre-existing vulnerabilities, a multiplicity of social, political and cultural factors influence the psychosocial outcomes of trauma exposure. Most individuals and their communities adapt to trauma without professional assistance, suggesting that there are natural restitutive mechanisms – biological, social and cultural – that foster recovery from even the most severe forms of trauma. A refocussing of attention thus seems warranted on the processes that promote post-traumatic adaptation both at an individual and at the communal level.

A proposed adaptational framework

The conceptual framework outlined hereunder aims to broaden the scope of traumatology in order to allow for greater coverage of the diverse experiences and types of response that occur following trauma exposure (Silove, 1999).

The aim of the model is to encourage greater convergence in the perspectives underlying clinical work and research, so that each area of activity might interact synergistically with the other. Importantly, the model tries to bring theoretical coherence to the eclectic array of interventions that are already used at various levels of practice (Cunningham & Silove, 1993): in models of debriefing and other forms of early intervention.

A focus on adaptive mechanisms, both in relation to individuals and communities as a whole, is grounded in several considerations. The approach draws on the observation that, as the most adaptable species on earth, human beings are likely to share universal mechanisms of survival in the face of the most threatening circumstances, even though the mode of expression of such adaptive mechanisms may differ substantially across different cultures and contexts. It is assumed that the core adaptive systems that will be described have reciprocal representations in the psychobiological make-up of individuals as well as in the social and cultural structures that they create collectively in order to foster the survival and propagation of the group. The model is therefore teleological in its focus, since it assumes that human reactions to trauma are governed by the drive towards survival and psychosocial development. Using the language of adaptation assists in bringing mental health strategies closer to the objectives of broader assistance initiatives aimed at achieving social reconstruction following disasters. Terms such as threat, loss, identity and justice are concepts that are familiar to social planners and the communities they serve. The model focuses attention on the inherent capacities of individuals and groups to repair their own institutions, given favourable support and judicious external assistance.

From a research perspective, clarification of the normative adaptive responses to trauma might assist in shifting the emphasis from the 'black box' model, that is, as mentioned earlier, a tendency to assume a linear relationship between trauma and a particular psychiatric outcome such as PTSD. By reinserting the individual and the community at the centre of the process, emphasis is given to the human construction of events and the capacity for affected communities to make active adaptations to external challenges.

An adaptive focus also is consistent with the overarching humanitarian mission of mental health workers in the field – by explicitly recognizing the capacities of trauma-affected individuals and their communities to adapt, the practitioner communicates a position of respect for the survivor and thereby encourages self-help strategies that avoid the trap of passivity and dependency. While most adaptations are directed at restoring the fundamentals of survival and stability, exposure to extreme situations may, in some instances, strengthen and transform survivors in ways that foster exceptional achievements in the period after exposure.

Five domains of stress and their adaptive systems

The five adaptive systems proposed herein are hypothetical constructs that are considered to subsume the functions of safety, attachment, identity and role, justice, and existential meaning (Silove, 1999). Although for simplicity, the postulated adaptive systems identified are described separately, it is assumed that they have evolved in an orchestrated manner to ensure that, under normal circumstances, the interaction of the individual and his or her society occurs in a way that promotes a degree of personal, social and cultural homeostasis. The systems and the challenges that stress them are not static but evolve according to several time continua. The refugee experience, for example, evolves over several defined phases, including the period of threat in the home country, the time of flight and asylum, and the stage of final resettlement or repatriation (Silove et al., 1991). Thus threats may occur concurrently or sequentially, and their nature, meaning and impact may vary over time, depending on the capacity of the individual and the group to adapt at key points in the process. Traumas may accumulate and compound one another, so that the final trigger of psychiatric disorder may, superficially, seem less threatening than preceding events. For example, the shock and disbelief associated with the threat of repatriation once they have reached a place of safety, may precipitate PTSD for the first time in asylum seekers who previously had weathered torture and other grievous abuses in their homelands. For many conflict-affected populations, the period of exposure to threat is prolonged so that it may span a substantial period of a person's life. Traumas that can be accommodated in childhood and adolescence may have different impacts in adulthood and on the elderly, and vice versa. A life course perspective is essential, therefore, in considering the effects of trauma and its impact on adaptive systems. The broader ecosystem, especially the sociopolitical arena in which threats of mass violence occur, often undergoes substantial flux during and after a period of mass upheaval. The uncertainties that are generated create another layer of uncertainty and challenge – especially because the final outcomes for survivor populations often depend on the vicissitudes of geopolitical policies.

The safety system

As indicated earlier, much of the recent focus of research into mass violence and displacement has been based on a narrow notion of trauma, which is defined by the *Diagnostic and Statistical Manual of Mental Disorders* (DSM-IV; American Psychiatric Association, 1994) system as events that threaten the physical survival or integrity of the self or those close to the victim. There is growing evidence that exposure to life threat may be specific in triggering psychobiological mechanisms, which may have an adaptive function. A period of arousal and hypervigilance, intrusive images following exposure to death, and the avoidance that accompanies such 'symptoms' can be regarded as adaptive, especially when there is a risk that the danger may reoccur (Silove, 1998). While many survivors are aroused, hypervigilant and fearful in the early stages, most should and will show a natural return to a state of psychological equilibrium.

Recognition that post-threat reactions generally are normative and self-limiting is critical to debates about the scale of psychological interventions needed after humanitarian crises. Aid agencies are preoccupied with the task of making rational allocations of scarce resources according to competing demands in a context where needs always exceed available funds and expertise. Priorities may be determined to some extent by logistics and opportunity costs: if a problem is too large, too complicated and too costly to solve, it may be forfeited on pragmatic grounds in favour of simple, constrained projects with circumscribed and achievable aims. Thus a conservative estimation of the numbers of trauma-exposed populations likely to need either acute psychological interventions or intensive treatment for PTSD may be more likely to win resources than extravagant proposals based on the assumption that the majority of survivor populations are 'traumatized'.

Broader, community-based psychosocial programmes may be justified as long as they focus on known risk and protective factors. Targeting of high-risk populations and stratification of interventions based on research-based evidence is essential, however, as is a demonstration of the effectiveness of any new initiatives in this area. Too many programmes have been based on nothing more than rhetoric, intuition or so-called good ideas. Although more needs to be known about the factors that influence PTSD outcomes, evidence already exists to support strategies that extend beyond simple notions of debriefing and instead focus on increasing the physical and psychological security of survivors, on providing conditions for communal reintegration and gainful activity, on facilitating religious practices where appropriate, and create a context that allows participation by survivors in self-governance and the pursuit of their ideals and causes. The creation of a genuine context of security in a humanitarian crisis may be a difficult task, given the multiple sources of real and perceived threats that trauma-affected and displaced communities face. The task of providing a secure recovery environment therefore involves a multidisciplinary effort in which mental health professionals provide only one component.

One possibility alluded to earlier, which requires much further investigation, is that particular cultures and their institutions may have especially potent mechanisms that restore a sense of individual and collective security once the immediate effects of threat have past. Modern traumatology may benefit greatly from the study of such culture-based mechanisms of adaptation (see Ober et al., Chapter 17).

The attachment–bonding system

The drive to form attachments and to maintain close interpersonal bonds is grounded in phylogenetically determined behaviours that are critical to the survival of the species (Bowlby, 1969). One of the key disruptions caused by torture, war trauma and refugee experiences is the impact on the survivor's interpersonal bonds. Separations and losses often are multiple and include actual and symbolic losses. The death of the loved one may be accompanied by extreme threat – family members may be killed in the presence of the survivor, often in horrific and terrifying ways. The circumstances of these deaths may be such as to engender self-doubt and a sense of responsibility for not 'doing more' to prevent what happened.

The impact of massive loss may be prolonged. For example, thousands of unaccompanied minors in refugee camps have never experienced a family life or the guidance of parental figures. The uncertain fate of relatives who are victims of 'disappearances', kidnapping and incarceration may make psychological resolution of losses by the bereaved more difficult. Family members may be unable to visit the graves of the deceased for either economic or political reasons. Apart from deceased or missing family, friends and colleagues, survivors of organized violence often experience massive material losses – of homes, property and other possessions. More subtle losses include those of a sense of belonging, of social cohesion, of connection with the land and ancestors, and of culture and traditions (Eisenbruch, 1991).

Normative reactions to such losses include grief, nostalgia and homesickness, and in some persons such psychological reactions can become extreme and disabling (van Tilberg et al., 1996). A revival in interest in describing the phenomenology of traumatic grief has been evident recently, with several expert groups publishing measures (or criteria) for the diagnosis of that category (Horowitz et al., 1997; Prigerson et al., 1997). Key features include: pining, yearning, or searching for the deceased; intrusive imagery, hallucinations, or illusions of the deceased's presence; sensitivity to triggers that revive memories of the deceased; and associated symptoms of social withdrawal, anxiety and depression. Although similar in several respects to the symptom constellations of PTSD, it is important to preserve the distinction between the two constellations (Raphael & Martinek, 1997). If unresolved, there is a substantial risk that grief will be complicated by frank depressive and/or anxiety disorders.

Other responses to bond ruptures have been described, for example a constellation of symptoms of separation anxiety in adulthood has been identified that is akin to the syndrome commonly seen in children and adolescents, and which may be provoked or exacerbated by traumatic separations (Manicavasagar et al., 1997). A more specific form of grief associated with the refugee experience has been termed cultural bereavement (Eisenbruch, 1991), an overwhelming nostalgia for the traditional way of life and culture of origin. Thus there appears to be a protean array of normal and maladaptive reactions to multiple, traumatic losses.

The threats to bonds experienced by trauma survivors can lead to some positive adaptations. Survivors may learn to cherish family bonds in a deeper way than before, and priorities may be reordered so that great energy is directed towards nurturing the young and towards preparing the way for their futures. At one extreme, such responses lead to excessive protectiveness and enmeshment; at the other, it may foster rich family ties that form a secure base for the succeeding generation.

Although the drive to restore and repair ruptured bonds appears to be universal, cultures may differ substantially in the approaches they employ to achieve these goals. Mourning rituals, in particular, are culture specific. Some groups, for example, find it particularly shameful if they are unable to pay respects at the burial sites of family members who have been slain. In mounting interventions for communities that have suffered mass losses, therefore, the specific religious, cultural and social traditions associated with grief need to be understood and supported.

The justice system

The human rights perspective adds a further dimension to the understanding of torture and mass abuses. Torture, for example, not only constitutes a threat to life and safety, but it is an extreme example of human rights violation in which the perpetrator actively seeks not only to threaten the victim, but to dehumanize, humiliate and degrade (Silove, 1996). The total environment may be engineered to achieve the goal of dehumanization, the concentration camp being the most blatant example. Once trapped within such environments, inmates may be compelled to act in ways that ordinarily would be reprehensible to them and survival may be possible only by sacrificing or exploiting others. Forced betrayal, denunciation and complicity commonly occur, victims often being obliged to make 'impossible choices' between equally reprehensible options.

Subsequent events may compound the sense of injustice engendered by torture, rape and acts of genocide. For example, survivors may find themselves living in a post-war society that remains riven by factionalism, plagued by corruption, and devoid of effective systems of justice; displaced communities confined in refugee camps may experience further exploitation and arbitrary treatment; and asylum seekers may endure prolonged periods of insecurity, living in societies that are hostile to their presence. Also, perpetrators may live with impunity in survivor societies, thus confronting victims daily with the inadequacies of international mechanisms for indicting those guilty of crimes against humanity.

Some survivors of persecution may adapt to their experiences by becoming fierce defenders of justice and human rights. Their personal experiences, however painful, may deepen their capacity for compassion for the suffering of others. Many great humanitarian leaders of this century themselves suffered persecution at some point in their careers. One pathway of adaptation to injustice is therefore to struggle for the creation of social structures that will prevent similar abuses in the future.

An important question, however, is whether the extreme sense of injustice provoked in survivors of human rights abuses may lead to difficulties in the control and expression of anger (Gorst-Unsworth et al., 1993). The importance of chronic anger, and problems in its modulation and expression, have been raised repeatedly as an area warranting further investigation in survivors of human-engendered trauma (Gorst-Unsworth et al., 1993; Lifton, 1993; Ochberg, 1993). A common feature of entrapment situations in which the victim is subjected repeatedly to human rights violations is the experience of outrage without the capacity to react (Davenport, 1991) – a state of 'frozen rage'. Clinical impressions support the notion that survivors who have been intensely humiliated or degraded and/or have been forced to betray their most cherished beliefs, may be left with feelings of ill-directed and unmitigated anger at the injustices they have suffered (Silove, 1996). Survivors may live in a chronic state of heightened and potentially overwhelming anger, often finding themselves oscillating between periods of suppression (dealt with by isolating from others, social withdrawal, avoiding interpersonal conflict) and loss of control, manifested as explosiveness, hostility and impulsive acts. Rage may be turned inwardly in acts of self-recrimination in which survivors denigrate themselves, often excessively, for not having reacted more forcefully against their persecutors. Thus survivors may become trapped in a vicious spiral in which loss of control of rage leads to enactment of the very aggression they detest, thereby intensifying their feelings of shame, guilt, desolation and despair.

The nosological status of anger and its manifestations in survivors warrants further examination. It is noteworthy that, unlike other affective reactions (depression, anxiety), there are no primary 'anger syndromes' in conventional typologies. In Korea, 'anger illness' is recognized as a reaction to the injustices suffered by women forced into sexual slavery during World War II (Summerfield, 1997a). Cambodia has instituted an annual Day of Anger, in which citizens are encouraged to express in socially acceptable ways the rage they feel when remembering the Khmer Rouge autogenocide. In the Western literature, it is usually assumed that anger is one manifestation of (and hence subsumed by) disorders such as PTSD, depression or grief. Further work is needed therefore to investigate whether the roots and phenomenology of anger in survivors of human rights violations are sufficiently discrete to warrant consideration of a separate affective category of 'traumatic anger disorder' (Silove, 1996).

The existential-meaning system

Exposure to inexplicable evil and cruelty can shake the foundations of the survivor's faith in the beneficence of life and humankind. The extreme violation of torture often leaves survivors with existential preoccupations in which they strive, often unsuccessfully, to find a coherent reason for the abuses they have suffered. They thus face a crisis of trust, faith and meaning, which may intensify feelings of alienation and emotional isolation (Gorst-Unsworth et al., 1993). Adherence to religious faith may help to mitigate such effects (Shrestha et al., 1998), as may a sense of ideological and political commitment in some contexts. Forms of debriefing that ignore such existential dilemmas risk provoking more intense feelings of self-doubt in survivors. In engaging survivor patients, therapists may therefore be obliged to enter into a wider domain of interaction in which values, ideology and faith are central to the discussion (Silove et al., 1991; Kinzie & Boehnlein, 1993).

The identity/role system

One of the key aims of torture is to undermine a person's sense of identity, agency and control. Many survivors report that they have 'never been the same person' after the experience of torture (Silove et al., 1991). Indoctrination, propaganda, ostracism and isolation are all techniques that oppressive regimes use to undermine the sense of cohesion and identity of individual dissidents as well as entire communities. Physical injury, mutilation and subsequent disability add to alterations in self-image and the sense of identity of survivors. Being divested of one's social position, role, possessions and employment represent not only a loss and a violation but also a potent threat to one's sense of empowerment, efficacy and individuality. Survivors may thus feel helpless, powerless and aimless. Forced displacement, loss of culture and land, and resettlement in an alien and, at times, forbidding environment further challenge the person's sense of identity and capacity to control his or her destiny.

Liminality and marginality are sociological terms that depict this state of being extruded from the mainstream of society. Adaptive responses may include an energetic adoption of new roles, such as leadership in rebuilding the community. Maladaptive social responses may include extreme passivity and an excessive abnegation of roles such as parenting responsibilities. In its extreme form, the gross alteration of roles observed may lead to the alienation and isolation described in the newly codified International Classification of Diseases (ICD) 10 category of 'enduring personality change after catastrophic events'.

Implications

The model proposed aims to encourage a process of abstraction in which crude 'trauma' events are organized according to their psychosocial meanings and their consequent impact on adaptation. In addition, the concepts used may have greater universal relevance

Table 25.1. Threats to adaptation

System	Challenge	Normative responses
Security/safety	Life threat	Hypervigilance, security-seeking
	Post-traumatic threats	
Attachment	Ruptured bonds	Grief, separation anxiety, 'searching'
	Threats to attachments	
Justice	Human rights violations	Anger, frustration, caution in trusting
Identity and role	Torture, disrupted institutions and	Role uncertainty and
	sociocultural structures	identity/cultural transitions
Existential meaning	Ruptured values, beliefs, worldview	Existential questioning/doubts

to the subjective experiences of survivors of mass trauma and violence than currently used diagnostic categories. For example, notions of safety, grief, injustice and faith may be more meaningful to trauma-affected people and their communities than categories such as traumatization, PTSD or depression. The model also may allow a more systematic examination of the transition points that lead from normative responses to pathological outcomes.

The model has been developed and described from the understandings relevant to the situations of mass trauma, conflict, violence, rape, human rights violations, torture and refugee experience. Nevertheless, its core domains or elements are relevant for many other situations of psychological trauma, particularly those linked to human violence and malevolence. The issues covered may also be pertinent to some major disasters, to warfare, to civilian incidents such as mass shootings, or even to some less obvious 'critical incidents'.

As discussed previously, in most people who experience circumstances of trauma, adaptation is the usual outcome. This model, both in its broadest sense and when applied to diverse incidents, sits across both the Western model of psychological trauma, and those understandings of experiences relevant to other contexts and cultures. Furthermore, it holds relevance for the most horrific and prolonged circumstances where other models may be at best simplistic and culturally inappropriate, at worst potentially damaging. Consideration of these issues is particularly important when the use of debriefing models is generalized to such contexts. How acute interventions may be rel-

evant to populations affected in this way, how decisions might be made as to whether or not they should be applied in view of the adaptations that occur for many, and what the implications may be for longer-term interventions all require close analysis from a contextual and cultural perspective (Table 25.1).

Acute intervention

The implications that may arise for acute interventions linked to the adaptive domains described could include the following:

1. *Safety/security*: Any acute interventions must ensure safety, provide a protective response, and reduce distress.
2. *Attachment domain*: Acute interventions would support the search for family members, for instance, or provide information about them, and give priority to kinship groups. If there is a loss or death of a loved one then comfort, and support for the appropriate rituals of grief, farewell and funeral would be appropriate.
3. *Justice domains*: Recognition of the affected person's human rights is critical, both in terms of the violations they have suffered and in relation to conditions in the post-traumatic environment (e.g. refugee camps, detention centres). Addressing core justice issues is not easy in acute responses apart from where there are evidentiary requirements – for instance in relation to violence, witnessing, rape and so forth. Supportive frameworks that recognize and

Table 25.2. Pathologies and treatments

System	Path responses	Intervention
Security/safety	PTSD/anxiety	Anxiety reduction, treat PTSD, prevent further threat/danger
Attachment	Traumatic/unresolved grief, separation anxiety, depression	Grief therapy, 'Interpersonal-style psychotherapy', assist in repairing networks and forming new ones
Justice	Pathological anger syndrome, 'Paranoia'	Social mechanisms for justice: e.g. Truth and Reconciliation Commissions
Identity and role	Role/identity confusion, loss of purpose, cultural bereavement	Practical assistance: language, training, work. Family interventions for role inversions; formulating new roles
Existential meaning	Loss of faith, incoherent belief systems, alienation	Links with religion Reconstructing cultures, Repairing/recreating meaning systems

PTSD, post-traumatic stress disorder.

acknowledge the victim's suffering without creating unrealistic expectations for immediate restitution is important.

4. *Identity and role*: Interventions explicitly recognize and reinforce valued identities other than victim status, including strengths, and should support and value the roles adopted by those affected in their attempts at adaptation and recovery.

5. *Existential meaning*: Acute interventions may include re-establishing contact with religious and spiritual leaders. At all levels meaning is not that provided by outsiders but rather is an evolving process of active searching by those affected. Most significant to many is re-establishing a sense of the value of life, and the value of survival for all it holds in relation to those who died.

There are some general issues that may be relevant to any acute or early intervention, but central to this endeavour is what is done to recognize and compassionately support individuals and populations in their search for safety, security, survival, the defence of human bonds and the restoration of human values.

How this model may be relevant in terms of pathologies and treatments is summarised in Table 25.2.

Thus this model provides a broader conceptual framework for understanding the field of psychological trauma and how it may be relevant to the burden of violence-induced suffering in developing worlds. The model attests to the importance of a multiplicity of issues, their complexity, and validity, against the critique of the irrelevance of concepts of psychological trauma and Western models. In addition, it provides both a reality-based and humanistic model that recognizes the primacy of self-directed adaptation in guiding context-relevant helping responses.

It obviates the application of 'debriefing' in inappropriate contexts – for instance, for refugees and victims of human rights violations, and for populations in disadvantaged and developing countries where safety, shelter and food may be primary needs. It recognizes the multiplicity of stressors for affected populations such as those experiencing major disasters and wars (see Wilson and Sigman, Chapter 4) or indigenous populations experiencing chronic trauma (see Ober et al., Chapter 17).

Although for convenience, the core adaptive systems identified in the proposed model were described independently, they clearly operate in concert, interacting with each other at multiple levels. The model is predicated on the notion that particular trauma events may have several meanings and hence exert diverse impacts on more than one adaptive system. Thus the mass rape of women may have manifold effects: such abuses may pose a mortal threat to the victims; they may erode the survivor's self-concept and feelings of integrity; they may disrupt marital functioning as a consequence of injury, stigma and unwanted pregnancy; and, as an instrument of 'ethnic cleansing', the abuses may constitute a massive threat to the identity, culture and the religious fabric of the whole community.

The model proposed may also assist in providing a coherent conceptual framework for strategies for intervention that extend beyond structured approaches to debriefing. Thus interventions as seemingly diverse as interpersonal forms of psychotherapy, assistance with tracing lost relatives, and encouragement of survivors to engage in culturally relevant mourning rituals, may all converge on the theme of loss and separation. Attempts to strengthen the sense of identity of individual survivors and their communities may range over multiple points of intervention, including assistance with work retraining, family therapy focussing on reconciling role changes and conflicts, and community development activities aimed at promoting group cohesion and the preservation of culture. Support for survivors and their communities in their pursuit of religious and political activities may assist in re-establishing a sense of meaning, purpose and faith, thus helping to overcome feelings of injustice, anger and existential despair. At a wider level, social mechanisms for reconciliation and forgiveness, as embodied, for example, in the Truth and Reconciliation Commission in South Africa, may serve a mass healing function by ensuring public acknowledgement of past injustices, vindicating the suffering of those who were subjected to cruelty, and offering amnesty that is conditional on full disclosure of past misdeeds by perpetrators (Summerfield, 1997b).

In examining this model, researchers face the challenge of operationalizing concepts that are commonly used, but rarely defined, in clinical practice. One of the potential limitations of the model proposed is that the concepts on which it is based may prove to be elusive to contemporary methods of research. Progress has been made, for example, in defining categories such as trau-

matic grief (Raphael & Martinek, 1997) and cultural bereavement (Eisenbruch, 1991), but measures of the sense of identity, existential meaning and religious commitment may be more difficult to define with accuracy.

Conclusions

This model provides a global context for considering the multiple traumata that may affect populations and for which solutions may be sought. It provides a framework for a humanistic and compassionate reponse that can be applied practically and systematically. It does so in a more holistic way than is implicit in contemporary concepts of debriefing since it recognizes and respects the natural tendency towards adaptation of those who will overcome such suffering. Like all models, it too requires empirical evaluation, a methodologically dificult task, yet one that is critical to resolving conflicting perspectives in the field.

REFERENCES

Allden, K., Poole, C., Chantavanich, S., Ohmar, K., Aung, N. N. & Mollica, R. F. (1996). Burmese political dissidents in Thailand: trauma and survival among young adults in exile. *American Journal of Public Health*, **86**, 1561–9.

American Psychiatric Association (1994). *Diagnostic and Statistical Manual*, 4th edn. Washington, DC: American Psychiatric Press.

Basoglu, M., Paker, M. & Paker, O., Ozmen, E., Marks, I., Incesu, C., Sahin, D. & Sarimurat, N. (1994). Psychological effects of torture: a comparison of tortured with non-tortured political activists in Turkey. *American Journal of Psychiatry*, **151**, 76–81.

Basoglu, M., Ozmen, E., Sahin, D., Paker, M., Tasdemir, O., Ceyhanli, A., Incesu, C. & Sarimurat, N. (1996). Appraisal of self, social environment, and state authority as a possible mediator of posttraumatic stress disorder in tortured political activists. *Journal of Abnormal Psychology*, **105**, 232–6.

Basoglu, M., Mineka, S., Paker, M., Aker, J., Livanou, M. & Gok, S. (1997). Psychological preparedness for trauma as a protective factor in survivors of torture. *Psychological Medicine*, **27**, 1421–33.

Beiser, M., Johnson, P. J. & Turner, R. J. (1993). Unemployment, underemployment and depressive affect among South East Asian refugees. *Psychological Medicine*, **23**, 731–43.

Bowlby, J. (1969). *Attachment and Loss*, vol. I *Attachment*. London: Penguin Books.

Chung, R. C. & Kagawa-Singer, M. (1993). Predictors of psychological distress among South East Asian refugees. *Social Science and Medicine*, **36**, 631–9.

Cunningham, M. & Silove, D. (1993). Principles of treatment and service development for refugee survivors of torture and trauma. In J. Wilson & B. Raphael (Eds.) *International Handbook of Traumatic Stress Syndromes* (pp. 751–62). New York: Plenum Press.

Davenport, D. S. (1991). The functions of anger and forgiveness: guidelines for psychotherapy with victims. *Psychotherapy*, **28**, 140–4.

Eisenbruch, M. (1991). From post-traumatic stress disorder to cultural bereavement: diagnosis of South East Asian refugees. *Social Science and Medicine*, **33**, 673–80.

Gorst-Unsworth, C. & Goldenberg, E. (1998). Psychological sequelae of torture and organised violence suffered by refugees in Iraq. Trauma-related factors compared with social factors in exile. *British Journal of Psychiatry*, **172**, 90–4.

Gorst-Unsworth, C., Van Velsen, C. & Turner, S. (1993). Prospective pilot study of survivors of torture and organised violence: examining the existential dilemma. *Journal of Nervous and Mental Disease*, **181**, 263–4.

Hauff, E. & Vaglum, P. (1993). Vietnamese boat refugees: the influence of war and flight traumatisation on mental health on arrival in the country of resettlement: a community cohort study of Vietnamese refugees in Norway. *Acta Psychiatrica Scandinavica*, **88**, 162–8.

Hinton, W. L., Chen, Y. C., Du, N., Tran, C. G., Lu, F. G., Miranda, J. & Faust, S. (1993). DSM-III-R disorders in Vietnamese refugees. Prevalence and correlates. *Journal of Nervous and Mental Disease*, **181**, 113–22.

Hinton, W. L., Tiet, Q., Tran, C. G. & Chesness, M. (1997). Predictors of depression among refugees from Vietnam: a longitudinal study of new arrivals. *Journal of Nervous and Mental Disease*, **185**, 39–45.

Horowitz, M. J., Siegal, B., Holen, A., Bonanno, G. A., Milbrath, C. & Stinson, C. H. (1997). Diagnostic criteria for complicated grief disorder. *American Journal of Psychiatry*, **154**, 904–10.

Kessler, R. C., Sonnega, A., Bromet, E., Hughes, M. & Nelson, C. B. (1995). Posttraumatic stress disorder in the national comorbidity survey. *Archives of General Psychiatry*, **52**, 1048–60.

Kinzie, J. D. & Boehnlein, J. K. (1993). Psychotherapy of the victims of massive violence: counter-transference and ethical issues. *American Journal of Psychotherapy*, **7**, 90–102.

Lavik, N. J., Hauf, E., Skrondal, A. & Solberg, O. (1996). Mental disorder among refugees and the impact of persecution on exile: some findings from an outpatient population. *British Journal of Psychiatry*, **169**, 726–32.

Lifton, R. J. (1993). From Hiroshima to the Nazi doctors: the evolution of psychoformative approaches to understanding traumatic stress syndromes. In J. P. Wilson & B. Raphael (Eds.) *International Handbook of Traumatic Stress Syndromes* (pp. 11–23). New York: Plenum Press.

Manicavasagar, V., Silove, D. & Curtis, J. (1997). Separation anxiety in adulthood: a phenomenological investigation. *Comprehensive Psychiatry*, **38**, 274–82.

Mollica, R. & Caspi-Yavin, Y. (1992). Overview: the assessment and diagnosis of torture events and symptoms. In M. Basoglu (Ed.) *Torture and its Consequences* (pp. 253–74). Cambridge: Cambridge University Press.

Mollica, R. F., Caspi-Yavin, Y., Bollini, P., Truong, T., Tor, S. & Lavelle, J. (1992). The Harvard Trauma Questionnaire: validating a cross-cultural instrument for measuring torture, trauma, and posttraumatic stress disorder in Indochinese refugees. *Journal of Nervous and Mental Disease*, **180**, 111–16.

Mollica, R. F., Donelan, K., Tor, S., Lavelle, J., Elias, C., Frankel, M. & Blendon, R. J. (1993). The effect of trauma and confinement on functional health and mental health status of Cambodians living in Thailand–Cambodia border camps. *Journal of the American Medical Association*, **270**, 581–6.

Mollica, R. F., McInnes, K., Pham, T., Smith Fawzi, M. C., Murphy, E. & Lin, L. (1998). The dose–effect relationships between torture and psychiatric symptoms in Vietnamese ex-political detainees and a comparison group. *Journal of Nervous and Mental Disease*, **186**, 543–53.

Mollica, R. F., McInnes, K., Sarajlic, N., Lavelle, J., Sarajlic, I. & Massagli, M. P. (1999). Disability associated with psychiatric comorbidity and health-status in Bosnian refugees living in Croatia. *Journal of the American Medical Association*, **282**, 433–9.

Ochberg, F. M. (1993). Posttraumatic therapy. In J. P. Wilson & B. Raphael (Eds.) *International Handbook of Traumatic Stress Syndromes* (pp. 773–83). New York: Plenum Press.

Prigerson, H. G., Shear, M. K., Frank, E., Beery, L. C., Silberman, R., Prigerson, J. & Reynolds, G. F. III (1997). Traumatic grief: a case of loss-induced trauma. *American Journal of Psychiatry*, **154**, 1003–9.

Raphael, B. & Martinek, N. (1997). Assessing traumatic bereavement and posttraumatic stress disorder. In J. P. Wilson & T. M. Keane (Eds.) *Assessing psychological trauma and PTSD* (pp. 373–95). New York: Guilford Press.

Shrestha, N. M., Sharma, B., van Ommeren, M., Regmi, S.,

Makaju, R., Kamproe, I., Sheshtha, G. B. & de Jong, J. T. (1998). Impact of torture on refugees displaced within the developing world. *Journal of the American Medical Association*, **280**, 443–8.

Silove, D. (1996). Torture and refugee trauma: implications for nosology and treatment of posttraumatic syndromes. In F. L. Mak & C. C. Nadelson (Eds.) *International Review of Psychiatry* (pp. 211–32). Washington, DC: American Psychiatric Press.

Silove, D. (1998). Is PTSD an overlearnt survival response? An evolutionary-learning hypothesis. *Psychiatry*, **61**, 181–90.

Silove, D. (1999). The psychosocial effects of torture, mass human rights violations and refugee trauma: toward an integrated conceptual framework. *Journal of Nervous and Mental Disease*, **187**, 200–1.

Silove, D., Tarn, R., Bowles, R. & Reid, J. (1991). Psychosocial needs of torture survivors. *Australian and New Zealand Journal of Psychiatry*, **25**, 481–90.

Silove, D., Sinnerbrink, I., Field, A., Mani Cavasagar, V. & Steel, Z. (1997). Anxiety, depression and PTSD in asylum seekers: associations with pre-migration trauma and post-migration stressors. *British Journal of Psychiatry*, **170**, 351–7.

Solomon, S. D. (1999). Interventions for acute trauma response. *Current Opinion in Psychiatry*, **12**, 175–80.

Steel, Z., Silove, D., Bird, K., McGorry, P. & Mohan, P. (1999). Pathways from war trauma to posttraumatic stress symptoms amongst Tamil asylum seekers, refugees and immigrants. *Journal of Traumatic Stress*, **12**, 421–35.

Summerfield, D. (1997a). Legacy of war: beyond 'trauma' to the social fabric. *Lancet*, **349**, 1568.

Summerfield, D. (1997b). South Africa: does a truth commission promote social reconciliation? *British Medical Journal*, **315**, 1393.

Summerfield, D. (1999). A critique of seven assumptions behind psychological trauma programmes in war-affected areas. *Social Science and Medicine*, **48**, 1449–62.

United Nations High Commissioner for Refugees (1997). *The State of the World's Refugees*. Oxford: Oxford University Press.

van Tilberg, M. A. L., Vingerhoets, A. J. J. M. & van Heck G. L. (1996). Homesickness: a review of the literature. *Psychological Medicine*, **26**, 899–912.

Conclusion: Debriefing – science, belief and wisdom

Beverley Raphael

Introduction

This volume combines the scientific face of debriefing and the powerfulness of belief, and reflects the wisdom of its contributors. Often these three elements are not dissected out but rather drive the presentations and the work of authors. It is useful to review each of these themes, and consider where, after reading these contributions and considering other available work in this field, our conclusions must lie. For ultimately how and if debriefing is taken forward will need to encompass these issues.

The science

Reviews presented by the contributors to this volume describe many of the available scientific studies and as well present their own substantial research efforts. They evaluate the effectiveness of debriefing broadly, as applied to: individuals affected by accident, illness or other life stresses; groups affected by disasters or emergency work; or as an element of a workplace or occupational health programme.

The findings reported include those provided by powerful advocates of debriefing, for instance Mitchell, and those whose research has shown no benefits, possibly even negative effects.

These may be usefully summarized as follows.

Studies investigating individualized one-off interventions

Bisson et al.'s (1997) study of psychological debriefing of victims of acute burns trauma showed that the de-

briefing group were worse at follow-up than the controls, although it must be noted that their burn trauma was more severe and their initial symptomatology higher. Hobbs et al.'s (1996) study of motor vehicle accident victims also involved random allocation to intervention and control groups, with independent follow-up. This study, described in Chapter 10, shows no benefit for manualized individual debriefing in preventing psychological morbidity. The recent *Cochrane Review* of debriefing for the treatment of immediate trauma-related symptoms and prevention of post-traumatic stress disorder (PTSD) concludes that these studies meet criteria for inclusion in terms of scientific quality (Wesseley et al., 1999). The *Review* also examined studies by Lee et al. (1996) on miscarriage, and other work with road crash victims, as well as two earlier studies that really sat in a crisis intervention framework. The *Review*'s authors concluded 'there is no current evidence that psychological debriefing is useful for prevention of post traumatic stress disorder after traumatic incidents' (Wesseley et al, 1999). To their findings might be added the positive report of Boyce and Condon (Chapter 19), but these authors suggest that psychological debriefing is part of good clinical care. The *Review* acknowledges the limitations of available studies in the whole field of debriefing in establishing its effectiveness of the technique in the full range of settings to which it is currently applied.

This form of debriefing could be most closely linked to crisis intervention (Raphael 1977; Bordow & Porritt, 1979; Viney et al., 1985) or to brief intervention for those at risk in relation to traumatic incidents. In these instances beneficial effects have been found for individually oriented intervention two weeks or more after the event, but usually with a number of sessions and frequently in a process of review, re-exposure and cognitive-behaviour therapy, for example rape victims (Foa et al., 1995) and after trauma in those with acute stress disorder (Bryant et al., 1998; Solomon, 1999). 'Debriefing' interventions could sit on a spectrum with these crisis interventions, or with other brief acute interventions that have preventive aims. They may also sit on a continuum with brief support and interventions such as psychological first aid (Foss, 1994). However, these latter techniques are only recently formulated and many have not yet been evaluated in research frameworks.

Studies investigating debriefing elements

Ursano et al.'s work (Chapter 2) examines two debriefing elements: talking and uptake of debriefing. Shalev (Chapter 1) investigates arousal and distress. Both these studies have the potential to contribute to theoretical understanding of debriefing, but obviously there is a need both to formulate and to investigate all potential influencing factors. These should include educational effects, timing, group process, debriefing and client variables, in fact anything that is potentially relevant. This of course also applies to other psychological and psychosocial interventions with which debriefing sits, including psychotherapies.

Studies investigating debriefing in response to disasters or major incidents

There are a number of contributions to this book that examine debriefing in these contexts. However, the chaos, complexity and breadth of the populations affected and the difficulties with screening, make for problems in establishing any sort of controlled intervention in such settings. These studies have been opportunistic, and even though using systematic measures, cannot fit with rigid criteria for controls. Studies include those of Watts (Chapter 9) group about major motor vehicle accidents, Kenardy et al.'s (1996, and se Chapter 12) research following an earthquake and Lundin's (Chapter 13) after multiple disasters in-

cluding one at sea. These acute debriefing interventions were provided to diverse populations in diverse disasters. They included affected populations (survivors), the bereaved, and emergency and rescue workers. The findings do not support a beneficial effect of debriefing in these diverse populations, even when it is perceived to be helpful. Nor do they establish it as being beneficial to the emergency workers so employed in the studies presented.

It should be noted, however, that delayed use of a debriefing intervention for a disaster-affected population was found to be effective in Chemtob's studies (Chapter 16). This followed closely a specific model with adaptations to cultural and individual needs and recognition of the developmental phase of the post-disaster response. There appears to be little to support the use of debriefing per se as an acute intervention for general disaster-affected populations. Indeed, there is even some suggestion that the greater exposure to debriefing is associated with, but not necessarily causative of, poorer outcomes. It might be argued that the intervention provided in such contexts did not maintain the integrity of debriefing, or may not have been delivered by appropriately qualified personnel. The difficulty with these issues is also the limitations of research rigour and quality control in overwhelming circumstances. Nevertheless, the lack of benefit for these broadly based interventions and the possibility of harm should mean a very cautious use of debriefing in these contexts, at least until the research has a stronger base. Clearly, if applied at all, psychological debriefing should never be compulsory. Debriefing in these settings merges with other psychosocial interventions in disaster settings, and few of these have been either applied or evaluated systematically. One follow-up of interventions with those bereaved in a disaster showed some benefits when this was integrated with other support (Singh & Raphael, 1981). There are many models of post-disaster mental health intervention developed and driven by goodwill and what is known of possible benefits, but the outcomes these achieve are not well recorded. Research in disaster intervention is complex and difficult.

Studies of debriefing in emergency, police and military service settings

These debriefing programmes reflect a much stronger commitment to a specific model, usually Mitchell's or a variant of this. As described in the overview they are more likely to be in an occupational health framework, and to have aims that are closer to those of stress management. They do not claim, and should not, to prevent PTSD. But they do claim to enhance feelings of competence, to reduce sick leave, job turnover and other indices of workplace stress. Mitchell and Everley's review (Chapter 5) suggests that there are considerable data to support these benefits, although much of it has not yet appeared in peer-review publications. Flannery et al.'s (1998) research also supports potential benefits of this stress management approach linked to a Critical Incident Stress Management (CISM) framework and these studies have been replicated. Alexander's work (Chapter 8) with body handlers supports this, although Deahl's (Chapter 7) with war graves soldiers does not. The former, however, used more of an integrated occupational health and safety approach. Deahl's study is controlled, but that study, like others, can also be criticized because of the inherent methodological difficulties imposed by its opportunistic framework.

The work of Avery and Ørner's group (Avery & Ørner, 1998a) has provided a further scientific challenge, as well as debate. They report data from the follow-up of an established critical incident programme for emergency workers in the UK. The debriefers were specially trained in the Mitchell model. The findings suggested that perceived helpfulness was inversely related to need, and that beneficial outcomes could not be established. The consensus group found no consistent evidence of the effectiveness of debriefing as a preventive intervention in terms of post-traumatic morbidity. They expressed specific concerns about Bisson et al's (1997) study and also that of Gerson et al. (1997), cited by Avery & Ørner (1998b), both of which reported higher risk for adverse outcomes in those debriefed, the latter with respect to police officers. This has lead to recommendations of a different method of staff mental health intervention and a discontinuation of Critical Incident Stress Debriefing (CISD) in this occupational health setting.

Mitchell & Everly (1998) reply to this challenge by presenting a further review, which covers many of the studies reported in their contribution to this volume, and that of Robinson (Chapter 6). They conclude from their studies and their meta-analysis of controlled group studies to which they have access, that there is a positive effect-size, particularly with studies of debriefing police (Bohl, 1995), medical workers after a mass shooting (Jenkins, 1996) and emergency workers of the *Estonia* ferry disaster (Nurmi, 1997). Also supporting their claims for benefit of their debriefing model is the work of Flannery (Chapter 20) as noted in this book, and other evaluations of CISD with nurses in Canada, including conference presentations and some publications. It appears that the benefits are those of stress management in an occupational health framework, i.e. decrease in sick leave, compensation claims, and job turnover, as well as some reports of lessened symptoms levels.

It is clear that this debate will continue, but, it is to be hoped, will bring a recognition of the methodological difficulties, the limitations of both positive and negative findings, and the grounds for caution. In particular, it is clear that one cannot claim prevention of PTSD, nor is this claimed by Mitchell's group. It may be that this is a potential effect, but a systematic research agenda would be needed to establish it. The debate is on both the science and its interpretation, as well as the views of the researchers. This is also reflected in the chapter on consensus development in another context (Morris, Chapter 23).

The other broad, inclusive debriefing format is of the military. Shalev (Chapter 1), Weisæth (Chapter 3), Lundin (Chapter 13) and Solomon et al. (Chapter 11) write specifically of military settings. They recommend a model that is more operational and historic and intended for those previously briefed, but the authors recognize the need to build on their data to better establish potential outcomes of this format. The decrease in arousal reported and the other impacts described in the model of military or 'forward treatment' suggest directions. These however, like other emergency service interventions, aim to preserve functioning of the soldier or worker. It will be critical that not only function but longer-term impacts are explored.

The beliefs

The powerfulness of the beliefs driving the debriefing movement is clear in the contributions to this book, as well as the challenges and debates. These beliefs are such that even those who have found no effect for debriefing in their research studies, for example Deahl (Chapter 7) and Watts (Chapter 9) believe it should continue to be provided.

The social movement of debriefing has such a momentum that there is a profound belief, even at a popular level, that it must be provided for all – for people experiencing sometimes even the most minor events or normal life transitions. While those powerfully committed to a debriefing model, such as Mitchell, do not claim that debriefing should be applied to all such instances or circumstances, it has nevertheless been extended to these. It has been taken up as an almost magical solution. Furthermore, the positive beliefs in the benefits are not easily set aside, even when research suggests that there could be grounds for caution and, indeed, for some potential capacity to make things worse. Certainly the research challenges to debriefing have lead to little diminution in its use, except perhaps for the changes outlined by Avery and Ørner.

As those most strongly committed to debriefing such as Mitchell, argue, it is widely perceived as helpful by those who receive it. And it is perceived as needed by those who do not. Mitchell and his followers have repeatedly emphasized its use is for emergency services; its aims are to deal with emergency service critical incident stress, and not trauma.

Both sides of the debate are bedevilled by the methodological weaknesses of the studies quoted, and the lack of a gold standard – the randomized controlled trial. Where trials with some degree of control have taken place, the groups may be arguably differently stressed, more highly reactive, previously traumatized, and not have received the debriefing interventions that are faithful to either the original hypotheses or specific theoretical constructs. Furthermore, when negative results are found they have not led to further detailed

analysis or indeed to more critical research. There are findings to support both arguments, but, as reviewed above, it can be seen that they may be referring to different stressors, populations or models of debriefing. Attempts at consensus seem to bring a consolidation of opposition rather than compromise or collaboration to address the key questions.

Why is the belief so strong? As Shalev (Chapter 1) and many contributors have pointed out, there is a very powerful and altruistic drive to assist those who have been subjected to trauma, and debriefing provides a socially sanctioned framework in which to do so. The word 'debriefing' itself suggests a taking away of something. It has been shifted into a taking away of the bad experience, an undoing. It is provided at a time of heightened arousal and focus, both in those traumatized and those wishing to help. This arousal and the altruism of the early helping response, are symbolically a drive to undo and take away the death and destruction.

There is perhaps a need to better separate these two issues of altruistic helping and debriefing. This may assist us in allowing, valuing and providing sanctions for the humane and caring response that is offered to others at times of stress or disaster. We can then use and test debriefing, as it was originated, as an intervention to diminish workplace stress in emergency workers, although here too it needs to be further evaluated.

There is likely to be a range of other interventions that may be effective in such settings including psychological first aid, education, information, group support, focussed counselling, practical assistance and so forth. Specific research questions addressing the potential for effect or harm need to clarify what can really help, and what may actually harm. However, repositioning debriefing as crisis intervention amongst these does not assist.

There is also the debate that debriefing, and indeed the concepts of psychological traumatization to which it is most frequently applied, are Western concepts, and inappropriate in the contexts of mass trauma, violence, and conflict in developing countries where it may now be applied, inappropriately as a model of response to these issues. Silove (Chapter 25) has conceptualized the needs and cultural relevance of intervention models and provided a broader framework of support and intervention that is relevant in these settings.

A further question that must arise about the power of this debriefing movement is to do with money. There are, in many instances, substantial sums to be made in the provision of debriefing. Providing a service in such demand can be good business, particularly with the ubiquity of situations to which it is now applied. There must be concern that in some instances this will be a powerful market force in the provision of such interventions.

Legal concerns may also be used to support this belief. For instance an organization may be determined as being negligent if it does not provide debriefing and there may be fears of litigation if PTSD develops. There is no evidence that debriefing can prevent this morbidity.

Organizations providing debriefing to their workers may see it as an indication that they have dealt with their workers' needs, and it is frequently perceived as an indication of managers' recognition of workers 'injury' or experience. Thus the symbolic meaning that is seen as being of value may also support the belief that debriefing is good and must be provided for all.

Wisdom

All of those contributing to the debriefing field, whether critics or concerned, acknowledge that 'debriefing' in its many forms may have the capacity to lead to learning. This may be learning of coping, learning for changes, learning for growth, learning for pathology, learning for victim-hood. It is vital that this issue takes into account learning for the individual, for the system, and for those providing assistance. This has been raised repeatedly by contributors, perhaps very specifically by Weisæth (Chapter 3). But this learning has to extend to those who believe in debriefing. The debate needs to continue but should deepen understanding by seeking new knowledge through further research and conceptualization.

Furthermore, there are major ethical issues. Providing a ubiquitous and broadly based intervention for a range of populations, where at the least it has failed to provide any demonstrable benefit for the majority, cannot be justified unless there is further research to determine that there is no harm or what form and components might be of benefit. Ethical issues are often brought forward to justify the failure to pursue research that is strongly scientifically based, for example with control groups. This can no longer be ethically justified in view of the many negative findings. Ethics also call for caution where there are negative findings and ethical considerations must also add to the debate when money is made from debriefing. What is the wisdom we need to distil from the contributions to this book and the work of others that has been reviewed?

Theories and conceptualization of debriefing

The theories behind debriefing and other interventions need to be more clearly delineated. They need to be far better linked to the rapidly advancing understandings of reactions to stressors in general, and to specific stresses including life threat and other experiences that are known to be linked to the development of post-trauma morbidity. The psychological adaptations, the neuroendocrine changes, the neurophysiological response and the whole phenomenology of reaction are key issues to be taken into account (see Stuhlmiller and Dunning, Chapter 22). The social frameworks and constructions of what is stress, what is a stressor and what are the expectations of reaction and adaptation, also need to be considered.

It has been previously noted that there is in some contexts a view of all of society as traumatized and stressed, rather than perceptions that stress is a necessary challenge with possibilities for learning and growth, although at times it may be overwhelming. The cultural prescriptions for what is a stressor, what it means and what is the response should also be understood. What variables might influence reaction, past, present and future in the person–environment interaction model described by Wilson and Sigman (Chapter 4)? What are the effects of gender? What are the effects of role? What is actually done, and by whom? These questions must form the basis for examining what an intervention might do, and how it might have effect. Inherent in this approach is the need to address and operationalize definitions of both stress and debriefing and to research potential effectiveness or otherwise of debriefing, rather than to reinvent it.

Research into debriefing

Building on such conceptualizations it is clear that research is needed: to identify potential active components, for instance in the model of Ursano; to examine the effects of debriefing interventions for specific purposes and specific populations and compare these to control groups to determine whether debriefing is an effective form of stress management for occupational health; to determine what effects debriefing-type interventions have and at which stages of response; and to examine developmental factors, for instance with children (Wraith, Chapter 14; Stallard, Chapter 15). How much, when, how, for whom, and with what effects does debriefing interact with other interventions and processes? Is there a place for debriefing in health contexts and in disaster contexts? What does the apparent benefit of historical debriefing in military situations suggest – and so forth. Many such questions have been raised in the chapters of this volume. Another urgent problem is whether or not debriefing can be harmful in delaying recovery, re-traumatizing, or negating normal adaptation and personal growth. Does the provision of debriefing lessen the likelihood of later and more appropriate interventions? There is much to suggest caution.

There is no question that research into debriefing is a challenge. But, as noted above, it seems most likely that benefits of debriefing lie in an integrated stress management approach for emergency and related services. Such groups, and the military are relatively controlled populations where pre- and post-test measures, cohort monitoring and measuring of interventions and outcomes could be readily implemented. It is now critical that scientific foundations to investigate the value or otherwise of debriefing and related interventions are established and rapidly commence activity. Furthermore prospective studies could more readily determine measures for potential and actual stressors to examine their effects. This research could be in a collaborative

framework with those researched – a 'we' project as suggested by Lundin (Chapter 13). This would allow both qualitative and quantitative assessments, with a bringing together of necessary methodologies to answer several questions, including those that might positively influence person–environment interactions to improve outcomes. Linkages of research groups with core methods and measures and agreements for collaboration could extend the databases and add to research strength (e.g. McFarlane, Chapter 24).

Ideally, research on debriefing should examine not only its aims, but, if it has a role, where it sits in the spectrum of interventions – for instance preventive or other. This could enable linkages between conceptualization from the trauma field and related effective interventions (e.g. Bryant et al., 1998) to inform research for debriefing interventions in relevant contexts.

Implementation or otherwise of research findings on debriefing

The translation of research to service frameworks is always a challenge – the more so if there are established beliefs about the value of interventions currently being provided. Implementation of what has been found to be effective needs to be supported by a range of other processes to ensure that benefit can be translated into broader reality to meet identified needs. This includes the defining of effective elements and ensuring programme integrity and fidelity. Education and training to demonstrably develop the necessary knowledge, attitudes and skills of the provider workforce are essential for effective implementation. Accreditation of such providers is also an issue. Quality improvement and continuous quality control measures then provide tools for monitoring the interventions. These may rely on evidence-based good practice guidelines or other manuals. Outcome monitoring of the achievement of desired aims, both individually and for populations served, and maintaining these across time are all further important elements. There are increasing requirements in the accountability of health and other systems and there is no reason to suggest that this should not be required for debriefing as a purchased intervention.

This leads to the further question of the use of debriefing when there has been limited demonstration of benefit and potential for negative outcomes.

Evaluation

Evaluation is a key part of the cycle of research and implementation and provides the necessary information to monitor the effectiveness of the service provided and what may need to be further researched, or modified, to do better. This of course requires (1) the identification of specific goals or targets, which can then be measured validly and reliably and monitored with relative ease, and (2) the information systems to support such processes. Clearly, the client population must be informed and involved at every level and this in itself is likely to be empowering, providing specific benefits of involvement.

Evaluation must involve comparisons: is this better than other things that may be done or simply better than doing nothing. Evaluation enables a detailed exploration of, and hopefully an answer to, the question of why debriefing is perceived so positively, often without benefits being clearly linked to this. Evaluation tests the realities of debriefing in the real world.

Linkages between briefing and debriefing can also be usefully explored, particularly in evaluation frameworks in service settings. This could provide the opportunity to answer questions such as those posed by Weisæth's work (Chapter 3) and to a degree that of Shalev (Chapter 1).

Special issues in research and evaluation

Social structures and systems should be examined to answer questions about what debriefing means and how these systems may explain or contribute to its effects or otherwise.

Cultural understandings are relevant not only for identifying stressors and their outcomes in different cultural settings, but in exploring the prescriptions and rituals that have evolved to deal with these, as indicated for instance by Weisæth (Chapter 3). Does debriefing as an intervention fit with holistic models and explana-tions of problems? Much can be learned that may inform responses to traditional groups as well as broader constituencies.

Acute or chronic stress or traumatization has been highlighted for indigenous peoples (Ober et al., Chapter 17), others who may be chronically affected and those affected by mass trauma and violence in global contexts (Silove, Chapter 25). This issue requires much further research, particularly when disadvantage and trauma effects are substantial, and often ongoing. Models appropriate to these cultural and psychosocial issues need to be developed in collaboration with these populations and tested in their frameworks.

Knowledge and information about debriefing, its effects, or lack thereof, needs wider dissemination. But information and community education may not be enough to test the magic of this belief. This is a very special research question that needs to be explored. Many effective interventions take years to disseminate and become a part of effective practice and service provision. Why has debriefing 'taken off', become so widely provided, and so powerfully believed in? How has it been so effectively marketed? Has the uptake reflected need? Is it more reflective of the desire for a way of helping? There is much to learn about these social processes and the sources and driving forces of this social movement.

The future of debriefing

Debriefing means many different things to many people. Overwhelmingly it seems to mean the possibility of help, the recognition of hurt, the reality of hope. As suggested by the authors in this volume, these are good reasons for providing such an intervention. But this cannot be done without critical appraisal, scientific research and the drawing together of wisdom in ongoing ways. Challenge and debate can drive new knowledge to lead to better practice, but their findings must be heard by all. From the work in this volume it is clear that debriefing is applied to too broad a constituency, that effectiveness appears to be in the direction of stress management, in an occupational health setting, or for emergency and related services. Even this can be challenged (Carlier et al., 1998; McNab et al., 1999). Its case may be argued in these settings but not more widely and not for effective prevention of post-trauma morbidity. Does it do harm? Then what should be provided?

There is one further vital issue which is central to the future of debriefing and the debriefing movement. Remembering, forgetting, meeting challenges, incorporating losses: these things are part of life. Debriefing must not disrupt these human processes nor diminish their value. Do we need debriefing at all? This is the real question – and it has not yet been fully answered.

The belief in debriefing must sit alongside knowledge and be informed by it. Its positive and hopeful aspects should be recognised and further developed. It is a powerful social movement that should be understood and assessed. Where it is not effective, practice must change and debriefing be set aside for the requirement is 'first, do no harm'. The debate about debriefing to find and use its truths must continue at both popular and scientific levels. The strength of the personal psyche and the social fabric to deal with stress, loss and trauma should be recognized and respected, while at the same time providing help to those at risk and in need. The core human and altruistic responses should be valued and developed for themselves, as the best of human nature and its ultimate hope for the future.

REFERENCES

Avery, A. & Ørner, R. (1998a). First report of psychological debriefing abandoned. The end of an era? *Traumatic Stress Points. International Society for Traumatic Stress Studies*, **12**(3), Summer.

Avery, A. & Ørner, R. (1998b). More on debriefing: report of psychological debriefing abandoned. The end of an era? *Australian Traumatic Stress Points*, Newsletter of the Australian Society for Traumatic Stress Studies, July, 4–6.

Bisson, J. I., Jenkins, J. A. & Bannister, C. (1997). Randomised controlled trial of psychological debriefing for victims of acute burn trauma. *British Journal of Psychiatry*, **171**, 78–81.

Bohl, N. (1995). The effectiveness of brief psychological interventions in police officers after critical incidents. In J. Reese, J. Horn, J. & C. Dunning (Eds.) *Critical Incidents in Policing*,

revised edn (pp. 31–8). Washington, DC: Department of Justice.

Bordow, S. & Porritt, D. (1979). An experimental evaluation of crisis intervention. *Social Science and Medicine*, **13**, 251–6.

Bryant, R. A., Harvey, A. G., Dang, S. T. & Sackville, T. (1998). Treatment of acute stress disorder: A comparison of cognitive-behavioural therapy and supportive counselling. *Journal of Consulting and Clinical Psychology*, **66**, 862–6.

Carlier, I., Lamberts, R., van Uchelen, A. & Gersons, B. (1998). Disaster-related post-traumatic stress in police officers: a field study of the impact of debriefing. *Stress Medicine*, **14**, 143–8.

Flannery, R. B., Hanson, M. A., Penk, W. E., Goldfinger, S., Pastva, G. J. & Navon, M. A. (1998). Replicated declines in assault rates after implementation of the Assaulted Staff Action Plan. *Psychiatric Services*, **49**, 241–3.

Foa, E. B., Hearst-Ikeda, D. & Perry, K. J. (1995). Evaluation of a brief cognitive-behavioural program for the prevention of chronic PTSD in recent assault victims. *Journal of Consulting and Clinical Psychology*, **63**, 948–55.

Foss, O. T. (1994). Mental first aid. *Social Science and Medicine*, **38**, 479–82.

Hobbs, M., Mayou, R., Harrison, B. & Worlock, P. (1996). A randomised control trial of psychological debriefing for victims of road traffic accidents. *British Medical Journal*, **313**, 1438–9.

Jenkins, S. R. (1996). Social support and debriefing efficacy among medical workers after a mass-shooting incident. *Journal of Social Behaviour and Personality*, **11**, 477–92.

Kenardy, J., Webster, R., Lewin, T., Carr, V. & Carter, G. (1996). Stress debriefing and patterns of recovery following natural disaster. *Journal of Traumatic Stress*, **9**, 37–49.

Lee, C., Slade, P. & Lygo, V. (1996). The influence of psychological debriefing on emotional adaptation in women following early miscarriage: a preliminary study. *British Journal of Medical Psychology*, **69**, 47–58.

McNab, A. J., Russell, J. A., Lowe, J. P. & Gagnon, F. (1999). Critical incident stress intervention after loss of an air ambulance: two-year follow up. *Prehospital Disaster Medicine*, **14**, 15–19.

Mitchell, J. T. & Everley, G. S. (1998). Critical incident stress management: a new era in crisis intervention. *Traumatic Stress Points*. International Society for Traumatic Stress Studies, **12**(4), Fall.

Nurmi, L. (1997). Experienced stress and the value of CISD among Finnish emergency personnel in the *Estonia* ferry disaster. Paper presented to the 4th World Congress on Stress, Trauma and Coping in the Emergency Service Professions, Baltimore, MD.

Raphael, B. (1977). Preventive intervention with the recently bereaved. *Archives of General Psychiatry*, **34**, 1450–4.

Singh, B. & Raphael, B. (1981). Postdisaster morbidity of the bereaved. *Archives of General Psychiatry*, **34**, 1450–4.

Solomon, S. D. (1999). Interventions for acute trauma response. *Current Opinion in Psychiatry*, **12**, 175–80.

Viney, L., Clarke, A., Bunn, T. & Benjamin, Y. (1985). An evaluation of three crisis intervention programs for general hospital patients. *British Journal of Medical Psychology*, **58**, 75–86.

Wessely, S., Rose, S. & Bisson, J. (1999). Brief psychological interventions ('debriefing') for immediate trauma related symptoms and the prevention of post traumatic stress disorder (Cochrane Review). *The Cochrane Library*, **4**. Oxford: Update Software.

Index